Neonatal Formulary 7

About the companion website

A free companion resources site for this book is available at:

www.neonatalformulary.com

The website lists each drug described in the book, with:

Updates and new material

New – Monographs on new drugs available since the publication of the book.

Updates – Revisions to monographs revised since the publication of the book.

Comments – Temporary postings, e.g., a change in usage.

Commentaries – Permanent website commentaries about a drug.

Web archive – Drug monographs for little-used drugs no longer included in the book.

Useful links

Cochrane reviews – Links to relevant Cochrane reviews for listed drugs.

UK guidelines – Links to UK management guidelines for listed drugs.

WHO – Identification of drugs classified as essential by the World Health Organisation.

E-mail alerting

Sign up for the e-mail alerting service and we will let you know whenever a new batch of updates is added to the site.

Feedback

If you would like to see any drug not currently mentioned appear in the next edition or to provide feedback on the text, please contact the editorial team using drug.information@neonatalformulary.com

Neonatal Formulary 7

Drug Use in Pregnancy and the First Year of Life

nnf7

WILEY Blackwell   BMJ|Books

Contents

Introduction

NNF7 has been designed to provide compact, up-to-date, referenced advice on the prescribing of drugs and their safe and accurate administration, during pregnancy, labour and the first year of life. While the book's main focus is on the baby, many drugs that are given to women during pregnancy or lactation have a potential impact on the fetus or baby in a way that is equally important. This compendium therefore also gives advice on maternal medications.

The number of drugs used in late pregnancy and the first few weeks of life continues to rise rapidly, although, in many cases, manufacturers have not yet sought market authorisation to recommend neonatal use. Globally the use of medications that are either not licensed or, if they are licensed, are used for indications out with the terms of their product license ('off label') is common in neonatal units. While a lot of general information on drugs may be given in the manufacturer's summary of product characteristics (SPC), advice on use in young children is often non-existent. Since advice in the SPC is all that has been seen and approved by regulatory bodies such as the Commission on Human Medicines in the United Kingdom, and since the British National Formulary (BNF) normally limits itself to summarising information that has been so validated, much drug use in the neonate occurs in a hazardous information vacuum. The same can be said for the use of many drugs during pregnancy and lactation. All this makes it increasingly important for midwives and nurses, as well as pharmacists and doctors, to be able to access a reference text that summarises the scattered but extensive therapeutic and pharmacokinetic information that *is* available on the safe and appropriate use of these products. Information on placental transfer and teratogenicity, and on the extent to which each drug appears in human milk (and the extent to which this matters), is provided for each drug. Where the text merely says that treatment during lactation is safe, it can be taken that the dose ingested by the baby is likely to be less than 5% of the dose taken by the mother on a weight for weight basis, and that no reports have appeared suggesting that the baby could be clinically affected.

Special attention has been paid to the rapid changes that occur in the renal and hepatic handling of some drugs in the first few weeks of life, and the impact of illness and severe prematurity on drug metabolism and drug elimination. Widespread use of therapeutic hypothermia in the treatment of asphyxiated newborn infants brought with it a need to understand the effects of temperature on the medications used in these infants. The symptoms associated with overtreatment are summarised, and the management of toxicity is outlined. Information is also included on the best way to use the few drugs so far known to be of therapeutic benefit to the fetus.

NNF7 also provides information on the main drugs used to modify the diet of babies with congenital enzyme deficiencies ('inborn errors of metabolism'), a monograph on breast milk fortifiers, and a monograph on the artificial milks ('formula' milks) for preterm infants most commonly used in the United Kingdom. A guide to some of the artificial milks used in babies with reflux, lactose intolerance and allergy is also included; however, no attempt has been made to list other dietary products or those artificial milks that are used as breast milk substitutes.

While the text predominantly reflects practice in the United Kingdom, medicine is increasingly international in its scope. Every section of the text has been revised with this in mind by a wide range of local, national and overseas collaborators. A wide range of journals have been searched in order to make the advice given in the latest revision as comprehensive and up-to-date as possible, and all relevant Cochrane reviews consulted. Input has also been sought from colleagues with a range of professional expertise in an attempt to ensure that the text reflects a distillate of current opinion. However, in deciding what should eventually find its way into print, it was the advice of those who could provide evidence to support their approach that carried most weight. A consensus driven text could, all too easily, merely reflect what most people are doing rather than what they ought to be doing! The references cited in each entry should make it easier for readers to make up their own minds on such issues.

Part 1 of the book contains important general information on drug storage, licensing and prescribing. Along with advice on drug administration, the care and use of intravascular lines, medication in renal failure and during therapeutic hypothermia, and the recognition, management and reporting of adverse reactions are also included. The information given on individual drugs in Part 2 needs to be interpreted in the light of this general advice; although it is tempting to skip this section the importance of understanding many of the concepts covered cannot be understated.

The *second* (and largest) part contains monographs on over 230 of the drugs most often used during labour and the first few months of life listed in alphabetical order. Information on a number of blood products and vaccines is included. Each monograph lists the drug's main uses, and the most appropriate dose to give, both in the term and the preterm baby. The neonatal half-life is noted where known, and a note made of those with an unusually large volume of distribution ($V_D > 1$ l/kg). A brief summary of the drug's discovery and development is usually included. Advice is also provided on how to measure accurately the small volumes frequently required, and how to administer bolus and IV infusions safely. The advice given can, in general, be used to guide management throughout the first year of life. Significant interactions between drugs included in the main section of the compendium are outlined. Adverse effects commonly encountered in infancy, and their management, receive attention, but the SPC should be consulted in respect of other, less common, adverse effects. Information under the heading 'supply' refers to the formulation most widely used in the United Kingdom. It is important to realise that other strengths and formulations may exist and essential to check the label on the container before giving medicine to any patient. The stated cost is the basic net price (normally quoted in the BNF) when the book went to press, rounded to two significant figures. This information has been included in order to make clinicians more cost conscious but should not be interpreted as representing the pricing policy of any particular hospital. Every monograph concludes with one or more recent key references to the obstetric, perinatal or neonatal literature (from which it is usually possible to identify other key reports).

Part 3 contains brief notes on a further 350 drugs, or groups of drugs, that may be taken by mothers during pregnancy, labour or the puerperium. The drugs mentioned include all the more commonly used products thought to affect the baby either because of placental transfer or because of excretion in human milk. Illicit drug use and legitimate self-medication both receive attention. Entries are almost always linked to two key references that can be used to access additional original studies and reports.

The *index* at the back of the compendium includes all the UK and US synonyms by which some drugs are occasionally known, and serves to identify more than 50 other drugs only referred to, in passing, within another drug monograph. Various common contractions are also spelt out.

A *website* was launched in January 2001 (www.neonatalformulary.com). New drugs continue to come onto the market at regular intervals, and further information relating to the use of many of the drugs already contained in the book continues to appear. As a result, the text remains under semi-continuous review. The website also provides longer, more fully referenced, commentaries on some important products, direct access to abstracts of all the relevant Cochrane Reviews and link access to the UK Government's current vaccination policy guidelines. It also contains monographs on a number of drugs that were included in earlier editions of this book, but which do not appear in the present print version (although their existence can still be traced using the index) because they are no longer used as often as they once were. While the publishers plan to continue producing new editions of this compendium approximately once every 3 years, the existence of the website makes it possible to alert readers to all the more important changes that are made to the text just as soon as they are issued.

Important advisory statement

This compendium discusses treatments and drug therapies in both mothers and their babies during the perinatal period. It is the responsibility of the treating clinician, relying on experience and knowledge, to determine dosages and the appropriateness of treatment in their patient. While every effort has been made to check the veracity of the information in this compendium, neither the publisher nor those responsible for compiling this edition assume any responsibility for the consequences of any remaining inaccuracy or for any injury and/or damage to persons or property.

The drugs included in this compendium are predominantly those in current use in neonatal units in the United Kingdom; however, recent updates have increasingly attempted to reflect international practise. Omission should not be taken to imply criticism of a drug's usefulness; neither should inclusion necessarily be seen as a recommendation either. Indeed a number of products are mentioned specifically to alert clinicians to some of the uncertainties or limitations associated with use in infancy. Personal preference and past experience must inevitably influence prescribing practice, and in neonatal practice, more than any other branch of medicine, it is better to use a limited number of carefully evaluated and widely used drugs knowledgeably than to use drugs with which the prescriber is not fully familiar.

Experience shows that it is also dangerous to uncritically use the latest product to reach the market. Too many drugs of proven efficacy in adult medicine have been widely and indiscriminately used during pregnancy and in the neonatal period before the potential hazards associated with their use ever became apparent, sometimes years after their introduction. Examples of these include diethylstilbestrol (given to millions of women to prevent miscarriage and premature delivery) leading to genital tract deformity and vaginal cancer in babies born to these women; chloramphenicol and sulphonamides widely used in the neonatal period some 50 years ago led to many hundreds of deaths that might have otherwise been avoided. Hexachlorophene baths and vitamin K injections also killed several hundred babies before anyone realised what was happening. A worrying number of babies died in the early 1980s before it was realised that preterm babies cannot metabolise one of the bacteriostatic excipients commonly used to ensure the sterility of the water used to 'flush' the line every time a blood sample is taken or a drug is given (as described in the archived entry on benzyl alcohol).

Sadly such inadvertent drug tragedies are not confined to the past. It took 10 years before people realised that cisapride did little to reduce the incidence of troublesome reflux 'posseting' and that such use risked triggering cardiac arrhythmia, and it then took another 8 years for many to realise that much the same could be true of domperidone. Evidence emerged some 15 years ago that using acetazolamide to control post-haemorrhagic hydrocephalus did more harm than good, and that the amount of aluminium that often gets infused when a baby is offered parenteral nutrition can cause permanent neurological damage. The harm that was being done to these patients only finally came to light when these forms of treatment were eventually subjected to controlled trial scrutiny. In the same way, concern over the near 'routine' use of insulin in babies thought to have an 'abnormally' high blood glucose level only surfaced, quite recently, when this strategy was also scrutinised for the first time in a controlled trial of meaningful size. Conversely however, because early neonatal trials only focused on short-term outcomes, it took 20 years for long-term benefits of early treatment with caffeine to be recognised.

Simultaneous use of several drugs increases the risk of harm from drug interaction. Examples include furosemide with an aminoglycoside, erythromycin with carbamazepine and ibuprofen or indometacin with dexamethasone or hydrocortisone. Errors in drug prescribing and administration occur more frequently when several products are in use at the same time. Almost all drugs are potentially harmful, and some of the drugs most frequently used in the neonatal period are potentially lethal when given in excess. It has been seriously suggested that every hospital drug cupboard should have the motto *'Is your prescription really necessary?'* pinned on the door.

Many paediatric and neonatal texts provide tabular drug lists and dosage guidelines. While these can be a useful *aide mémoire,* they can give the false impression that all you need to know about a drug is how much to give. These reference tables should *never* be used on their own, except by somebody who is already fully familiar with all the drug's indications and contraindications, and with all aspects of the drug's pharmacokinetic behaviour (including its behaviour in the sick preterm baby). Information also becomes dated quite quickly, so any text that is more than 2 years old should be used with great caution.

All important amendments made to this regularly revised text after the present edition went to press can be found on the web at: www.neonatalformulary.com.

Contact can be made with the team responsible for the current text and for keeping it up-to-date using the following e-mail address for all such contact: drug.information@ neonatalformulary.com.

Further reading

Many good books about drug use in children now exist, but detailed up-to-date neonatal information is harder to find. The world's first neonatal reference text published by Roberts in 1984 was never updated, while the slim American reference booklet by Young and Mangum is not widely available in the United Kingdom and only covers a limited range of drugs. Recently the comprehensive paediatric text by Taketomo was expanded to include the neonatal period; this is updated annually, but is only thinly referenced. *Martindale* remains a mine of useful information, and there is more specific information relating to pregnancy and the neonatal period available in the *British National Formulary* (BNF and BNFC) than is generally realised (although the BNFC is the only text to include information on dosage other than that suggested in the manufacturer's Summary of Product Characteristics). These books and the local Formularies produced by the Hammersmith Hospital in London, by the Hospital for Sick Children in Toronto and by the Royal Women's Hospital in Melbourne were all consulted during the preparation of the latest edition of the present text. For books relating to drug use during pregnancy and lactation see page 558.

Aronoff GR, Bennet WM, Berns JS, *et al.* eds. *Drug prescribing in renal failure. Dosing guidelines for adults and children*, 5th edn. Philadelphia: American College of Physicians, 2007.

Guy's, St Thomas' and Lewisham Hospitals. *Paediatric formulary*, 9th edn. London: Guy's Hospital Pharmacy, 2012.

Isaacs D, ed. *Evidenced-based pediatric infectious diseases*. Oxford: BMJ Books, 2007.

Jacqz-Aigrain E, Choonara I, eds. *Paediatric clinical pharmacology*. Switzerland: FontisMedia SA, 2006.

Paediatric Formulary Committee. *British National Formulary for Children 2013–2014 (BNFC)*. London: Pharmaceutical Press, 2013.

Pagliaro LA, Pagliaro AM, eds. *Problems in pediatric drug therapy*, 4th edn. Hamilton IL: Drug Intelligence Publications, 2002.

Pickering LK, Baker CJ, Kimberlin DW, eds. *Red Book*. 2012. *Report of the committee on infectious disease*, 29th edn. Elk Grove Village, IL: American Academy of Pediatrics, 2012.

Sweetman SC, ed. *Martindale. The complete drug reference*, 37th edn. London: Pharmaceutical Press, 2011.

Taketomo CK, Hodding JH, Kraus DM. *Pediatric & Neonatal Dosage Handbook*, 20th edn. Hudson, OH: Lexi-Comp Inc., 2013.

Trissel L. *Handbook of injectable drugs*, 17th edn. Bethesda, ML: American Society of Health-System Pharmacists, 2012.

World Health Organisation. *WHO model formulary 2008*. Geneva: WHO, 2008.

Yaffe SJ, Aranda JV. *Neonatal and pediatric pharmacology. Therapeutic principles in practice*, 4th edn. Philadelphia: Lippincott Williams and Wilkins, 2010.

Young TE, Mangum B. *Neofax 2011. A manual of drugs used in neonatal care*, 24th edn. Montvale, NJ: Thomson Reuters, 2011. [Subsequent editions available in electronic format.]

Zenk KE, Sills JH, Koeppel RM. *Neonatal medications and nutrition. A comprehensive guide*, 3rd edn. Santa Rosa, CA: NICU Ink, 2003 [Not since updated.]

Many drugs in common use have never been shown to achieve what is claimed for them. Others, when subjected to rigorous evaluation in a randomised controlled trial, have eventually been shown to cause unexpected adverse problems. An increasingly complete tally of all such studies and overviews is now available in *The Cochrane*

Library, an electronic database published for the international Cochrane Collaboration by John Wiley and Sons Ltd. and updated quarterly.

A ⟳ (Cochrane collaboration) symbol has been used to highlight those drugs or topics for which there is at least one review relating to use in pregnancy or the neonatal period. Links to the whole text of these systematic reviews can now be viewed on the NNF7 website (www.neonatalformulary.com). The symbol **DHUK** identifies those drugs and vaccines for which there is a useful and relevant UK management guideline (documents that can also be accessed in the same way).

Acknowledgements

This neonatal pharmacopoeia started life in 1978 as a loose-leaf A4 reference folder of commonly used drugs for the neonatal surgical intensive care unit at the Hospital for Sick Children (Fleming Hospital) in Newcastle upon Tyne. It was prepared by Dr. John Inkster, the Fleming Hospital's first Consultant Paediatric Anaesthetist, and Dr. Edmund Hey, the Paediatrician from the adjoining Princess Mary Maternity Hospital. It has been updated many times since then and has now expanded considerably, but the format and the basic layout have not changed.

The 1987 and 1989 revisions reflected practice in all the Newcastle units, and the 1991 and 1993 revisions, which drew on the accumulated experience of all the units in the region, were made widely available in pocketbook format by the Northern Regional Health Authority. Both of the hospitals where this book first originated have since closed, and the Regional Health Authority is also now no more. The local Neonatal Network was pleased to find a national publisher for a new pocket version in 1996 and for further new print editions since then.

Since then, input has become progressively more international in scope, as is reflected by the inclusion of drugs for the treatment of malaria in this new update. Nurses, midwives and staff pharmacists have continued to play a part by asking for the inclusion of further new information, and by criticising, firmly but constructively, any lack of clarity in the text. Developments in neonatal medicine are continually occurring; therapeutic hypothermia has become a standard of care for infants with hypoxic–ischaemic encephalopathy and this modality of treatment impacts on how many of the drugs are metabolised, newborn screening programmes are expanding, and, coupled with better prospects for antenatal diagnosis, many inherited metabolic conditions are now being treated earlier and earlier.

Change continues apace, and several important amendments make their appearance with the arrival of this latest update. The book is now available in both paper and electronic formats. Regular updates can be found on the book's website, where an increasing range of supplementary information can also be found. The book's scope has also been expanded to include a number of drugs generally needed only in the management of tropical diseases such as malaria, and the book's contributors come from an increasing number of different countries.

Sadly two of the major driving forces behind previous editions have since died – Edmund Hey in 2009 and Sam Richmond in 2013 however the formulary continues to honour its original vision but at the same time providing up-to-date information about the drugs to which the fetus, neonate and infant may be exposed.

Doctors, midwives, pharmacists, nurses and others who made a significant contribution to the preparation of this and the most recent editions include:

M. Alam, B. Anderson, J. van den Anker, R. Appleton, D. Azzopardi, E. Banda, D. Barker, P. Baxter, A. Bedford-Russell, I. Begg, J. Berrington, A. Bint, E. Boyle, R. Bray, P. Brocklehurst, C. Brook, J. Bunn, T. Cheetham, I. Choonara, J. Clark, M. Coulthard, S. Craig, A. Curley, B. Darlow, T. David, J. Davison, D. Dhawan, L. Duley, D. Elbourne, N. Embleton, A. Emmerson, N. Evans, A. Ewer, A. Fenton, D. Field, T. Flood, P. Fowlie, D. Gardner-Medwin, D. Gibb, R. Gilbert, H. Halliday, A. Hallman, F. Hampton, J. Hawdon, R. Hearns, P. Heath, D. Isaacs, K. Ives, L. Jones, S. Jones, C. Kennedy, S. Kenyon, H. Kirpalani, W. Lamb, H. Lambert, A. Lander, P. Loughnan, J. Lumley, N. Marlow, A. Macleod, C. Macpherson, J. Madar, N. McIntosh, P. McKiernan, A. McNinch, P. Midgley, D. Milligan, D. Mitchell, N. Modi, E. Molyneux, J. Morrice, A. Morris, N. Murray, M.-L. Newell, S. Oddie, A. Ogilvie Stuart, A. Ohlsson, S. Pedler, P. Powell, S. Rahman, M. Reid, J. Rennie, I. Roberts, M. Robinson, S. Robson, H. Russell, M. Rutter, S. Ryan, D. Salisbury, B. Schmidt, N. Shaw, D. Sims, S. Sinha, J. Skinner, J. Smith, N. Subhedar, A. Taylor, D. Taylor, W. Tin, G. Toms, P. Tookey, G. Tydeman, I. Verber, P. Vermeer-de Bondt, S. Walkinshaw, S. Wardle, M. Ward Platt, U. Wariyar, R. Welch, B. Wharton, A. Whitelaw, A. Wilkinson, C. Wren and J. Wyllie.

The future of the compendium rests in the hands of those who use it; anyone spotting an error or ambiguity in the text, or identifying an important omission or a drug in development but worthy of inclusion in future editions, is urged to contact the editorial team using the email address on *page xii*, so that the reference value of the various drug monographs can be sustained and further improved.

Any reader would like to see any medications not currently mentioned appear in the next edition please contact the editorial team via the e-mail address drug.information@neonatalformulary.com.

PART 1

Drug prescribing and drug administration

This part of NNF7 covers important aspects of safely prescribing and administering drugs. It also explains what happens when renal failure is present or the infant is undergoing therapeutic hypothermia.

Staff should never prescribe or administer any drug without first familiarising themselves with the way it works, the way it is handled by the body and the problems that can arise as a result of its use. Most of the essential facts relating to use in adults are summarised by the manufacturer in the 'package insert' or Summary of Product Characteristics (SPC). Many are also summarised in a range of reference texts such as the *British National Formulary* (BNF) and the *BNF for Children* (BNFC). However manufacturers seldom provide much information about drug handling *in infancy*. Although *BNFC* now offers more advice on dosage in childhood than can be obtained from the manufacturer's package insert, it stresses that the use of any unlicensed medicine (or licensed medicine in an unlicensed manner) should only be undertaken by those who have also first consulted *other appropriate and up-to-date literature*. This edition of *Neonatal Formulary* aims to summarise and to provide a referenced guide to that literature.

While many texts offer advice on the best dose to use in infancy – often in tabular form – very few provide much information on the idiosyncrasies associated with neonatal use. Such dosage tables can be a useful *aide mémoire*, but they should **never** be relied upon, on their own, to help the staff decide what to use when, what works best or what potential adverse effects are commonly encountered during use in infancy. Lists summarising common side effects and potential drug interactions are seldom of much help in identifying which problems are common or likely to be of clinical importance in the neonate, and access to this more detailed information is as important for the staff responsible for drug administration as it is for those prescribing treatment in the first place.

Similar challenges relate to the safe use of drugs during pregnancy and lactation because standard texts (such as the BNF) offer very little information as to what is, and is not, known about use in these circumstances. Such information is available in a range of specialised reference texts (see p. 558) and Part 3 of this compendium summarises what is currently known about the use of most of the more commonly used drugs.

Never use any other reference text except the most recent edition of this or any other formulary. Copies of earlier editions of this or any other formulary should not be left where they might be used in error.

Terms, symbols, abbreviations and units

Post-menstrual age: The term post-menstrual age, as used in this book, refers to the child's total age in weeks from the start of the mother's last menstrual period (LMP). Thus a 7-week old baby born at 25 weeks' gestation is treated as having a post-menstrual age of 32 weeks.

The term 'post-conceptional age' is sometimes incorrectly used to describe this combination, although technically, conception occurs about 2 weeks after the start of the LMP. The term 'post-conceptional age' is best avoided. Where the date of conception is determined during assisted reproductive techniques, the convention for calculating gestation at birth is to add 2 weeks to the 'conceptual age'.

Giving intravenous drugs: Intravenous (IV) drugs should *always* be given slowly, with a few notable exceptions. This universal good practice is not reiterated in each drug monograph. A simple way of achieving slow administration is described in p. 8. Where previous dilution or a particularly slow rate of infusion is important, this is specified in the relevant drug monograph, and the reason given. Drugs should also be given separately. Where two different IV drugs have to be given at the same time, the best way to stop them mixing is described in p. 22. Intramuscular (IM) drugs should never be mixed, except as described in the individual drug monographs.

Continuous co-infusion: Special problems arise when it is necessary to give more than one drug continuously and vascular access is limited. Here terminal co-infusion (the mixing of two different infusates using a tap or Y connector sited as close to the patient as possible) is sometimes known to be safe. In the most frequently encountered situations where such co-infusion is safe, a comment to that effect occurs in the relevant drug monograph. In all other situations two different infusion sites should be used unless advice to the contrary has been obtained from the local hospital pharmacy. Advice relating to Parenteral Nutrition (TPN) *only* applies to formulations similar to the one described in this compendium.

Drug names: Drugs are, in general, referred to by their non-proprietary ('generic') name, following the usage currently adopted by the BNF. Where, for clarity, a proprietary name has been used, the symbol ® has been appended the first time it is used. Where the British Approved Name (BAN) or the United States Adopted Name (USAN) differ from the recommended International Non-proprietary Name (rINN), these alternatives are also given. All synonyms are indexed.

Symbols and abbreviations: Cross references between monographs are marked by the Latin phrase *quod vide* (contracted to q.v.). Drugs vary in the extent to which they are distributed within the body. Some only accumulate in the extracellular tissues. Others are taken up and concentrated in some or all body tissues, the total amount in

Neonatal Formulary 7: Drug Use in Pregnancy and the First Year of Life, Seventh Edition. Sean B Ainsworth.
© 2015 John Wiley & Sons, Ltd. Published 2015 by John Wiley & Sons, Ltd.
Companion website: www.neonatalformulary.com

the body being more than would be presumed from a measure of that present in the blood. This is referred to as the drug's apparent volume of distribution – summarised by the symbol V_D. References to a randomised controlled trial are marked by the symbol [RCT]; those referring to a systematic review or meta-analysis are marked [SR]. Drugs for which the Cochrane Collaboration has produced a systematic review are marked with ⊙, and vaccines for which one can access official UK guidance *via* this book's website are marked with **DHUK**. Other abbreviations have been kept to a minimum and are explained in the index.

UNITS

1 kilogram (kg)	=	1000 grams
1 gram (g)	=	1000 milligrams
1 milligram (mg)	=	1000 micrograms
1 microgram (µg)*	=	1000 nanograms
1 nanogram (ng)*	=	1000 picograms

A 1% weight for volume (w/v) solution contains 1 g of substance in 100 ml of solution

It follows that:
a 1:100 (1%) solution contains 10 mg in 1 ml
a 1:1000 (1‰)* solution contains 1 mg in 1 ml
a 1:10,000 solution contains 100 micrograms in 1 ml

* The contractions (µg, ng and ‰) should be avoided as they can be misread when handwritten.

Drug storage and administration

Safe drug administration is every bit as important as safe and effective drug prescribing.

Neonatal prescribing: It is important to consider the practicalities of drug administration when prescribing, and to avoid prescribing absurdly precise doses that cannot realistically be measured. Such problems arise with particular frequency when body weight enters into the calculation. It is difficult to measure volumes of less than 0.05 ml even with a 1 ml syringe, and anyone who prescribes a potentially dangerous drug without first working out how to give it must inevitably carry much of the responsibility if such thoughtlessness results in an administrative error. Guidance on this is given in the individual drug monographs, with advice on prior dilution where necessary.

Equal thought should also be given to the timing and frequency of drug administration. Because many drugs have a relatively long neonatal elimination 'half-life', they only need to be given once or twice a day. More frequent administration only increases the amount of work for all concerned and increases the risk of errors creeping in. Parents are also more likely to give what has been prescribed after discharge if they are not asked to give the medicine more than twice a day!

Length of treatment: Remembering to stop treatment can be as important as remembering to start it. Neonatal antibiotic treatment seldom needs to be continued for very long. Treatment should always be stopped after 36–48 hours or sooner if the initial diagnosis is not confirmed. Babies with meningitis, osteitis and staphylococcal pneumonia almost always need 2–3 weeks' treatment, but 10 days is usually enough in septicaemia. Few babies need to go home on treatment; even anticonvulsants can usually be stopped prior to discharge (cf. the monograph on phenobarbital). Babies are often offered respiratory stimulants like caffeine for far longer than is necessary. Few continue to need such treatment when they are more than 32 weeks gestation: it should, therefore, usually be possible to stop all treatment at least 3 weeks before discharge. In the case of some widely used nutritional supplements (such as iron and folic acid), there was probably never any indication for starting treatment in the first place given the extent to which most artificial milks are now fortified (cf. the monograph on pre-term milk).

Storage before use: Most drugs are perfectly stable at room temperature (i.e. at between 5 and 25 °C) and do not require specialised storage facilities. Temperatures above 25 °C can be harmful, however, and some drugs are damaged by being frozen, so special thought has to be given to transport and dispatch. Some drugs are best protected from direct daylight, and, as a general rule, all drugs should be stored in a

Neonatal Formulary 7: Drug Use in Pregnancy and the First Year of Life, Seventh Edition. Sean B Ainsworth.
© 2015 John Wiley & Sons, Ltd. Published 2015 by John Wiley & Sons, Ltd.
Companion website: www.neonatalformulary.com

cupboard and kept in the boxes in which they were dispensed and dispatched. Indeed, in a hospital setting, all drugs are normally kept under lock and key.

Hospital guidelines usually specify that drugs for external use should be kept in a separate cupboard from drugs for internal use. Controlled drugs, as specified in the regulations issued under the UK Misuse of Drugs Act 1971, must be kept in a separate cupboard. This must have a separate key, and this key must remain under the control of the nurse in charge of the ward at all times. A witnessed record must be kept of everything placed in, or taken from, this cupboard and any loss (e.g. due to breakage) should be accounted for. Medical and nursing staff must comply with identical rules in this regard.

Special considerations apply to the storage of vaccines. Many of these are damaged if they are not kept at between 4 and 8 °C at all times – even during transit and delivery (no mean feat in many resource poor or underdeveloped countries). A range of other biological products, such as the natural hormones desmopressin, oxytocin, tetracosactide and vasopressin, need to be stored at 4 °C. The same goes for cytokines, such as erythropoeitin (epoetin) and filgrastim, and surfactants of animal origin. The only other widely used neonatal drugs that need to be stored at 4 °C are amphotericin, atracurium, dinoprostone, soluble insulin, lorazepam and pancuronium, and even here the need to maintain such a temperature *all* the time is not nearly as strict as it is with vaccine storage. Many oral antibiotic preparations have only a limited shelf life after reconstitution. The same goes for a number of oral suspensions prepared for neonatal use 'in house'. The 'shelf life' of all these preparations can be increased by storage at 4 °C. Drugs that do not *need* to be kept in a ward refrigerator should *not* be so stored.

All the drugs mentioned in this compendium that require special storage conditions have their requirements clearly indicated in the relevant drug monograph – where no storage conditions are specified it can be taken that no special conditions exist.

Continued retention of open vials: Glass and plastic ampoules must be discarded once they have been opened. Drug vials can generally be kept for a few hours after they have been reconstituted, as long as they are stored at 4 °C but, because they often contain no antiseptic or preservative, it becomes increasingly more hazardous to insert a fresh needle through the cap more than two or three times, or to keep any open vial for more than 6–8 hours. It is, therefore, standard practice to discard all vials promptly after they have been opened (with the few exceptions specifically mentioned in the individual monographs in Part 2).

Drug dilution: Many drugs have to be diluted before they can be used in babies because they were formulated for use in adults. In addition, dilution is almost always required when a drug is given as a continuous infusion. Serious errors can occur at this stage if the dead space in the hub of the syringe is overlooked. Thus if a drug is drawn into a 1 ml syringe up to the 0.05 ml mark, the *syringe* will then contain between 0.14 and 0.18 ml of drug. If the syringe is then filled to 1 ml with diluent, the syringe will contain **three times** as much drug as was intended!

To dilute any drug safely, therefore, draw some diluent into the syringe first, preferably until the syringe is about half full, and then add the active drug. Mix the drug and diluent if necessary at this stage by one or two gentle movements of the plunger, and then finally make the syringe up to the planned total volume with further diluent.

In this way the distance between two of the graduation marks on the side of the syringe can be used to measure the amount of active drug added.

While this may be adequate for 10-fold dilution, it is not accurate enough where a greater dilution than this is required. In this situation it is necessary to use two syringes linked by a sterile three-way tap. The active drug is drawn up into a suitable *small* syringe and then injected into the larger syringe through the side port of the tap. The tap is then turned so as to occlude the side port and diluent added to the *main* syringe until the desired total volume is reached.

Detailed guidance is given in Part 2 of this compendium on how to reconstitute each drug prior to administration, and how to handle drug dilution whenever this is called for. This can be found under the heading 'Supply' or 'Supply and administration' in each drug monograph.

Giving drugs by mouth: Oral medication is clearly unsuitable for babies who are shocked, acidotic or otherwise obviously unwell because there is a real risk of paralytic ileus and delayed absorption. Babies well enough to take milk feeds, however, are nearly always well enough to take medication by mouth, and many drugs are just as effective when given this way. Antibiotics that can be given by mouth to any baby well enough to take milk feeds without detriment to the blood levels that are achieved include amoxycillin, ampicillin, cephalexin, chloramphenicol, ciprofloxacin, co-trimoxazole, erythromycin, flucloxacillin, fluconazole, flucytosine, isoniazid, metronidazole, pyrimethamine, rifampicin, sodium fusidate and trimethoprim. Oral administration is often quicker, cheaper and safer than intravenous (IV) administration. Oral administration is also much more easily managed on the postnatal wards, and treatment can then be continued by the parents after discharge where appropriate.

Remember that if medicine is passed down an orogastric or nasogastric feeding tube, much of it will be left in the tube unless it is then flushed through. It used to be standard practice to formulate drugs given by mouth so that the neonatal dose was always given in 5 ml aliquots (one teaspoonful), but this practice has now been discontinued. Dilution often reduced stability and shortened the drug's 'shelf life', while dilution with a syrup containing glucose threatened to increase the risk of caries in recently erupted teeth in later infancy. Small quantities are best given from a dropper bottle (try to avoid the pipette touching the tongue) or dropped onto the back of the tongue from the nozzle of a syringe.

Additives to milk: Vitamins are often added to milk. Sodium, phosphate and bicarbonate can also be given as a dietary supplement in the same way. It is important to remember that if only half the proffered feed is taken, only half the medicine is administered. Where possible all of a day's supplements should be added to the first feed of the day, so the baby still gets all that were prescribed even if feeding is later curtailed. The giving of any such dietary supplement must be recorded either on the feed chart or on the drug prescription sheet, and, to avoid confusion, each unit needs to develop a consistent policy in this regard.

Intravenous drugs: IV drugs should be given slowly and, where possible, through a secure established IV line containing glucose and/or sodium chloride. Drugs should never be injected or connected into a line containing blood or a blood product. Since the volume of the drug to be given seldom exceeds 2 ml in neonatal practice, abrupt administration can be avoided by siting a three-way tap so there is only 10–25 cm of narrow-bore tubing containing about 2 ml of fluid between the tap and the patient. Give the drug over about 5 seconds as described under the heading IV injections, but do not, except in special circumstances, flush the drug through. The adoption of this practice as a *routine* ensures that any 'bolus' of drug reaches the patient slowly over a period of 5–20 minutes after being injected into the fluid line without staff having to stand by the patient throughout the period of administration, or set up a special mechanical infusion system.

On the rare occasions when a small rapid bolus injection *is* called for (as, for example, when adenosine is used in the management of a cardiac arrhythmia), the drug infusion should be followed by a 2 ml 'chaser' of 0.9% sodium chloride from a second syringe in order to flush the active drug through the IV line as rapidly as possible. Do not flush the drug through by changing the basic infusion rate: several deaths have resulted from a failure to handle this manoeuvre correctly. Giving a routine chaser by hand ties up valuable senior nursing time, tends to result in over-rapid administration when staff time is at a premium, and can, if repeated frequently, result in the baby getting a lot of undocumented water, sodium or glucose.

Particular care must be taken not to mix potentially incompatible fluids. This issue is dealt with, in some detail, in the final part of the monograph on the Care and Use of Intravascular Lines (see pp. 17–21). Staff must also remain alert to the very real risks of air embolism, infection, inflammation, thrombosis and tissue extravasation (as set out in the earlier parts of that monograph). They should also be familiar with the management of anaphylaxis (see p. 267).

IV injections: The standard procedure for using a three-way tap to give a slow IV 'stat' dose is to:
- Connect the pre-loaded syringe to the free tap inlet
- Turn the tap so the syringe is connected to the patient and give the injection
- Turn the tap so the syringe is connected to the giving set, draw up about 0.2 ml of infusion fluid, turn the tap back so the syringe is reconnected to the patient and flush this fluid through so that it just enters the giving set
- Where two drugs are scheduled for simultaneous administration proceed as outlined in p. 22.

While the above method is adequate for most purposes, it always results in the administration of too much medicine because it causes the baby to get the medicine that was trapped in the hub of the syringe. A slightly more complex (and expensive) procedure that avoids this problem is preferable when the amount of drug to be given is less than 0.3 ml, and essential whenever a potentially toxic drug such as digoxin, chloramphenicol or an aminoglycoside is given intravenously. Proceed as above but modify the third of the three stages listed by using a second small syringe containing water for injection or 0.9% sodium chloride, instead of fluid from the drip line, and flush just 0.2 ml of fluid through the tap. Do not give more than this or you will end up giving the drug as a relatively rapid bolus.

Slow intermittent IV infusions: Drugs that need to be given by slow intermittent IV infusion (such as phenobarbital, sodium bicarbonate or trometamol) can, if necessary, be given by hand through a three-way tap as a series of 2 ml bolus doses every few minutes, but aciclovir, amphotericin B, ciprofloxacin, cotrimoxazole, erythromycin, fluconazole, flucytosine, phenytoin, rifampicin, sodium fusidate, vancomycin and zidovudine are best injected into an existing IV line through a three-way tap using a programmable syringe pump. Slow infusion has been recommended for a range of other antibiotics without the support of any justificatory evidence. Manufacturers recommend slow aminoglycoside administration in North America, but not in Europe. Inconsistencies abound. The continued unquestioning acceptance of any time consuming policy of this type without a critical review of its justification limits the time staff can give to other potentially more important tasks.

Continuous IV infusions: Drugs for continuous infusion such as adrenaline, atracurium, atosiban, diamorphine, dobutamine, dopamine, doxapram, enoximone, epoprostenol, glyceryl trinitrate, hydrocortisone, insulin, isoprenaline, labetalol, lidocaine, lipid emulsions, magnesium sulphate, midazolam, milrinone, morphine, noradrenaline, nitroprusside, oxytocin, prostaglandin E, streptokinase, thiopental and tolazoline should be administered from a second carefully labelled infusion pump connected by a three-way tap into the main infusion line. Remember to readjust the total fluid intake. Great care is needed to ensure that patients never receive even a brief surge of one of the vasoactive drugs accidentally, and the same is true of many inotropes. Never load the syringe or burette with more of the drug than is likely to be needed in 12–24 hours to limit the risk of accidental over infusion. Also check and chart the rate at which the infusion pump is actually operating by looking at the amount of fluid left once an hour. The guidelines relating to the administration of intermittent IV injections also apply when a continuous infusion is first set up.

Intramuscular administration: Intramuscular (IM) medication is more reliable than oral medication in a baby who is unwell, but drug release from the IM 'depot' is sometimes slow (a property that is used to advantage during treatment with naloxone, procaine penicillin and vitamin K). It may also be unreliable if there is circulatory shock. Bulky injections are also painful, but it should not necessarily be assumed that permanent attachment to an IV line is without its frustrations either, especially if this involves limb splinting! Prior cleaning of the skin is largely a token ritual. The main hazard of IM medication is the risk that the injection will accidentally damage a major nerve. Small babies have little muscle bulk and the sciatic nerve is easily damaged when drugs are given into the buttock, even when a conscious effort is made to direct the injection into the outer upper quadrant. The anterior aspect of the quadriceps muscle in the thigh is the *only* safe site in a small wasted baby, and this is the only site that should be used routinely in the first year of life.

Try to alternate between the two legs if multiple injections are required. Multiple large injections into the same muscle can, very rarely, precipitate an ischaemic fibrosis severe enough to cause muscle weakness and a later disabling contracture. IM injection should also be avoided in any patient with a severe uncorrected bleeding tendency. A superficial injection may result in the drug entering subcutaneous fat rather than muscular tissue causing induration, fat necrosis, delayed drug release and a palpable subcutaneous lump that may persist for many weeks. An intradermal injection can also leave a permanent scar. With certain drugs, such as bupivacaine, the accidental injection of drug into a blood vessel during deep tissue infiltration is toxic to the heart, and it is essential to pull back the plunger each time the needle is moved to ensure that a vessel has not been entered. It is also wise to give any dose slowly while using a pulse oximeter in order to get early warning of any possible adverse cardiorespiratory effect.

Intradermal and subcutaneous administration: BCG vaccine has to be given *into* the skin (intradermally). The best technique for achieving this is outlined in pp. 98–99. A number of other products, including insulin and the cytokines filgrastim and erythropoietin, are designed to be given into the fatty tissue just below the skin (subcutaneously). Vaccines were often given subcutaneously in the past, but it is now generally accepted that IM injection actually causes less pain at the time and less discomfort afterwards. IM injection also improves the immune response. It is wrong to assume that a long needle makes any injection more painful – there are many pain receptors just below the skin but relatively few in muscle tissue. Approach the skin vertically when giving an IM injection, and at 45° when giving a subcutaneous injection. Use a needle at *least* 15 mm long for any IM injection, even in the smallest baby.

Rectal administration: This can be a useful way of giving a drug that is normally given by mouth to a baby who is not being fed. Chloral hydrate, codeine phosphate and paracetamol are sometimes given this way. So are some anticonvulsants such as carbamazepine, diazepam and paraldehyde. However, absorption is usually slower, often less complete, and sometimes less reliable than with oral administration. Suppositories have usually been used in the past, but liquid formations are more appropriate in the neonatal period. Absorption is always more rapid and often more complete when a liquid formulation is used. It is also much easier to administer a precise, weight related, dose. Half a suppository does not necessarily contain half the active ingredient even when accurately halved.

Intrathecal and intraventricular administration: Streptomycin was the first effective antituberculous drug. Because it does not cross the blood–brain barrier well, a policy of repeated intrathecal injection soon evolved to cope with the scourge of TB meningitis. It then quickly became common to treat other forms of meningitis the same way. Penicillin, in particular, was quite often injected into the cerebrospinal fluid (CSF), even though good levels can be achieved with high dose IV treatment. This approach is now seldom adopted because a range of antibiotics are available that penetrate CSF well. Gentamicin and vancomycin are, however, still occasionally injected into the CSF in babies with ventriculitis, particularly if the ventricles need to be tapped diagnostically, or therapeutically, because of obstructive hydrocephalus. Diagnostic needling of a thick-walled intracerebral abscess can also usefully be followed by the direct injection of a suitable antibiotic into the abscess cavity. The use of an intraventricular reservoir is often recommended when repeated intrathecal treatment is called for, but implanted plastic can increase the difficulty of eliminating bacterial infection because there is a strong risk of the catheter itself becoming colonised.

The intrathecal dose is always much smaller than the IV or IM dose because of the smaller volume of distribution. Gentamicin is still sometimes given into the cerebral ventricles, but the only published controlled trial suggested that children so treated actually did worse than children given standard IV treatment. Many antibiotics are irritant and the preservatives even more so. Special intrathecal preparations of benzylpenicillin and gentamicin should always be used. Dilute the preparation before use, and check whether there is free flow of CSF before injecting the drug.

Intraosseous administration: This can be a valuable way of providing fluid in an emergency. Any drug that can be given IV can also be given by this route. Insert the needle into the upper end of the tibia a little below the tuberosity, using a slight

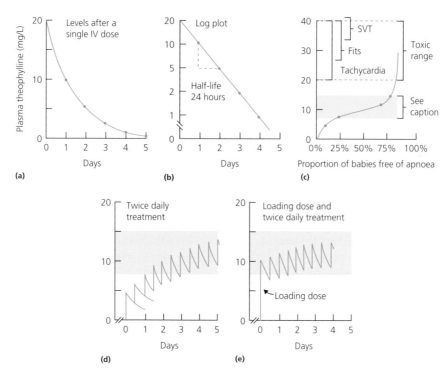

Fig. 1 Baby with a theophylline half-life of 24 hours. The therapeutic range (8–15 mg/L) is shaded. SVT, supraventricular tachycardia.

elimination only changes slowly, therefore, in the weeks after birth. Other drugs, like the penicillins, are excreted with increasing rapidity after delivery as renal tubular secretion becomes more active. The actual dose required depends on the extent of the drug's distribution within the body, and dose frequency on its speed of elimination. This is usually proportional to the amount present, unless saturation occurs (as with phenytoin). It can be described by the time it takes for the blood level to halve (elimination *half-life* or $t_{1/2}$), a relationship (Fig. 1a) that is linear when plotted on a log scale (Fig. 1b). The challenge is to achieve and sustain levels in the safe therapeutic range. The response to the drug may improve as levels increase (Fig. 1c), but toxic effects may also appear, and the ratio of the toxic to the therapeutic level (*therapeutic index*) may be quite small. A drug has to be given for a time equal to four half-lives before levels stabilise (Fig. 1d), unless a *loading dose* is given (Fig. 1e).

Drugs and the law

Licensing

While the UK laws that control the prescribing and the supply of medicines may seem complex, they actually impose few constraints on staff working in a hospital setting. The Medicines Act of 1968, passed in the wake of the thalidomide disaster, regulates the activity of the pharmaceutical industry, making it illegal for any medicine to be marketed for human use in the United Kingdom without a product licence (marketing authorisation). These are issued by the Licensing Authority (the Ministers of Health) on the advice of the Medicines and Healthcare products Regulatory Agency (MHRA). The MHRA also oversees the manufacture, promotion and distribution of medicines, while the Committee on Safety of Medicines (CSM) advises the agency on their efficacy, quality and safety. While these licences are not published, the relevant provisions, including indications for use, recommended precautions and dose ranges, are summarised in the manufacturer's Summary of Product Characteristics (SPC). These summaries can now be accessed via the Internet (www.medicines.org.uk), as can copies of the manufacturer's Patient Information Leaflet (PIL) be drafted to make key information available in a more accessible format.

However, the 1968 Act was deliberately framed in such a way that it did not restrict 'clinical freedom', and it exempts doctors and dentists from many of the constraints placed on drug companies. It is, therefore, perfectly in order for a doctor to recommend, or administer, a drug for which no product licence exists. The Act, and EC Directive 89/341/EEC, also made it clear that a doctor could use an unlicensed drug in clinical trials, or give an unlicensed product that has been specially prepared or imported, for a particular ('named') patient. It is also acceptable for a doctor to use, or recommend the use of, a drug in a dose, by a route, for a condition or for a group of patients, which differs from those mentioned in the manufacturer's product licence (so-called 'off label' or 'off licence' use). It is also legal for such a drug to be dispensed by a pharmacist or administered by a nurse or midwife. Legislation in America, and in many other countries, has adopted a broadly similar approach.

This legal freedom placed doctors under a heavy legal, moral and professional obligation to ensure that the recommendations they make about drug use are well founded. Such problems become acute when a manufacturer offers no advice with regard to the use of a drug for children of less than a certain age, as is, for example, currently true of almost all drugs used to manage hypotension and hypertension in childhood. Such problems can turn children into 'therapeutic orphans'. Manufacturers are often reluctant to bear the cost of sponsoring the trials necessary to support a change to the original marketing licence or the cost of collating all the information published in the scientific

Neonatal Formulary 7: Drug Use in Pregnancy and the First Year of Life, Seventh Edition. Sean B Ainsworth.
© 2015 John Wiley & Sons, Ltd. Published 2015 by John Wiley & Sons, Ltd.
Companion website: www.neonatalformulary.com

literature after a product's first commercial launch so the licence can be updated. Here it becomes particularly important for the doctor to be sure that the use to which they are putting a product is reasonable and prudent in the light of such scientific information as *is* available in print. This compendium is one aid to that end. The *BNF for Children* (BNFC) offers similar guidance on how to handle some of the many situations in which older children may need to be treated in ways not covered by the manufacturer's recommendations, but it is not a referenced text. In addition, it only provides limited information on how to manage drug treatment in the ill preterm baby, and it provides very little useful guidance on drug use during pregnancy and lactation.

Prescribing

The 1968 Act classifies medicines into those available for general sale (a General Sale List or GSL drug), those only available for retail sale through a pharmacy (P) and those that can only be dispensed from a pharmacy against a prescription (a Prescription Only Medicine or POM). Additional rules apply to Controlled Drugs (CD). All medicines, other than GSL drugs, have to be sold from a registered pharmacy *unless* they are being sold or supplied by a hospital or health centre, and are being administered in accordance with the directions of a doctor. The only POM products that could be dispensed by a community pharmacist without a doctor's prescription (except in an emergency) were, until now, the few products in the Nurse Prescribers' and Dental Practitioners' Formularies, as listed in the British National Formulary (BNF) and its counterpart for children (BNFC).

Non-medical prescribing: New legislation came into force in the United Kingdom in May 2006, which made it possible for senior, experienced, first level nurses, midwives, specialist community public health nurses and some pharmacists, to acquire almost exactly the same prescribing rights as doctors. Staff put forward for such training will need to be working in an area where this skill could be put to use. They will also need the background to be able to study at level 3 (degree level), to have acquired at least 3 years' post-registration clinical experience and to have been working for at least the last year in the clinical area in which they are expecting to prescribe once trained. Their register will be annotated to record the successful completion of this training, and they will then be in a position where they can legally prescribe any licensed drug, even for 'off label' use, as long as it is not a controlled drug (where some, slightly ambiguous, restrictions still operate). Any borderline food product, dressing or appliance listed in the BNF can also be prescribed. Staff so qualified should all be at least as aware as any doctor of the need to work within the limits of their sphere of professional competence and within any guidelines laid down by their employing authority. These developments should, once such training becomes more generally available, make it much easier for senior midwifery and nursing staff to start treatment when it is called for without first having to get a doctor to authorise this. They will also make it possible for experienced nurses and midwives to manage urgent inter-hospital transfers appropriately even when there is not a doctor on the transfer team.

There are, however, a few residual restrictions and uncertainties. The indications for which a limited range of CD can now be prescribed are not always very precisely specified either (an area where legislation is as much a matter for the UK Home Office as for the Department of Health). Morphine can be given for suspected myocardial infarction, for 'post-operative pain relief' and for 'pain caused by trauma', but it is not clear whether this includes the pain associated with childbirth, or the trauma associated with many aspects of neonatal intensive care. Staff can also give morphine to a baby with severe necrotising enterocolitis but only, it would seem, after surgery. Diazepam, lorazepam and midazolam can be used to control 'tonic-clonic seizures' and can also be used, like morphine and diamorphine, to provide 'palliative care', but that phrase is often used to mean simply the terminal care of a patient with an untreatable condition rather than the palliation of the stress associated with the sudden urgent need to initiate artificial respiratory support. Doubtless most of these residual uncertainties will be clarified in time.

Patient group directions: Because legislation in the United Kingdom does not allow most nurses to prescribe, alternative and more flexible strategies have been developed in the past 8 years to enable appropriately trained staff to assume greater personal responsibility for administering a range of POM products. An *ad hoc* system of 'Group Protocols' was recognised as having much merit by the Crown Report in 1998, and legislation was subsequently passed in 2000 making it legal for nurses to supply and administer any licensed medicine (even 'off label') to specific groups of patients under a formal agreement with a prescribing doctor. The work of pharmacists, physiotherapists and other 'paramedic' groups can be covered in a similar way. Such agreements (known as Patient Group Directions or PGDs) need to conform to the guidance given in HSC 2000/026 (England), HDL (2001) 7 (Scotland) and WHC (200) 116 (Wales), and any direction has to be prepared by a multidisciplinary group involving a senior doctor, pharmacist and nurse or midwife, in consultation with the local Drug and Therapeutics Committee and then approved by the Hospital or Primary Care Trust.

While the introduction of PGDs is restricted to situations where such administration 'offers an advantage to patient care without compromising patient safety', there are many aspects of maternity care where it is clearly possible to improve the delivery of care by making better use of these, as yet very inconsistently applied, arrangements. Vaccine administration (including hepatitis B vaccine) has been the aspect of primary care most often covered by the development of PGDs. However, the administration of rhesus D immunoglobulin, the initiation of antenatal steroid treatment and the provision of prophylactic antibiotic cover to any mother (and/or baby) where there has been significant pre-labour rupture of membranes are the three further important aspects of maternity care that can often be improved by the development of an appropriate PGD at unit level. Unfortunately, because PGDs cannot be used to initiate treatment with a controlled drug, pethidine still remains, very inappropriately, one of the few controlled drugs that a midwife can prescribe and administer on her own authority. There is a widespread belief that these directions can only be used to administer a single dose of some licensed medicinal product; this is incorrect. A PGD can certainly, for example, be used in appropriate circumstances to initiate a course of antibiotic treatment.

Supplementary prescribing: This provides an alternative strategy for involving nurses, midwives and allied healthcare professionals more productively in the management of conditions where treatment needs may vary over time, allowing staff to prescribe from within the elements of a previously agreed joint management plan. Some hospitals in the United Kingdom have used this option to allow bedside intensive care staff to adjust treatment hour by hour as the patient's condition dictates, but the option has been more widely adopted in the community management of long-term medical conditions such as asthma or diabetes.

The care and use of intravascular lines

Intravascular lines serve a number of vital functions. They make it possible to give fluids, including glucose and a range of other nutrients, when oral nutrition is impossible or inappropriate. They also make it possible to monitor both arterial and central venous pressure directly and continuously, to collect blood specimens without causing pain or disturbance, and to give drugs reliably and painlessly.

These very real advantages have to be balanced against a range of very real disadvantages. Of these, infection due to localised vasculitis or insidious low-grade septicaemia is perhaps the most common. Vascular thrombosis is a hazard, and thrombi can also shed emboli. Even reactive arterial vasospasm can cause significant ischaemia. Bleeding from an arterial line can cause serious blood loss, life threatening air embolism can occur into any central venous line and fluid extravasation can cause severe ischaemia or chemical tissue damage with subsequent necrosis. Any baby with an intravascular line in place is at risk of sudden fluid overload if steps are not taken to make the unintentional and uncontrolled infusion of more than 30 ml/kg of fluid technically impossible (see the Section on Minimising IV Infusion and Other Drug Hazards). There is also a risk of reactive hypoglycaemia if any glucose infusion is stopped (or the rate changed) too abruptly (see p. 241).

Line care

Thrombosis: Relatively little can be done to reduce the risk of thrombosis. A small amount of heparin (q.v.) may reduce the risk of catheter occlusion, but this has little effect on the formation of mural thrombi. Whether the benefit of full heparinisation outweighs the risk remains unclear. Clinical vigilance can speed the recognition of problems when they occur, and the routine use of a lateral X-ray to identify where any central catheter has lodged can help to ensure that the tip is optimally sited (a lateral X-ray is more easily interpreted than an antero-posterior or AP view). An attempt is usually made to site any central venous catheter in a major vein or at the entrance to the right atrium. The larger the vessel, the less the risk of occlusion (or extravasation), but the greater the hazard should this occur. Similarly, it is standard practice to site any aortic catheter either above the diaphragm (T6) or below the two renal arteries (L4) to minimise the risk of a silent renal or mesenteric artery thrombosis. There is now good evidence that there are fewer recognisable complications associated with high placement (although there may be a marginally increased risk of necrotising enterocolitis). Case controlled studies suggest, however, that intraventricular haemorrhage may be commoner when aortic catheters are positioned above the diaphragm, and

Neonatal Formulary 7: Drug Use in Pregnancy and the First Year of Life, Seventh Edition. Sean B Ainsworth.
© 2015 John Wiley & Sons, Ltd. Published 2015 by John Wiley & Sons, Ltd.
Companion website: www.neonatalformulary.com

when heparin is used to prolong catheter patency. Only a very large properly conducted randomised controlled trial is likely to resolve some of these uncertainties.

Limb ischaemia is usually readily recognised, but by the time it is identified much of
the damage has often been done. Thrombosis of the abdominal vessels is often silent,
but may be a significant cause of renal hypertension. Central venous thrombosis is also
under-diagnosed but can cause a chylous ascites by occluding the exit of the thoracic
duct. Occlusion of a small vein is seldom a problem because of the nature of the anas-
tomotic venous plexus, but occlusion of even a small artery can cause severe ischaemia
if it is an 'end-artery' (i.e. the only vessel supplying a particular area of the body). Even
occlusion of the radial artery can sometimes cause vascular compromise if there is no
significant terminal anastomosis between the radial and ulnar arteries. Every baby with
an intravascular line in place should be examined regularly by the nursing staff for evidence of any of the above complications. There are good grounds for particular vigilance
in the first few hours after an arterial line has been sited but, with this one exception,
all lines merit equal vigilance. Treatment options are reviewed in a commentary linked
to the monograph on the use of alteplase (see p. 68).

Vasospasm: Arteries are particularly likely to go into spasm shortly after cannulation.
This may make it necessary to withdraw the catheter, but a single small dose of tolazoline can sometimes correct the acute 'white leg' seen after umbilical artery catheterisation, and a continued low-dose infusion may work when a single bolus dose is only
transiently effective. Papaverine has also been used experimentally in the same way.

Extravasation: Never give a drug into a drip that has started to 'tissue'. Delivery cannot
be guaranteed once this has happened, and some drugs (as noted in the individual drug
monographs) can also cause severe tissue damage. Fluids containing calcium cause particularly severe scaring. Serious damage can also be caused by the fluids used in providing
parenteral nutrition. Such problems will only be noticed promptly if every drip is so
strapped that the tissue around the cannula tip can be inspected at any time. The best
line of management, if extravasation is starting to cause tissue damage, involves early
tissue irrigation, as outlined in the monograph on hyaluronidase in p. 258. Hot or cold
compresses are of no measurable value. Neither is limb elevation.

Infection: Localised or generalised infection is probably the commonest complication
of the use of intravascular lines. Indolent, usually low grade, but occasionally life
threatening, blood borne infection (septicaemia) has been reported in more than 20%
of all babies with 'long lines' in some units. Infection can be devastating in a small baby,
and it is a clear indictment of unit policy if the way in which a baby is cared for puts it
unnecessarily at increased risk of infection. The risk of such iatrogenic infection can
only be minimised by scrupulous attention to hygiene. Inadequate attention to skin
sterility (see p. 469) is probably the most common reason why cannulae and catheters
have later become colonised. Access should always be achieved using an aseptic
approach. A gown, mask and surgical drape should also be used whenever a long line
is being inserted. The risk of infection is not reduced by the use of an antiseptic or antibiotic cream. Indeed there is evidence that such use can actually increase the risk of
fungal infection. Covering the insertion site with a transparent occlusive dressing helps

even though increased humidity under such a dressing can speed the multiplication of skin bacteria. An impregnated chlorhexidine disc may help prevent this.

Infection most frequently enters where the catheter pierces the skin. This is why most infusion-related infections are caused by coagulase-negative *Staphylococci* and why Broviac® lines that are surgically 'tunnelled' under the skin are less prone to infection. Complications, including infection, seem more common in neonates if the line is inserted into an arm rather than a leg. Bacterial colonisation of the catheter hub (where the catheter connects to the giving set) can also be the precursor of overt septicaemia. Stopcocks often become contaminated, but there is no evidence that such contamination causes catheter-related infection. The risk of generalised infection is increased by the use of a long line rather than a short line. Independently of this, parenteral nutrition may, and intralipid certainly does, further increase the risk of systemic infection. Antibiotic treatment for this can, in turn, greatly increase the risk of life-threatening fungal septicaemia. These are strong reasons for avoiding the unnecessary use of long lines and for only using parenteral nutrition when oral feeding is impracticable. Catheters impregnated with an antimicrobial agent have started to become available, but their use is no substitute for proper attention to other aspects of catheter hygiene. Heparin fusions may decrease the risk of thrombosis and infections where use is unavoidable.

It was thought that the risk of infection could be reduced by resiting all infusions at regular intervals, and short cannulas are still often resited in adults once every 2–3 days to reduce the risk of phlebitis and catheter colonisation. There is, as yet, no good evidence that this approach is justified in children. It was also said that fluids and administration sets should be changed daily to minimise the risk of in-use fluid contamination, but this practice is *not* now endorsed by the American Centers for Disease Control (CDC) in Atlanta, Georgia. Such routines generate a lot of work, increase costs and have not been shown to reduce the risk of blood stream infection. Unnecessary interference with the infusion line could actually increase the risk. There is, however, one small controlled trial (in urgent need of confirmation) suggesting that the regular use of an in-line filter does reduce the risk of septicaemia in the preterm baby, and that this remains true even if the giving set is changed only once every 4 days. There are also good grounds for changing the administration set each time the infusion fluid is changed (although infusion with insulin may be an exception to this generalisation as explained in p. 274). This is particularly important after any blood or blood product has been given because the presence of a thin thrombin film increases the chance of bacteria then colonising the giving set. Lipid solutions are also particularly likely to become infected, and it is probably good practice to change these once every 48 hours. In addition, some continuously infused drugs are only stable for a limited time (as outlined in the individual drug monographs) and need to be prepared afresh once every 12–24 hours. There is no evidence that other fluids (or giving sets) need to be changed more than once every 3–4 days. The catheter *must* be removed promptly once bacteraemia is documented if complications are to be minimised (a single coagulase-negative staphylococcal blood culture being the only exception to this general rule).

Air embolism: An air embolus can kill a patient very rapidly. Air is so much more compressible than blood that once it enters the heart it tends to stay there instead of being pumped on round the body, especially if the baby is lying flat. This air then completely stops the circulation unless immediately aspirated. Umbilical vein catheters are particularly dangerous; air can easily be drawn into the heart when the baby takes a breath if there is not a three-way tap or syringe on the end of any catheter at all times (especially during insertion). Similarly, if air gets into a giving set (through, for example, a cracked syringe), it can easily be pumped into the blood stream.

Blood loss: Babies can easily die of blood loss. Serious loss from the cord has become rare since the invention of the modern plastic umbilical clamp, but haemorrhage can still occur if no clamp has been placed on the umbilical vessels so that they can be cannulated (especially if the baby is then wrapped up for warmth with, perhaps, a 'silver swaddler', through which tell-tale blood cannot seep). Death can also occur from haemorrhage if an intravascular line becomes disconnected. To minimise this latter risk, all connections in any intravascular line should always have Luer-Lok® fittings.

Use of lines

There has been a lot of confused thought as to what may, and may not, be put into what sort of intravascular line. Policy varies widely from unit to unit, and all the policies cannot possibly be right. There is equal uncertainty over who has the necessary authority to put drugs into, or take blood out of, what sort of line. True 'authority' comes with training and experience, not with the mere possession of a medical qualification.

A midwife or nurse who has been trained in the care and use of intravascular catheters will often be in a better position to give safe care than a 'qualified' but untrained and inexperienced doctor. With proper training, all qualified staff working in any neonatal unit ought to be equally competent in all aspects of intravascular catheter care and use. Anyone experienced enough to give drugs into an established line should have enough experience to sample blood from such a line, and anyone who has been trained to give drugs or sample from a venous catheter has all the knowledge necessary to use a properly inserted arterial line.

What you can safely put *into* a line depends not only on what sort of line it is but also on what sort of fluid is already in the line (see below). This is also true of what you can reliably take *out* of a line. Any line can, in theory, be used for blood sampling, but care needs to be taken to clear the 'dead space' first. Sodium levels can only be measured from a line being infused with 0.9% sodium chloride after a volume equal to three times the dead space has been withdrawn first. Blood glucose levels cannot be measured in a blood sample taken from *any* line through which glucose is being infused, even if the catheter dead space is first cleared by temporarily withdrawing 5 ml of blood before collecting the sample for analysis. Nor can reliable blood coagulation test results be obtained from any line that has ever contained heparin. False-positive evidence of infection can also result if blood is drawn for blood culture from an already established intravascular line. Where septicaemia is suspected it is always best to collect blood direct into a culture medium from a fresh venous 'needle stab'.

Peripheral veins: These can be used for collecting blood samples and for giving almost any drug, although care should be taken when infusing a number of vasoactive drugs (as indicated in the relevant drug monographs). Drugs such as dopamine and isoprenaline are better delivered through a central venous line. Where there is no need to give a continuous infusion, a cannula can be inserted and left 'stopped off' with a rubber injection 'bung'. There is no good evidence that these benefit from heparinisation and, in any strict interpretation of the regulations, both the drug *and* the heparinised flush solution would need to be prescribed, and each administration signed for separately each time (although it has not, as yet, generally been considered necessary to record the giving of every 'flush' of saline or water).

Central veins: Drugs can be given safely into any central venous line once ultrasound, or an X-ray, has shown where the catheter tip has lodged. This is the best route for giving any drug or infusion that tends to damage the vascular endothelium (such as solutions containing more than 10% glucose). Keep the tip away from the right atrium and mediastinal vessels since, if wall damage *does* occur, the resultant pleural or pericardial effusion will kill if not recognised promptly. Anchor the exposed end of the catheter firmly to the skin – serious complications can arise if the catheter migrates further into the body after insertion. Only give drugs into an umbilical vein catheter as a last resort if the tip has lodged in a portal vein. Any midwife or nurse who has been trained to give drugs into a peripheral vein should be competent to give drugs into a central vein. However, because of the greater risk of infection when a central line is in place, such lines should not be 'broken into' either to give drugs or to sample blood unnecessarily. It will often be difficult to sample blood from a central venous line because of its length and narrow bore. Furthermore, if blood is allowed to track back up a central venous catheter, there is a serious risk of a clot developing, blocking the line.

Peripheral arteries: Such lines are almost always inserted in order to monitor blood pressure or sample arterial blood. They should never be used for giving drugs. The right radial artery is the most frequently used. It may be safe to use a continuous infusion of glucose saline into a peripheral artery, but it is probably best to limit any infusion to as small a volume of heparinised 0.18% (or 0.9%) sodium chloride as is compatible with maintaining catheter patency (see p. 253).

Central arteries: These will almost always be aortic catheters positioned through an umbilical artery. Such lines are usually sited in order to monitor blood pressure or sample post-ductal arterial blood, but they can safely be used to give glucose or total parenteral nutrition once the site of the catheter tip has been checked radiologically. Take care that this is not close to the coeliac axis, because exposing the pancreas to an infusion of concentrated glucose can cause hypoglycaemia by stimulating an excessive release of insulin. Because blood flow down the aorta is high, it is also perfectly safe to give most drugs (other than some of the vasoconstrictive drugs such as adrenaline, dopamine and isoprenaline) as a slow continuous infusion into the aorta. Bolus infusions should be avoided, however, unless there is no realistic alternative (particularly if the drug is a vascular irritant) because of the risk that an excessive amount of drug will be delivered into a single vulnerable 'end artery'. Severe tissue necrosis in the area served by the internal iliac artery has been documented quite frequently when drugs such as undiluted sodium bicarbonate have been administered as a bolus into an umbilical artery during emergency resuscitation after circulatory collapse.

Compatible and incompatible fluids

All the drugs mentioned in the main section of this compendium as being suitable for intravenous (IV) use are capable of being injected into, or piggy-backed onto, any existing IV infusion containing up to 0.9% sodium chloride and/or up to 10% glucose unless otherwise stated (amphotericin B, enoximone, phenytoin and erythromycin [unless buffered] being the main exceptions). Do not add drugs to any line containing blood or blood products.

Different drugs should never be mixed together however, except as specified in the various drug monographs, without consulting with an experienced pharmacist. Where a single infusion line *has* to be used to give more than one drug, and it is not practicable to delay the administration of the second drug for at least 10 minutes, different products must be separated by 1 ml of glucose saline, 0.9% sodium chloride or sterile water for injection (less will do with very narrow bore tubing). Adherence to these guidelines is particularly important where a very alkaline product such as sodium bicarbonate or trometamol is being infused. Use the technique described under IV injection in the review of 'Drug Storage and Administration' (see p. 8), and give the separating 1 ml bolus *slowly* over at least 2 minutes to ensure that the drug already in the IV line does not reach the patient as a sudden, dangerously rapid, surge. This is particularly important if the line contains an inotrope or vasoactive product, or a drug, such as aminophylline, cimetidine, phenytoin, or ranitidine, which can cause a cardiac arrhythmia if infused too fast.

Special problems arise when it is necessary to give more than one drug continuously, and intravascular access is limited. Here terminal co-infusion (the brief mixing of two different infusates using a three-way tap or Y connector sited as close to the patient as possible) is sometimes known to be safe. In this situation the two drugs are only in contact for a relatively short time (although with slow infusion rates in a very small baby contact may last longer than is generally appreciated). In the most frequently encountered situations where such co-infusion is thought to be safe, a statement to this effect has been added to one of the two relevant drug monographs. The documentary evidence for this practice comes (unless otherwise stated) from *Trissel's Handbook of Injectable Drugs*. Note that, even here, compatibility will have only been formally assessed for a limited range of drug concentrations.

Special considerations apply to the administration of any drug into a line containing an amino acid solution when a baby requires parenteral nutrition. Terminal co-infusion, using any product that approximates fairly closely to the formulation described in this compendium, is probably safe for certain drugs, as outlined in the various drug monographs. It is not, however, safe to assume that this is true for other formulations. *No* drug (other than Vitlipid®) should ever be added to any infusion containing emulsified fat (Intralipid®), nor should lipid be co-infused with any fluid containing any other drug (other than heparin, insulin, isoprenaline, noradrenaline or vancomycin). The use of a double, or triple, lumen umbilical catheter makes it possible to give drugs to a baby receiving parenteral nutrition through a single infusion site.

References

Ainsworth SB, Clerihew L, McGuire W. Percutaneous central venous catheters versus peripheral cannulae for delivery of parenteral nutrition in neonates. *Cochrane Database of Systematic Reviews* 2007, Issue 3. Art. No. CD004219. [SR]

American Academy of Pediatrics. Committee on Drugs. 'Inactive' ingredients in pharmaceutical products: update (subject review). *Pediatrics* 1997;**99**:268–78.

Benjamin DK, Miller W, Garges H, *et al.* Bacteremia, central catheters, and neonates: when to pull the line. *Pediatrics* 2001;**107**:1272–6.

Birch P, Ogden S, Hewson M. A randomised, controlled trial of heparin in total parenteral nutrition to prevent sepsis associated with neonatal long lines: the Heparin in Long Line Total Parenteral Nutrition (HILLTOP) trial. *Arch Dis Child Fetal Neonatal Ed* 2010;**95**:F252–7. [RCT]

Burn W, Whitman V, Marks VH, *et al.* Inadvertent over administration of digoxin to low-birth-weight infants. *J Pediatr* 1978;**92**:1024–5.

Buttler-O'Hara M, Buzzard CJ, Reubens L, *et al.* A randomized trial comparing long-term and short-term use of umbilical venous catheters in premature infants with birthweights of less than 1251 grams. *Pediatrics* 2006;**118**:e25–36. [RCT]

Dann TC. Routine skin preparation before injection: unnecessary procedure. *Lancet* 1969;**ii**:96–8.

Davies MW, Mehr S, Morley CJ. The effect of draw-up volume on the accuracy of electrolyte measurements from neonatal arterial lines. *J Paediatr Child Health* 2000;**36**:122–4.

Gillies D, O'Riordan L, Wallen M, *et al.* Optimal timing for intravenous administration set replacement. *Cochrane Database of Systematic Reviews* 2005, Issue 4. Art. No. CD003588.

Golombek SG, Rohan AJ, Parvez B, *et al.* 'Proactive' management of percutaneously inserted central catheters results in decreased incidence of infection in the ELBW population. *J Perinatol* 2002;**22**:209–13.

Hoang V, Sills J, Chandler M, *et al.* Percutaneously inserted central catheter for total parenteral nutrition in neonates: complications rates relating to upper versus lower extremity insertion. *Pediatrics* 2008;**121**:e1152–9.

Hodding JH. Medication administration via the umbilical arterial catheter: a survey of standard practices and review of the literature. *Am J Perinatol* 1990;**7**:329–32.

Leff RD, Roberts RJ. Methods for intravenous drug administration in the pediatric patient. *J Pediatr* 1981;**98**:631–5.

van Lingen RA, Baerts W, Marquering ACM, *et al.* The use in-line intravenous filters in sick newborn infants. *Acta Paediatr* 2004;**89**:658–62.

MacDonald MG, Chou MM. Preventing complications from lines and tubes. *Semin Perinatol* 1986;**10**:224–33.

MacDonald MG, Ramasethu J, Rais-Bahrami K. *Atlas of procedures in neonatology*, 5th edn. Philadelphia, PA: JB Lippincott, 2012.

Marlow AG, Kitai I, Kirpalani H, *et al.* A randomised trial of 72- versus 24-hour intravenous tubing set changes in newborns receiving lipid therapy. *Infect Control Hosp Epidemiol* 1999;**20**:487–93. [RCT]

Moore TD, ed. *Iatrogenic problems in neonatal intensive care*. Sixty-ninth Ross Conference on Pediatric Research, 4–7 May, 1975. Columbus, OH: Ross Laboratories, 1976.

O'Grady NP, Alexander M, Dellinger EP, *et al.* Guidelines for the prevention of intravascular catheter-related infections. *Pediatrics* 2002;**110**:e51.

Phillips I, Meers PD, D'Arcy PF. *Microbiological hazards of infusion therapy*. MTP Press, Lancaster, 1976.

Orlowski JP. Emergency alternatives to intravenous access. *Pediatr Clin North Am* 1994;**41**:1183–99.

Salzman MB, Rubin LG. Intravenous catheter-related infections. *Adv Pediatr Infect Dis* 1995;**10**:337–68.

Sinclair JC, Bracken MB, eds. *Effective care of the newborn infant*. Oxford: Oxford University Press, 1992. (See especially Chapter 10, pp. 188–9; Chapter 19, pp. 440–1; and Chapter 23, p. 582.)

Shah PS, Kalyn A, Satodia P, *et al.* A randomized, controlled trial of heparin versus placebo infusion to prolong the usability of peripherally placed percutaneous central venous catheters (PCVCs) in neonates: the HIP (Heparin Infusion for PCVC) study. *Pediatrics* 2007;**119**:e284–91. [RCT]

Trissel LA. *Handbook of injectable drugs*, 17th edn. Bethsda, MA: American Society of Health System Pharmacists, 2012.

Minimising IV infusion and other drug hazards

Errors of intravenous (IV) fluid and drug administration are common. Reporting of such is important, but should never be made the pretext for disciplinary action unless there has been obvious negligence. The prescriber shares responsibility for any administrative error that occurs when prescribing in an unclear or unnecessarily complex way. Staff new in place, at all levels, frequently find themselves working under considerable pressure, and low staffing levels often impose further stress. Management share responsibility for protecting staff from excessive pressure, for ensuring that unit policies are such as to minimise the risk of any error occurring and (even more importantly) for seeing that the potential danger associated with any error is minimised by the use of 'fail-safe' routines like those outlined below. If senior staff and managers over-react when mistakes occur, errors may simply go unreported, increasing the risk of a recurrence.

It is important to retain a sense of proportion in considering the issues raised by the rule that every error of drug prescribing has to be reported. While any error of **commission** is generally looked upon as a potentially serious disciplinary issue, serious errors of **omission** often go unremarked. Inadvertent reductions in IV fluid administration due to tissue extravasation, failure to resite an infusion line promptly or failure to set up the syringe pump correctly, are more likely to put a baby at hazard (from reactive hypoglycaemia) than a transient period of excess fluid administration. Note that hypoglycaemia is particularly likely to occur where a maintenance infusion of glucose saline IV is cut back or stopped abruptly so that blood can be given (for guidance on this, see the monograph on blood transfusion). Similarly, failure to give a dose of medicine may sometimes be just as hazardous as the administration of too big a dose.

Drug prescribing and drug administration call for close teamwork between the medical, midwifery and nursing staff. When an error does occur it is seldom one person's sole fault, and this needs to be acknowledged if disciplinary action is called for. Where it is clear that a doctor and a midwife or nurse both share responsibility for any untoward incident, natural justice demands that any necessary disciplinary action is handled in an equable and equitable way.

Minor medication errors (i.e. any deviation from the doctor's order as written on the patient's hospital chart) are extremely common. Rates of between one per patient day and two per patient week have been reported in the United States. Prescribing errors are also common. Anonymous self-reporting schemes have been initiated in a few hospitals, as part of a more general risk management strategy, in an attempt to identify high risk situations. Dilutional errors are particularly common in neonatal

---

Neonatal Formulary 7: Drug Use in Pregnancy and the First Year of Life, Seventh Edition. Sean B Ainsworth.
© 2015 John Wiley & Sons, Ltd. Published 2015 by John Wiley & Sons, Ltd.
Companion website: www.neonatalformulary.com

practice, and the individual drug guidelines in this compendium have been carefully framed so as to minimise these.

Ten golden rules

Attention to the following 10 rules will help to minimise error and, even more importantly, ensure that when an error does occur the impact is minimised:

1 Keep the prescribing of medication to a minimum, and use once or twice daily administration where this is possible.

2 Never have more than two IV infusion lines running at the same time unless this is absolutely necessary.

3 Never put more than 30 ml of fluid at any one time into any syringe used to provide continuous IV fluid or milk for a baby weighing less than 1 kg.

4 Record the amount of fluid administered by every syringe pump by inspecting the movement of the syringe and by inspecting the infusion site once every hour. Do not rely merely on any digital electronic display.

5 In an analogous way, where the infusion of fluid from any large (half litre) reservoir is controlled by a peristaltic pump (or by a gravity operated system with a gate valve and drop counter), it is always wise to interpose a burette between the main reservoir and the control unit. Limiting the amount of fluid in the burette limits the risk of accidental fluid overload, and recording the amount of fluid left in the burette every hour speeds the recognition of any administrative error.

6 Do not change the feeding or IV fluid regime more than once or, at most, twice a day except for a very good reason. Try to arrange that such changes as do have to be made are made during the morning or evening joint management rounds.

7 Those few drugs that have to be administered over 30 minutes or more should be administered using a separate programmable syringe pump 'piggy-backed' onto an existing IV Line. As an extra precaution, the syringe should never be set up containing more than twice as much of the drug as it is planned to deliver. Do not adjust the rate at which the main IV infusion fluid is administered unless there is a serious risk of hyperglycaemia, or it is necessary to place an absolute restriction on the total daily fluid intake.

8 Do not routinely flush drugs or fluids through an established IV line except in the rare situations where this is specifically recommended in this compendium. To do so can expose the baby to a dangerously abrupt 'bolus' of drug. Using fluid from the main IV line to do this can also make the baby briefly and abruptly hyperglycaemic.

9 Beware giving a small newborn baby excess sodium unintentionally. The use of flush solutions of Hep-lok®, Hepsal® or 0.9% sodium chloride can expose a baby to an unintended excess of IV sodium. The steady infusion of 1 ml/hour of heparinised 0.9% sodium chloride (normal saline) to maintain catheter patency is sometimes enough to double a very small baby's total daily sodium intake. So too can intra-tracheal sodium chloride administration during tracheal 'toilet'.

10 Treat the prescribing of potentially toxic or lethal drugs (such as chloramphenicol and digoxin) with special care. There are relatively few situations where it is really necessary to use such potentially dangerous drugs.

If something *does* go wrong

Report any significant error of omission or commission promptly so that appropriate action can be taken to minimise any possible hazard to the baby. Nine times out of ten a senior member of staff with pharmacological expertise will be able to determine that no harm has been done quite quickly and offer much needed reassurance to all concerned. If malfunction of a pump or drip regulator is suspected, switch the equipment off and replace it *without touching* the setting of the rate control switches, pass the equipment to medical electronics for checking without delay and record the serial number of the offending piece of equipment on the incident form.

CHECK AND DOUBLE CHECK

1 **Have you got the right drug?** *Check the strength of the formulation and the label on the ampoule as well as the box.*
2 **Has the shelf-life expired?** *Check the 'use by' date.*
3 **Has it been reconstituted and diluted properly?** *Check the advice given in the individual drug monograph in this compendium.*
4 **Have you got the right patient?** *Check the name band.*
5 **Have you got the right dose?** *Have two people independently checked steps 1–4 with the prescription chart?*
6 **Have you picked up the right syringe?** *Deal with one patient at a time.*
7 **Is the IV line patent? Have you got the right line?** *Is it correctly positioned? Could the line have tissued?*
8 **Is a separate flush solution needed?** *Have two people checked the content of the flush syringe?*
9 **Are all the 'sharps' disposed of?** *What about any glass ampoules?*
10 **Have you 'signed up' what you have done?** *Has it been countersigned?*

Patient safety initiatives

Background

Drug errors are an avoidable cause of iatrogenic injury in neonatal patients. Most (71%) medication errors are due to poor prescribing. The most common example of this in many studies is an incorrect dose (unexplained deviation of >10% from the neonatal unit formulary) or an incorrect dose interval; this is something particularly seen with gentamicin and vancomycin. To counter this particular aspect, many units now employ a 'gentamicin safety bundle', and there are similar ones for vancomycin (see below).

Dosing errors may also become a factor when staff are making up individualised infusion – more common in neonatal and paediatric practice than in adults because of many different factors such as changes in weight over the course of a neonatal stay and age-related maturational changes in drug pharmacokinetics and pharmacodynamics. Many infusions are, out of necessity, made up after undertaking sometimes complex calculations and dilutions that have the potential for errors in the placing of decimal points leading to $\times 10$ dosing errors. Standardising the composition of the infusion and using a 'constant concentration variable rate' method of administration often in conjunction with Intelligent Infusion Pump Systems (sometimes referred to as Smart Pumps) may take away a lot of the cot-side calculation that currently occurs.

The similarity of some drug names can cause the wrong medication to be administered, particularly if the prescription is also barely legible. In North America, one initiative that has been introduced to counter this is the 'Tall man' system of writing drug names. This uses a mix of UPPERCASE and lowercase letters in the name of the medication such that it becomes easier to see differences between drug names that would otherwise look very similar.

Gentamicin bundle

In 2010, the National Patient Safety Agency (NPSA) developed a Patient Safety Alert around a care bundle for the safer use of IV gentamicin for neonates. Data collected by the NPSA had shown that 15% of all neonatal medication errors involved the prescription, administration and monitoring of gentamicin. A number of factors were implicated in these errors including:

1 Medication error
2 Interruptions and distractions to those involved in drug administration
3 Incorrectly calculating doses
4 Incorrectly calculating dosing intervals – especially a problem when the dose interval is 36 hours (as can be the case in neonates)

Neonatal Formulary 7: Drug Use in Pregnancy and the First Year of Life, Seventh Edition. Sean B Ainsworth.
© 2015 John Wiley & Sons, Ltd. Published 2015 by John Wiley & Sons, Ltd.
Companion website: www.neonatalformulary.com

5 Lack of any double-checking by staff preparing and administering the drugs
6 Training, education and communication

The resulting neonatal gentamicin care bundle incorporates the following four elements:

1 Any prescribing of gentamicin should use the 24-hour clock and any unused time slots in the prescription administration record should be blocked out to prevent wrong time dosing.
2 Interruptions during the preparation and administration of gentamicin should be minimised by the wearing of a disposable coloured apron by staff.
3 A double-checking prompt (available to download from www.nrls.npsa.nhs.uk/alerts) being used during the preparation and administration of gentamicin.
4 The prescribed dose of gentamicin should be given within an hour either side of the administration time.

Constant concentration variable rate and 'smart pumps'

Until recently, the majority of neonatal infusions have been made up according to the baby's weight and the infusion run at a constant rate for a given dose. The infused solution is, in many cases, made up by the nurses who are looking after the baby rather than in some standardised manner either by the manufacturer or in a pharmacy. This practice is prone to many of the same errors seen with gentamicin (see above). Such infusions are described as having a 'variable concentration' and a 'constant rate'. A variation of this which many perceive to be safer is to have a 'constant concentration' of the drug (which may be that supplied by the manufacturer or made up in a standardised way by the hospital's pharmacy) and which are given at a 'variable rate' (which varies from baby to baby according to their weight). Although such infusions – called constant concentration variable rate because the concentration (or strength) of the infusion remains constant and the rate is adjusted according to the baby's weight – can be used with any pump, they are frequently used in conjunction with 'smart pumps' which remove some of the need to make calculations about which rate needs to be used to achieve which dose. If a 'smart pump' is not used, a computer spreadsheet-based programme such as Microsoft® Excel has been shown to be helpful in calculating the required rate for a given dose.

Smart pumps or intelligent infusion pump systems are increasingly becoming available. Such pumps incorporate sophisticated computer technologies for storing drug information, for example, a drug library with doses, pre-programmed concentrations, automating calculations and checking information entered against agreed administration parameters (i.e. providing a safety net). The implementation of smart pump technology can therefore reduce the incidence of errors in the administration of IV drugs. The initial stages involve developing a drug library for the specific needs of the population, and setting hard and soft limits for each drug. The needs of a neonatal unit will be different from that of a paediatric intensive care unit. Beginning to build a library requires input from clinicians as well as pharmacists and can seem like a lot of hard work. Support from the local IT department is essential as any subsequent changes (e.g. in the concentrations of the infusate brought about perhaps by a change in manufacturer) need to be implemented across all the smart pumps in use simultaneously (wireless technology can be helpful here).

No one size fits all in term of drug libraries, particularly in a population of neonatal patients whose weight can vary from less than 500 g to over 5 kg. A major perceived barrier is that of possible fluid overload particularly in lower weight patients or in those whose overall fluids are restricted for clinical reasons. The Vermont Oxford Network and Institute of Safe Medication Practices (ISMP) in America have produced a list of standard concentrations of neonatal drug infusions (see http://www.ismp.org/Tools/PediatricConcentrations.pdf) that could be used in about 80% of cases.

Tall man lettering

The ISMP also advocate the use of 'Tall man' lettering (see http://www.ismp.org/tools/tallmanletters.pdf). Use of a mix of UPPERCASE and lowercase letters can help, particularly with printed labels, differentiate between drugs with very similar names, for example 'DOBUTamine' and 'DOPamine'. The ISMP list is fairly specific to North American practice and the full list contains many proprietary as well a generic names.

References

Conroy S, Appleby K, Rostock D, *et al*. Medication errors in a children's hospital. *Paediatr Perinatal Drug Ther* 2007a;**8**:18–25.

Conroy S, Sweis D, Planner C, *et al*. Interventions to reduce dosing errors in children: a systematic review of the literature. *Drug Saf* 2007b;**30**:1111–25. [SR]

Filik R, Purdy K, Gale A, *et al*. Drug name confusion: evaluating the effectiveness of capital ("Tall Man") letters using eye movement data. *Soc Sci Med* 2004;**59**:2597–601.

Grissinger M. 'Smart pumps' are not smart on their own. *P T* 2010;**35**:489–529.

Irwin A, Mearns K, Watson M, *et al*. The effect of proximity, tall man lettering, and time pressure on accurate visual perception of drug names. *Hum Factors* 2013;**55**:253–66.

Irwin D, Vaillancourt R, Dalgleish D, *et al*. Standard concentrations of high-alert drug infusions across paediatric acute care. *Paediatr Child Health* 2008;**13**:371–6.

Kaushal R, Bates DW, Landrigan C, *et al*. Medication errors and adverse drug events in pediatric inpatients. *JAMA* 2001;**285**:2114–20.

Lemoine JB, Hurst HM. Using smart pumps to reduce medication errors in the NICU. *Nurs Womens Health* 2012;**16**:151–8.

Manrique-Rodríguez S, Sánchez-Galindo A, Fernández-Llamazares CM, *et al*. Developing a drug library for smart pumps in a pediatric intensive care unit. *Artif Intell Med* 2012;**54**:155–61.

Mooney J. The safer use of intravenous gentamicin for neonates. *Infant* 2010;**6**:134–7.

Raju TNK, Thornton JP, Kecskes S, *et al*. Medication errors in neonatal and pediatric intensive-care units. *Lancet* 1989;**2**(8659):374–6.

Scanlon M. The role of "smart" infusion pumps in patient safety. *Pediatr Clin North Am* 2012;**59**:1257–67.

Wilson K, Sullivan M. Preventing medication errors with smart infusion technology. *Am J Health Syst Pharm* 2004;**61**:177–83.

Writing a hospital prescription

Comprehensive guidance on how to 'write up' (or transcribe) a prescription is given for those working in the United Kingdom in the introduction to the British National Formulary, but many of the points in this bear repetition. While the formal constraints that operate in the community do not apply in a hospital setting (see p. 14), the following guidelines still represent good practice:

Block capitals: Always use UPPERCASE letters when prescribing drug names to ensure legibility (one exception to this is where the Tall man system is in use). A poorly written prescription is, at best, discourteous to nurses and pharmacists who may have to spend time checking what has been written. Illegibility can also be dangerous.

Approved names: These should always be used to ensure consistency between vials, ampoules, bottles and other labels. Proprietary names ('trade names') should only be used for compound preparations when a generic name does not exist (e.g. Gaviscon® Infant – half a dual sachet), or where bioavailability of the drug may be affected by changing brands (e.g. anticonvulsants). Avoid abbreviations and contractions other than those universally used and recognised.

The dose: This should be given in grams (g), milligrams (mg), micrograms or, exceptionally, nanograms. Do not use abbreviations for anything other than grams (g) or milligrams (mg).

Units: When the dose is in 'UNITS', write this word out in full. Avoid the symbol 'U' because it is too easily misread, and avoid the term 'microunits'. Oxytocin (see p. 383) is one exception to this rule. Some drug companies still use the term 'international units' (IU) but, since international agreement has now been reached as to the meaning of all such terms, this terminology is unnecessary, and best avoided.

Volumes: Volumes should always be prescribed in millilitres. This can be abbreviated to ml (but it should not be contracted to cc or cm³).

Decimal places: Carelessness in use of decimals is a major cause of potentially lethal overtreatment. Decimals should be avoided where possible and, where unavoidable, always prefaced by a zero. Write 500 mg not 0.5 g. If a decimal has to be used, write 0.5 ml not .5 ml. Do not use a comma, use a full stop (0.5 ml not 0,5 ml).

Time: This is best written using the 24-hour clock when prescribing for patients in hospital.

Route of administration: This must always be indicated. The following abbreviations are generally acceptable:

IV	Intravenous	**IM**	Intramuscular
NEB	Nebuliser	**PO**	Oral (per Os)
PR	Rectal (per rectum)	**SC**	Subcutaneous

Neonatal Formulary 7: Drug Use in Pregnancy and the First Year of Life, Seventh Edition. Sean B Ainsworth.
© 2015 John Wiley & Sons, Ltd. Published 2015 by John Wiley & Sons, Ltd.
Companion website: www.neonatalformulary.com

All other methods of administration should be written in full (e.g. intradermal and intra-tracheal).

Continuous IV administration: Drugs for continuous intravenous (or, rarely, umbilical arterial) infusion can be prescribed on an IV infusion chart, and signed for on this chart in the usual way. Full details do not then need to be written up and signed for in duplicate on the main inpatient medicine chart, but the front of this chart does, as a minimum, need to be marked to show clearly what other charts are in use.

Reconstitution and dilution: Drugs frequently have to be reconstituted and/or diluted before they can be given to babies. It is not necessary to write down how this should be done when prescribing a drug listed in this compendium and where all staff routinely follow these guidelines because it will be assumed that reconstitution and dilution will be carried out as specified in the relevant drug monograph. Indeed, it would only cause confusion to give any instruction that was unintentionally at variance with the advice given here. Instructions *must* be given however where this is not the case, or if a drug is prescribed that is not in this compendium.

Limits of precision: Do not ask for impossible precision. A dose prescribed by weight will almost always have to be given to a child by volume (often after dilution, as above), and it is not generally possible to measure or administer a volume of less than 0.1 ml with any precision (as noted on p. 6).

Flexible dosage: Some drugs (such as insulin) are regularly prescribed on a 'sliding scale'. Where this is the case it may not be necessary or appropriate for a doctor to write up each individual dose given. In the same way, detailed authorisation for hour-by-hour dose variation within a prescribed range (such as the use of labetalol or an inotrope to control blood pressure) does not require a doctor's signature each time treatment is adjusted as long as each change in dosage is recorded and signed for on the IV chart by the relevant responsible nurse.

Management at delivery: Drugs commonly given to the baby at birth (such as vitamin K or naloxone) do not need to be written up on a medicine chart as long as their administration is fully documented in a fixed and standardised position in the maternity notes.

Emergency resuscitation: Where drugs are given in an acute emergency by a doctor or nurse during cardiorespiratory resuscitation they do not need to be recorded in duplicate in the medicine chart as long as they are accurately recorded in the narrative record in the medical notes (along with dosage and timing) when this is subsequently written up.

Blood products and vaccines: While these are not traditionally recorded on the medicine chart, administration must be recorded somewhere in the clinical notes along with the relevant batch number.

Dietary supplements: Vitamins, and other dietary supplements for which no prescription is necessary, and once daily additions to milk feeds (such as supplemental sodium) need not be prescribed on the medicine chart. Administration does, however, need to be recorded each time on the child's feed chart.

Self-administration: Parents may be encouraged to give certain drugs (such as eye drops) on their own, especially where they are likely to have to continue giving such treatment after discharge from hospital. This can be done by writing *'self-administered'* in the space labelled 'notes' on some medicine charts.

Midwife authorised prescriptions: Drugs given by a midwife on her own responsibility in the United Kingdom must be properly recorded and 'signed up' on the medicine chart. Some units ask staff to add the symbol 'M' after their signature.

Patient group directions: Patient safety makes it very important for all medication administered under the terms of a Patient Group Direction (PGD) to be documented on the same chart as is being used to record all the *other* drugs the patient is being given. Just transcribing such a directive onto a medicine chart is *not* an act of 'prescribing' that occurred when the PGD was drawn up.

'As required' prescriptions: Be specific about how much may be taken, how often and for what purpose. Do not *only* write 'as required' or 'PRN' (*pro re nata*). Specify a minimum time interval before another such dose can be given. It will often be important to indicate a maximum cumulative daily (24-hour) dose. Patients offered analgesics 'PRN' often end up undertreated. A flexible prescription (see above) can often be more appropriate.

Medication on discharge: Hospitals in the United Kingdom generally instruct staff not to issue a prescription for more of any drug than the minimum needed to continue treatment until such time as the family can get a further prescription from their general practitioner unless, as with a small minority of drugs used in the neonatal period, the drug is only obtainable from a hospital pharmacy. It should not, in other circumstances, be necessary to dispense more than 2 week's treatment. The same guidelines apply to the dispensing of drugs for outpatients.

Telephone messages: Hospital rules vary. Most accept that under exceptional circumstances a telephone message may be accepted from a doctor by two nurses (one of whom must be a Registered Nurse and one of whom acts as witness to receipt of the message). It is not acceptable to prescribe controlled drugs in this way, and any other drug so prescribed should be given only once. The doctor must then confirm and sign the prescription within 12 hours. Faxed prescriptions should also be confirmed in writing within 72 hours.

Signature: Each entry must be signed for, separately, in full by a registered doctor or by a nurse with independent prescribing rights (except, in the United Kingdom, as covered by the PGD provisions outlined above). In all cases, the signature should be followed by the name of the prescriber in 'UPPERCASE' letters. The date that the entry was signed must also be recorded.

Cancellation: Drugs should not be taken for longer than necessary. Stop dates for short course treatments (such as antibiotics) can often be recorded on the medicine chart when first prescribed. The clearest way to mark the chart is to draw a horizontal line through the name of the drug, and the date, and then date and initial the 'Date Discontinued' space. Many drugs are given for much longer than is truly clinically necessary.

Adverse reactions and overtreatment

Adverse reactions

Any drug capable of doing good is also capable of doing harm, and unwanted reactions may be unexpected. Some of these adverse reactions are dose-related, but others are idiosyncratic. Problems may relate to the drug's main pharmacological action in the body, or to some secondary action ('side effect'). The recognition of adverse reactions is of vital importance, but their proper documentation and reporting is frequently neglected. The Commission on Human Medicines operates a simple 'Yellow Card' reporting system in the United Kingdom for the Medicines and Healthcare Regulatory Agency (MHRA) that is designed to make it easier for staff to initiate such notifications. Copies of the prepaid lettercard can be found in the back of the British National Formulary. The MHRA website (www.mhra.gov.uk) offers advice on what to report and how to complete a 'Yellow Card'. Reporting of adverse reactions can be made via the related website (www.yellowcard.mhra.gov.uk) or by telephone (0808 100 3352).

All prescribers have a professional duty to report all serious suspected reactions even if they are already well recognised, especially if they are fatal, life-threatening, disabling or incapacitating. This is necessary so that reports can be prepared comparing the risk/benefit ratio seen with other drugs of a similar class. Prescribers should also report any adverse or unexpected event, *however minor*, where this could conceivably be a response to a drug that has only been on the market for a relatively short time. Pharmacists also have a responsibility to report all important adverse reactions coming to their attention. Nurses and midwives are often the first to suspect an adverse reaction: they have a duty to see that any such reaction is brought to the attention of the appropriate doctor or pharmacist, and to initiate a report themselves if necessary. Deaths have, by law, to be reported to the coroner (Procurator Fiscal in Scotland).

The Commission on Human Medicines are interested in hearing about adverse reactions caused by *any* therapeutic agent (including any drug, blood product, vaccine, dental or surgical material, X-ray contrast medium, intra-uterine device, etc.). Reactions observed as a result of self medication should be reported in the same way as those seen with prescribed drugs. Drug interactions of a serious nature should also be reported. Drugs can sometimes have a delayed effect, causing problems such as later anaemia, jaundice, retroperitoneal fibrosis or even cancer. Any suspicion of such an association should always be reported. Whenever a baby is miscarried, is aborted or is born with a congenital abnormality, healthcare professionals should always consider whether this might have been an adverse drug reaction and report all the drugs (including any self-medication) taken during the pregnancy.

Neonatal Formulary 7: Drug Use in Pregnancy and the First Year of Life, Seventh Edition. Sean B Ainsworth.
© 2015 John Wiley & Sons, Ltd. Published 2015 by John Wiley & Sons, Ltd.
Companion website: www.neonatalformulary.com

Adverse reactions are particularly common when drugs are given at the extremes of life. This is, in part, because the liver and the kidneys handle drugs less efficiently, both in the first weeks of life, and in old age. Nevertheless, although the MHRA receives many reports relating to drug medication in the elderly, relatively few reports are received in relation to adverse events in the neonatal period. This is not because such events are uncommon, as many of the individual drug monographs in this compendium bear testimony, but because a proper tradition of reporting never seems to have become established. Yet, without such reporting, the identification of many important side effects is avoidably delayed. Because, in particular, some of the most important side effects seen in the neonatal period differ from those normally seen later in life, failure to report can also delay the recognition, and quantification, of a very real drug hazard.

Defective medicines constitute a related but different problem. Problems can occur either during manufacture, or during distribution, rendering the product either dangerous or ineffective. Whenever such a problem is suspected it should be reported *at once* to the hospital pharmacy who will, in turn, notify the MHRA's Defective Medicines Report Centre in London if the suspicions are confirmed. Contact may be made by telephone (020 3080 6574 or out of office hours 07795 641532) or using the on-line form on the MHRA website (www.mhra.gov.uk under the header 'Safety Information').

Overtreatment

Identifying the right dose of medicine to give a newborn baby is never easy, and the problem is made even more difficult if kidney or liver immaturity is compounded by illness or organ failure. Progressive drug accumulation is a very real possibility in these situations. A major error can easily arise during the drawing up of the small dose needed in a small preterm baby, particularly if prior dilution is involved. Few of these events ever get widely reported. Indeed, where the baby is already ill, the cause of death may go unrecognised. Tenfold administration errors are not unheard of.

Luckily even after serious overtreatment, most babies recover with supportive or symptomatic care (although this is not always true where drugs such as atropine, chloramphenicol, digoxin, lidocaine and potassium chloride are concerned). If the drug has been given by mouth, it may be worth giving a stomach washout. A 1 g/kg oral dose of activated charcoal (repeatable every 4 hours until charcoal appears in the stool) may also be of some help, especially if it is started within 4 hours. Do not try to make the baby sick. Other forms of forced elimination such as exchange transfusion, haemoperfusion, dialysis and forced diuresis are only of limited value for a small number of drugs taken in severe excess. Whole bowel irrigation with a polyethylene glycol-electrolyte solution (such as Klean-Prep®) may occasionally be appropriate. Always seek the immediate help and advice of the nearest Poisons Centre (see below) if there are severe symptoms. For a limited number of drugs, specific antidotes, antagonists or chelating agents are available; these are mentioned briefly, where appropriate, under the name of the drug for which they are of use, in the various monographs in the main section of this compendium. Specific antagonists include naloxone for opioid drugs, DigiFab® for digoxin, and flumazenil for benzodiazepines. Acetylcysteine is of value after paracetamol over-dosage, methylthioninium chloride (methylene blue) is used to control methaemoglobinaemia and the chelating agent desferrioxamine mesylate is used in iron poisoning. Following are the main components of supportive care.

Respiration: Airway obstruction is a real hazard in patients who become unconscious. Vomiting is not uncommon and inhalation a real risk. Most poisons that impair consciousness also depress breathing, so artificial respiratory support may well be required. While specific opioid and benzodiazepine antagonists can be helpful, respiratory stimulants should not be used. Correct any serious metabolic acidosis (pH < 7.2) with sodium bicarbonate or trometamol.

Fluid and glucose intake: Reduce fluid intake to a minimum and monitor urine output while retaining normoglycaemia until it is clear that kidney function is unaffected. Stop all oral feeds if there is acidosis, hypotension and/or suspected ileus.

Blood pressure: Do not use vasopressor drugs without first getting expert advice. Cautious plasma volume expansion may help if there is serious hypotension.

Arrhythmia: Do not give drugs, especially if output is tolerably well maintained, before defining the nature of the arrhythmia and seeking advice as outlined in the monograph on adenosine. A beta-blocker (such as propranolol) may help to moderate the tachyarrhythmia sometimes seen with excess theophylline, chloral hydrate, quinine, amfetamine or some of the antihistamines, and may improve cardiac output. These drugs do not seem to cause an arrhythmia in children as often as they do in adults.

Convulsions: While short-lived seizures do not require treatment, prolonged seizures should be controlled, especially if they seem to be impeding respiration. A slowly infused intravenous dose of diazepam (preferably the emulsified formulation) is the anticonvulsant most often used in older patients, but phenobarbital is more usually used in the neonatal period. Either drug can, in itself, cause further respiratory depression.

Temperature control: Poisoning can cause both hypo- and hyperthermia. The rectal temperature should be measured to monitor deep body temperature, using a low reading thermometer if necessary so as not to miss hypothermia, and appropriate environmental measures taken.

NATIONAL POISONS INFORMATION SERVICES

United Kingdom National Poisons Information Centre 'hot-line'
0844 892 0111
Republic of Ireland National Poisons Information Centre 'hot-line'
01 809 2566

Maternal drug abuse

Drug misuse (abuse) is common, but only a minority of misuse is associated with dependence (or addiction). Society currently displays a schizophrenic attitude to drug abuse. We seem to accept alcohol intake and, to a lesser extent, smoking during pregnancy even though we know that these drugs can be addictive, and that regular use can affect the baby. There is a puritanical (and paternalistic) streak, that is particularly strong amongst legislators in America, that would ban all alcohol intake in pregnancy, but there is no evidence that an intake of less than 10 units a week is harmful unless it is consumed in one go (one 'unit' of alcohol being a single pub measure of spirits, a small glass of wine or half a pint of ordinary strength beer or cider). In addition, smoking in pregnancy is now seen as one of those 'facts of life' that the medical and midwifery professions can do little to change. The attitude to other recreational drug use is more censorious, even though we know that many healthcare professionals occasionally take drugs themselves.

Opiate addiction presents the most serious challenge, and IV injection further increases the risk to the mother's health. Indeed the main reason for offering these mothers methadone is that it may help them to avoid the hazards associated with giving any drug IV. Access to oral methadone may, by limiting the woman's urge to acquire other costly drugs of doubtful purity, also help stabilise her lifestyle. Attitudes change over time. Opium and laudanum were widely used by the middle classes in Europe and North America in the 19th century. Opium was even added in many infant 'soothing syrups'. Now it has been estimated that, when no legal source is available, the average UK addict gets through £20,000 worth of heroin a year. Diet may become inadequate, and alcohol intake may rise. Judgmental attitudes can deter addicts from seeking help until problems escalate. Users may seem to have neglected their condition when the health services have actually, by their attitude, effectively excluded them from care. Despite this, many manage to lead apparently normal lives, running a family or holding down a job.

Few areas of maternity care are more in need of a collaborative, team-based, approach. Little can be achieved until the woman's trust and confidence have been won. Antenatal care should identify those most in need of support. Intravenous drug users should always be tested, with their informed consent, for sexually transmitted infection, and for hepatitis B, hepatitis C and HIV infection, both to optimise the scope for treatment and to minimise the risk that the baby will also become infected. Plans for post-delivery care should also be made ahead of delivery, and the mother should know what these are.

Neonatal Formulary 7: Drug Use in Pregnancy and the First Year of Life, Seventh Edition. Sean B Ainsworth.
© 2015 John Wiley & Sons, Ltd. Published 2015 by John Wiley & Sons, Ltd.
Companion website: www.neonatalformulary.com

Many heroin users also take other drugs. While recreational use of drugs such as cannabis, lysergic acid diethylamide (LSD), phencyclidine (PCP), amfetamine (amphetamine), ecstasy or cocaine on their own do not usually cause neonatal withdrawal symptoms serious enough to require treatment, the same is not true for high-dose benzodiazepine use. Transferring from heroin to methadone may actually make matters worse because this does not give the immediate 'high' obtained when heroin is smoked, inhaled or injected. Cocaine may then be turned to for the 'lift' that it

W	Wakefulness
I	Irritability
T	Tachypnoea (>60/minutes)
H	Hyperactivity
D	Diarrhoea
R	Rub marks
A	Autonomic dysfunction
W	Weight loss
A	Alkalosis (respiratory)
L	Lacrimation (tears)

gives and a benzodiazepine, such as temazepam, used to reduce the 'low' that tends to follow. Fashions change, but combined addiction to heroin and temazepam is common in the United Kingdom.

Most people who misuse drugs are not drug dependent. The problem only becomes an addiction if abrupt discontinuation causes serious physical and mental symptoms to appear. This is, however, what can happen to the baby after birth. Babies exposed to opiates throughout pregnancy, or to high sustained benzodiazepine usage, often exhibit a range of symptoms (see box) 12–72 hours after birth. *None* of these, on their own, need treatment, but treatment is called for if sucking is so in-coordinate that tube feeding is required, if there is profuse vomiting, or watery diarrhoea or the baby remains seriously unsettled after two consecutive feeds despite gentle swaddling and the use of a pacifier.

Many units currently admit such babies to special care for observation and then 'score' the child's condition once every 4 hours. However, experience shows that an observer's views and their 'attitude' to drug misuse can influence the score awarded. Scores ask the observer to say how 'severe' the symptoms are. If the nurse or doctor has not cared for such a baby before, how can they decide on the severity of the symptoms? Scoring systems, though popular, can also have the perverse effect of suggesting that an increasingly sedated baby is 'improving' when the real need is to get the baby feeding normally and sleeping normally.

A better approach is to make the mother aware before delivery that her baby will need to be watched for a period, to involve the mother in this and to care for both mother and baby. Most mothers already feel guilty about their drug habit and fear having their children taken from them. Knowledge of antenatal drug intake (even if accurate) is only of limited value in predicting whether the baby will develop symptoms, and mothers need to be aware of this. If mother and baby have been cared for together, both can be discharged home after 72 hours if no serious symptoms have developed.

If symptoms serious enough to make the baby unwell do develop, then the logical approach is to wean the baby slowly from the drug to which the mother is habituated, rather than introducing yet another drug. Babies of mothers taking an opiate should be weaned using a slowly decreasing dose of morphine or methadone. Morphine is widely used, and the dose can be easily and rapidly adjusted up or down, but methadone may provide smoother control. Weaning should not normally take more than 7–10 days. The same approach can be used where the mother is addicted to buprenorphine, codeine or dihydrocodeine. The use of paregoric for the baby, or tincture of opium, lacks any rational justification. Benzodiazepine dependency is harder to manage using this strategy, because nearly all these drugs have such a long half-life. Some use chloral hydrate in this situation but this can over-sedate the baby, and chlorpromazine may be a better choice. For the occasional mother with barbiturate dependency, phenobarbital should be considered but, while this may provide sedation, it does nothing to control gastrointestinal symptoms.

Although there have been many small controlled trials looking at strategies for managing neonatal withdrawal, assessors have generally merely looked to see how many symptoms there were rather than how distressing and disabling the symptoms were. In addition, the assessors have usually been aware of how the babies were being treated. There is scope for some useful nursing research here.

Breastfeeding can be generally encouraged in the period immediately after birth even if the mother has been taking several drugs, since these babies seem to show fewer features of withdrawal. There is no need to place any arbitrary limit on the length of time the mother is 'permitted' to breastfeed. It should, however, be explained that weaning needs to be gradual. No baby should be left in the care of anyone taking a hallucinogen, and few would condone the possible exposure of a baby to such a drug in breast milk. The place of breastfeeding in mothers taking other drugs is summarised in pp. 560–607.

Screening urine, or meconium, for drugs serves little purpose unless serious thought is being given to care proceedings, since it is unlikely to influence management. If you tell the mother you plan to do this, you imply that you do not believe what she has told you about her drug history. If you tell her later, she will merely conclude that you are another person she cannot trust. The decision of any child protection conference, or court, will be influenced purely by what is best for the child, and by the mother's ability to provide that care. Drug misuse is not in itself a sufficient reason to separate mother and child.

Babies can also become addicted to opiates and benzodiazepines *after* birth. Fentanyl and midazolam are the drugs that most often cause problems. Continuous use for even a few days can produce tolerance (the need for a progressively larger dose) and dependency (addiction). Management is the same as for addiction acquired *in utero* – a slow tapered withdrawal of treatment. Perhaps we should do what we tell mothers to do and avoid sustained use all together.

DRUGSCOPE

DrugScope, a registered and independent charity, is a national membership organisation for the drug sector and the UK's leading independent centre of expertise on drugs and drug use. It was formed in 2000 from the merger of the Institute for the Study of Drug Dependence (ISDD), established in 1968, and the Standing Conference on Drug Abuse (SCODA), established in 1973.

DrugScope can be contacted at:
  DrugScope, 4th Floor, Asra House, 1 Long Lane, London SE1 4PG
  Telephone: 020 7234 9730
  Fax: 020 7234 9773
  Website: www.drugscope.org.uk

Renal failure

Since the kidney is responsible for the elimination of most drugs from the body (either before or after inactivation by the liver), an assessment of how well the kidney is functioning is an essential part of the daily care of any patient on medication. Kidney function can fluctuate rapidly in the neonatal period so it should be assessed at the time treatment is first prescribed and monitored daily.

Deterioration occurs because blood flow has decreased (*pre-renal failure*), because the kidney has suffered damage (*intrinsic renal failure*) or because urine flow has been obstructed (*post-renal failure*) – although both pre- and post-renal failure can also cause secondary kidney damage. Clinical examination, and knowledge of the other problems involved, will often suggest where the problem lies. In babies with normal renal function, sodium excretion is driven by intake, and therefore varies widely. The proportion filtered that appears in urine (fractional excretion, FE_{Na}) is equally variable.

$$FE_{Na}(\%) = \frac{\text{Urinary sodium}}{\text{Plasma sodium}} \times \frac{\text{Plasma creatinine}}{\text{Urinary creatinine}} \times 100$$

Check whether all concentrations are expressed in the same units. Babies with pre-renal failure (who are typically oliguric and hypotensive) conserve sodium avidly under the control of aldosterone. They will have a $FE_{Na} \leq 3\%$ (<5% when <32 weeks gestation and <2 weeks old) regardless of the intake and the plasma level, except after a large dose of furosemide. Babies with established failure have a high FE_{Na} excretion because reabsorption is impaired by tubular damage.

Weigh all ill babies at least once a day because weight change is a sensitive index of fluid balance. Babies normally lose weight for 3–5 days after birth as they shed extracellular fluid (including sodium) following the loss of the placenta through which they were 'dialysed' before birth. Weight gain at this time is either a sign of excessive fluid intake or of early renal failure. Even healthy growing babies gain weight only by 2% a day. Gain in excess of this is a very useful sign of kidney failure. Urine output will vary with fluid intake, but any baby putting out less than 1 ml/kg of urine per hour is almost certainly in failure. A rising plasma creatinine or a level above 88 µmol/l (>1 mg%) in a baby more than 10 days old suggests some degree of renal failure, but the plasma level should never be relied on to identify failure because it rises six times more slowly after any insult than it does in an older child or adult.

Early diagnosis is vital because the elimination of some commonly used but potentially toxic drugs, such as gentamicin, is entirely dependent on excretion in the urine. Furthermore, most acute renal failure in the neonatal period is, at least initially, pre-renal in origin – often as a result of sepsis, intrapartum stress or respiratory

Neonatal Formulary 7: Drug Use in Pregnancy and the First Year of Life, Seventh Edition. Sean B Ainsworth.
© 2015 John Wiley & Sons, Ltd. Published 2015 by John Wiley & Sons, Ltd.
Companion website: www.neonatalformulary.com

difficulty – and early diagnosis makes early treatment possible. Trouble can often be anticipated. The later the problem is recognised, the more difficult management becomes.

The frequency with which it is necessary to rescue a baby from metabolic chaos by dialysis is inversely related to the promptness with which such a threat is recognised. A strategy for the conservative management of hyperkalaemia in p. 464 (and p. 420).

Reduce all medication to the minimum as soon as there is evidence of definite renal failure to minimise the risk of toxic drug accumulation and of unpredictable interactions. Antibiotics should be given as indicated in Table 1. Flucytosine, vancomycin and

Table 1 Drugs used to combat infection, and their clearance from the body in babies with severe renal failure before or during peritoneal dialysis (PD).

Drug	Dose adjustment needed	Comment
Aciclovir	Major	Quadruple the dose interval. Removal by PD is poor
Amikacin	Measure	Judge dose interval from trough serum level. Removal by PD is slow
Amoxicillin	Some	Increase dose interval or give one IV dose and put 125 mg/l in the PD fluid
Amphotericin	None	Give IV treatment as normal. The drug is not removed by PD
Ampicillin	Some	Increase dose interval or give one IV dose and put 125 mg/l in the PD fluid
Azithromycin	None	Give as normal. The drug is not removed by PD
Aztreonam	Major	Halve the dose. The drug is not removed by PD
Cefotaxime	Some	Increase dose interval or give one IV dose and put 125 mg/l in the PD fluid
Cefoxitin	Major	Double the dose interval or give one IV dose and put 125 mg/l in the PD fluid
Ceftazidime	Major	Double the dose interval or give one IV dose and put 125 mg/l in the PD fluid
Ceftriaxone	Some	Reduce dose if there is both renal and liver failure. Removal by PD is poor
Cefuroxime	Major	Increase dose interval or give one IV dose and put 125 mg/l in the PD fluid
Chloramphenicol	None	Use with caution – metabolites accumulate. The drug is not removed by PD
Ciprofloxacin	Major	Halve the dose. Crystalluria may occur. The drug is not removed by PD
Clindamycin	Minimal	Give IV treatment as normal. The drug is not removed by PD
Erythromycin	None	Give IV as normal. The drug is not removed by PD
Flucloxacillin	Minimal	Give IV as normal or give one dose IV and put 250 mg/l in the PD fluid
Fluconazole	Major	Double the dose interval or, in babies on PD, put 7 mg/l in the PD fluid
Flucytosine	Measure	Monitor the serum level or, in babies on PD, put 50 mg/l in the PD fluid
Gentamicin	Measure	Judge dose interval from trough serum level. Removal by PD is slow
Isoniazid	None	Give oral or IV treatment as normal. The drug is removed by PD
Meropenem	Major	Double the dose interval. It is not known if the drug is removed by PD
Metronidazole	Minimal	Give oral or IV treatment as normal. The drug is removed by PD
Netilmicin	Measure	Judge dose interval from trough serum level. Removal by PD is slow
Penicillin	Substantial	Use with caution – penicillin is neurotoxic. Removal by PD is poor
Rifampicin	None	Give oral or IV treatment as normal. The drug is not removed by PD
Teicoplanin	Moderate	Give if IV level can be measured, or give one IV dose and put 20 mg/l in PD fluid
Trimethoprim	Moderate	Halve the IV dose after 2 days. Removal by PD is slow
Vancomycin	Measure	Monitor serum level or give one IV dose and put 25 mg/l in the PD fluid

Table 2 Solutions for neonatal PD.

Solution	Preparation	Final concentration		
		Sodium (mmol/l)	Bicarbonate (mmol/l)	Glucose (%)
A	500 ml 5% glucose modified by removing 60 ml of fluid and adding 60 ml of 8.4% sodium bicarbonate	120	120	4.4
B	500 ml 0.9% sodium chloride	150	0	0
C	500 ml 0.9% sodium chloride modified by removing 50 ml of fluid and adding 50 ml of 50% glucose and 1.5 ml of 30% (strong) sodium chloride	150	0	5.0
Potential combinations:				
1/3 A plus 2/3 B		140	40	1.47
1/3 A plus 1/2 B plus 1/6 C		140	40	2.30
1/3 A plus 1/3 B plus 1/3 C		140	40	3.13
1/3 A plus 2/3 C		140	40	4.80

cefuroxime are sometimes added to dialysis fluids to prevent peritonitis. A first dose of the appropriate antibiotic should always be given IV (if the baby is not already on treatment) before utilising the peritoneal dialysis (PD) fluid to sustain an appropriate blood level if there are signs of systemic infection. Sustained high aminoglycoside levels are not bactericidal (as explained in p. 237) so these drugs should not be put in PD fluid. Pancuronium should be replaced by atracurium if the baby requires paralysis. Morphine may accumulate because it is renally excreted. The half-life of heparin seems unaffected, but that of low molecular weight heparin is reduced. The clearance of the drugs commonly used to control arrhythmia, seizures, hypertension and hypotension are (luckily) unaffected by renal failure.

PD is the most effective strategy in most small babies, but surgical problems may occasionally make haemodialysis necessary. Commercial dialysis fluids usually contain lactate, but some ill neonates metabolise this poorly. A flexible range of fluids can be prepared containing bicarbonate by combining three different basic solutions as outlined in Table 2. Use an in-line IV burette, and adjust the glucose concentration by varying ingredients B and C in order to control ultrafiltration and the removal of water. Because these dialysis fluids cannot contain calcium, it is necessary to give supplemental calcium IV. Start with 1 mmol/kg a day and adjust as necessary. Magnesium may occasionally be needed. Add heparin (1 unit/ml) if the dialysis fluid is cloudy or bloodstained to stop fibrin and clots obstructing the catheter. Watch for peritonitis by microscoping and culturing the effluent fluid daily.

Body weight and surface area

Basal metabolic rate (BMR) has a fairly fixed relationship to body surface area throughout childhood and adult life. For this reason, it was once common practice to use body surface area when calculating drug dosage in childhood. However, while this works reasonably well for children more than a few months old, it is not appropriate in early infancy because BMR rises rapidly in the first 2 or 3 weeks after birth, even though little growth takes place, and BMR is only one of the many factors influencing drug metabolism at this time. Changes in kidney and liver function are of much more relevance, and all the treatment recommendations given in this book are based on what we know of the variable way that these two factors interact to affect how long each drug remains active in the body.

Most paediatric reference texts have, until recently, provided nomograms that allow derivation of surface area from a knowledge of height and weight, but height (or length) is seldom measured with any real accuracy in children who cannot yet stand,

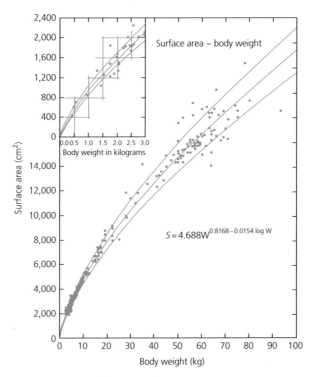

Fig. 2 Relationship between body weight and surface area.

Neonatal Formulary 7: Drug Use in Pregnancy and the First Year of Life, Seventh Edition. Sean B Ainsworth.
© 2015 John Wiley & Sons, Ltd. Published 2015 by John Wiley & Sons, Ltd.
Companion website: www.neonatalformulary.com

and further errors often creep in when nomograms are used without due care. What is more, as Edith Boyd showed in her book on *The Growth of the Surface Area of the Human Body* (University of Minnesota Press, 1935), is that surface area can be predicted as accurately in very young children from a knowledge of weight alone.

The table relating weight to surface area given in earlier editions of this book utilised Boyd's data, but the revised figures given here have also made use of the additional data collected by Meban in 1983 (*J Anat* **137**:271–8) (Fig. 2; Table 3). In truth however, in young children more than 1–2 months old, it is nearly always best to simply use body weight to calculate the most appropriate dose to employ (see Johnson, *Arch Dis Child* 2008;**93**:207–11).

Table 3 Relationship between body weight (kg) (full units down left side and part units across the top) and surface area (m²), for example a baby weighing 2.3 kg will have a surface area of 0.17 m².

Kilograms	0.0	0.1	0.2	0.3	0.4	0.5	0.6	0.7	0.8	0.9
0	–	–	0.04	0.04	0.05	0.06	0.07	0.08	0.08	0.09
1	0.10	0.10	0.11	0.11	0.12	0.12	0.13	0.14	0.14	0.15
2	0.15	0.16	0.17	0.17	0.18	0.18	0.19	0.19	0.20	0.21
3	0.21	0.22	0.22	0.23	0.23	0.24	0.24	0.25	0.25	0.26
4	0.26	0.27	0.27	0.27	0.28	0.28	0.29	0.29	0.30	0.30
5	0.31	0.31	0.32	0.32	0.32	0.33	0.33	0.34	0.34	0.35
6	0.35	0.35	0.36	0.36	0.36	0.37	0.37	0.38	0.38	0.38
7	0.39	0.39	0.39	0.40	0.40	0.40	0.41	0.41	0.41	0.42
8	0.42	0.43	0.43	0.43	0.44	0.44	0.44	0.45	0.45	0.45
9	0.46	0.46	0.46	0.47	0.47	0.48	0.48	0.48	0.49	0.49

Effects of therapeutic hypothermia on medications

Background

Prolonged mild-to-moderate hypothermia has been shown to be efficacious in reducing post-ischaemic neurological injury in the term newborn population. Infants subjected to a hypoxic insult demonstrate variable multi-organ impairment which may impact on drug pharmacokinetics and pharmacodynamics, for example drugs excreted by the kidneys may accumulate due to the renal impairment. However, hypothermia itself may impact on the responses to drugs.

Hypothermia causes the redistribution of regional blood flow, which may significantly impact on both drug distribution and clearance. It has been associated with decreased GFR in a number of animal studies, and may, therefore, impair the renal excretion of drugs in humans.

Many drugs, especially those metabolised in the liver, are modulated by enzymes that exhibit a temperature dependency that can be affected by therapeutic hypothermia. Depending on the action of the enzyme on the drug metabolism, therapeutic hypothermia can lead to lack of action of some drugs and accumulation of others. The additional difficulty is that whilst drug metabolism may be affected by hypothermia, it can also change during re-warming 72 hours after hypothermia has elapsed. Drugs with a large volume of distribution given before the start of hypothermia can be sequestered in peripheral tissues at the onset of hypothermia and may undergo recirculation upon re-warming, exposing the patient to higher serum concentrations and a greater risk of toxicity. It should not be forgotten that the baby undergoing therapeutic hypothermia will have, in many cases, suffered hepatic and renal injuries and that this too can greatly impact on how the baby handles the drugs that are given.

Table 4 lists most of the drugs that are used in asphyxiated infants undergoing therapeutic hypothermia; it explains where there is a known significant effect on that drug's efficacy due to altered metabolism. This list is not exhaustive but instead reflects merely those drugs in frequent use in this population and also those drugs for which information is available. Further information is available on the website commentary.

Neonatal Formulary 7: Drug Use in Pregnancy and the First Year of Life, Seventh Edition. Sean B Ainsworth.
© 2015 John Wiley & Sons, Ltd. Published 2015 by John Wiley & Sons, Ltd.
Companion website: www.neonatalformulary.com

Table 4 Effects of therapeutic hypothermia on medications.

Drug	Effect of hypothermia	Suggested dose adjustments during hypothermia
Antibiotics		
Gentamicin	Conflicting reports because of co-existing renal injury. Data suggest a 25–33% reduction in renal clearance	Give a dose of 4 mg/kg every 36 hours Measure serum levels
Vancomycin	No data in neonates (in adults undergoing cardiac by-pass, there appears to be no effect). It is unusual for this drug to be used in treating early onset sepsis.	No data in neonates
Penicillin and other β-lactam antibiotics	The pharmacokinetics of these antibiotics during hypothermia have not yet been studied, however, because of their safe profiles, any effect, if there is one, is unlikely to be of any clinical significance.	No dose adjustment necessary
Anticonvulsants		
Phenobarbital	Reduced clearance during hypothermia, some reports suggest a doubling of the half-life; however, this does not appear to have a clinically relevant effect. **NOTE**: Phenobarbital has an effect on the amplitude integrated EEG (aEEG) and it is generally not recommended to give more than a single loading dose of 20 mg/kg before cerebral function monitoring is initiated.	Give single loading dose of 20 mg/kg A second dose (10–20 mg/kg) should probably be considered before other anticonvulsants but avoid maintenance if possible
Phenytoin	The pharmacology of phenytoin is already complicated in the neonate due to a variable rate of elimination and a highly variable volume of distribution. It exhibits non-linear (saturable) metabolism via hepatic cytochromes P450 2C9 and 2c139 and levels are higher during hypothermia.	Use the same (or slightly lower) loading dose of 20 mg/kg given IV over 10–20 minutes and to closely monitor levels
Midazolam	Midazolam is exclusively metabolized by hepatic cytochromes P450 3A4 and 3A5. Use in hypothermic adults is associated with a fivefold increase in serum levels.	Dosing not established in hypothermia. Use with caution, ensure access to appropriate monitoring and respiratory support in non-ventilated patients.
Clonazepam	Clonazepam is metabolized extensively by cytochrome P450 enzymes. The half-life in normothermic neonates is 24–48 hours, and although it has yet to be studied in a population being treated with hypothermia, it is likely that this half-life is extended during treatment.	Dosing not established in hypothermia. Use with caution, ensure access to appropriate monitoring and respiratory support in non-ventilated patients.
Lidocaine (lignocaine)	Lidocaine is metabolised by hepatic cytochrome P450 1A2 and 3A4. During therapeutic hypothermia in neonates, clearance of lidocaine is reduced by 24%.	Use modified regime as suggested in lidocaine monograph (q.v.)
Topiramate	Experience with topiramate in neonates is limited and pharmacokinetic data even more so. Very limited data from infants undergoing hypothermia suggest a slower absorption and elimination.	5 mg/kg on the first day and then a **lower dose** (3 mg/kg daily) for the next 2 days

Continued

Table 4 *Continued*

Drug	Effect of hypothermia	Suggested dose adjustments during hypothermia
Levetiracetam	The predominantly renal excretion of levetiracetum should mean that hypothermia *per se* should not impact on dosing; however excretion is affected by renal impairment which is commonly seen in these infants as a result of their initial hypoxic insult.	Use modified regime as suggested in levetiracetum monograph (q.v.)

Sedatives/analgesics

Drug	Effect of hypothermia	Suggested dose adjustments during hypothermia
Morphine	There are potentially two effects of hypothermia on morphine to be considered; firstly, that the affinity of morphine for the μ-opioid receptors is reduced in hypothermia rendering it less effective, and secondly, that clearance of morphine is reduced.	50 micrograms/kg loading dose over 30 minutes followed by an infusion started at 10 micrograms/kg/hour. The rate of infusion is titrated according to the response of the infant. If the infant is adequately sedated, the dose should be **reduced after 24–48 hours** to lessen the risk of accumulation and toxicity.
Fentanyl	Fentanyl is primarily metabolized by cytochrome P450 3A4. The half-life of fentanyl is already very variable in the neonate (6–30 hours). Hypothermia can lead to a 25% increase in plasma fentanyl concentrations. There are currently insufficient data from hypothermic newborns to recommend any specific dosing schedule; however, it would seem sensible to begin by halving the 'normothermic' doses.	Give a loading dose of 5 micrograms/kg and then infuse starting at 0.75 microgram/kg/hour and titrating according to the response of the infant. As with morphine, consider **reducing at 24–48 hours** to lessen the risk of accumulation and toxicity
Remifentanil	Remifentanil has a short half-life due to rapid hydrolysis by non-specific blood and tissue esterases. The metabolite is renally excreted through the kidneys. N-dealkylation of remifentanil by cytochrome P450 also occurs. Data from adults undergoing hypothermia suggested that for each degree fall in temperature below 37 °C, there is a proportional decrease of 6.37% in remifentanil clearance. But there are no published data of use in neonatal therapeutic hypothermia.	No data in neonates

Neuromuscular blocking agents

Drug	Effect of hypothermia	Suggested dose adjustments during hypothermia
Atracurium	Atracurium is primarily metabolized by non-enzymatic decomposition in the blood (Hoffman elimination); however, an alternative elimination pathway involving enzymatic ester hydrolysis also operates. In healthy individuals, mild hypothermia (34 °C) results in an approximate 1.5-fold increase in the duration of action of atracurium.	No dose adjustment necessary. Duration of action may be longer.

Table 4 *Continued*

Drug	Effect of hypothermia	Suggested dose adjustments during hypothermia
Pancuronium	Pancuronium is primarily (~80%) excreted by the kidneys, with some biliary excretion. Studies in hypothermic adults show an initial increased requirement during early stages of hypothermia and then, when hypothermia is established, increased plasma concentrations. There is no data in neonates.	No dose adjustment necessary. The baby may seem to require more frequent dosing to begin with but once hypothermic the duration of action may be longer.
Rocuronium	In children undergoing hypothermia for a variety of reasons, for every degree Celsius decrease in core body temperature the duration of action of rocuronium increased by 5 minutes.	No dose adjustment necessary. Duration of action may be longer.
Vercuronium	Vecuronium is primarily eliminated via the liver by carrier-mediated transport (via p-glycoprotein) and P450-mediated metabolism. Risks of accumulation, particularly with infusions, increase as hypothermia is established.	No initial dose adjustment is necessary but titrate the dose after 6–12 hours according to the need. Avoid infusion if possible.
Inotropic agents		
Adrenaline	There is no evidence to suggest that a different dosing strategy for inotropic support is needed during or following neonatal therapeutic hypothermia.	No dose adjustment necessary. Titrate according to response
Dopamine	As above	No dose adjustment necessary. Titrate according to response
Dobutamine	As above	No dose adjustment necessary. Titrate according to response
Milrinone	There is very limited data regarding milrinone in therapeutic hypothermia. However, milrinone, being 80–85% excreted unchanged in urine, is unlikely to be significantly affected by hypothermia *per se*. The renal impairment in these babies may have some effect.	No dose adjustment thought to be necessary. Titrate according to response

Useful websites

American Academy of Pediatrics (AAP)

The AAP makes a wealth of well-formulated advice available on its website. The e-Archive of the AAP's official journal, *Pediatrics*, provides a browse and search ability for all papers published since 1948. Abstracts and some of the articles are available free of charge, otherwise a subscription is required.

- www.aap.org
- http://pediatrics.aappublications.org

British Association of Perinatal Medicine

The BAPM is a UK association of healthcare professionals from various specialties involved in the delivery of perinatal care. It has been responsible for the development of neonatal guidelines and standards as well as supporting neonatal and perinatal research.

- www.bapm.org

British National Formulary

This formulary, sponsored jointly by the British Medical Association and the Royal Pharmaceutical Society of Great Britain, aims to provide authoritative and practical information on the selection and use of all UK-licensed medicines in a clear, concise and accessible manner. It is semi-continuously updated and published afresh in book form every 6 months, but it can also be accessed on line, and has grown over the years to become one of the world's most authoritative reference texts. A separate publication, the BNF for Children (or BNFC), was launched in September 2005 jointly with the Royal College of Paediatrics and Child Health, and updates of this version appear annually.

- www.bnf.org
- www.bnfc.org

Clinical Evidence

Clinical Evidence is an '*international database of high-quality, rigorously developed systematic overviews assessing the benefits and harms of treatments*'. Relatively few perinatal issues are covered, but the number covered is increasing steadily. Regularly updated full text is available on the web. The text is also currently available in Italian, German, Hungarian, Portuguese, Russian and Spanish. A summary of each monograph is also published by the BMJ Publishing Group in book form twice a year under the title *BMJ Clinical Evidence Handbook*.

- www.clinicalevidence.com

The Cochrane Library

The Cochrane Collaboration is an international not-for-profit organisation whose aim is to provide up-to-date information about the effects of health

Neonatal Formulary 7: Drug Use in Pregnancy and the First Year of Life, Seventh Edition. Sean B Ainsworth.
© 2015 John Wiley & Sons, Ltd. Published 2015 by John Wiley & Sons, Ltd.
Companion website: www.neonatalformulary.com

care. The library contains the Cochrane Database of Systematic Reviews, the Database of Abstracts of Reviews of Effectiveness, and the Cochrane Central Register of Controlled Trials. Access to the full text of all the reviews that have something useful to say about drugs mentioned in the main section of this compendium can be assessed directly from this Formulary's website, while the National Institutes of Health (NIH) website in America provides access to all existing and currently planned neonatal reviews.

- www.cochrane.org
- www.nichd.nih.gov/cochrane

Communicable disease centres

Many countries maintain a national communicable disease centre. Two that make a particularly wide range of information publicly available are the Health Protection Agency (HPA) – formerly the Public Health Laboratory Service (PHLS) – in the United Kingdom, and the Communicable Disease Centre (CDC) in the United States.

- http://www.hpa.org.uk/HPAwebHome
- www.cdc.gov

Contact a Family

When families are told that their child has a rare, possibly inherited, disorder they often feel bereft of good quality advice and information. Contact a Family in the United Kingdom and National Organization for Rare Disorders (NORD) in the United States bridge that gap. They can also offer help to those who want to contact other families facing a similar challenge.

- www.cafamily.org.uk
- www.rarediseases.org

Contraception

The website managed by the Faculty of Sexual and Reproductive Healthcare (formerly the Faculty of Family Planning and Reproductive Health Care) in the United Kingdom provides authoritative advice on all aspects of contraception and family planning.

- http://www.fsrh.org

Controlled clinical trials

Registration of all interventional trials, using International Standard Randomised Controlled Trial Number (ISRCTN), is considered to be a scientific, ethical and moral responsibility. It is also an essential requirement if the results are to be published in many journals. Information about trials is now becoming available through a number of sites listed below.

- www.trialscentral.org
- www.clinicaltrials.gov
- www.controlled-trials.com
- www.crncc.nihr.ac.uk

Drug abuse

Drugscope is an independent registered UK charity that undertakes research, and provides authoritative advice, on all aspects of drug abuse and drug addiction.

- www.drugscope.org.uk

Drugs and Lactation Database (LactMed)

The National Library of Medicine hosts a peer-reviewed and fully referenced database of drugs to which breastfeeding mothers may be exposed. The site provides data on maternal and infant levels of drugs, possible effects on breastfed infants and on lactation, and alternate drugs to consider.

- www.toxnet.nlm.nih.gov/cgi-bin/sis/htmlgen?LACT

Drugs in Lactation Advisory Service

This is a joint service provided by the West Midlands and Trent Drug Information Services providing advice about medicines use during lactation.

* www.ukmicentral.nhs.uk/drugpreg/ guide.htm

Drug use during pregnancy

The perinatology website has a useful alphabetical list summarising how most drugs commonly used in pregnancy and breastfeeding are classified by the American Food and Drug Administration (FDA). It also provides links to a number of similar websites that provide information about drugs, vaccines and diagnostic agents that might be used. See also the two websites giving information on teratogenicity (see below).

* www.perinatology.com/exposures/ druglist.htm

First Steps Nutrition Trust

This organisation, a registered charity, provides nutrition information and resources to support women who may become pregnant, pregnant women and parents of children under 5 years. The Trust offers freely available evidence-based, objective information that is free from influence and sponsorship by food manufacturers or retailers.

* www.firststepsnutrition.org

Genetic disease

The National Institutes of Health (NIH) in America supports an ever expanding register of known human genetic disorders (22,031 conditions at the last count). This register 'Online Mendelian Inheritance in Man' provides a wealth of constantly updated information.

* www.ncbi.nlm.nih.gov/omim

History of controlled trials

For an insight into the way in which objectivity was eventually brought to bear on the many claims that doctors (and others) have always made for the drugs and treatments that they had on offer see

* www.jameslindlibrary.org

HIV and AIDS

An authoritative website, AIDSinfo, supported by the National Institutes of Health provides extensive and very up-to-date information on the treatment of HIV and AIDS in patients of all ages, together with information on clinical trials currently in progress. The British HIV Association (BHIVA) also has an active medical website, whilst its sister organisation, the Children's HIV Association (CHIVA) caters for those caring for children. The independent group NAM (which originally stood for National AIDS Manual) supports a more general website (aidsmap), and the University of Liverpool in the United Kingdom provides a website giving information on drug interactions.

* www.aidsinfo.nih.gov
* www.bhiva.org
* www.aidsmap.com
* www.chiva.org.uk
* www.hiv-druginteractions.org

Immunisation

NHS Choices website has information for parents and professionals alike about the UK immunisation schedule. It also offers advice on travel vaccinations and travel issues. A further useful website is supported by Great Ormond Street Hospital in London

- http://www.nhs.uk/Conditions/ vaccinations/Pages/vaccination-schedule-age-checklist.aspx
- www.gosh.nhs.uk/parents-and-visitors/ general-health-advice/immunisation

Immunisation (Nation Immunisation Schedules)

Originally compiled in 1996, the UK Government's official publication 'Immunisation against infectious disease' has undergone progressive updating. It is currently hosted on the UK Government's website. Access to the fully revised text is available from the following website, while all the individual chapters relating to those vaccines covered in this book can also be accessed direct from this Formulary's website. Other countries' immunisation schedules differ and much of the vaccine information is often just as useful. The World Health Organisation (WHO) maintains a searchable website that allows comparison not only of immunisation schedules but also the numbers of reported cases of these preventable diseases.

- **United Kingdom:**
  www.gov.uk/government/organisations/ public-health-england/series/immunisation-against-infectious-disease-the-green-book
- **United States:**
  www.immunize.org
  www.cdc.gov/vaccines
- **Australia:**
  www.immunise.health.gov.au
- **Canada:**
  www.immunize.cpha.ca
- **New Zealand:**
  http://www.immune.org.nz

- **World Health Organisation:**
  http://apps.who.int/immunization_ monitoring/globalsummary

Malaria

The malarial parasite is becoming progressively more resistant to many of the drugs usually used for prophylaxis and treatment. For area-specific advice on management of malaria from the World Health Organisation (WHO), and from the Communicable Disease Centre (CDC) in the United States, see

- www.who.int/ith/en
- http://www.cdc.gov/malaria

Medicines compendium

The information issued by the manufacturer of every product licensed in the United Kingdom – the manufacturer's Summary of Product Characteristics (SPC) and Patient Information Leaflets (PILs) – can be accessed electronically on the web. Access is free.

- www.medicines.org.uk/emc

Medicines for Children

Medicines for Children is a partnership between the Royal College of Paediatrics and Child Health (RCPCH), Neonatal and Paediatric Pharmacists (NPPG) and WellChild that produces information for parents about an increasing number of medicines.

- www.medicinesforchildren.org.uk

Medicine use during lactation

Thomas Hale, the pharmacist at the Tech University School of Medicine in Texas is the author of the valuable and frequently updated book *Medications and Mothers Milk* which is a mine of information on drug use during lactation. He also maintains an active and useful website. The UK Breastfeeding Network, who run an invaluable support and advice line [0300 100 0212], has issued a series of useful fact sheets about drug use during lactation that can be accessed from their website. For those interested in learning more about this subject, 'NHS Education for Scotland' has developed a very useful eLearning resource covering drug use during lactation

- www.medsmilk.com
- www.breastfeedingnetwork.org.uk
- www.breastfeeding.nes.scot.nhs.uk

Midwifery Digest

MIDIRS is a UK-based not-for-profit organisation. The website provides extensive regularly updated information on all issues relating to childbirth. It also supports a very active inquiry service and publishes a quarterly digest containing original articles and overviews of recent medical, midwifery and neonatal research taken from over 500 international journals. Subscribers also, for a fee, enjoy online access to regularly updated standard reading lists, and to over 100,000 articles on pregnancy, midwifery and childbirth issues.

- www.midirs.org

Motherisk program

The Motherisk program, backed by the expertise of the Department of Clinical Pharmacology and Toxicology at the Hospital for Sick Children in Toronto, maintains a very authoritative website dealing with the safety of drug use during pregnancy and lactation. The site provides links to areas designed for mothers and professionals as well as a specific site for foetal alcohol syndrome research.

- www.motherisk.org/women/index.jsp
- www.motherisk.org/FAR/index.jsp

National and International Associations for Neonatal Nurses

A number of national and international neonatal nurse organisations exist:

The Healthy Newborn Network (HNN)
- www.healthynewbornnetwork.org
  Council of International Neonatal Nurses (COINN)
- www.coinnurses.org
  National Association of Neonatal Nurses (NANN) in the United States
- www.nann.org
  Neonatal Nurses Association (NNA) in the United Kingdom
- www.networks.nhs.uk/nhs-networks/neonatal-nurses-association
  Australian College of Neonatal Nurses (ACNN)
- www.acnn.org.au
  Canadian Association of Neonatal Nurses (CANN)
- www.neonatalcann.ca
  Neonatal Nurses College of Aotearoa (NNCA) in New Zealand
- www.nzno.org.nz/groups/colleges/neonatal_nurses_college
  Sociedad Española de Enfermería Neonatal (SEEN) in Spain
- www.seen-enfermeria.com
  Neonatal Nursing Association of Southern Africa (NNASA)
- www.nnasa.org.za/cms/
  Scottish Neonatal Nurses Group
- www.snng.org.uk

National Institute for Health and Care Excellence

This organisation was originally set up in 1999 as the National Institute for Clinical Excellence (NICE), a special health authority, to reduce variation in the availability and quality of NHS treatments and care. This merged with the Health Development Agency in 2005 and began developing public health guidance. The website has separate sections on patient and public involvement, medicines and prescribing and guidance development. The medicines and prescribing section allows access to the BNF and BNFC as well as new, unlicensed and off-label medicines.

- www.nice.org.uk

Neonatal and Paediatric Pharmacy Group

The NPPG is a UK-based organisation with a website providing extensive advice for pharmacists on neonatal and paediatric pharmacy issues.

- www.nppg.scot.nhs.uk

Neonatology on the Web

This site contains an absorbing selection of classic papers and historical reports. The 'New Stuff' link takes you to a roundup of recently updated features. There is a useful collection of bibliographies on a wide range of topics.

- www.neonatology.org

Renal failure

There are no published guidelines that relate specifically to the safe prescribing of drugs to children in renal failure, but the American College of Physicians in Philadelphia publishes an extremely useful book on *'Drug Prescribing in Renal Failure: Dosing Guidelines for Adults and Children'*. The most recent (fifth) edition was published in 2007. An outline summary of its current advice on individual

drugs can be accessed from the following university website.

- www.kdp-baptist.louisville.edu/renalbook/

Royal College of Obstetricians and Gynaecologists

This London-based college has published a small series of clinical practice guidelines (so-called 'Green Top' Guidelines) in the Guidance section of their website that cover some of the management issues mentioned in this book.

- www.rcog.org.uk

Royal College of Paediatrics and Child Health

This London-based college also has a website where a number of management guidelines can be found. The British Association of Perinatal Medicine has also issued a number of important guidelines. For details see:

- www.rcpch.ac.uk

UNICEF UK Baby Friendly Initiative

The Baby Friendly Initiative is a global UNICEF (United Nations Children's Fund) programme which works to improve practice so that parents are helped and supported in making an informed choice over the way they feed and care for their babies by health professionals. For details see:

- www.unicef.org.uk/babyfriendly

Teratogens

Two large collaborative groups collate information and disseminate advice on drugs that may be teratogenic (i.e. cause fetal damage) if taken during pregnancy. The European Network of Teratology Information Services (ENTIS) covers not only Europe but also Israel and Latin America. The Organisation of Teratogen Information Specialists (OTIS) covers North America:

* www.entis-org.com
* www.mothertobaby.org

This book

BMJ Books have a website maintained by Wiley-Blackwell Publishing where detailed, and regularly updated, commentaries are posted on a number of the individual drug entries in this Formulary. The site does *not* provide direct access to the main monographs themselves, but all monographs added or updated after the latest print edition went to press can be found and downloaded from this site. It also provides access to archived monographs of those drugs that are no longer included in the printed version of the most recent edition (although they do still receive recognition in the index). It also provides a cross link to all relevant Cochrane Reviews.

* www.neonatalformulary.com

Travel advice

A number of sites provide advice for members of the public thinking of travelling abroad. The following are provided by the World Health Organisation (WHO), by the Communicable Disease Centre (CDC) in America, and by the National Health Service (NHS) in the United Kingdom respectively:

* www.who.int/ith/
* wwwnc.cdc.gov/travel
* www.fitfortravel.scot.nhs.uk

US Food and Drug Administration

The FDA (which is responsible for licensing all drug products in America) maintains a full and very informative website with good search facilities.

* www.fda.gov

World Health Organisation

The WHO has long had the provision and dissemination of reliable information on a core of essential drugs *'that satisfy the priority healthcare needs of the population, selected with due regard to public health relevance, efficacy and safety, and comparative cost-effectiveness'* as one of its major briefs. This website provides links to a large number of relevant documents and resources, including a model formulary for both children and adults (now also published in book form).

* www.who.int/selection_medicines/ list/en/

PART 2
Drug monographs

This part of NNF7 provides information on the use, dosages, supply and administration of drugs used in the neonatal period and later infancy, as well as some of the more commonly used maternal medications.

The staff should never prescribe or administer any drug without first familiarising themselves with the way it works, the way it is handled by the body and the problems that can arise as a result of its use. Most of the essential facts relating to use in adults are summarised by the manufacturer in the 'package insert' or summary of product characteristics (SPC). Many are also summarised in a range of reference texts, such as the *British National Formulary* (BNF) and the related text *BNF for Children* (BNFC). However, manufacturers seldom provide much information about drug handling *in infancy*, and although *BNFC* now offers more advice on dosage in childhood than can be obtained from the manufacturer's package insert, it stresses that the use of any unlicensed medicine (or licensed medicine in an unlicensed manner) should only be undertaken by those who have also first consulted 'other appropriate and up-to-date literature'. This book aims to summarise and to provide a referenced guide to that literature.

While many texts have long offered advice on the best dose to use in infancy – often in tabular form – very few provide much information on the idiosyncrasies associated with neonatal use. Such dosage tables can be a useful *aide-mémoire*, but they should **never** be relied upon, on their own, to help the staff decide what to use when, what works best or what potential adverse effects are commonly encountered during use in infancy. In addition, lists summarising common side effects and potential drug interactions are seldom of much help in identifying which problems are common or likely to be of clinical importance in the neonate, and access to this more detailed information is as important for the staff responsible for drug administration as it is for those prescribing treatment in the first place.

Similar challenges relate to the safe use of drugs during pregnancy and lactation because standard texts (such as the BNF) offer very little information as to what is, and is not, known about use in these circumstances. Such information is available in a range of specialised reference texts (see p. 258), and Part 3 of this compendium summarises what is currently known about the use of most of the more commonly used drugs.

Never use anything except the most recent edition of this or any other reference text. Indeed, copies of earlier editions should not be left where they might get used in error.

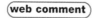
Use

Acetylcysteine is the first-line therapy for paracetamol overdose in all age groups.

There are also a number of avenues of research where acetylcysteine use is being explored as a means of reducing oxidative stress in patients of all ages; the results of these studies, however, merit further scrutiny before acetylcysteine can be recommended.

Background

Acetylcysteine is the N-acetyl derivative of the amino acid L-cysteine and is a precursor in the formation of the antioxidant glutathione. It was originally introduced as a mucolytic agent for chronic pulmonary diseases some 50 years ago. Its effect is based on breaking of disulphide bridges of high molecular weight glycoproteins of mucus, resulting in reduced viscosity. In many countries, it is prescribed for this purpose, but in the United Kingdom, for example, it is perceived to be ineffective.

Indications

Paracetamol overdose: The toxicity of paracetamol overdose has long been recognised, and neonates may potentially be at greater risk than older children with reports of 10-fold overdoses from intravenous (IV) paracetamol (propacetamol) use. Hepatotoxicity is caused by the formation of a toxic metabolite, N-acetyl-p-benzoquinone imine (NAPQI). When paracetamol is used in therapeutic doses, most of it is metabolised via glucuronidation and sulphation; a very small amount of paracetamol is metabolised to NAPQI by the hepatic enzyme cytochrome P450 2E1 (CYP2E1). NAPQI is then conjugated by glutathione to form the benign metabolite, mercapturic acid, which is excreted in the urine. Hepatotoxicity develops when large doses of paracetamol saturate the typical conjugation pathways and overwhelm available glutathione stores leading to reduced clearance of NAPQI, and as it accumulates, it can cause untoward effects on cellular structures and functions. Acetylcysteine reduces the hepatotoxic effects of paracetamol overdose by replenishing glutathione stores, thereby enhancing production of the non-toxic metabolites.

Other uses: Acetylcysteine has been used or is under investigation in neuroprotection (as an adjunct to therapeutic hypothermia), in chronic lung disease, as a mucolytic in ventilated babies, as a supplement to parenteral nutrition and to treat meconium ileus/inspissated meconium. Details regarding these uses – none of which can be routinely recommended – are discussed in the web commentary.

Treatment of paracetamol overdose

Give 150 mg/kg of IV acetylcysteine during the first hour and then 50 mg/kg over the next 4 hours followed by 100 mg/kg over 16 hours as described below:

Initial infusion: Take one 10 ml vial of acetylcysteine and dilute with 30 ml of 5% glucose to give a 50 mg/ml solution. Infuse at a rate of 3 ml/kg/hour for **1 hour only**.

Subsequent infusion: Take one 10 ml vial of acetylcysteine and dilute with 310 ml of 5% glucose to give a 6.25 mg/ml solution. When the initial infusion has finished, infuse this solution at a rate of 2 ml/kg/hour for **4 hours** and then at a rate of 1 ml/kg/hour for **16 hours**.

Supply

10 ml ampoules of N-acetylcysteine (200 mg/ml) cost £2.

References

(see also the relevant Cochrane reviews)

Ahola T, Fellman V, Laaksonen R, *et al*. Pharmacokinetics of intravenous N-acetylcysteine in pre-term newborn infants. *Eur J Clin Pharmacol* 1999;**55**:645–50.

Freeman R. MHRA recommendations on the use of intravenous acetylcysteine in paracetamol overdose. *Arch Dis Child Educ Pract Ed* 2014;**99**:37–40.

Isbister GK, Bucens IK, Whyte IM. Paracetamol overdose in a preterm neonate. *Arch Dis Child Fetal Neonatal Ed* 2001;**85**:F70–2.

Nevin DG, Shung J. Intravenous paracetamol overdose in a preterm infant during anesthesia. *Paediatr Anaesth* 2010;**20**:105–7.

Porta R, Sánchez L, Nicolás M, *et al*. Lack of toxicity after paracetamol overdose in an extremely preterm neonate. *Eur J Clin Pharmacol* 2012;**68**:901–2.

de la Pintiére A, Beuchée A, Bétrémieux PE. Intravenous propacetamol overdose in a term newborn. *Arch Dis Child Fetal Neonatal Ed* 2003;**88**:F351–2.

Use
Aciclovir is used to treat herpes simplex virus (HSV) infection. It is also used, along with varicella zoster immunoglobulin (q.v.), to treat those with varicella zoster (chickenpox) who are immuno-incompetent.

Pharmacology
Aciclovir is converted by viral thymidine kinase to an active triphosphate compound which inhibits viral DNA polymerase. It was first marketed in 1957. It has no effect on dormant viruses and needs to be given early to influence viral replication. Oral uptake is limited and delayed and, at high doses, progressively less complete (bioavailability 10–20%). Aciclovir is preferentially taken up by infected cells (limiting toxicity) and cleared by a combination of glomerular filtration and tubular secretion. Slow intravenous (IV) administration is important to prevent drug crystals precipitating in the renal tubules. Monitor for signs of progressive neutropenia. Oral treatment is not recommended in the neonatal period. Signs of CNS toxicity, with lethargy, tremor and disorientation, will develop if poor renal function causes aciclovir to accumulate. The neonatal half-life is about 5 hours, but it is 2½ hours in adults and in children over 3 months old. Aciclovir enters the CSF and ocular fluids well. It also crosses the placenta, but there are no reports of teratogenicity. Treatment during lactation only results in the baby receiving 2% of the weight-related maternal dose.

Herpes simplex infection
Neonatal illness is less common in the United Kingdom (1:40,000 births) than in North America, but overt infection can follow vaginal exposure to the HSV after a variable latent period. Lesions of the skin, eyes and mouth are usually the first signs, but an encephalitic or a generalised illness with pneumonia and hepatitis may develop without warning even, rarely, after some weeks. The virus grows readily in cell culture, and a positive diagnosis is often possible within 2–3 days. Scrapings from a skin vesicle can be used to provide rapid diagnosis by immunofluorescence. Isolates from specimens collected greater than 36 hours after birth suggest genuine infection rather than transient colonisation. A polymerase chain reaction (PCR) test can be used to detect viral DNA in the CSF in cases of suspected encephalitis. Congenital (transplacental) infection is rare but has been documented. Babies born to women with an active genital infection at delivery are at significant risk of infection, the risk being very much lower (well <5%) with reactivated infection. Unfortunately, differentiation can be difficult, maternal infection is often silent, and routine cervical culture is unhelpful. Caesarean delivery can prevent the baby becoming infected but is of limited value if the membranes have been ruptured more than 6 hours. Only one small trial has yet assessed whether oral aciclovir (400 mg once every 8 hours from 36 weeks' gestation) can reduce the need for caesarean delivery or risk of neonatal infection in mothers becoming infected for the first time during pregnancy. Babies who survive a generalised or encephalitic illness are often disabled, but long-term oral treatment (up to 6 months) improves neurodevelopmental outcomes in the survivors.

A mother with recurrent facial cold sores (labial herpes) will not infect her own baby because both will have the same high viral antibody titre. Ward staff with lesions need to apply topical 5% aciclovir cream every 4 hours as soon as the first symptoms develop (2 g quantities are available without prescription), adhere to a careful hand washing routine and wear a mask until the lesions dry. Staff with an active herpetic whitlow should not have direct hands-on responsibility for babies.

Treatment
Dose: 20 mg/kg IV once every 8 hours. The dosing interval must be at least doubled if there is renal failure.

Duration: Treat chickenpox for 1 week and disseminated neonatal herpes simplex infection for 3 weeks (especially if there could be CNS involvement). Long-term oral suppression treatment in surviving infants with CNS herpes simplex can be given 300 mg/m^3 of body surface area orally three times daily for 6 months.

Eye ointment: Apply five times a day under ophthalmic supervision until 3 days after resolution is complete.

Supply and administration
Aciclovir is available in 250 mg vials of powder costing £9.10 (Na$^+$ content 1.16 mmol). To prepare a solution for IV use, reconstitute the 250 mg vial with 10 ml of water or 0.9% sodium chloride, and dilute to 50 ml with 5% dextrose to give an alkaline solution containing 5 mg/ml.

Continued on p. 59

Extravasation causes marked tissue damage (fluid pH 11). Do not refrigerate or keep for more than 12 hours after reconstitution. 100 ml of the 40 mg/ml sugar-free oral syrup costs £24.00 and 200 mg dispersible tablets cost 20p each. 4.5 g of 3% eye ointment costs £10.

References

(see also the Cochrane reviews and the UK guideline on genital herpes in pregnancy **DHUK**)

Caviness AC, Demmler GJ, Almendarez Y, *et al*. The prevalence of neonatal herpes simplex virus infection compared with serious bacterial illnesses in hospitalized neonates. *J Pediatr* 2008;**153**:164–9. (See also commentaries 155–8.)

Jones CA. Vertical transmission of genital herpes. Prevention and treatment options. *Drugs* 2009;**69**:421–34.

Kimberlin DW, Lin C-Y, Jacobs RF, *et al*. Safety and efficacy of high-dose intravenous acyclovir in the management of neonatal herpes simplex virus infection. *Pediatrics* 2001a;**108**:230–8.

Kimberlin DW, Lin Y-C, Jacobs RF, *et al*. Natural history of neonatal herpes simplex virus infections in the acyclovir era. *Pediatrics* 2001b;**108**:223–9.

Kimberlin DW, Whitley RJ, Wan W, *et al*. Oral acyclovir suppression and neurodevelopment after neonatal herpes. *N Engl J Med* 2011;**365**:1284–92.

Malm G. Neonatal herpes simplex virus infection. *Semin Fetal Neonat Med* 2009;**14**:204–8.

Tiffany KF, Benjamin DK, Palasanthiran P, *et al*. Improved neurodevelopmental outcomes following long-term high-dose acyclovir therapy in infants with central nervous system and disseminated herpes simplex disease. *J Perinatol* 2005;**25**:156–61.

Tod M, Lokiec F, Bidault R, *et al*. Pharmacokinetics of oral acyclovir in neonates and in infants: a population analysis. *Antimicrob Agents Chemother* 2001;**45**:150–7.

Use

Adenosine is the drug of choice in the management of neonatal supraventricular tachycardia (SVT).

Physiology

In infants, SVT is usually an atrioventricular (AV) re-entry tachycardia and presents with a heart rate of 260–300 bpm. A strong vagal stimulus may be enough to re-establish a normal rhythm especially in the very young baby, and one very effective way of triggering this is to wrap the baby in a towel and then submerge the baby's face in a bowl of ice-cold water for about 5 seconds. Even a cold face flannel may occasionally suffice. There is no need to obstruct the mouth or nose as submersion will cause reflex apnoea. Other approaches are, however, generally more effective in older children, and a bolus dose of adenosine is now accepted as the approach of choice if intravenous (IV) access can be achieved.

Pharmacology

Adenosine is a short-acting purine nucleoside with a serum half-life of about 10 seconds, first marketed commercially in 1992. It has the potential to slow the conduction through the AV node and suppress the automaticity of atrial and Purkinje tissues. It has no negative inotropic effects and does not cause significant systemic hypotension and can therefore be used safely in children with impaired cardiac function or early post-operative arrhythmia. Transient flushing may occur. There is no evidence that its use is dangerous in pregnancy or lactation (although respiratory side effects may occur in mothers with asthma). It has even been given to the fetus by cordocentesis. There are limited animal and human data to suggest that a continuous infusion of adenosine into the right atrium might, by causing pulmonary vasodilatation, be of some value in babies with persistent pulmonary hypertension.

Adenosine is the drug of choice in the initial management of any SVT that fails to respond to vagal stimulation. The arrival of this rapidly effective drug has greatly reduced the need for synchronised DC cardioversion, although this remains the treatment of choice for the shocked, collapsed infant. If the tachycardia persists or recurs, other drugs such as propranolol (q.v.), flecainide (q.v.) and amiodarone (q.v.) may be needed, but the true diagnosis needs confirmation first. Seek the advice of a paediatric cardiologist, and arrange, if necessary, to fax an electrocardiograph (ECG) trace for assessment. An unsynchronised DC shock remains the only effective treatment for ventricular fibrillation, but this is very rare in infancy, even in babies with congenital heart disease.

Monitoring treatment

Try to connect an ECG (and, if available, a multichannel recorder) before starting and during treatment so it is possible to record and review the trace to establish what caused the tachycardia. Following successful interruption of AV conduction, there may be a period of no electrical activity ('flat line') until such time that nodal escape and then bradycardia occur before eventual restoration of normal sinus rhythm.

Treatment

Arrhythmia: Give 150 micrograms/kg IV (0.15 ml/kg of a dilute solution made up as specified below) as rapidly as possible into a central or large peripheral vein, followed by a bolus of 0.9% sodium chloride. A larger dose is sometimes needed; repeat the injection every 1–2 minutes while increasing the dose by 50–100 micrograms/kg until either the tachycardia is terminated or the maximum single dose of 300 micrograms/kg (in neonates) or 500 micrograms/kg (in older infants) is reached.

Lowering pulmonary vascular tone: Adenosine has very occasionally been given as a continuous IV infusion. Some have used a catheter positioned in the right atrium or (preferably) the pulmonary artery, but it is not clear how necessary this is. Start with a dose of 30 microgram/kg/minute and double (or even treble) this if there is no response within half an hour. Treatment may be needed for 1–5 days.

Supply and administration

2 ml vials are available containing 3 mg/ml of adenosine (costing £4.90). To obtain a dilute solution for accurate 'bolus' use containing 1 mg/ml, take 1 ml of this fluid and dilute to 3 ml with 0.9% sodium chloride.

Continued on p. 61

To administer a continuous infusion of 30 micrograms/kg/minute, infuse the undiluted solution at a rate of 0.6 ml/kg/hour. 10 ml vials (cost £11.70), also containing 3 mg/ml of adenosine, are available and may be more suited for use as an infusion. Check the strength of the ampoule carefully because some hospitals stock non-proprietary ampoules of a different strength. Discard the ampoule once it has been opened. Do not refrigerate.

References

Dixon J, Foster K, Wyllie JP, *et al*. Guidelines and adenosine dosing in supraventricular tachycardia. *Arch Dis Child* 2005;**90**:1190–1. (See also *Arch Dis Child* 2005;**91**:373.)

Kothari DS, Skinner JR. Neonatal tachycardias: an update. *Arch Dis Child Fetal Neonatal Ed* 2006;**91**:F136–44.

Motti A, Tissot C, Rimensberger PC, *et al*. Intravenous adenosine for refractory pulmonary hypertension in a low-weight premature newborn: a potential new drug for rescue therapy. *Pediatr Crit Care Med* 2006;**7**:380–2.

Patole S, Lee J, Buettner P, *et al*. Improved oxygenation following adenosine infusion in persistent pulmonary hypertension of the newborn. *Biol Neonate* 1998;**74**:345–50.

Paul T, Bertram H, Bökenkamp R, *et al*. Supraventricular tachycardia in infants, children and adolescents. *Paediatr Drugs* 2002;**2**:171–81.

Skinner JR, Sharland G. Detection and management of life threatening arrhythmias in the perinatal period. *Early Hum Dev* 2008;**84**:161–72.

Sreeram N, Wren C. Supraventricular tachycardia in infants: response to initial treatment. *Arch Dis Child* 1990;**65**:127–9.

Wren C. Adenosine in paediatric arrhythmias. *Paediatr Perinat Drug Ther* 2006;**7**:114–7.

Use
'Bolus' doses of adrenaline are widely used during cardiopulmonary resuscitation in adults, but there has never been much evidence to support their use during neonatal resuscitation. Continuous infusions of adrenaline, or noradrenaline (q.v.), are increasingly used to treat cardiac dysfunction and septic shock.

Pharmacology
Adrenaline, first isolated in 1901, is the main chemical transmitter released by the adrenal gland. It has a wide range of α and β receptor effects. Metabolism is rapid; the half-life is less than 5 minutes. *Low* doses (<500 nanograms/kg/minute) usually cause systemic and pulmonary vaso-dilatation, with some increase in heart rate and stroke volume. *High* doses cause intense systemic vasoconstriction; while blood pressure rises as a result, the effect on cardiac output depends on the heart's ability to cope with a rising afterload (see web commentary). Combined support with a corticosteroid may help, at least in the neonatal period. Adrenaline acts as a bronchodilator and respiratory stimulant; it also causes increased wakefulness, reduced appetite and reduced renal blood flow (partly from juxtaglomerular renin release). Excessive doses cause tachycardia, hypertension and cardiac arrhythmia.

   Adrenaline is one of the few drugs used in newborn resuscitation; however, very few babies truly *require* drugs during resuscitation, and most of those who do have a bad outlook. Reports to the contrary usually come from centres that use drugs so frequently that they must have often been given unnecessarily. Adrenaline also features prominently in cardiac arrest treatment algorithms for non-shockable and shockable rhythms in children and adults. By inducing vasoconstriction and increasing diastolic pressure, it improves coronary artery perfusion pressure, enhances myocardial contractility, stimulates spontaneous contractions and increases the amplitude and frequency of VF, thus increasing the likelihood of successful defibrillation. Adrenaline can exceptionally be given down an endotracheal tube, although there is almost no evidence that this is effective especially in the newborn lung that retains some fetal lung fluid. This route no longer features in resuscitation of older children.

Treatment
Anaphylaxis: See the monograph on immunisation. *Never* give more than a 1 microgram/kg intravenous (IV) bolus.
Newborn resuscitation: The IV dose is 10–30 micrograms/kg (0.1–0.3 ml/kg of 1:10,000 solution). Only a rough estimate of weight is needed. There is no evidence that a higher IV dose is better. Tracheal administration is of doubtful efficacy and should be tried *only* if IV access is unavailable – a higher dose (50–100 micrograms/kg) is suggested.
Resuscitation (infants and older children): Give 10 micrograms/kg (0.1 ml/kg of 1:10,000 solution) every 3–5 minutes via the IV or intraosseous routes.
Croup and bronchiolitis: Giving 3 ml of a 1:1000 solution through a nebuliser does very little to reduce symptoms in babies with bronchiolitis but reduced the number admitted in one study. It provides 1–2 hours of symptomatic relief in croup, but an oral or intramuscular dose of dexamethasone (q.v.) provides more sustained relief.
Cardiac dysfunction: Continuous IV infusions of 30–300 nanograms/kg/minute, made up as described under 'Supply and administration', can increase output without causing vasoconstriction; higher doses should only be used if facilities exist to monitor cardiac output, especially in the first day of life.

Compatibility
It can be added (terminally) to a line containing dobutamine and/or dopamine, doxapram, fentanyl, heparin, midazolam, milrinone, morphine or standard TPN (but not lipid).

Supply and administration
Stock 1 ml ampoules containing 1 mg of L-adrenaline (1:1000) cost 39p each. To give a 100 nanograms/kg/minute infusion, place 3 mg of adrenaline for each kilogram the baby weighs in a syringe, dilute to 50 ml with 10% glucose saline, and infuse at 0.1 ml/hour. A less concentrated dextrose (or dextrose saline) solution can be used, as can 0.9% saline. These solutions are stable and do not need to be prepared afresh every 24 hours. Protect ampoules from light and always check their strength, because 100 micrograms/ml (1:10,000) ampoules also exist. Tissue extravasation can be dangerous.

Continued on p. 63

References

(see also the relevant Cochrane reviews and UK anaphylaxis guideline **DHUK**)

Barber CA, Wyckoff MH. Use and efficacy of endotracheal versus intravenous epinephrine during neonatal cardiopulmonary resuscitation in the delivery room. *Pediatrics* 2006;**118**:1028–34.

Bjornson CL, Johnson DW. Croup. *Lancet* 2008;**371**:329–39. [SR]

Germanakis I, Bender C, Hentschel R, *et al.* Hypercontractile heart failure caused by catecholamine therapy in premature neonates. *Acta Paediatr* 2003;**92**:836–8.

Heckmann M, Trotter A, Pohlandt F, *et al.* Epinephrine treatment of hypotension in very low birthweight infants. *Acta Pediatr* 2002;**91**:566–70.

McLean-Tooke APC, Bethune CA, Fay AC, *et al.* Adrenaline in the treatment of anaphylaxis: what is the evidence? *Br Med J* 2003;**327**:1332–5. [SR]

Pellicer A, Valverde E, Elorza MD, *et al.* Cardiovascular support for low birth weight infants and cerebral haemodynamics: a randomized, blinded, clinical trial. *Pediatrics* 2005;**115**:1501–12. [RCT]

Perondi MBM, Reis AG, Paiva EF, *et al.* A comparison of high-dose and standard-dose epinephrine in children with cardiac arrest. *N Eng Med J* 2004;**350**:1722–30. [RCT]

Sicherer SH, Simons FER. Self-injectable epinephrine for first-aid management of anaphylaxis. *Pediatrics* 2007;**119**:638–46.

Wyckoff MH, Wyllie J. Endotracheal delivery of medications during neonatal resuscitation. *Clin Perinatol* 2006;**33**:153–60. [SR]

Use
Albendazole is used to treat a range of parasitic diseases including hookworm, roundworm, threadworm and whipworm infection. It also has a role in the treatment of some tapeworm (cestode) infections and is the drug of choice to treat symptomatic microsporidiosis (*Enterocytozoon bieneusi* and *E. intestinalis* infection).

Pharmacology
The drug benzimidazole was first studied for its antiviral properties between 1947 and 1953, and it was then discovered that the related thiabendazole was active against many roundworms. Further exploratory work with a range of related products finally led to the patenting of mebendazole by Janssen in 1971 and the development of albendazole, which was thought to have fewer side effects, 4 years later.

Intestinal parasitic infestation is so prevalent in young children in many developing countries that it generally goes unnoticed unless it produces acute florid ill health. Indeed, a quarter of the world's population probably currently harbours roundworm, hookworm or whipworm infection. Forty million pregnancies are affected by hookworm infection each year.

The oral absorption of albendazole is very limited in man (although improved by a simultaneous fatty meal), and what is absorbed is rapidly metabolised by the liver into the active drug, albendazole sulphoxide, which is then cleared from the body with a half-life of 8–12 hours. The active metabolite shows little toxicity in animals but is rapidly lethal to most nematode worms because of tubulin binding. High-dose treatment has been teratogenic in some animals; although fetal damage has not been identified in man, treatment should, where possible, be avoided in the first trimester of pregnancy. Use during lactation is probably safe.

Two hundred million people in Africa have schistosomiasis (bilharziasis), and this contributes to the death annually of a quarter of a million people from complicated nephrosis and portal hypertension even though the infection is cheaply and easily treated with two 20 mg/kg oral doses of praziquantel (q.v.) 6 hours apart (three such doses for *Schistosoma japonicum* infection). The balance of risk supports *including* pregnant and lactating women in mass treatment programmes with praziquantel even if breastfeeding cannot be safely substituted for 48 hours after administration.

Intestinal nematode parasites
Hookworm: *Ancylostoma duodenale* and *Necator americanus* are the most common causes of this usually asymptomatic hookworm infection. Heavy infection can cause serious microcytic anaemia in young children.

Roundworm: Infection with *Ascaris lumbricoides*, the most common of all the roundworm infections, is normally asymptomatic, but heavy infection can cause malnutrition. It is large enough to cause intestinal obstruction in some small children, while migration out of the bowel can cause a protean range of symptoms.

Threadworm: Infection with the small white roundworm, *Enterobius vermicularis*, causes threadworm (or pinworm) which is the most common worm infection in the United Kingdom.

Whipworm: Infection with *Trichuris trichiura* is commonly asymptomatic, but severe infection can affect growth and lead to bloody diarrhoea or an inflammatory colitis. Mature worms, which are 3–5 cm long, attach themselves to the wall of the large bowel, but diagnosis is usually made by identifying eggs in the stool.

Maternal treatment
Community-based studies in an area where severe anaemia from hookworm infection is extremely common have shown that a 400 mg oral dose of albendazole given in the second and the third trimester can reduce the incidence of severe anaemia, boost birthweight and improve infant survival.

Treatment in infancy
A single 400 mg oral dose of albendazole will effectively 'deworm' children who are 2 or more years old (although 3 days' treatment is advisable for whipworm infection). Children less than a year old should only be treated if symptomatic, and the WHO tentatively suggests a 200 mg dose for such children. There is, as yet, no evidence on the safety of treatment in children less than 6 months old.

Continued on p. 65

Supply

While albendazole (as a 400 mg tablet and 40 mg/ml suspension) and praziquantel (as a 150 or 600 mg tablet) are both licensed for sale in the United States, they are, at the moment, only available on a named-patient basis in the United Kingdom from IDIS, Weybridge, Surrey. GlaxoSmithKline (which has donated large quantities of albendazole to the WHO) is the main manufacturer in the United States.

References (see also the relevant Cochrane reviews)

Bethony J, Brooker S, Albonico M, *et al.* Soil-transmitted helminth infections: ascariasis, trichuriasis and hookworm. *Lancet* 2006;**367**:1521–32.

Christian P, Khatry SK, West KP. Antenatal anthelmintic treatment, birthweight, and infant survival in rural Nepal. *Lancet* 2004;**364**:981–3.

Kalra V, Dua T, Kumar V. Efficacy of albendazole and short-course dexamethasone treatment in children with 1 or 2 ring-enhancing lesions of neurocysticercosis: a randomized controlled trial. *J Pediatr* 2003;**143**:111–4. [RCT]

Keiser J, Utzinger J. Efficacy of current drugs against soil-transmitted helminth infections: systematic review and meta-analysis. *JAMA* 2008;**299**:193748. [SR]

Montresor A, Awasthi S, Crompton DWT. Use of benzimidazoles in children younger than 24 months for the treatment of soil-transmitted helminthiasis. *Acta Trop* 2003;**86**:223–32 (see also 141–59).

Tremoulet AH, Avila-Aguero ML, Paris MM, *et al.* Albendazole therapy for *Microsporidium* diarrhea in immunocompetent Costa Rican children. *Pediatr Infect Dis J* 2004;**23**:915–8.

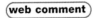

Use

Alginate compounds, like Gaviscon®, are used to control some of the symptoms of gastro-oesophageal reflux. The preparations for use in older children and adults are different from that used in babies (Gaviscon® Infant), and care should be taken when prescribing to specify the correct formulation.

Pharmacology

A range of antacid preparations containing magnesium salts (which have a mild laxative effect) and aluminium salts (which have the opposite tendency) are commercially available 'over the counter'. There are no contraindications to use during pregnancy or lactation. Magnesium trisilicate and magnesium or aluminium hydroxide are commonly chosen, because they are retained rather longer in the stomach. Alginates are often added when reflux is a problem, because they react with gastric acid to form a viscous gel or 'raft' that then floats to the top of the stomach, acting as a mechanical barrier to oesophageal reflux.

Each sachet of Gaviscon Infant, the formulation most widely used in infancy, contains 225 mg of sodium alginate, and 87.5 mg of magnesium alginate, with colloidal silica and mannitol. Unlike adult formulations, it does not contain bicarbonate (and no longer contains aluminium). It does, however, contain 21 mg (0.9 mmol) of sodium chloride per dose which may contribute to hypernatraemia if there is dehydration or poor renal function. Other formulations contain even more sodium. Gaviscon is specifically contraindicated in the treatment of gastroenteritis and of suspected intestinal obstruction. Gaviscon Infant has, on occasion, formed a solid intra-gastric mass or 'bezoar' which can lead to obstruction but which, if detected early, will dissolve as long as the Gaviscon is discontinued.

Gastro-oesophageal reflux

Art plays a larger role than science in the feeding of the small preterm baby, and experienced neonatal nurses are the acknowledged artists. Many babies 'posset' a few mouthfuls of milk and some swallow a lot of air while feeding, bringing back milk when winded. Many smaller babies regurgitate some milk back into the lower oesophagus after feeding because of poor sphincter tone, but only a few aspirates, and very few develop oesophagitis because milk is an excellent antacid. Nevertheless, silent reflux can cause serious lung damage; babies with a post-menstrual age less than 35 weeks have no effective cough reflex.

Some preterm babies with reflux also have episodes of apnoea. Distinguishing apnoea due to reflux from apnoea of prematurity is not easy. Placing the baby prone (face down), or on its left side, may help, but such a strategy should only be adopted with monitored babies in a hospital setting because of the increased risk of cot death. Tilting the head of the cot up 30° was once thought to help but may increase abdominal pressure, and one trial suggests that a semi-upright posture can make matters worse. While severe symptoms may merit oesophageal impedance–pH monitoring, this is seldom needed in milder cases. Gaviscon only reduces reflux slightly but may be helpful where oesophagitis is suspected, or growth is affected, and probably works by thickening the feed. While it may lessen the reflux, it does little for the apnoeic spells which many associate with the condition.

Treatment

Term babies: Babies less than 5 kg should be offered one dose of the Gaviscon Infant dual sachet with feeds. Babies over 5 kg may be offered both doses with each feed.

Preterm babies: The manufacturer does not recommend the use of Gaviscon Infant in preterm babies although it is widely used. It may be appropriate to give a proportionate dose (see below) with each feed.

Supply and administration

Gaviscon Infant comes made up in paired sucrose- and lactose-free sachets (cost 24p) containing enough powder for *two* standard doses. They can be purchased from pharmacies without a doctor's prescription, but such use is not to be encouraged. Gaviscon Infant is one of the few commercial products, marketed specifically for use in the treatment of reflux vomiting in infancy, which can be prescribed on the NHS.

Continued on p. 67

Take the powder from one section of a paired sachet of Gaviscon Infant, mix with 5 ml (1 teaspoon) of fresh tap water, and add 1 ml of this thin paste to each 25 ml of artificial milk. Breastfed babies can be offered a similar quantity after each feed on a spoon. Do not give the liquid formulation to babies.

References

(see also the Cochrane review of reflux)

Carroll AE, Garrison MM, Christakis DA. A systemic review of nonpharmacological and nonsurgical therapies for gastroesophageal reflux in infants. *Arch Pediatr Adolesc Med* 2002;**156**:109–13. [SR]

Corvaglia L, Spizzichino M, Zama D, *et al.* Sodium Alginate (Gaviscon®) does not reduce apnoeas related to gastro-oesophageal reflux in preterm infants. *Early Hum Dev* 2011;**87**:775–8.

Del Buono R, Wenzl TG, Ball G, *et al.* Effect of Gaviscon Infant on gastro-oesophageal reflux in infants assessed by combined intraluminal impedance/pH. *Arch Dis Child* 2005;**90**:460–3. [RCT] (See also 2006;**91**:93.)

Hegar B, Dewanti NR, Kadim M, *et al.* Natural evolution of regurgitation in healthy infants. *Acta Paediatr* 2009;**98**:1189–93.

James ME, Ewer AK. Acid oro-pharyngeal secretions can predict gastro-oesophageal reflux in preterm infants. *Eur J Pediatr* 1999;**158**:371–4.

Sorbie AL, Symon DN, Stockdale EJ. Gaviscon bezoars. *Arch Dis Child* 1984;**59**:905–6.

Tighe MP, Afzal NA, Bevan A, *et al.* Current pharmacological management of gastro-esophageal reflux in children: an evidence-based systematic review. *Pediatr Drugs* 2009;**11**:185–202. [SR]

Use

Alteplase is a fibrinolytic drug used to dissolve intravascular thrombi. Streptokinase (q.v.) is cheaper.

Pharmacology

All fibrinolytic drugs work by activating plasminogen to plasmin, which then degrades fibrin, causing the break-up of intravascular thrombi. Treatment should always be started as soon as possible after any clot has formed. Streptokinase and alteplase both have an established role in the management of myocardial infarction, but controlled trials show that benefit is limited if treatment is delayed for more than 12 hours. Alteplase, a human tissue plasminogen activator first manufactured by a recombinant DNA process in 1983, is a glycoprotein that directly activates the conversion of plasminogen to plasmin. It became commercially available in 1988. When given intravenous (IV), it remains relatively inactive in the circulation until it binds to fibrin, for which it has a high affinity. It is, however, rapidly destroyed by the liver, with a plasma half-life of only 5 minutes. As a result, adverse effects (including excess bleeding) are uncommon in adults and usually controlled without difficulty by stopping treatment. There is little experience of use during pregnancy. The high molecular weight makes placental transfer unlikely. There is no evidence of teratogenicity, but placental bleeding is a theoretical possibility. Use during lactation seems unlikely to pose any serious problem.

There have been many reports of the use of alteplase to lyse arterial and intracardiac thrombi in the neonatal period, but it is not clear whether it is any safer or more effective than streptokinase and the drug is considerably more expensive. There is, however, probably rather less risk of an adverse effect and less theoretical risk of an allergic reaction. Visualise the clot and take advice from a vascular surgeon before starting treatment, remembering that ultrasound review has shown that the great majority of catheter-related thrombi never give rise to symptoms. Use can certainly speed the resolution of infective endocarditis. There is a risk of bleeding, especially if the platelet count is less than 100×10^9/l or the fibrinogen level falls below 1 g/l. Intracranial bleeding was a common complication with sustained use in one recent neonatal case series, so risk assessment is important before starting treatment. Combined use with heparin (q.v.) optimises outcome in adults with myocardial infarction, but the value of such dual treatment in babies has not been properly studied. Try and avoid venepuncture and intramuscular injections during treatment. See the website for a commentary on the slim evidence base that currently underpins the management of clots and emboli in early infancy.

Alteplase (0.5 mg/kg) has been instilled experimentally into the cerebral ventricles of babies with severe intraventricular bleeding to reduce post-haemorrhagic hydrocephalus. The **DR**ainage, **I**rrigation and **F**ibrinolytic **T**herapy (**DRIFT**) procedure is complicated and probably should be restricted to centres where neurosurgical support is available. While neither of the first two trials of this strategy showed any evidence of early benefit and some risks of further bleeding, a 2-year follow-up showed a reduction in survivors affected by severe cognitive disability and reduced overall risk of death or severe disability.

Prophylaxis

A 1 mg/ml solution of alteplase is better (if more expensive) than heparin at maintaining patency of 'stopped-off' long lines. Slightly overfill the line. Aspirate before reuse to stop dispersal of small emboli into the lung.

Treatment

Blocked catheters: Instil a volume of alteplase (1 mg/ml) slightly greater than the catheter dead space. Other strategies, as outlined in the monograph on urokinase, may sometimes work better in lines that have been used to infuse parenteral nutrition.

Thrombi: Give a continuous infusion of 100–600 micrograms/kg/hour for 6 hours. The optimal dose has not been established; some patients require lower doses and shorter periods of treatment; therefore, consider starting treatment at 100 micrograms/kg/hour. Use Doppler ultrasound assessment to monitor the effect before considering a second course of treatment.

Monitoring

Monitor the fibrinogen level regularly during sustained treatment, and adjust the dose if the level falls below 1 g/l. Give cryoprecipitate or fresh frozen plasma (q.v.) at once if a bleeding tendency develops.

Continued on p. 69

Supply and administration

10 mg (5.8 megaunits) vials of powder suitable for reconstitution using 10 ml of water for injection (as provided) cost £144. The resultant solution (containing 1 mg/ml of alteplase) must be used within 24 hours, even if stored at 4 °C, but small pre-prepared syringes can be kept for 3 months at −20 °C. To give 100 micrograms/kg/hour, dilute the reconstituted solution with an equal volume of 0.9% sodium chloride and infuse at a rate of 0.2 ml/kg/hour. Do not dilute the reconstituted solution with anything except 0.9% sodium chloride. 2 mg (1.16 megaunits) vials of powder costing £45 are available for the restoration of catheter patency. These are reconstituted using 2 ml of water for injection (supplied with the powder).

References   (see also the Cochrane review on interventions to restore the patency of central venous catheters)

Gittins NS, Hunter-Blair YL, Matthews J, *et al.* Comparison of alteplase and heparin in maintaining the patency of pediatric central venous haemodialysis lines: a randomised controlled trial. *Arch Dis Child* 2007;**92**:499–501. [RCT] (See also pp. 516–7.)

Gupta AA, Leaker M, Andrew M, *et al.* Safety and outcomes of thrombolysis with tissue plasminogen activator for treatment of intravascular thrombosis in children. *J Pediatr* 2001;**139**:682–8.

Hartmann J, Hussein A, Trowitzsch E, *et al.* Treatment of neonatal thrombus formation with recombinant tissue plasminogen activator: six years experience and review of the literature. *Arch Dis Child Fetal Neonatal Ed* 2001;**85**:F18–22. (See also pp. F66–72.)

Jacobs BR, Haygood M, Hingl J. Recombinant tissue plasminogen activator in the treatment of central venous catheter occlusion in children. *J Pediatr* 2001;**139**:593–6.

Monagle P, Chalmers E, Chan A, *et al.* Antithrombotic therapy in neonates and children: American College of Chest Physicians Evidence-Based Clinical Practice Guidelines (8th Edition). *Chest* 2008;**133**(Suppl):887S–968S.

Whitelaw A, Aquilina K. Management of posthaemorrhagic ventricular dilatation. *Arch Dis Child Fetal Neonatal Ed* 2012;**97**:F229–33.

Whitelaw A, Evans D, Carter M, *et al.* Randomized clinical trial of prevention of hydrocephalus after intraventricular hemorrhage in preterm infants: brain-washing versus tapping fluid. *Pediatrics* 2007; **119**:e107–18. [RCT]

Whitelaw A, Jary S, Kmita G, *et al.* Randomized trial of drainage, irrigation and fibrinolytic therapy for premature infants with posthemorrhagic ventricular dilatation: developmental outcome at 2 years. *Pediatrics* 2010;**125**:e852–8.

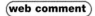
Use

Amikacin is commonly used to treat suspected neonatal infection in some countries, but it is usually held in 'reserve' in the United Kingdom for use against Gram-negative bacteria that are resistant to gentamicin, as well as all the other commonly used antibiotics, and should only be used on the advice of a consultant microbiologist.

Pharmacology

Amikacin is a semi-synthetic aminoglycoside antibiotic first developed in 1972. It can be particularly useful in the treatment of Gram-negative bacteria resistant to gentamicin (such as certain *Enterobacter* species).

Significant placental transfer occurs and, although the drug has not been documented as causing fetal damage, it would seem wise to monitor blood levels when amikacin is used in pregnancy to minimise the risk of fetal ototoxicity because drug accumulation has been documented in the fetal lung, kidney and placenta. Only small amounts appear in human milk, and as absorption from the gut is minimal, the breastfed infant is unlikely to suffer from adverse effects.

The drug, like its parent compound, kanamycin, is largely excreted through the renal glomerulus. The half-life is 7–14 hours in babies with a post-menstrual age of less than 30 weeks and 4–7 hours at a post-menstrual age of 40 weeks (the adult half-life being about 2 hours). Nephrotoxicity and cochlear or vestibular damage can occur if 'trough' blood levels in excess of those generally recommended go uncorrected, as with all aminoglycosides. The risk is increased if amikacin is prescribed for more than 10 days, follows treatment with another aminoglycoside or is given at the same time as a diuretic such as furosemide (q.v.). Amikacin is less toxic to the neonatal kidney than gentamicin or netilmicin, however, and also probably less ototoxic. Absorption is said to be somewhat unpredictable after intramuscular (IM) administration in very small babies. CSF penetration is limited.

For a justification of the dose regimen recommended under 'Treatment', see the monograph on gentamicin, and for a more general discussion of the prescribing of aminoglycosides in infancy, see the associated web commentary. The dosage interval should be increased in patients with renal failure and adjusted according to serum antibiotic levels.

Treatment

Dose: Give 15 mg/kg Intravenous (IV) or IM to babies less than 4 weeks old and 20 mg/kg to babies older than this.
Timing: Give a dose once every 36 hours in babies less than 28 weeks' gestation in the first week of life. Give all other babies a dose once every 24 hours unless renal function is poor. Check the trough serum level just before the fourth dose is due and increase the dosage interval if this level is more than 5 mg/l.

Blood levels

The trough level is all that usually needs to be monitored in babies on high-dose treatment once every 24–36 hours, and this is probably only necessary as a *routine* in babies less than 10 days old or with possible renal failure. Aim for a trough level of less than 5 mg/l (1 mg/l = 1.71 μmol/l). The 1 hour peak level, when measured, should be 20–30 mg/l. Collect specimens in the same way as for gentamicin.

Supply and administration

Amikacin is available in two strengths: a non-proprietary 2 ml vial containing 500 mg (250 mg/ml) costing £9.60 and a proprietary 2 ml vial containing 100 mg (50 mg/ml) costing £2.10 (Na$^+$ content ~0.5 mmol). Material should not be stored after dilution. Do not mix amikacin with any other drug. IV doses do *not* need to be given slowly over 30 minutes.

References

Allegaert K, Cossey V, Langhendries JP, *et al*. Effects of co-administration of ibuprofen-lysine on the pharmacokinetics of amikacin in preterm infants during the first days of life. *Biol Neonat* 2004;**86**:207–11.
Allegaert K, Anderson BJ, Cossey V, *et al*. Limited predictability of amikacin clearance in extreme premature neonates at birth. *Br J Clin Pharmacol* 2006;**61**:39–48.

Continued on p. 71

Allegaert K, Scheers I, Cossey V, *et al*. Covariates of amikacin clearance in neonates: the impact of postnatal age on predictability. *Drug Metab Lett* 2008;**2**:286–9.

Kenyon CF, Knoppert DC, Lee SK, *et al*. Amikacin pharmacokinetics and suggested dosage modifications for the preterm infant. *Antimicrob Agents Chemother* 1990;**34**:265–8.

Kotze A, Bartel PR, Sommers DK. Once versus twice daily amikacin in neonates: prospective study on toxicity. *J Paediatr Child Health* 1999;**35**:283–6. [RCT]

Labaune JM, Bleyzac N, Maire P, *et al*. Once-a-day individualized amikacin dosing for suspected infection at birth based on population pharmacokinetic models. *Biol Neonate* 2001;**80**:142–7.

Langhendries JP, Battisti O, Bertrand JM, *et al*. Once a day administration of amikacin in neonates: assessment of nephrotoxicity and ototoxicity. *Dev Pharmacol Ther* 1993;**20**:220–30. [RCT]

Langhendries JP, Battisti O, Bertrand JM, *et al*. Adaptation in neonatology of the once-daily concept of aminoglycoside administration: evaluation of a dosing chart for amikacin in an intensive care unit. *Biol Neonate* 1998;**74**:351–62.

Marik PE, Lipman J, Kobilski S, *et al*. A prospective randomized study comparing once-versus twice-daily amikacin in critically ill adult and paediatric patients. *J Antimicrob Chemother* 1991;**28**:753–64. [RCT]

Prober CG, Yeager AS, Arvin AM. The effect of chronologic age on the serum concentration of amikacin in the sick term and premature infant. *J Pediatr* 1981;**98**:636–40.

Sherwin CM, Svahn S, Van der Linden A, *et al*. Individualised dosing of amikacin in neonates: a pharmacokinetic/pharmacodynamic analysis. *Eur J Clin Pharmacol* 2009;**65**:705–13.

Vásquez-Mendoza MG, Vargas-Origel A, Ramos-Jiménez A del C, *et al*. Efficacy and renal toxicity of one daily dose of amikacin versus conventional dosage regime. *Am J Perinatol* 2007;**24**:141–6.

Use

Amiodarone is increasingly used to control persisting troublesome supraventricular, and junctional ectopic, tachycardia. It is also used to manage those fetal cardiac arrhythmias that do not respond to digitalisation or flecainide (q.v.). Use should *always* be initiated and supervised by a paediatric cardiologist because adverse reactions are not uncommon, and the manufacturers have not yet endorsed use in children. Treatment can usually be discontinued after 9–12 months.

Pharmacology

Amiodarone, a class III antiarrhythmic agent first developed in 1963, is used in the management of certain congenital or post-operative re-entry tachycardias, especially where there is impaired ventricular function. It prolongs the duration of the action potential and slows atrioventricular (AV) nodal conduction. It also increases the atrial, AV nodal and ventricular refractory periods, facilitating re-entrant rhythm suppression. Blood levels are of no value in optimising treatment or in avoiding toxicity. Combined treatment with oral propranolol (q.v.) may be needed at first, but the use of propranolol can usually be discontinued after a few months. Flecainide is probably a better first choice for automatic arrhythmias. Amiodarone has largely replaced lidocaine as the antiarrhythmic agent of choice in cardiac arrest situations. It is given, along with adrenaline, in pulseless ventricular fibrillation and tachycardias after the third DC shock has been given.

Tissue levels greatly exceed plasma levels (V_D ~40–80 l/kg). Amiodarone also has an extremely long half-life (several weeks), and treatment usually has to be given for several days before a therapeutic response is achieved. Intravenous (IV) treatment can be used, when necessary, to speed the achievement of a response as long as the consequent exposure to benzyl alcohol is judged acceptable. Most of the adverse effects associated with amiodarone treatment are reversible once treatment is withdrawn. Skin photosensitivity (controlled by using a sunblock cream), skin discolouration, corneal microdeposits (easily seen with a slit lamp), liver disorders (with or without jaundice), pneumonitis and peripheral neuropathy have all been reported, but such complications have not yet been seen in infancy.

Amiodarone is thought to be hazardous in pregnancy because of its iodine content, and the manufacturer has not endorsed the drug's use in children under three. Such a risk may have to be accepted, however, if no other treatment can be found for maternal (or fetal) arrhythmia. For the same reason, most texts recommend that patients on long-term treatment should also be monitored for hypo- and hyperthyroidism. In addition, since breast milk contains a substantial amount of amiodarone, there are important reasons why a mother on treatment who wishes to breastfeed should only do so under close medical supervision. While absorption is incomplete, experience suggests that the baby can receive, on a weight-for-weight basis, a dose equivalent to about a third of that taken by the mother.

Drug interactions

Joint medication can prolong the half-life of flecainide, digoxin, phenytoin and warfarin. Treatment with these drugs *must* be monitored, since the dose of these drugs may have to be reduced if toxicity is to be avoided. Amiodarone can prolong the QT interval and cases of torsades de pointes have been reported.

Treatment

Resuscitation: In management of 'shockable' cardiopulmonary arrest, amiodarone 5 mg/kg is administered after the third DC shock while CPR is continued. A further 5 mg/kg is given if the rhythm is unchanged after the fifth shock.

Intravenous: Only give this drug IV in an intensive care setting and when a rapid response is essential. Give 5 mg/kg over 30 minutes and a second similar dose if the first is ineffective. Watch for bradycardia and hypotension. Further 5 mg/kg maintenance doses can be given IV every 12 or 24 hours if necessary. Change to oral administration as soon as possible.

Oral: Give a 15 mg/kg loading dose (unless the baby has already had IV treatment) and then a maintenance dose of between 5 and 12 mg/kg once a day depending on the response achieved.

Supply and administration

Amiodarone is available in two strengths: a non-proprietary 10 ml pre-filled syringe containing 300 mg (30 mg/ml) of amiodarone hydrochloride costing £13.50 and both non-proprietary vials and proprietary vials containing 50 mg/ml of amiodarone hydrochloride (and 20 mg/ml of benzyl alcohol) (costing £1.50 for a 3 ml vial and £2.90 for a 6 ml vial).

Continued on p. 73

Use the 50 mg/ml vials to give 5 mg/kg of amiodarone IV by placing 0.5 ml (25 mg) of amiodarone for each kilogram the baby weighs in a syringe, dilute to 25 ml with 5% glucose (***NOT*** sodium chloride), and give 5 ml of this dilute preparation over 30 minutes. Watch for extravasation because the excipient, Tween 80, is very irritant and the solution quite acidic (pH ~4). Try to avoid giving a continuous infusion to a child under three because it can leach the plasticiser out of an IV giving set. Prepare a fresh solution each time. An oral suspension in syrup containing 20 mg/ml with a 14-day shelf life can be prepared on request. It must be protected from light.

References

Biarent D, Bingham R, Eich C, *et al*. European Resuscitation Council Guidelines for Resuscitation 2010. Section 6. Paediatric life support. *Resuscitation* 2010;**81**:1364–88.

Burri S, Hug MI, Bauersfeld U. Efficacy and safety of intravenous amiodarone for incessant tachycardias in infants. *Eur J Pediatr* 2003;**162**:880–4.

Etheridge SP, Craig JE, Compton SJ. Amiodarone is safe and highly effective therapy for supraventricular tachycardia in infants. *Am Heart J* 2001;**141**:105–10. (See also pp. 3–5.)

Magee LA, Downar E, Sermer M, *et al*. Pregnancy outcome after gestational exposure to amiodarone in Canada. *Am J Obstet Gynecol* 1995;**172**:1307–11.

Perry JC, Fenrich AL, Hulse JE, *et al*. Pediatric use of intravenous amiodarone: efficacy and safety in critically ill patients from a multicenter protocol. *J Am Coll Cardiol* 1996;**27**:1246–50.

Pézarda PG, Boussion F, Sentilhes L, *et al*. Fetal tachycardia: a role for amiodarone as first- or second-line therapy? *Arch Cardiovasc Dis* 2008;**101**:619–27.

Ramusovic S, Läer S, Meibohm B, *et al*. Pharmacokinetics of intravenous amiodarone in children. *Arch Dis Child* 2013;**98**:989–93.

Saul JP, Scott WA, Brown S, *et al*. Intravenous amiodarone for incessant tachyarrhythmias in children: A randomized, double-blind, antiarrhythmic drug trial. *Circulation* 2005;**112**:3470–7. [RCT]

Trudel K, Sanatani S, Panagiotopoulos C. Severe amiodarone-induced hypothyroidism in an infant. *Pediatr Crit Care Med* 2011;**12**:e43–5.

Ward RM, Lugo RA. Cardiovascular drugs for the newborn. *Clin Perintol* 2006;**32**:979–97.

Use

Amodiaquine is generally effective against most strains of *Plasmodium falciparum* that are chloroquine sensitive (q.v.) and some that are not. Toxicity can sometimes develop with long-term use, so it is only used to treat episodes of overt infection. To stop drug resistance developing, it is used together with an artemisinin such as artesunate.

History

The search for a drug that can prevent, rather than cure, infection with the malaria parasite began in 1917 with the testing of a range of compounds on deliberately infected patients with terminal paralytic syphilis, before it was shown, in 1924, that canaries could be used instead. Knowing that the plasmodia parasite takes up methylene blue, work initially focused on quinoline/methylene blue hybrids, and clinical trials soon showed that one such drug, pamaquin, could cure naturally acquired falciparum malaria. It kills the sporozoites in the liver but not the merozoites liberated by cyclical liver cell rupture into the blood as quinine does. A number of 4- and 8-aminoquinoliness were studied during World War II by the American Army's Malaria Research Programme before chloroquine, and then amodiaquine, came into use in the late 1940s. The artemisinin drugs artemether (q.v.) and artesunate have now emerged as the most potent drugs for combating malaria, and, to prevent the emergence of drug resistance yet again, these are now routinely given together with an antimalarial such as amodiaquine or lumefantrine (as outlined in the monograph on artemether).

Pharmacology

Amodiaquine hydrochloride is a 4-aminoquinoline structurally related to chloroquine. It is well absorbed when taken orally and rapidly converted by hepatic cytochrome CYP2C8 to an active metabolite, *N*-desethyl amodiaquine. This metabolite is excreted by the kidney in a relatively slow and variable way (mean plasma half-life 2–3 days). Amodiaquine is no longer used to *prevent* infection (it was withdrawn from the WHO Essential Drugs List in 1988 due to major side effects associated with long-term use) but has, since 2003, been used to *treat* infection when a number of reviews concluded that it was safe. Overdose of amodiaquine can cause seizures and loss of consciousness, but it does not appear to cause any of the life-threatening cardiovascular complications often seen after an overdose of chloroquine. Amodiaquine was reintroduced for the treatment of uncomplicated malaria and recommended as partner drug in both artemisinin-based combinations and non-artemisinin-based combinations.

Malaria in the last 6 months of pregnancy can seriously affect maternal health and jeopardise fetal survival. Treatment with amodiaquine ideally with one dose of pyrimethamine (q.v.) and sulphadoxine (as Fansidar®) seems very safe, though it can briefly exacerbate tiredness, dizziness and nausea. Little is known about use during lactation, but use of the closely related drug chloroquine is extremely safe. Artesunate is not known to cross into maternal milk.

Treatment

During pregnancy: Give two 600 mg doses 24 hours apart and then one 300 mg dose. Co-treatment with a single 75 mg dose of pyrimethamine and 1.5 g of sulphadoxine on the first day minimises treatment failure.

During infancy: Give two 10 mg/kg doses of amodiaquine base 24 hours apart and then one 5 mg/kg dose after a further 24 hours. Artesunate/amodiaquine combination tablets may be used in the following doses (where the first number is the amount of artesunate, and the second is the amount of amiodaquine):

Weight of infant	
4.5 to <9 kg	One 25 mg/67.5 mg tablet crushed with water daily for 3 days
9 to <18 kg	One 50 mg/135 mg tablet daily for 3 days

Rectal artesunate: Early rectal artesunate before transit to more distant facilities is helpful in those too ill to take oral medication. A 10 mg/kg rectal dose seems ideal, but a 100 mg suppository, given as soon as the child is ill, seems safe in children between the ages of 6 months and 6 years. Move to oral treatment as soon as possible.

Continued on p. 75

Supply

Amodiaquine with or without artesunate is not currently marketed in the United Kingdom or the United States, but is available from Parke-Davis as a 200 mg tablet (Camoquin®) costing 65p. This can be crushed, suspended in water and given by spoon. A commercial suspension has also been supplied for research purposes. It is normally described in terms of the amount of amodiaquine base (260 mg of hydrochloride = 200 mg of base).

WHO-promoted artesunate/amodiaquine combination packs are increasingly available in a variety of strengths: 25 mg/67.5 mg, 50 mg/135 mg and 100 mg/270 mg. A range of artesunate products suitable for intravenous, intramuscular or rectal use are available in many countries where malaria is endemic.

References

(see also the relevant Cochrane reviews)

Clerk CA, Bruce J, Affipunquh PK, *et al*. A randomized, controlled trial of intermittent preventive treatment with sulfadoxine-pyrimethamine, amodiaquine, or the combination in pregnant women in Ghana. *J Infect Dis* 2008;**198**:1202–11. [RCT]

Falade CO, Oqundele AO, Yusuf BO, *et al*. High efficacy of two artemisinin-based combinations (artemether-lumefantrine and artesunate plus amodiaquine) for acute uncomplicated malaria in Ibadan, Nigeria. *Trop Med Int Health* 2008;**13**:635–43. [RCT]

Gomes MF, Faiz MA, Gyapong JO, *et al*. Pre-referral rectal artesunate to prevent death and disability in severe malaria: a placebo controlled trial. *Lancet* 2009;**373**:557–66. [RCT]

Massaga JJ, Kitua AY, Lemnge MM, *et al*. Effect of intermittent treatment with amodiaquine on anaemia and malarial fevers in infants in Tanzania: a randomised placebo-controlled trial. *Lancet* 2003;**361**:1853–60. [RCT]

Nosten F, McGready R, d'Alessandro U, *et al*. Antimalarial drugs in pregnancy: a review. *Curr Drug Saf* 2006;**1**:1–15.

Olliaro P, Nevill C, Le Bras J, *et al*. Systematic review of amodiaquine treatment in uncomplicated malaria. *Lancet* 1996;**348**:1196–201. [SR] (See also pp. 1184–5.)

Rijken MJ, McGready R, Jullien V, *et al*. Pharmacokinetics of amodiaquine and desethylamodiaquine in pregnant and postpartum women with Plasmodium vivax malaria. *Antimicrob Agents Chemother* 2011;**55**:4338–42.

Schramm B, Valeh P, Baudin E, *et al*. Efficacy of artesunate-amodiaquine and artemether-lumefantrine fixed-dose combinations for the treatment of uncomplicated Plasmodium falciparum malaria among children aged six to 59 months in Nimba County, Liberia: an open-label randomized non-inferiority trial. *Malar J* 2013;**12**:251. [RCT]

Staedke SG, Kamya MR, Dorsey G, *et al*. Amodiaquine, sulfadoxine/pyrimethamine, and combination therapy in treatment of uncomplicated falciparum malaria in Kampala, Uganda: a randomised trial. *Lancet* 2001;**358**:368–74. [RCT]

Tagbor H, Bruce J, Browne E, *et al*. Efficacy, safety and tolerability of amodiaquine plus sulphadoxine-pyrimethamine used alone or in combination for malaria treatment in pregnancy: a randomised trial. *Lancet* 2006;**368**:1349–56. [RCT] (See also pp. 1306–7.)

Tagbor HK, Chandramohan D, Greenwood B. The safety of amodiaquine use in pregnant women. *Expert Opin Drug Saf* 2007;**6**:631–5.

Use

Amoxicillin has similar properties to ampicillin (q.v.), and there is little to choose between the two when given by the intravenous (IV) route to treat *Listeria*, β-lactamase-negative *Haemophilus* or enterococcal infection.

Pharmacology

Amoxicillin is a semi-synthetic broad-spectrum, bactericidal, aminopenicillin that is active against a wide range of organisms including *Listeria, Haemophilus,* enterococci, streptococci, pneumococci and many coliform organisms and is also active against *Salmonella, Shigella* and non-penicillinase-forming strains of *Proteus*. It remains, 50 years after its introduction in 1964, the drug recommended by the WHO when treating bacterial respiratory tract illness in young children.

The half-life in the term baby is about 4 hours (but very variable) falling to a little over 1 hour in later infancy as renal excretion improves, and because efficacy depends on keeping the blood level continuously above the minimum inhibitory dose (as with all β-lactam antibiotics), dosing frequency must reflect this. Amoxicillin readily crosses the placenta, but use during lactation exposes the baby to less than 1% of the weight-adjusted maternal dose.

The dosage policy recommended here is more than adequate but is designed to achieve high CSF levels in the face of early subclinical meningitis and in the knowledge that the drug is very non-toxic. A combination of amoxicillin with clavulanic acid, marketed as co-amoxiclav (q.v.), extends the activity to cover β-lactamase-producing organisms.

There is little to choose between ampicillin and amoxicillin when given parenterally, although amoxicillin is said to be more rapidly bactericidal at doses close to the minimum inhibitory concentration. Both antibiotics are well absorbed when taken by mouth, widely distributed in body tissues (including bronchial secretions) and rapidly excreted in the urine. Although amoxicillin shows better bioavailability when taken by mouth, it can still be quite variable in young children. Adverse effects are similar to those seen with ampicillin but rare, and diarrhoea may be slightly less common.

Prophylaxis

Mothers: While ascending infection may be an occasional cause of spontaneous preterm labour, the only antibiotic that has yet been shown to delay labour or improve outcome is clindamycin (q.v.) in women with overt bacterial vaginosis in early pregnancy. See the monograph on ampicillin for a comment on antibiotic use when labour starts before 35 weeks and the membranes ruptured before there were overt signs of labour.

Children: Give babies with structural heart disease (excluding those with isolated ASD, fully repaired VSD or PDA or fully epithelialised closure device) 50 mg/kg of amoxicillin IV or intramuscular (IM) half an hour before and 6 hours after any surgical procedure involving a site where infection is suspected to reduce the risk of bacterial endocarditis. Some would give gentamicin as well to those at very high risk. It may be better to give azithromycin or clindamycin (q.v.) rather than amoxicillin in a baby who has had more than one dose of a penicillin class antibiotic in the preceding month.

Measles: Pre-emptive antibiotic treatment may prevent complicating bacterial pneumonia, especially in countries where measles remains a dangerous illness.

Treatment

Dose: Give 100 mg/kg IV or IM if meningitis is a possibility. In all other situations, a dose of 50 mg/kg is more than adequate, given (if the patient is well enough) by mouth. Otitis media only needs 25 mg/kg.

Timing: Give one dose every 12 hours in the first week of life, every 8 hours in babies 1–3 weeks old and every 6 hours in babies 4 or more weeks old. Increase the dosage interval if there is severe renal failure. Treat otitis media for 5–7 days, septicaemia for 10–14 days, meningitis for 3 weeks and osteitis for 4 weeks. Even severe pneumonia can usually be managed by treatment three times a day for 5–7 days. Oral medication can nearly always be used to complete any sustained course of treatment.

Continued on p. 77

Supply

Stock 250 mg vials cost 32p. Add 2.4 ml of water for injection to the 250 mg vial (or 4.6 ml to the 500 mg vial) to get a solution containing 100 mg/ml and always use this at once. A 100 mg/kg dose contains 0.33 mmol/kg of sodium. A sugar-free oral suspension (25 mg/ml) is available which costs £1.20 for 100 ml. It can be kept at room temperature after reconstitution but should be used within 2 weeks.

References

(see the relevant Cochrane reviews)

Addo-Yobo E, Chisaka N, Hassan M, *et al*. Oral amoxicillin versus injectable penicillin for severe pneumonia in children aged 3 to 59 months: a randomised multicentre equivalency study. *Lancet* 2004;**364**:1141–8. [RCT] (See also pp. 1104–5.)

Gras-Le Guen C, Boscher C, Godon N, *et al*. Therapeutic amoxicillin levels achieved with oral administration in term neonates. *Eur J Clin Pharmacol* 2007;**63**:657–62.

Muller-Pebody B, Johnson AP, Heath PT, *et al*. Empirical treatment of neonatal sepsis: are the current guidelines adequate? *Arch Dis Child Fetal Neonatal Ed* 2011;**96**:F4–8.

National Institute for Health and Clinical Excellence. CG64 prophylaxis against infective endocarditis: full guidance. 2008.

Pichichero ME, Reed MD. Variations in amoxicillin pharmacokinetic/pharmacodynamic parameters may explain treatment failure in acute otitis media. *Pediatr Drugs* 2009;**11**:243–9.

Pullen J, Driessen M, Stolk LML, *et al*. Amoxicillin pharmacokinetics in (preterm) infants aged 10 to 52 days: effect of postnatal age. *Ther Drug Monit* 2007;**29**:376–80.

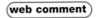
Use

Amphotericin B is a valuable treatment in the management of suspected or proven systemic fungal infection. A liposomal formulation can be used if toxicity develops, but these are more costly. The liposomal formulation is also used to treat leishmaniasis (kala-azar) as outlined in the web commentary.

Pharmacology

Amphotericin B is a polyene antifungal derived from *Streptomyces nodosus*. It has been widely used to treat aspergillosis, candidiasis, coccidioidomycosis and cryptococcosis since it was first isolated in 1953. It works by binding to a cytoplasmic membrane ergosterol on the organism's surface, causing cell death by increasing cell membrane permeability. The half-life, volume of distribution and clearance are highly variable in infants. The clinical response does not always correlate with the result of *in vitro* testing. Because CSF penetration of amphotericin is poor, synergistic co-treatment with flucytosine (q.v.) may be required.

Amphotericin is a potentially toxic drug with many common adverse effects including a dose-dependent and dose-limiting impairment of renal function. Drug elimination is poorly understood, unrelated to renal function and extremely unpredictable in the neonatal period. Significant drug accumulation is thought to occur in the liver (V_D ~4 l/kg). A low salt intake increases the risk of nephrotoxicity. Anaemia and leucopenia are not uncommon, and hypokalaemia can occur. Fever, vomiting and rigors can occur during or after intravenous (IV) infusion. Anaphylaxis in older patients (but rarely seen in neonates) can be avoided by giving a 'test' dose of 100 micrograms/kg over 10 minutes before the first full dose. Rapid infusion can cause hyperkalaemia and an arrhythmia, while an overdose has occasionally caused death. Over 80% of adults given amphotericin experience some renal impairment, but such problems seem much less common in infancy. Liposomal preparations are generally used when there is renal impairment or intolerance of the standard preparation. They have less impact on the kidney due in part to poor renal tissue penetration and can be given in higher doses of the parent drug. The poor renal tissue penetration, in turn, makes them a poor option for renal fungal disease. Amphotericin crosses the placenta, but does not seem to be toxic or teratogenic to the fetus, so treatment does not need to be withheld during pregnancy. No information is available on amphotericin use during lactation; however, poor oral absorption means the infant is unlikely to absorb significant amounts.

Treatment

Standard formulation: Give 1 mg/kg IV over 4 hours once a day for 7 days and then 1 mg/kg once every 48 hours. Incremental treatment is not appropriate, and a first 'test' dose is not necessary in a neonate. Ensure a sodium intake of at least 4 mmol/kg/day. Treatment is usually continued for 4 weeks.

Liposomal formulation: AmBisome® and Abelcet® are the most widely studied products in neonates, but there appears to be no clinical advantage of one preparation over the other. Start by giving 1 mg/kg IV over 30–60 minutes once a day especially if there is renal impairment. Increase the dose by 1 mg/kg every day up to 5 mg/kg once a day. This dose has been used in deep-seated neonatal infection involving bone or the CNS without causing recognisable toxic side effects and is often used in older children with proven infection.

Supply and administration

Ready-to-use pre-filled syringes (which should be stored in the dark and used within 48 hours but which do not need to be protected from light during administration) may be dispensed by some pharmacies. The different preparations of amphotericin vary in their pharmacodynamics, pharmacokinetics, dosage and administration and should not be considered interchangeable. Specify the formulation to be used when prescribing.

Standard formulation: 50 mg vials of dry powder (which should be stored at 4 °C) cost £3.90 (Na⁺ content <0.5 mmol). Prepare the powder immediately before use by adding 10 ml of sterile water for injection into the vial through a wide bore needle to give a solution containing 5 mg/ml. Shake until the colloidal solution is clear. Then further dilute the drug by adding 1 ml of this colloidal solution to 49 ml of 5% glucose to give a solution containing 100 micrograms/ml. Do not employ a less than 1 μm filter, expose to bright light or mix with any other drug.

Continued on p. 79

Liposomal formulations: 50 mg vials of AmBisome cost £97. Add 12 ml of water for injection to obtain a solution containing 4 mg/ml and shake vigorously until the powder is completely dispersed. Take 20 mg (5 ml) from the vial using the 5 μm filter provided, dilute to 10 ml with 5% glucose to give a solution containing 2 mg/ml, and infuse the prescribed amount over 30–60 minutes. 20 ml vials containing 100 mg of Abelcet suspension cost £78. Remove the required volume of the suspension and dilute to a concentration of 2 mg/ml using 5% glucose. Administer by infusion at a rate not exceeding 1.25 ml/hour.

Compatibility: Do not let any of these product come into contact with *any* fluid other than 5% glucose. If using a pre-existing cannula, this must be flushed with 5% glucose before and after the infusion.

References

(see also the relevant Cochrane reviews)

Bailey JE, Meyers C, Kleigman RM, *et al*. Pharmacokinetics, outcome of treatment, and toxic effects of amphotericin B and 5-fluorocytosine in neonates. *J Pediatr* 1990;**116**:791–7.

Blyth CC, Palasanthiran P, O'Brien TA. Antifungal therapy in children with invasive fungal infection: a systematic review. *Pediatrics* 2007;**119**:772–84. [SR]

Linder N, Klinger G, Shalit I, *et al*. Treatment of candidaemia in premature infants: comparison of three amphotericin B preparations. *J Antimicrob Chemother* 2003;**52**:663–7. [RCT]

Moen MD, Lyseng-Williamson KA, Scott LJ. Liposomal amphotericin B: a review of its use in empirical therapy in febrile neutropenia and in the treatment of invasive fungal infections. *Drugs* 2009;**69**:361–92. [SR]

Sobel JD. Use of antifungal drugs in pregnancy: a focus on safety. *Drug Saf* 2000;**23**:77–85.

Tripathi N, Watt K, Benjamin DK Jr. Treatment and prophylaxis of invasive candidiasis. *Semin Perinatol* 2012;**36**:416–23.

Weitkamp TJ, Poets CF, Sievers R, *et al*. Candida infection in very low birth-weight infants: outcome and nephrotoxicity of treatment with liposomal amphotericin B (AmBisome). *Infection* 1998;**26**:11–5.

Wurthwein G, Groll AH, Hempel G, *et al*. Population pharmacokinetics of amphotericin B lipid complex in neonates. *Antimicrob Agents Chemother* 2005;**49**:5092–8.

Use
Ampicillin is a widely used antibiotic with similar properties to amoxicillin (q.v.).

Pharmacology
Ampicillin is a semi-synthetic broad-spectrum aminopenicillin that crosses the placenta. A little appears in human milk, but it can safely be given to a lactating mother since the baby is known to receive less than 1% of the weight-related maternal dose. Maculo-papular drug rashes are *not* a sign of serious drug sensitivity and are relatively rare in the neonatal period. The drug is actively excreted in the urine and, partly as a result of this, the plasma half-life falls from about 6 to 2 hours during the first 10 days of life. Penetration into the CSF is moderately good particularly when the meninges are inflamed.

Ampicillin was, for many years, the most widely used antibiotic for treating infection with *Listeria*, β-lactamase-negative *Haemophilus*, enterococci, *Shigella* and non-penicillinase-forming *Proteus* species. It is also effective against streptococci, pneumococci and many coliform organisms. Ampicillin has frequently been used prophylactically to reduce the risk of infection after abdominal surgery (including caesarean delivery). Ampicillin is resistant to acids and moderately well absorbed when given by mouth, but oral medication can alter the normal flora of the bowel (causing diarrhoea), and the absorption and 'bioavailability' of ampicillin when taken by mouth do not approach that achieved by amoxicillin. The arrival of ampicillin on the market before amoxicillin probably explains the former's continued common use, even though most authorities now consider amoxicillin the better product for this and a range of other reasons.

Preterm pre-labour rupture of membranes (PPROM)
Prophylactic antibiotic treatment can delay delivery enough to measurably reduce the risk of neonatal problems after birth. Ampicillin has been widely used, but erythromycin (q.v.) may be a better option.

Care in spontaneous preterm labour
Similar prophylaxis does *not* delay delivery, or improve outcome, when labour threatens to start prematurely before the membranes rupture, but high-dose penicillin *during* delivery can reduce the risk of early-onset neonatal group B streptococcal infection. Ampicillin is sometimes given instead in the hope that this will prevent coliform sepsis as well, but as such organisms are increasingly resistant to ampicillin, all women going into unexplained spontaneous labour before 35 weeks' gestation are best given both intravenous (IV) penicillin and IV gentamicin. Even in pregnancies more mature than this, there are grounds for giving IV penicillin (q.v.) throughout labour to reduce the risk of group B streptococcal infection if the membranes are known to have ruptured more than 6 hours before labour starts. One recent study has suggested that a combination of these two strategies would result in 80% of all the babies currently dying of *any* bacterial infection of intrapartum origin (i.e. babies developing symptoms within 48 hours of birth) receiving appropriate antibiotic treatment during delivery. It means giving antibiotics to between 40 and 60 women during labour to provide optimum treatment for one baby with bacterial sepsis of intrapartum origin. Many policies treat even more patients than this, and it seems possible that this could increase the risk of *late-onset* infection.

Neonatal treatment
Dose: The neonatal dose when meningitis is suspected is 100 mg/kg IV or intramuscular (IM). In other situations, a dose of 50 mg/kg is more than adequate, given (when the patient is well enough) by mouth.
Timing: Give every 12 hours in the first week of life, every 8 hours in babies 1–3 weeks old and every 6 hours in babies 4 or more weeks old. Increase the dosage interval if there is severe renal failure. Sustain treatment for 10–14 days in proven septicaemia, for 3 weeks in babies with meningitis and for 4 weeks in osteitis. Oral medication can sometimes be used to complete treatment even though absorption is limited.

Supply
500 mg vials cost £7.80. Add 4.6 ml of sterile water for injection to the dry powder to get a solution containing 100 mg/ml and always use at once after reconstitution. A 100 mg/kg dose contains 0.3 mmol/kg of sodium. The oral suspension (25 mg/ml) costs £7.88 per 100 ml. Use within

Continued on p. 81

1 week if kept at room temperature (2 weeks if kept at 4 °C). No sugar-free oral suspension is currently available (a sugar-free oral suspension of amoxicillin is available and is a suitable alternative).

References

(see also the relevant Cochrane reviews and UK guideline on managing PPROM **DHUK**)

Bizzarro MJ, Dembry L-M, Baltimore RS, *et al*. Changing patterns in neonatal *Escherichia coli* sepsis and ampicillin resistance in the era of intrapartum antibiotic prophylaxis. *Pediatrics* 2008;**121**:689–96.

Egarter C, Leitich H, Karas H, *et al*. Antibiotic treatment in preterm and premature rupture of membranes and neonatal morbidity: a meta-analysis. *Am J Obstet Gynecol* 1996;**174**:589–97. [SR]

Gilbert RE, Pike K, Kenyon SL, *et al*. The effect of prepartum antibiotics on the type of neonatal bacteraemia: insights from the MRC ORACLE trials. *BJOG* 2005;**112**:830–2.

Glasgow TS, Young PC, Wallin J, *et al*. Association of intrapartum antibiotic exposure and late-onset serious bacterial infections in infants. *Pediatrics* 2005;**116**:696–702.

Kenyon SL, Taylor DJ, Tarnow-Mordi W, for the ORACLE Collaborative Group. Broad-spectrum antibiotics for preterm, prelabour rupture of fetal membranes: the ORACLE I randomised trial. *Lancet* 2001;**357**:979–88. [RCT] (See also **358**:502–4.)

Lamont RF, Sobel J, Mazaki-Tovi S, *et al*. Listeriosis in human pregnancy: a systematic review. *J Perinat Med* 2011;**39**:227–36. [SR]

Schuchat A, Zywicki SS, Dinsmoor MJ, *et al*. Risk factors and opportunities for prevention of early-onset neo-natal sepsis: a multicenter case-control study. *Pediatrics* 2000;**105**:21–6.

Use

Bevacizumab and **ranibizumab** are two of a number of anti-vascular endothelial growth factor (anti-VEGF) therapies that have emerged since the late 1990s. As a group, anti-VEGF drugs are used to treat a number of different conditions. Ophthalmic interest in this group of drugs arose because of the importance of VEGF in the pathogenesis of proliferative retinal vascular diseases in adults and, more recently, retinopathy of prematurity (ROP). Intra-vitreal injection of bevacizumab or ranibizumab has been used to treat ROP, particularly in infants too ill to undergo ablative laser treatment.

Retinopathy of prematurity

ROP is one of the most common preventable causes of childhood blindness and is due to mal-adaptation of the immature retinal vessels to changing availability of oxygen between the fetal and neonatal environments. There are two phases in the development of ROP: the first phase consists of delayed retinal blood vessel development. *In utero* retinal blood vessel development is partly driven by 'physiological hypoxia' and the avascular retina produces VEGF which stimulates physiological angiogenesis. The preterm neonate is exposed to much more oxygen and as a result VEGF production ceases. At about 32 weeks' post-menstrual age, the growing avascular peripheral retina begins to produce high levels of VEGF that lead to the abnormal growth of vessels seen in ROP. The posterior retinal blood vessels become dilated and tortuous ('plus' disease), and abnormal blood vessels grow out of the retina and into the vitreous.

The mainstay of treatment for severe ROP is diode laser ablation of the peripheral retina. Not only does this usually require sedation or anaesthesia, but it is difficult to perform and results in destruction of the peripheral retina. Interest in anti-VEGF drugs arose out of the need for an alternative to the current treatment, particularly in those infants too sick to undergo anaesthesia. Caution is advised, and VEGF has been implicated in glomerular, brain and alveolar development; thus, systemic leakage of either of these drugs can have major implications for the developing organs. Studies in adults and neonates show that small, but nevertheless clinically important, amounts enter the systemic circulation and in the only randomised comparative trial of use in the treatment of ROP there was an increased incidence of adverse events across many organ systems in the bevacizumab arm, the significance of which remains unclear.

Pharmacology

Bevacizumab is a recombinant humanised monoclonal antibody produced by DNA technology from Chinese hamster ovary cells. Ranibizumab is a smaller monoclonal antibody fragment derived from the same parent antibody as bevacizumab and is considerably more expensive. Both drugs are injected into the vitreous humour under local anaesthesia and sedation. In adult studies, there is less systemic leakage of ranibizumab and the potential for the adverse effects on other developing organs is, theoretically at least, lower.

Reactivation of ROP is a potential feature of treatment with both drugs and prolonged monitoring for signs of ROP is required after treatment and needs to continue until such time that the retina is fully vascularised.

Treatment

Bevacizumab: The BEAT-ROP study used an intra-vitreal dose of 0.625 mg in each eye.
Ranibizumab: Most experience has been gained with an intra-vitreal dose of 0.25 mg in each eye.

There is some evidence to suggest that these doses may be excessive; the doses above are half the doses used in adult retinopathies and are those reported to have been used in most studies. Lower doses may be as effective and have less potential for systemic effects; in adults with retinopathies, a bevacizumab dose of 1.25 mg is normally used, but evidence of effect is seen with doses as low as 6.25 micrograms in preterm infants with ROP.

Continued on p. 83

Supply

There is no ocular formulation for bevacizumab as it does not have a licence. A 4 ml vial for its licensed intravenous use costs £243.00. Many doses for ocular use can be produced from a single vial and therefore can be supplied for a much lower cost of approximately £50–100. Ranibizumab is available in 0.23 ml vials containing 2.3 mg of ranibizumab at a cost of £742.00.

References (see also the relevant Cochrane reviews)

Avery RL. Bevacizumab (Avastin) for retinopathy of prematurity: wrong dose, wrong drug, or both? *J AAPOS* 2012;**16**:2–4.

Avery RL, Pearlman J, Pieramici DJ, *et al.* Intravitreal bevacizumab (Avastin) in the treatment of proliferative diabetic retinopathy. *Ophthalmology* 2006;**113**:1695.e1–15.

Bakri SJ, Snyder MR, Reid JM, *et al.* Pharmacokinetics of intravitreal bevacizumab (Avastin). *Ophthalmology* 2007;**114**:855–9.

Castellanos MA, Schwartz S, García-Aguirre G, *et al.* Short-term outcome after intravitreal ranibizumab injections for the treatment of retinopathy of prematurity. *Br J Ophthalmol* 2013;**97**:816–9.

Darlow BA, Ells AL, Gilbert CE, *et al.* Are we there yet? Bevacizumab therapy for retinopathy of prematurity. *Arch Dis Child Fetal Neonatal Ed* 2013;**98**:F170–4.

Fierson WM, American Academy of Pediatrics Section on Ophthalmology, American Academy of Ophthalmology, *et al.* Screening examination of premature infants for retinopathy of prematurity. *Pediatrics* 2013;**131**:189–95.

Hård AL, Hellström A. On safety, pharmacokinetics and dosage of bevacizumab in ROP treatment – a review. *Acta Paediatr* 2011;**100**:1523–7.

Hu J, Blair MP, Shapiro MJ, *et al.* Reactivation of retinopathy of prematurity after bevacizumab injection. *Arch Ophthalmol* 2012;**130**:1000–6.

Mintz-Hittner HA, Kennedy KA, Chuang AZ. Efficacy of intravitreal bevacizumab for stage 3+ retinopathy of prematurity. *N Engl J Med* 2011;**364**:603–15. [RCT]

Patel RD, Blair MP, Shapiro MJ, *et al.* Significant treatment failure with intravitreous bevacizumab for retinopathy of prematurity. *Arch Ophthalmol* 2012;**130**:801–2.

Sato T, Wada K, Arahori H, *et al.* Serum concentrations of bevacizumab (avastin) and vascular endothelial growth factor in infants with retinopathy of prematurity. *Am J Ophthalmol* 2012;**153**:327–33.e1.

Use

L-Arginine is an essential nutritional supplement for patients with inborn errors of metabolism affecting the urea cycle, other than arginase deficiency, in which dietary restriction of arginine is required. In some urea cycle disorders, L-arginine also facilitates nitrogen excretion, along with sodium phenylbutyrate and sodium benzoate (q.v.).

Two small randomised studies suggest that L-arginine supplementation of 1.5 mmol/kg/day (261 mg/kg/day) may reduce the risk of necrotising enterocolitis in premature very low birthweight infants. However, further studies are required before this can be recommended routinely.

Biochemistry

Arginine is a naturally occurring amino acid needed for protein synthesis. Since it is produced in the body by the 'urea cycle', it is not, ordinarily, an essential nutrient. Dietary supplementation becomes essential, however, in most patients with urea cycle disorders because the enzyme defect limits arginine production, while dietary protein restriction limits arginine intake. Further supplementation also aids nitrogen excretion in citrullinaemia and argininosuccinic aciduria because excess arginine is metabolised to citrulline and argininosuccinic acid, incorporating nitrogen derived from ammonia and aspartic acid. As citrulline and argininosuccinic acid can be excreted in the urine, treatment with arginine can lower the plasma ammonia level in both these conditions. Treatment with arginine needs to be combined with a low-protein diet and supervised by a consultant experienced in the management of metabolic disease. Treatment with oral sodium phenylbutyrate and/or sodium benzoate is also usually necessary.

Specialist advice

Specialist advice on a range of inborn errors of metabolism is available from the British Inherited Metabolic Disease Group (BIMDG), and detailed guidance on the management of hyperammonaemia is available on this Group's website (www.bimdg.org.uk). Click on the red box to access a range of emergency protocols.

Treatment

> Note: Treatment with L-arginine should be initiated only after consultation with a specialist metabolic diseases centre.

Ornithine transcarbamoylase and carbamoyl phosphate synthetase deficiency: Give 25–35 mg/kg of arginine by mouth four times a day to meet the basic need for protein synthesis. Patients with acute hyperammonaemia should be given 6 mg/kg an hour as a continuous intravenous (IV) infusion.

Citrullinaemia and argininosuccinic aciduria: Up to 175 mg/kg of arginine four times a day can be given by mouth to promote nitrogen excretion. During acute hyperammonaemia, an IV loading dose of 300–600 mg/kg is given over 90 minutes followed by a continuous infusion of 12.5–25 mg/kg/hour.

Monitoring

Vomiting and hypotension have occasionally been reported as a result of treatment with IV arginine. Hyperchloraemic acidosis can occur in patients on high-dose arginine hydrochloride: pH and plasma chloride concentrations should be monitored and bicarbonate given if necessary. High arginine levels are thought to contribute to the neurological damage in arginase deficiency, and it is recommended that plasma arginine levels should be monitored during long-term use and kept between 50 and 200 µmol/l.

Supply and administration

L-Arginine can be made available (as hydrochloride) in powder form for oral use; 100 g costs £12. This is a chemical, not a pharmaceutical, product. Regular supplies can be made available on prescription to patients with urea cycle disorders in the United Kingdom, as long as these are marked Advisory Committee on Borderline Substances (ACBS). L-Arginine is also available as a

Continued on p. 85

sugar-free medicine in 200 ml bottles. Add 185 ml of purified water to the contents of the bottle to obtain 200 ml of a 100 mg/ml liquid which remains stable for 2 months. This can be mixed with milk, fruit juice or food.

A 200 ml IV infusion pack containing 20 g (200 mg/ml) of L-arginine (as the hydrochloride) is available, as are 10 ml (500 mg/ml) ampoules costing £3. These should be diluted to 20 mg/ml before use with 0.9% sodium chloride or 10% glucose. Most pharmacies can obtain supplies from 'special-order' manufacturers or specialist importing companies.

References (see also the relevant Cochrane reviews)

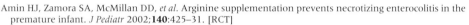

Amin HJ, Zamora SA, McMillan DD, *et al*. Arginine supplementation prevents necrotizing enterocolitis in the premature infant. *J Pediatr* 2002;**140**:425–31. [RCT]

Brusilow SW. Arginine, an indispensable amino acid for patients with inborn errors of urea synthesis. *J Clin Invest* 1984;**74**:2144–8.

Brusilow SW, Horwich AL. Urea cycle enzymes. In: Scriver CR, Beaudet AL, Sly WS, *et al.*, eds. *The metabolic and molecular bases of inherited disease*, 8th edn. New York: McGraw-Hill, 2001: pp. 1909–64.

Häberle J, Boddaert N, Burlina A, *et al*. Suggested guidelines for the diagnosis and management of urea cycle disorders. *Orphanet J Rare Dis* 2012;**7**:32.

Polycarpou E, Zachaki S, Tsolia M, *et al*. Enteral L-arginine supplementation for prevention of necrotizing enterocolitis in very low birth weight neonates: a double-blind randomized pilot study of efficacy and safety. *JPEN J Parenter Enteral Nutr* 2013;**37**:617–22. [RCT]

Wijburg FA, Nassogne M-C. Disorders of the urea cycle and related enzymes. In: Saudubray J-M, van den Berghe G, Walter JH, eds. *Inborn metabolic diseases. Diagnosis and treatment*, 5th edn. Berlin: Springer-Verlag, 2012: pp. 297–310.

Use

Artemether is a methyl ether derivative of artemisinin now widely used in countries where many *Plasmodium falciparum* and some *Plasmodium vivax* parasites have become resistant to most other antimalarials. The World Health Organization (WHO) recommends artemisinin-based combination therapy to treat uncomplicated falciparum malaria during the second and third trimesters of pregnancy and quinine plus clindamycin during the first trimester.

Pharmacology

Extracts of the herb *Artemisia annua* (sweet wormwood) have been used to treat fever in China for many centuries. The key ingredient seems to be the sesquiterpene lactone called qinghaosu (or artemisinin), which was first isolated by Chinese chemists in 1971. Artemisinin and its derivatives, artemether and artesunate, have since been shown to clear malarial parasites from the blood more rapidly than other drugs. Parasitic recrudescence is common unless a second antimalarial is taken at the same time, or the drug is taken for at least 7 days. They also reduce gametocyte carriage (the sexual form of the parasite capable of infecting any blood-sucking mosquito), but they have no sporontocidal activity. Artemisinin and its derivatives are all hydrolysed quite rapidly in the body to the active metabolite dihydroartemisinin which then accumulates within the cytoplasm of the parasite, disrupting calcium homeostasis. Treatment with a single dose is unreliable because the half-life is much shorter than that of most other antimalarial drugs. Combined treatment with a second antimalarial is generally considered essential to stop the parasite becoming as resistant to this new drug as it has already become to most of the other drugs used in the past. A product containing 20 mg of artemether and 120 mg of lumefantrine (Coartem®) is the most widely studied combination. Artesunate with amiodarone (q.v.) is a second widely used combination.

Published reports of the use of artemisinin in over 900 pregnancies have not identified any adverse treatment-related pregnancy outcomes, but animal experiments suggest that use can cause the early embryo to die and be resorbed. Nothing has yet been published in the use of these drugs during lactation.

Managing severe malaria

Additional supportive care is necessary in any seriously ill child, as outlined in the monograph on quinine.

Oral treatment

Dose: Give children weighing 5–15 kg one tablet of Coartem crushed, if necessary, in a little water. Quinine (q.v.) is still, at the moment, the only well-studied treatment for any child weighing <5 kg.
Timing: Give six doses over 3 days (at 0, 8, 24, 36, 48 and 60 hours). Repeat the dose if it is vomited within an hour.

Children too ill to take a drug by mouth

Early treatment is critically important and, in rural settings where it may take more than 6 hours to get definite care started, a strategy for giving a rectal suppository before the child reaches medical care can halve the risk of death or long-term disability.
Artemether: Rectal artemether seems at least as effective as intravenous (IV) quinine in infants with cerebral malaria. Give babies under 9 kg one 40 mg suppository daily until oral treatment can be started. Babies over 9 kg should have a loading dose of 80 mg (two suppositories) on the first day and 40 mg/day thereafter.

Supply

Tablets of Coartem containing 20 mg of artemether and 120 mg of lumefantrine are now widely available from the WHO and are also available in North America. A dispersible tablet has also been developed to aid administration to young children. Similar tablets (costing €1) are available in Europe under the trade name Riamet®. Counterfeit products are currently known to be circulating in SE Asia. Suppositories containing 40 mg of artemether are available from Dafra Pharma in Belgium.

Continued on p. 87

References

(See also the relevant Cochrane reviews)

Abdulla S, Sagara I. Dispersible formulation of artemether/lumefantrine: specifically developed for infants and young children. *Malar J* 2009;**8**(Suppl 1):S7.

Abdulla S, Sagara I, Borrmann S, *et al*. Efficacy and safety of artemether-lumefantrine dispersible tablets compared with crushed commercial tablets in African infants and children with uncomplicated malaria: a randomised, single-blind, multicentre trial. *Lancet* 2008;**372**:1819–27. [RCT] (See also pp. 1786–7.)

Aceng JR, Byarugaba JS, Tumwine JK. Rectal artemether versus intravenous quinine for the treatment of cerebral malaria in children in Uganda: randomised controlled trial. *Br Med J* 2005;**330**:334–6. [RCT] (See also pp. 317–8.)

Barnes KI, Mwenechanya J, Tembo M, *et al*. Efficacy of rectal artesunate compared with parenteral quinine in initial treatment of moderately severe malaria in African children and adults: a randomised study. *Lancet* 2004;**363**:1598–605. [RCT]

Dellicour S, Hall S, Chandramohan D, *et al*. The safety of artemisinins during pregnancy: a pressing question. *Malaria J* 2007;**6**:15.

Dorsey G, Staedke S, Clark TD, *et al*. Combination therapy for uncomplicated falciparum malaria in Ugandan children. *JAMA* 2007;**297**:2210–9. [RCT]

Fanello CI, Karema C, van Doren W, *et al*. A randomised trial to assess the safety and efficacy of artemether-lumefantrine (Coartem) for the treatment of uncomplicated Plasmodium falciparum malaria in Rwanda. *Trans R Soc Trop Med Hyg* 2007;**101**:344–50. [RCT]

Gomes MF, Faiz MA, Gyapong JO, *et al*. Pre-referral rectal artesunate to prevent death and disability in severe malaria: a placebo-controlled trial. *Lancet* 2009;**373**:557–66. [RCT] (See also pp. 522–3.)

Hamed K, Grueninger H. Coartem®: a decade of patient-centric malaria management. *Expert Rev Anti Infect Ther* 2012;**10**:645–59.

Karunajeewa HA, Mueller I, Senn M, *et al*. A trial of combination antimalarial therapies in children from Papua New Guinea. *N Engl J Med* 2008;**359**:2545–57. [RCT] (See also pp. 1601–3.)

Kiang KM, Bryant PA, Shingadia D, *et al*. The treatment of imported malaria in children: an update. *Arch Dis Child Educ Pract Ed* 2013;**98**:7–15.

Manyando C, Mkandawire R, Puma L, *et al*. Safety of artemether-lumefantrine in pregnant women with malaria: results of a prospective cohort study in Zambia. *Malar J* 2010;**9**:249.

Manyando C, Kayentao K, D'Alessandro U, *et al*. A systematic review of the safety and efficacy of artemether-lumefantrine against uncomplicated Plasmodium falciparum malaria during pregnancy. *Malar J* 2012;**11**:141. [SR]

McGready R, Tan SO, Ashley EA, *et al*. A randomised controlled trial of artemether-lumefantrine versus artesunate for uncomplicated *Plasmodium falciparum* treatment in pregnancy. *PLoS Med* 2008;**5**:e253. [RCT]

Ratcliff A, Siswantoro H, Kenangalem E, *et al*. Two fixed-dose artemisinin combinations for drug-resistant falciparum and vivax malaria in Papua, Indonesia: an open-label randomised comparison. *Lancet* 2007;**369**:757–65. [RCT]

SEAQUAMAT Trial Group. Artesunate versus quinine for treatment of severe falciparum malaria: a randomised trial. *Lancet* 2005;**366**:717–25. [RCT] (See also **367**:110–2.)

Shingadia D, Ladhani S. UK treatment of malaria. *Arch Dis Child Educ Pract Ed* 2011;**96**:87–90.

Use

Aspirin is now seldom given to children because it is thought that use during a viral illness can trigger Reye's syndrome (an acute life-threatening encephalopathy with fatty liver degeneration). It is still used in Kawasaki disease, in children with severe rheumatoid arthritis and to limit clot formation after cardiac surgery. The web commentary reviews aspects of safe use during pregnancy and lactation.

Pharmacology

Aspirin has been better studied in pregnancy than almost any other drug. Self-treatment to relieve headache around the time of conception seems, as with all NSAIDs, to increase the risk of miscarriage, but a 75 mg daily dose started shortly after conception *reduces* the risk of repeated miscarriage in women with phospholipid antibodies. Early low-dose use also produces a 10% reduction in the risk of pre-eclampsia and of perinatal death. Low-dose use for 3 days before and on the day of any long-haul flight also probably reduces the risk of deep vein thrombosis. Even high-dose use does not seem to be teratogenic, but sustained high-dose use may increase the risk of bleeding and has been associated with premature duct closure and a rise in perinatal mortality. Episodic use during lactation seems harmless because the baby only ingests ~3% of the weight-related maternal dose, but little is known about continuous high-dose treatment. Ibuprofen (q.v.) is a much safer alternative.

Kawasaki disease

Kawasaki disease, first described in 1967, is a systemic vasculitis predominantly affecting children under the age of 5 years (peak incidence at 9–11 months). It has a number of classic clinical features required for diagnosis. Features include high fever for at least 5 days with a variable rash, conjunctivitis, inflamed oral mucosa, swollen neck glands and redness and swelling of the hands and feet with later desquamation. Other common features include abdominal pain, vomiting, diarrhoea, aseptic meningitis, arthritis and mild liver dysfunction.

The exact aetiology has not yet been established, but there is considerable support for it to be due to an infectious agent. Mild cases may go unrecognised, but nearly a third of children with overt disease develop serious inflammation of the coronary arteries, sometimes leading to aneurysm formation, if treatment is not started early. A high platelet count during convalescence further increases the risk of coronary thrombosis and myocardial infarction. However, 90% respond to a single 2 g/kg dose of human immunoglobulin (q.v.) given intravenously over 12 hours, if this is given within a week of the onset of symptoms, and this greatly reduces the risk of secondary complications. Aspirin is given, because of the drug's antithrombotic properties. There is no clear evidence that high doses (80–100 mg/kg/day) are better than low doses. Patients with severe or progressive vasculitis should be referred promptly to a paediatric cardiologist.

Treatment

Kawasaki disease: Give 8 mg/kg (neonatal patients) or 7.5–12.5 mg/g (older children) by mouth four times a day for 2 weeks to control acute symptoms and then 5 mg/kg once daily for 6–8 weeks. If there is no evidence of coronary lesions after 8 weeks, it may be discontinued; if coronary artery lesions persist, then the child should remain on treatment.
Thrombus prophylaxis: A dose of 1–5 mg/kg is used after Fontan and Blalock–Taussig shunt surgery and is also often given for 3 months after certain other forms of cardiac surgery to minimise the risk of clot formation until endothelial lining cells finally cover all post-operative scar tissue.

Monitoring

Oral absorption can be variable during the acute inflammatory phase of Kawasaki disease. Monitoring salicylate levels is not usually required unless the child is receiving high doses.

Supply

To obtain a 5 mg/ml sugar-free solution for oral use, add one 75 mg tablet of dispersible aspirin to 15 ml of water, and use immediately. Tablets cost 3p each.

Continued on p. 89

References

(See also the relevant Cochrane reviews)

Akagi T, Kato H, Inoue O, *et al*. Salicylate treatment in Kawasaki disease: high dose or low dose? *Eur J Pediatr* 1991;**150**:642–6.

Askie LM, Duley L, Henderson-Smart DJ, *et al*. Antiplatelet agents for prevention of pre-eclampsia: a meta-analysis of individual patient data. *Lancet* 2007;**369**:1791–8. [SR] (See also pp. 1791–2 and **370**:1685–6.)

Council on Cardiovascular Disease in the Young, American Heart Association. Diagnosis, treatment and long-term management of Kawasaki disease. *Pediatrics* 2004;**114**:1708–33.

Farquharson RG, Quenby S, Greaves M. Antiphospholipid syndrome in pregnancy: a randomised, controlled trial of treatment. *Obstet Gynecol* 2002;**100**:408–13. [RCT]

Kozer E, Nikfar S, Costei A, *et al*. Aspirin consumption during the first trimester of pregnancy and congenital anomalies: a meta-analysis. *Am J Obstet Gynecol* 2002;**187**:1623–30. [SR]

Li D-K, Liu L, Odouli R. Exposure to non-steroidal anti-inflammatory drugs during pregnancy and risk of miscarriage: population based cohort study. *Br Med J* 2003;**327**:368–71. (See also 2004;**328**:108–9.)

Li JS, Yow E, Berezny KY, *et al*. Clinical outcomes of palliative surgery including a systematic-to-pulmonary artery shunt in infants with cyanotic congenital heart disease. Does aspirin make a difference. *Circulation* 2007;**116**:293–7. (See also pp. 236–7.)

Luca NJ, Yeung RS. Epidemiology and management of Kawasaki disease. *Drugs* 2012;**72**:1029–38.

Roberge S, Giguère Y, Villa P, *et al*. Early administration of low-dose aspirin for the prevention of severe and mild preeclampsia: a systematic review and meta-analysis. *Am J Perinatol* 2012;**29**:551–6. [SR]

Use

Atosiban, a synthetic peptide and a competitive antagonist of oxytocin, is used to arrest preterm labour. It is one of a number of drugs that are used for this purpose; other agents include beta-mimetics (such as ritodrine), magnesium sulphate, prostaglandin inhibitors (e.g. indometacin), calcium channel blockers (e.g. nifedipine and nicardipine) and nitrates (e.g. nitroglycerine).

Pharmacology

Oxytocin and vasopressin (q.v.) are closely related nonapeptides secreted by the posterior part of the pituitary gland. Oxytocin, secreted by the pituitary in a pulsatile manner, is also produced by the ovaries, the placenta, the fetal membranes and the myometrium and has long been recognised to have an important role in the initiation of labour. Binding of oxytocin to receptors on uterine muscle is thought to initiate uterine contractility by increasing the myometrial intracellular calcium. Oxytocin further stimulates uterine contractility and initiates cervical ripening by stimulating the release of prostaglandins in the decidual and fetal membranes. Because of this, attention was turned to synthesising compounds that structurally mimicked oxytocin and which blocked the action of oxytocin on its receptors (having a so-called 'tocolytic' effect).

Atosiban was introduced into use in 1998 and can inhibit labour at least as effectively as any betamimetic. It can sometimes cause nausea and headache but seldom causes the tachycardia or the other unpleasant maternal side effects associated with betamimetics. It has a large volume of distribution (V_D ~18 l/kg) and is cleared in a biphasic manner – the effective half-life being about 18 minutes. Despite its low molecular weight, relatively little seems to cross the placenta, and there is no reason to think that its appearance in breast milk is of any clinical significance. The European manufacturers have only been authorised, as yet, to recommend use when labour looks likely to cause delivery at 24–33 weeks' gestation, but a single intravenous (IV) 6.75 mg dose may be useful in controlling the fetal distress that can be caused by uterine hyperstimulation.

Choice of tocolytic agent

The choice of tocolytic agent is not straightforward; the ideal agent should delay delivery by 48 hours, reduce neonatal mortality and neonatal respiratory distress syndrome and have few maternal side effects. As a group, betamimetics have a high frequency of adverse effects. Two randomised comparisons involving 207 women given either atosiban or nifedipine (q.v.) suggested a marginal advantage for atosiban during the initial 48 hours but that babies born after nifedipine tocolysis may have marginally better outcomes. That nifedipine is cheaper and can be given orally was seen as an advantage for that drug. There are no head-to-head comparisons between atosiban and prostaglandin inhibitors, and the effects of the latter on fetal renal function and closure of the arterial duct are a concern. Unfortunately, while tocolytics have been shown to delay labour, none has been shown to improve perinatal outcome; hence, their use remains contentious and variable.

Sustained drug use to prevent preterm labour

Although a number of drugs are capable of delaying delivery in mothers in early preterm labour for long enough to give betamethasone (q.v.) and, if necessary, arrange hospital transfer, there is no evidence that *sustained* treatment with any of these drugs is capable of delaying delivery for more than a few days.

Treatment

Give an initial 6.75 mg IV dose of atosiban base over 1 minute. Then infuse a solution made up as described below at a rate of 12 ml/hour (18 mg/hour) for 3 hours; thereafter, continue the infusion at a rate of 4 ml/hour (6 mg/hour) for 45 hours. The total duration of treatment should not exceed 2 days.

Supply and administration

0.9 ml vials of atosiban acetate (which contain 6.75 mg of atosiban base) cost £19 and are used to initiate treatment. 5 ml vials containing 37.5 mg of atosiban base cost £53; draw the contents from two such vials into a syringe and dilute to 50 ml with 0.9% sodium chloride or 5% glucose to give a solution containing 1.5 mg/ml, and infuse this as described earlier under 'Treatment'. Store vials at 4 °C and use promptly once opened.

Continued on p. 91

References

(See also the relevant Cochrane reviews and UK guidelines on tocolytic use) **DHUK**

Coomarasamy A, Knox EM, Gee H, *et al.* Effectiveness of nifedipine *versus* atosiban for tocolysis in preterm labour: a meta-analysis with an indirect comparison of randomised trials. *Br J Obstet Gynaecol* 2003;**110**:1045–9. [SR]

Haas DM, Caldwell DM, Kirkpatrick P, *et al.* Tocolytic therapy for preterm delivery: systematic review and network meta-analysis. *Br Med J* 2012;**345**:e6226. [SR]

Haas DM, Imperiale TF, Kirkpatrick PR, *et al.* Tocolytic therapy: a meta-analysis and decision analysis. *Obset Gynecol* 2009;**113**:585–94. [SR]

Husslein P, Roura L, Duden hausen J, *et al.* Clinical practice evaluation of atosiban in preterm labour management in six European countries. TREASURE study group. *Br J Obstet Gynaecol* 2006;**113**(Suppl 3);105–10. [RCT] (See also **114**:1043–4.)

Sanchez-Ramos L, Huddleston JF. The therapeutic value of maintenance tocolysis: an overview of the evidence. *Clin Perinatol* 2003;**30**:841–54.

Shim J-Y, Park YW, Yoon BH, *et al.* Multicentre, parallel-group, randomised, single-blind study of the safety and efficacy of atosiban versus ritodrine in the treatment of acute preterm labour in Korean women. *Br J Obstet Gynaecol* 2006;**113**:1228–34. [RCT]

Tsatsaris V, Carbonne B, Cabrol D. Atosiban for preterm labour. *Drugs* 2004;**64**:375–82.

Valenzuela GJ, Sanchez-Ramos L, Romero R, *et al.* The Atosiban PTL-089 Study Group. Maintenance treatment of preterm labour with the oxytocin antagonist atosiban. *Am J Obstet Gynecol* 2000;**182**:1184–90. [RCT]

Worldwide Atosiban versus Beta-agonists Study Group. Effectiveness and safety of the oxytocin antagonist atosiban versus beta-adrenergic agonists in the treatment of preterm labour. *Br J Obstet Gynaecol* 2001;**108**:133–42. [RCT]

Use

Atracurium besylate is a relatively short-acting alternative to pancuronium (q.v.). In the United Kingdom, suxamethonium (q.v.) is more commonly used when only brief paralysis is necessary.

Pharmacology

Atracurium is a non-depolarising muscle relaxant that competes with acetylcholine at the neuromuscular junction's receptor site; thus, its action can be reversed with anticholinesterases such as neostigmine (q.v.). It is a mixture of 10 stereoisomers and was first developed as an analogue of suxamethonium and patented in 1977. Atracurium was particularly popular in anaesthetic practice because it has no vagolytic or sympatholytic properties and is eliminated by non-enzymatic Hofmann degradation at body temperature independently of liver or kidney function. It is non-cumulative and only effective for about 20 minutes (30 minutes in older children). Weight-for-weight young children do not need as high a dose as adults. Little seems to cross the placenta, and no concerns have been identified as a result of use during pregnancy, delivery or lactation. Atracurium (400 micrograms/kg injected into the umbilical vein or 1 mg/kg injected into the fetal buttock) has been shown to reliably abolish all fetal movement for about half an hour.

The manufacturer has not yet endorsed the use of atracurium in neonates. As a tetrahydroisoquinolinium neuromuscular-blocking agent, atracurium, like most other drugs in this class, is associated with histamine release upon rapid administration of a bolus intravenous (IV) injection. This has caused a number of allergic and anaphylactic reactions in adults and may be responsible for four serious adverse reactions in neonates that were reported in 2000 after staff gave atracurium while preparing babies for tracheal intubation. Three babies became so hypoxic, bradycardic and unventilatable that they died.

Cisatracurium is a more potent single-isomer refinement of atracurium. It takes rather longer (2–3 minutes) to cause muscle paralysis, but it is less likely to trigger histamine release. The usual bolus dose is 150 micrograms/kg IV, but there is only limited experience of use in very young children and even less in neonates.

Treatment

Pre-intubation paralysis: A 300 micrograms/kg IV dose of atracurium causes almost complete paralysis after 2 minutes. A 500 micrograms/kg dose will almost always provide sustained muscle relaxation for 15–35 minutes in babies less than a year old. Always flush the bolus through into the vein.

Continuous infusion: IV infusions of 300–400 micrograms/kg/hour of atracurium can provide sustained neuromuscular blockade in neonates. Older patients may need 500 micrograms/kg/hour. Babies requiring paralysis should always be sedated as well and provided with pain relief where necessary.

Compatibility

A continuous infusion of atracurium can, if necessary, be given (terminally) into a line containing adrenaline, dobutamine, dopamine, fentanyl, heparin, isoprenaline, midazolam, milrinone or morphine.

Antidote

Most of the effects of atracurium can be reversed by giving a combination of 50 micrograms/kg of neostigmine and either 10 micrograms/kg of glycopyrronium or 20 micrograms/kg of atropine, although reversal is seldom called for given atracurium's short half-life.

Supply and administration

Atracurium: 2.5 ml ampoules containing 25 mg (10 mg/ml) cost £1.70; larger ampoules are also available. Multi-dose vials are available in North America but are best avoided in young children because they contain benzyl alcohol. Store at 2–8 °C. To give a bolus injection of atracurium, take 0.5 ml from a 10 mg/ml ampoule and dilute to 5 ml with 5% glucose or glucose saline to obtain a preparation containing 1 mg/ml (1000 micrograms/ml) for accurate administration. To give a continuous infusion of 500 micrograms/kg/ hour, draw 2.5 ml of atracurium besylate for each kilogram the baby weighs from the ampoule into a syringe, dilute to 50 ml with 0.9% sodium chloride or 10% glucose in 0.18% sodium chloride, and infuse at 1 ml/hour. A less concentrated solution of glucose or glucose saline can be used. Make up a fresh solution daily.

Continued on p. 93

Cisatracurium: 10 ml ampoules containing 20 mg of cisatracurium cost £7.50. Both the single dose and the multi-dose ampoules available in North America contain benzyl alcohol. Store at 2–8 °C.

References

Bryson HM, Faulds D. Cisatracurium besilate: a review of its pharmacology and clinical potential in anaesthetic practice. *Drugs* 1997;**53**:848–68.

Clarkson A, Choonara I, Martin P. Suspected toxicity of atracurium in the neonate. *Paediatr Anaesth* 2001;**11**:631–2.

Flynn PJ, Frank M, Hughes R. Use of atracurium in caesarean section. *Br J Anaesth* 1984;**56**:599–604.

Martin LD, Bratton SL, O'Rourke PP. Clinical uses and controversies of neuromuscular blocking agents in infants and children. *Crit Care Med* 1999;**27**:1358–68.

Piotrowski A. Comparison of atracurium and pancuronium in mechanically ventilated neonates. *Intensive Care Med* 1993;**19**:401–5.

ShangGuan W, Lian Q, Li J, *et al.* Clinical pharmacology of cisatracurium during nitrous oxide-propofol anesthesia in children. *J Clin Anesth* 2008;**20**:411–4.

Sparr HJ, Beuafort TM, Fuchs-Buder T. Newer neuromuscular blocking agents. How do they compare with established agents? *Drugs* 2001;**61**:919–42.

Use

Atropine was once widely used as a premedication prior to surgery but is used less often these days. It is still used during and after surgery to the eye. Atropine features in several drug combinations used to premedicate infants undergoing elective intubation. It is sometimes used to treat intra-operative bradycardia.

Pharmacology

The medicinal properties of the Solanaceae group of plants have been known for many centuries, and pure atropine was first isolated from deadly nightshade root in 1833. Venetians called this plant 'herba bella donna' because ladies used water distilled from the plant as a cosmetic to beautify the eye (by dilating the pupil). Linnaeus later gave the plant its Latin botanical name *Atropa belladonna* in recognition of its toxicity and use as a poison (Atropos being the name of one of the Greek fates who could 'cut the slender thread of life').

Atropine blocks the muscarinic effects of acetylcholine on the postganglionic autonomic nerve fibres and produces a vagal block that can abolish the sudden bradycardia caused by operative vagal stimulation. The half-life in adults is 4 hours but is longer in infants. While use prior to anaesthesia reduces oropharyngeal secretions, it also reduces lower oesophageal sphincter tone and does nothing, directly, to reduce the risk of laryngospasm. Bronchial secretions become more viscid and less copious; gastrointestinal secretions and motility are reduced.

Atropine is moderately well absorbed by the small intestine ($V_D \sim 3\,l/kg$). It crosses the placenta with ease and can affect the fetal heart rate. Small amounts are thought to appear in breast milk, but no neonatal symptoms have ever been reported. It has a role in heart block due to digoxin poisoning and in patients with serious reflex (vagal) bradycardia. Atropine eye drops are used to achieve sustained dilatation of the pupil after ocular surgery (as described in the monograph on eye drops), but excess usage can lead to ileus and other problems, especially when the standard 1% drops are used.

Atropine use to make surgery unnecessary in babies with pyloric stenosis merits evaluation through properly conducted randomised trials; case series suggest atropine has a success rate of less than 75% (surgery has at least a 95% success rate), longer hospital stays than when surgery is used and the potential for children who fail to respond to be sicker when surgery is eventually undertaken.

Treatment with atropine

Oral premedication: Some doubt the need to use *any* drug prior to the induction of anaesthesia in most neonates as long as there is intravenous (IV) access. If a 'premed' is judged appropriate, an intramuscular (IM) injection can be avoided by giving 20–40 micrograms/kg of atropine by mouth 2 hours before induction as long as gut motility is normal.
Parenteral premedication: A 10 micrograms/kg IV bolus produces an effect within 30 seconds and lasts at least 6 hours. A subcutaneous or IM dose will be maximally effective after 30–60 minutes.
Premedication for intubation: A 20 micrograms/kg bolus of atropine is given before the sedation/analgesia and paralytic drugs used for non-emergency intubation.
Pyloric stenosis: A 10 micrograms/kg dose IV every 4 hours before feeds can often check the contractile spasm of the pyloric muscle. Treatment should be continued for 3 weeks but can be undertaken at home after a few days, once vomiting has stopped, using twice this dose by mouth every 4 hours.
Reversing neuromuscular blockade: Give 20 micrograms/kg of atropine IV followed by a 40 microgram/kg dose of IV neostigmine.
Digoxin toxicity: Give 25 micrograms/kg IV for AV block. Ten times as much is occasionally given.

Toxicity

Check the dose of atropine carefully – even a moderate overdose will cause tachycardia, flushing and dilatation of the pupils. A severe overdose will cause respiratory depression, convulsions and coma requiring sedation, ventilatory support for respiratory depression and steps to control hyperpyrexia. Neostigmine (q.v.) will counteract some of the effects of a severe overdose.

Continued on p. 95

Supply and administration

1 ml ampoules containing 600 micrograms cost 60p each. Dilute 0.1 ml of the ampoule with 0.9 ml of 0.9% saline in a 1 ml syringe to obtain a solution containing 60 micrograms/ml. Prefilled disposable 5 ml syringes of atropine are also available in different strengths: 100 micrograms/ml (cost £4.60), 200 micrograms/ml (cost £6.80), 300 micrograms/ml (cost £6.50) and 600 micrograms/ml (cost £6.80).

References

Bonthala S, Sparks JW, Musgrove KH, *et al*. Mydriatics slow gastric emptying in preterm infants. *J Pediatr* 2000;**127**:327–30.

Carbajal R, Eble B, Anand KJ. Premedication for tracheal intubation in neonates: confusion or controversy? *Semin Perinatol* 2007;**31**:309–17.

Kawahara H, Imura K, Yagi M, *et al*. Motor abnormality in the gastroduodenal junction in patients with infantile hypertrophic pyloric stenosis. *J Pediatr Surg* 2001;**36**:1641–5.

Mercer AE, Phillips R. Can a conservative approach to the treatment of hypertrophic pyloric stenosis with atropine be considered a real alternative to surgical pyloromyotomy? *Arch Dis Child* 2013;**98**:474–7.

Shorten GD, Bissonnette B, Hartley E, *et al*. It is not necessary to administer more than 10 µg·kg^{-1} of atropine to older children before succinylcholine. *Can J Anaesth* 1995;**42**:8–11. (see also pp. 1–7.)

Use

Azithromycin is a macrolide antibiotic related to erythromycin and clarithromycin (q.v.) that is increasingly used to treat neonatal *Chlamydia, Mycoplasma* and *Ureaplasma* infections and to reduce whooping cough cross infection. A single dose can also speed up recovery in children with severe cholera (*Vibrio cholerae* infection).

Pharmacology

Azithromycin is an azalide developed in 1988 by structurally modifying the erythromycin molecule. It works by interfering with bacterial protein synthesis. Although it is slightly less potent against Gram-positive organisms, it demonstrates superior *in vitro* activity against a wide variety of Gram-negative bacilli, including *Haemophilus influenzae*. A single dose is a more effective way of treating childhood cholera than a 3-day course of erythromycin and probably as effective as a single dose of ciprofloxacin (c.v.). Azithromycin is moderately well absorbed when taken by mouth (40% bioavailability) and better tolerated than erythromycin because it triggers fewer gastrointestinal side effects. It has a very low peak serum level and a very high volume of distribution ($V_D \sim 23$ l/kg) consistent with data showing extensive tissue distribution and intracellular accumulation. This makes it particularly effective against intracellular microorganisms such a *Chlamydia* and *Legionella*. CSF levels are low but there is substantial penetration into brain tissue. Much of the drug undergoes biliary excretion (terminal half-life ~ 5 days), and the rest is inactivated in the liver – properties that make once a day treatment more than adequate, but can also make it important to give a first loading dose. The interactions with other drugs sometimes seen with erythromycin do not seem to occur with azithromycin. The manufacturers have not yet recommended use in children less than 6 months old, and unconfirmed epidemiological evidence suggests an increased risk of hypertrophic pyloric stenosis in exposed infants.

Like other macrolides, azithromycin has been used to treat *Ureaplasma urealyticum* infection in the hope that it would reduce bronchopulmonary dysplasia in preterm infants, unfortunately although the organism responds very well – and the drug is safe and well tolerated – there appears to be limited effect on the lung disease.

There is little published information relating to use in pregnancy, but the macrolide antibiotics are not, as a class, considered teratogenic. Less than 3% of maternally administered azithromycin crosses the placenta, and no adverse effects have been reported in the human fetus. A breast-fed baby only ingests ~5% of the weight-adjusted maternal dose.

Maternal treatment

A single 1 g dose by mouth eliminates maternal genital infection due to *Chlamydia trachomatis*. A 2 g dose has been used as an alternative to intramuscular benzathine or procaine benzylpenicillin in adults with early syphilis, but the efficacy of such an approach has not yet been assessed in women who are pregnant.

Prophylaxis

Trachoma: Endemic disease can be much reduced in the whole community by giving all children under 11 years a single 20 mg/kg dose, once every 3 months.

Pertussis prophylaxis: In neonates and young infants, give 10 mg/kg orally once a day for 3 days.

Treatment in infancy

Bacterial infection: Give a single 10 mg/kg dose once a day. Authorities in the United Kingdom suggest that treatment should not be continued for more than 3 days, but those in North America favour a 5-day course. There is almost no information on use in the first month of life. There is limited experience of parenteral azithromycin in infants and most will tolerate oral medication.

Conjunctivitis: A single oral 20 mg/kg dose is an effective treatment for chlamydial conjunctivitis, including chronic follicular trachoma. Giving 1.5% eye drops twice a day for 3 days is also very effective.

Supply and administration

Small 600 mg packs of powder costing £4 are normally reconstituted with 9 ml of water to give 15 ml of a fruit-flavoured sucrose-sweetened oral suspension containing 40 mg/ml of azithromycin which is stable for 5 days after reconstitution. Further dilution in order to give a very low dose accurately should only be done just before use. Vials containing 500 mg of azithromycin

Continued on p. 97

powder for infusion costing £9.50 are available from Aspire Pharma Ltd. Add 4.8 ml of water for injection to the 500 mg vial and shake to ensure the powder is dissolved. Make up the infusion to a volume of 250 ml by adding to 0.9% sodium chloride or 5% glucose/0.45% sodium chloride to give a solution containing 2 mg/ml. Infuse 5 ml of this for every kilogram the infant weighs over at least 60 minutes. Single use azithromycin dihydrate 1.5% eye drops (costing £1.20) are available.

References

(See also the relevant Cochrane reviews)

Atik B, Thanh T, Luong VQ, *et al*. Impact of annual targeted treatment of infectious trachoma and suscepti-bility to infection. *JAMA* 2006;**296**:1488–97. [RCT]

Cochereau I, Meddeb-Ouertanu A, Khairallah M, *et al*. 2-day treatment with azithromycin 1.5% eye drops versus 7-day treatment with tobramycin 0.3% for purulent bacterial conjunctivitis: multicentre, randomised and controlled trial in adults and children. *Br J Ophthalmol* 2007;**91**:465–9. [RCT]

Gebre T, Ayele B, Zerihun M, *et al*. Comparison of annual versus twice-yearly mass azithromycin treatment for hyperendemic trachoma in Ethiopia: a cluster-randomised trial. *Lancet* 2012;**379**:143–51.

Hassan HE, Othman AA, Eddington ND, *et al*. Pharmacokinetics, safety, and biologic effects of azithromycin in extremely preterm infants at risk for ureaplasma colonization and bronchopulmonary dysplasia. *J Clin Pharmacol* 2011;**51**:1264–75.

House JI, Ayele B, Porco TC, *et al*. Assessment of herd protection against trachoma due to repeated mass antibiotic distributions: a cluster-randomised trial. *Lancet* 2009;**373**:1111–8. [RCT] (See also **373**:1061–3, and **374**:449; author reply 449–50.)

Khan WA, Saha A, Rahman A, *et al*. Comparison of single-dose azithromycin and 12-dose 3-day erythro-mycin for childhood cholera: a randomised, double-blind trial. *Lancet* 2002;**360**:1722–7. [RCT]

Morrison W. Infantile hypertrophic pyloric stenosis in infants treated with azithromycin. *Pediatr Infect Dis J* 2007;**26**:186–8.

Rieder G, Rusizoka M, Todd J, *et al*. Single-dose azithromycin versus penicillin G benzathine for the treatment of early syphilis. *N Engl J Med* 2005;**353**:1236–44. [RCT] (See also pp. 1291–3.)

Sorensen HT, Skriver MV, Pedersen L, *et al*. Risk of infantile hypertrophic pyloric stenosis after maternal post-natal use of macrolides. *Scand J Infect Dis* 2003;**35**:104–6.

Srinivasan R, Yeo TH. Are newer macrolides effective in eradicating pertussis? *Arch Dis Child* 2005;**90**:322–4. [SR]

Viscardi RM, Othman AA, Hassan HE, *et al*. Azithromycin to prevent bronchopulmonary dysplasia in urea-plasma-infected preterm infants: pharmacokinetics, safety, microbial response, and clinical outcomes with a 20-milligram-per-kilogram single intravenous dose. *Antimicrob Agents Chemother* 2013;**57**:2127–33.

West SK, Muroz B, Mkocha H, *et al*. Infection with Chlamydia trachomatis after mass treatment of a trachoma hyperendemic community in Tanzania: a longitudinal study. *Lancet* 2005;**366**:1296–300.

Woodrow CJ, Planche T, Krishna S. Artesunate versus quinine for severe falciparum malaria. *Lancet* 2006;**367**:110–1; author reply 111–2.

Wright HR, Turner A, Taylor HR. Trachoma. *Lancet* 2008;**371**:1945–54. [SR]

Zar HJ. Neonatal chlamydial infections. Prevention and treatment. *Paediatr Drugs* 2005;**7**:103–10.

Use

Bacillus Calmette–Guérin (BCG) vaccine is used to reduce the risk of tuberculosis (TB) in children without evidence of cell-mediated immunity to *Mycobacterium tuberculosis* or *M. bovis*. TB is a notifiable illness.

Product

BCG vaccine contains a live-attenuated strain of *M. bovis*. It was developed after 13 years of research involving 200 serial subcultures and was first used in France in 1921. Since then, it has been widely used in the international control of TB. TB remains a severe illness, especially in infants, and there is clear evidence that correctly administered neonatal BCG vaccination greatly reduces the risk of serious infection in early childhood without obscuring the diagnosis of active infection by intradermal testing. Immunity probably wanes after 10–15 years, but revaccination is not considered appropriate. The protection conferred is not absolute, but a review of prospective studies shows a mean protective efficacy of 75% against serious early infection.

BCG vaccination forms part of the WHO's global immunisation programme, but it is not routinely offered in countries where the community prevalence is low. Recent studies have also suggested that use in resource-poor countries may improve all-cause infant mortality in some non-specific (as yet unexplained) way.

Indications

Babies being cared for in a family or household where there is a patient with active respiratory TB under treatment should be given prophylactic isoniazid (q.v.) for 6 months from birth and then vaccinated at 6 months if the Mantoux test remains negative.

Current policy in the United Kingdom is that BCG should also be offered to all children born in (or likely to spend a considerable time in) an area where prevalence currently exceeds 40/100,000 and to any child whose parents or grandparents were born in a country where prevalence is that high. Information about a country's prevalence can be obtained at www.who.int/tb/country/data/profiles/en/index.html.

Prior tuberculin testing is *not* necessary before giving BCG to children less than 6 years old. Tuberculin-negative children of any age should be offered BCG if there is a clear history of contact exposure or a case in the family in the last 6 years, and vaccination should also be offered, as opportunity permits, to those who were born in, or lived for several months in, a country where the prevalence of TB is high. Vaccination is probably best delayed in the very preterm baby until shortly before discharge, because this may improve conversion. However, postponing it longer than this runs the risk that vaccination will never get offered until the period of greatest vulnerability is past.

Drug interactions

BCG can be given at the same time (but not into the same arm) as another vaccine. Leave a 4-week interval after giving any live vaccine before giving BCG. Do not give any other vaccine into the arm into which BCG was given for 3 months to minimise the risk of lymphadenitis.

Contraindications

BCG vaccine should not be given to anyone who is immunodeficient, immunosuppressed or on high dose corticosteroid treatment (any dose equivalent to more than 1 mg/kg of prednisolone per day, as summarised in the monograph on hydrocortisone). In countries where the prevalence of TB is low, BCG (unlike other live vaccines) should not be given to babies who are HIV positive or to babies born to mothers who are HIV positive (in the latter group, BCG can be given if required after two 'negative' PCR results are available). In high prevalence countries, the balance of risk is very different. Avoid administration in any area of skin actively affected by eczema.

Administration

Infants should receive 0.05 ml intradermally; older children should receive 0.1 ml.

Strict attention **must** be paid to the technique used if 'conversion' is to be achieved and complications are to be avoided. Injections are normally given into the left upper arm over the point where the deltoid muscle is attached to the humerus to minimise the risk of scarring. This point is only a little above the middle of the upper arm: vaccination is often inappropriately administered higher than this (over the bulk of the deltoid muscle). The skin only needs to be cleaned first if it is overtly dirty. If spirit is used, it must be allowed to dry. Soap and water is better.

Continued on p. 99

Do not use an antiseptic. Use a 1 ml syringe and a 10 mm long 26 gauge short-bevel needle (with the bevel facing upwards). A separate syringe and needle must be used for each child to avoid transmitting infection. Stretch the skin between the thumb and finger and insert the needle parallel with the surface about 3 mm into the superficial layers of the dermis. The tip should remain visible through the skin, and a raised blanched 3 mm bleb will appear if the injection has been given correctly. If no resistance is encountered, the tip is almost certainly too deep and needs to be repositioned. Give the injection slowly and leave the injection site uncovered to facilitate healing. Successful administration will usually, but not invariably, cause a papule to appear at the injection site after 2–4 weeks which may ulcerate before healing to leave a small flat scar after 1–3 months. Babies should become tuberculin positive within 6 weeks if vaccination was effective (routine testing to confirm this is not generally thought necessary).

Adverse reactions
Early reactivity: A very early response to BCG administration that progresses to pustule formation within 3–5 days (Koch phenomenon) strongly suggests that the subject has active TB.
Other problems: If the slow local reaction generally expected eventually turns into a discharging ulcer, this should be covered with a simple dry non-occlusive dressing (occlusive dressings can delay healing). The lesion will still heal over 1–2 months and should still only leave a small scar if the injection technique has been sound. Lymphadenitis may occur. More serious local reactions should be referred to the doctor responsible for the local TB contact clinic. If disseminated infection does occur, anti-tubercular treatment may need to be given (the Danish strain of BCG [1331] being sensitive *in vitro* to isoniazid and rifampicin). For the management of anaphylaxis (an extremely rare occurrence), see the monograph on immunisation (q.v.).

Documentation
The identification of high-risk babies remains poorly organised in many UK maternity units at present. Parents need to be approached in the antenatal period so that babies likely to benefit can be identified before birth and an agreement reached regarding the need for early vaccination. Early post-delivery discharge and the fragmentation of postnatal care have further damaged the systems that used to exist for delivering and documenting such prophylaxis reliably in many Health Districts. Vaccination *must* be documented in the child's personal health record (red book) and in the computerised community child health record – failure to do this can render later interpretation of the child's tuberculin status very difficult. Make a note of the batch number and the expiry date, as well as the date of administration.

Mantoux testing
Tuberculin (tuberculin PPD) is a purified protein made from sterile heat-treated products of the growth and lysis of *M. tuberculosis* that produces induration of the skin after intradermal injection. The peak extent of any induration induced (ignoring any associated erythema or redness) is documented to the nearest millimetre.
Testing for active tuberculosis: Inject 0.1 ml of tuberculin PPD containing 20 units/ml intradermally into the middle third of the flexor surface of the previously cleaned forearm producing a 'bleb' about 7 mm in diameter (using the same technique as described earlier for giving BCG). Induration on review 48–72 hours later that extends more than 5 mm indicates a positive response, and induration extending 15 mm or more at this time is a strong reaction probably indicative of active infection. Interpretation is unreliable after 96 hours.
Tests for cellular immunity: A more concentrated (100 unit/ml) preparation of PPD can be used, in the same way, to document the existence of cellular immunity if the response to the low-dose test is negative.

Supply
BCG: 1 ml vials of lyophilised material (containing enough vaccine for 7–8 children) are manufactured by the Danish Statens Serum Institut (SSI). Supplies are distributed within the United Kingdom by Farillon for the Department of Health. Vials should be stored at 2–8°C, protected from light and used within 18 months. Do not allow the vaccine or associated diluent (in vials labelled 'Diluted Sauton SSI') to freeze. Reconstitute the vials using this diluent. Do **not** use water for injection. Draw up 1 ml of the diluent using a long needle and transfer this to the BCG vial without attempting to clean the rubber stopper with any antiseptic, detergent or alcohol-impregnated swab. Invert the vial a few times but do not shake it. Swirl the vial round

Continued on p. 100

gently to resuspend the material before drawing up each dose. Discard any material not used within 4 hours.

Tuberculin: 1.5 ml vials of tuberculin PPD (in 20 units/ml and 100 units/ml vials) are available from SSI in Denmark. Store at 2–8°C, and protect from light. Do not freeze. A Patient Group Direction cannot currently be used to authorise use because the product's European marketing authorisation does not cover the United Kingdom.

References

(see also the full UK website guidelines **DHUK**)

Aaby P, Roth A, Ravn H, *et al*. Randomized trial of BCG vaccination at birth to low-birth-weight children: beneficial nonspecific effects in the neonatal period? *J Infect Dis* 2011;**204**:245–52.

Abubakar I, Laundry MT, French CE, *et al*. Epidemiology and treatment outcome of childhood tuberculosis in England and Wales 1999–2006. *Arch Dis Child* 2008;**93**:1017–21.

Bergamini BM, Losi M, Valenti F, *et al*. Performance of commercial blood tests for the diagnosis of latent tuberculosis infection in children and adolescents. *Pediatrics* 2009;**123**:e419–24.

Bothamley GH, Cooper E, Shingadia D, *et al*. Tuberculin testing before BCG vaccination. *Br Med J* 2003;**327**:243–4. (See also p. 932.)

Hawkridge A, Hatherill M, Little F, *et al*. Efficacy of percutaneous versus intradermal BCG in the prevention of tuberculosis in South African infants: randomised trial. *Br Med J* 2008;**337**:a2052. [RCT] (See also p. a2086.)

National Institute for Health and Clinical Excellence. *NICE Guideline CG117: Tuberculosis. Clinical management and diagnosis of tuberculosis, and measures for its prevention and control*, 2011.

Pollock L, Basu Roy R, Kampmann B. How to use: interferon γ release assays for tuberculosis. *Arch Dis Child Educ Pract Ed* 2013;**98**:99–105.

Roth A, Jensen H, Garly M-L, *et al*. Low birth weight infants and Calmette-Guérin bacillus vaccination at birth. *Pediatr Infect Dis J* 2004;**23**:544–50.

Soysal A, Millington KA, Bakir M, *et al*. Effect of BCG vaccination on risk of *Mycobacterium tuberculosis* infection in children with household tuberculosis contact: a prospective community-based study. *Lancet* 2005;**366**:1443–51.

Thayyil-Sudhan S, Kumar A, Singh M, *et al*. Safety and effectiveness of BCG vaccination in preterm babies. *Arch Dis Child Fetal Neonatal Ed* 1999;**81**:F64–6.

Trunz BB, Fine PEM, Dye C. Effect of BCG vaccination on childhood tuberculosis and miliary tuberculosis worldwide: a meta-analysis and assessment of cost-effectiveness. *Lancet* 2006;**367**:1173–80. [SR] (See also pp. 1122–4.)

Use
Betaine is used in the management of a number of metabolic diseases associated with homocystinuria.

Biochemistry
Homocysteine is an intermediate in the breakdown of the amino acid methionine. Homocysteine has toxic effects on the brain (causing developmental delay, seizures and psychiatric disease) and predisposes to lens dislocation, thromboembolism, osteoporosis and marfanoid habitus. Betaine (N,N,N-trimethylglycine) is a small N-trimethylated amino acid that acts as a methyl group donor, allowing hepatic methyltransferases to convert homocysteine to the less toxic methionine.

Causes of homocystinuria
Homocystinuria is a heterogeneous group of disorders.
Classical homocystinuria: This autosomal recessive disorder results from cystathionine β-synthase deficiency. A few patients are detected by neonatal screening programmes, but most patients present with developmental delay, dislocated lenses, skeletal abnormalities or thromboembolic disease. Betaine is used in patients who do not respond to pyridoxine (q.v.) and who either cannot comply with or are inadequately controlled by a low-methionine and low-protein diet. Betaine lowers plasma and urine homocysteine concentrations and usually improves symptoms such as behaviour and seizures. Women with homocystinuria should continue with treatment during pregnancy to minimise the risk of thromboembolic disease and, possibly, the risk of fetal loss.
Other causes: Homocystinuria can also be caused by deficiency of methylenetetrahydrofolate reductase (MTHFR) or disorders of cobalamin metabolism (which may be accompanied by methylmalonic aciduria or megaloblastic anaemia). Patients with these rare disorders can present in many different ways, including acute neonatal encephalopathy and developmental delay. Betaine is the best available treatment for MTHFR deficiency; such patients should also be given 5 mg/day of folic acid. Betaine is also used in defects of cobalamin metabolism if homocystinuria persists despite pharmacological doses of vitamin B_{12} (q.v.).

Treatment
Start by giving 50 mg/kg by mouth twice a day. The dose is then adjusted by monitoring the plasma homocysteine level, but doses in excess of 150 mg/kg/day seldom confer additional benefit.

Monitoring
Plasma methionine concentrations rise during treatment in classical homocystinuria, and monitoring is recommended to ensure that potentially toxic levels (>1000 μmol/l) do not develop. Clinicians need to be aware that acute cerebral oedema has (very rarely) been reported a few weeks after starting treatment.

Supply
A palatable strawberry-flavoured medicine is now available as a 'special' from Special Products Ltd; 100 ml costs £40. Reconstitute the dry powder with 55 ml of purified water to obtain a liquid containing 50 mg/ml, and use within 28 days.

A pharmaceutical product (Cystadane® powder) is available from Orphan Europe. It comes with three spoons allowing measurement of 1 g, 150 mg or 100 mg of powder. The required amount of powder is mixed with water, juice or milk (including formula milk) until completely dissolved and taken immediately. The cost of 100 g from this supplier is £347.

References
(See also the Cochrane review of newborn screening for homocystinuria)

Devlin AM, Hajipour L, Gholkar A, *et al.* Cerebral edema associated with betaine treatment in classical homocystinuria. *J Pediatr* 2004;**144**:545–8.
Mudd SH, Levy HL, Kraus JP. Disorders of transsulfuration. In: Scriver CR, Beaudet AL, Sly WS, *et al.*, eds. *The metabolic and molecular bases of inherited disease*, 8th ed. New York: McGraw-Hill, 2001: pp. 2007–56.
Mudd SH, Skovby F, Levy HL, *et al.* The natural history of homocystinuria due to cystathionine beta-synthase deficiency. *Am J Hum Genet* 1985;**37**:1–31.

Continued on p. 102

Ogier de Baulny H, Gérard M, Saudubray J-M, *et al.* Remethylation defects: guidelines for clinical diagnosis and treatment. *Eur J Pediatr* 1998;**157**(Suppl 2):S77–83.

Ronge E, Kjellman B. Long term treatment with betaine in methylenetetrahydrofolate reductase deficiency. *Arch Dis Child* 1996;**74**:239–41.

Rosenblatt DS, Fenton WA. Inherited disorders of folate and cobalamin transport and metabolism. In: Scriver CR, Beaudet AL, Sly WS, *et al.*, eds. *The metabolic and molecular bases of inherited disease*, 8th ed. New York: McGraw-Hill, 2001: pp. 3897–934.

Schiff M, Blom HJ. Treatment of inherited homocystinurias. *Neuropediatrics* 2012;**43**:295–304.

Watkins D, Rosenblatt DS, Fowler B. Disorders of cobalamin and folate transport and metabolism. In: Saudubray J-M, van den Berghe G, Walter JH, *et al.*, eds. *Inborn metabolic diseases. Diagnosis and treatment*, 5th ed. Berlin: Springer-Verlag, 2012: pp. 385–404.

Wilken DEL, Wilken B, Dudman NPB, *et al.* Homocystinuria – the effects of betaine in the treatment of patients not responsive to pyridoxine. *N Engl J Med* 1983;**309**:448–53.

Use

Maternal treatment with betamethasone accelerates surfactant production by the fetal lung, reducing the incidence of neonatal respiratory distress syndrome, a property it shares with dexamethasone (q.v.).

Pharmacology

The pharmacology of betamethasone and dexamethasone is very similar. See the website commentary for a discussion of the relative merits of betamethasone and dexamethasone.

Indications for antenatal use

The seminal paper that first identified a strategy for preventing, rather than curing, surfactant deficiency was published >40 years ago. The first clue came from the observation that experimental lambs delivered prematurely failed to develop the respiratory problems seen in control animals if exposed to corticosteroids before delivery. A randomised placebo-controlled trial that eventually recruited more than a thousand mothers from New Zealand soon confirmed that two 12 mg intramuscular (IM) doses of betamethasone caused a significant reduction in the incidence of respiratory distress in babies born >8 weeks early and a fall in neonatal mortality in all babies born >3 weeks early. Doubling this dose brought about no further improvement in outcome. No study has ever looked to see if a smaller dose might be equally effective.

It took 20 years for this strategy to gain general acceptance and, in the interim, a further 11 trials were mounted to replicate the original findings. The most recent Cochrane review of all the 21 trials ever done shows that antenatal treatment with 24 mg of betamethasone *or* dexamethasone is associated with a 40–60% reduction in the risk of neonatal respiratory distress and with a similar reduction in cerebroventricular haemorrhage, in necrotising enterocolitis and in early systemic infection and that this, in turn, results in fewer deaths and in a reduction in the cost and duration of neonatal care. Benefit 'appears to apply to babies born at *all* gestational ages at which respiratory distress syndrome may occur', and one recent trial showed that it also reduced problems for babies electively delivered at 37–38 weeks' gestation. Babies delivered <24 hours after prophylaxis is started derive only limited benefit, and it is now clear that benefit wanes after a week. Twins seem to benefit just as much as singleton babies, but because they were not separately identified in many trials, the available sample size is currently too small to establish this. Giving one more dose once a week to women not delivered within 7 days further reduced the number of babies troubled by respiratory problems after birth in the Australasian trial (ACTORDS), and there were no detectable adverse effects in the 2-year survivors. Only long-term follow-up will show if there are any late consequences. Giving more than this delivers no additional benefit and may further retard fetal growth, while fortnightly repetition (as in the MACS trial) delivered no benefit. Delaying further prophylaxis until delivery again seems imminent can also work well (as long as delivery can then be delayed for at least 36 hours) as the Obstetrix trial showed in March 2009.

No adverse late consequence of exposure to a single course of betamethasone could be detected when the children of the mothers recruited into the first trial in New Zealand were recontacted after 30 years. Women with hypertension and fetal growth retardation were excluded from many early trials, but we now know that these babies benefit too. Use (under prophylactic antibiotic cover) was also beneficial where there has been pre-labour rupture of membranes, but use in mothers with diabetes remains less well established, since treatment could affect diabetic control. Repetitive antenatal treatment slows fetal growth, but the effect was too small to be detectable at discharge in most trials and non-existent in the most recent trial.

Maternal prophylaxis

First course of treatment: Give 12 mg of betamethasone *base* as a deep IM injection and a second dose after 24 hours while trying to delay delivery for 48 hours. Oral treatment cannot be recommended on the basis of the only small trials conducted to date. While prophylaxis is of no proven benefit when delivery threatens before 24 weeks' gestation, it should not be denied to those at risk of delivery at 23 weeks if requested.

Repeat treatment: If delivery does not occur for 7 days and then again becomes likely in the next 7 days, consider giving another 12 mg dose and try to delay delivery for 24 hours, since respiratory problems and their complications can be serious after delivery before 30 weeks' gestation (and a reducible risk before 33 weeks).

Continued on p. 104

Supply

Celestone®, a product that contains both betamethasone sodium phosphate and the longer-acting ester betamethasone acetate, was used in all the more important perinatal trials, but this product is still not on sale in the United Kingdom. The only formulation routinely available in the United Kingdom is a 1 ml ampoule containing 5.3 mg of betamethasone sodium phosphate (4 mg of betamethasone base) costing £1.20, and the ampoules provided by some manufacturers contain sodium metabisulphite. 500 micrograms (5p) tablets are also available.

References

(See also the relevant Cochrane reviews and UK guideline)

Crowther CA, Doyle LW, Haslam RR, *et al.* Outcomes a 2 years of age after repeat doses of antenatal corticosteroids. *N Engl J Med* 2007;**357**:1179–89. [RCT] (See also pp. 1191–8, and editorial pp. 1248–50.)

Garite TJ, Kurtzman J, Maurel K, *et al.* Impact of a 'rescue course' of antenatal corticosteroids: a multicenter randomized placebo-controlled trial. *Am J Obstet Gynecol* 2009;**200**:248.e1–9. [RCT] (See also pp. 217–8.)

Joseph KS, Netta F, Scott H, *et al.* Prenatal corticosteroid prophylaxis for women delivering at late preterm gestation. *Pediatrics* 2009;**124**:e835–43.

Murphy KE, Hannah ME, Willan AR, *et al.* Multiple courses of antenatal corticosteroids for preterm birth (MACS): a randomised controlled trial. *Lancet* 2008;**372**:2143–51. [RCT] (See also pp. 2094–5.)

Wapner R, Jobe AH. Controversy: antenatal steroids. *Clin Perinatol* 2011;**38**:529–45.

Use
Two rare, recessively inherited, metabolic diseases respond to biotin treatment.

Biochemistry
Biotin is one of the water-soluble group B vitamins. It is found in a wide range of foods including eggs, liver, kidneys and some vegetables. Nutritional deficiency is extremely rare. Biotin is a cofactor for four carboxylases: propionyl-CoA carboxylase, pyruvate carboxylase, 3-methylcrotonyl-CoA carboxylase and acetyl-CoA carboxylase. Holocarboxylase synthetase catalyses the covalent attachment of biotin to these proteins. When carboxylases are degraded, biotin is liberated by the action of biotinidase and recycled.

Pathology
Deficiency of either holocarboxylase synthetase or biotinidase leads to 'multiple carboxylase deficiency'. Holocarboxylase synthetase deficiency is caused by mutations in the HLCS gene (21q22.1), and biotinidase deficiency is caused by one of >150 identified mutations in the BTD gene (3p25). Both conditions are inherited as autosomal recessive traits.

Holocarboxylase synthetase deficiency: These children present as neonates or infants with feeding problems, encephalopathy, metabolic acidosis and urinary organic acids compatible with the four carboxylase deficiencies. Lymphocytes and fibroblasts can be used to confirm the enzyme deficiency. Mothers of patients are sometimes given 10 mg of biotin a day during any subsequent pregnancy, although it is not clear whether such prenatal treatment is actually necessary.

Biotinidase deficiency: Children with this rare condition present in the first 2 years of life, usually with seizures or developmental delay. Rashes and alopecia are common. Biotinidase can be measured in blood.

In both conditions, there is a good response to pharmacological doses of biotin, but if treatment is delayed, irreversible brain damage will often have occurred. Although screening at birth has not yet been initiated in the United Kingdom (as it has in some countries), it does have the potential to prevent most of these problems. Screening also brings to light cases of *partial* biotinidase deficiency. It is not yet clear whether these children benefit from routine supplementation, but supplementation seems harmless enough in itself. There have been no convincing reports of benefit from biotin in patients with an isolated carboxylase deficiency.

Treatment
Patients with either holocarboxylase synthetase or biotinidase deficiency usually respond to 5–10 mg of biotin a day (irrespective of weight or age), but doses of up to 100 mg a day may be needed in a few patients. Treatment can usually be given by mouth, but a parenteral preparation is available.

Supply
The need for high-dose biotin treatment is so uncommon that there is no regular pharmaceutical preparation on the market. It is possible for hospital pharmacies to get 5 mg tablets in packs of 30 (cost £19) and ampoules containing 5 mg/ml (cost £6.70) intended for intramuscular use through John Bell and Croyden, 54 Wigmore Street, London W1H 0AU (telephone 020 7935 5555), by special request on a named-patient basis from Roche Products Ltd. A suspension can be prepared on request. A 5 mg/5 ml suspension of biotin is available from The Specials Laboratory with a 14-day expiry date.

References

Baumgartner MR, Suormala T. Biotin-responsive disorders. In: Saudubray J-M, van den Berghe G, Walter JH, *et al.*, eds. *Inborn metabolic diseases. Diagnosis and treatment*, 5th ed. Berlin: Springer-Verlag, 2012: pp. 375–84.

McVoy JR, Levy HL, Lawler M, *et al.* Partial biotinidase deficiency: clinical and biochemical features. *J Pediatr* 1990;**116**:78–83.

Moslinger D, Stockler-Ipsiroglu S, Scheibenreiter S, *et al.* Clinical and neuropsychological outcome in 33 patients with biotinidase deficiency ascertained by nationwide newborn screening and family studies in Austria. *Eur J Pediatr* 2001;**160**:277–82. (See also **161**:167–9.)

Packman S, Cowan MS, Golbus MS, *et al.* Prenatal treatment of biotin-responsive multiple carboxylase deficiency. *Lancet* 1982;**i**:1435.

Salbert BA, Pellock JM, Wolf B. Characterization of seizures associated with biotinidase deficiency. *Neurology* 1993;**43**:1351–5.

Continued on p. 106

Suormala T, Fowler B, Duran M, *et al*. Five patients with biotin-responsive defect in holocarboxylase formation. *Pediatr Res* 1997;**41**:667–73.

Tammachote R, Janklat S, Tongkobpetch S, *et al*. Holocarboxylase synthetase deficiency: novel clinical and molecular findings. *Clin Genet* 2010;**78**:88–93.

Thuy LP, Jurecki E, Nemzer L, *et al*. Prenatal diagnosis of holocarboxylase synthetase deficiency by assay of the enzyme in chorionic villus material followed by prenatal treatment. *Clin Chim Acta* 1999;**284**:59–68.

Wastell HJ, Bartlett K, Dale D, *et al*. Biotinidase deficiency: a survey of 10 cases. *Arch Dis Child* 1988;**63**:1244–9.

Weber P, Scholl S, Baumgartner ER. Outcome in patients with profound biotinidase deficiency: relevance of newborn screening. *Dev Med Child Neurol* 2004;**46**:481–4.

Wolf B. Biotinidase deficiency: "if you have to have an inherited metabolic disease, this is the one to have". *Genet Med* 2012;**14**:565–75.

Wolf B. Disorders of biotin metabolism. In: Scriver CR, Beaudet AL, Sly WS, *et al*., eds. *The metabolic and molecular bases of inherited disease*, 8th ed. New York: McGraw-Hill, 2001: pp. 3935–64.

Zempleni J, Kuroishi T. Biotin. *Adv Nutr* 2012;**3**:213–4.

Use

Red cell concentrates, or 'plasma-reduced cells' (previously called 'packed cells'), and red cell suspensions are used to correct serious symptomatic anaemia.

Products

Blood is not sterile, and viruses can be transmitted during transfusion, although the risk of cell-associated virus transmission is now routinely minimised by prior leucodepletion (i.e. the removal of virtually all white cells). Vigorous action has also been taken to minimise the risk from variant Creutzfeldt–Jakob disease (vCJD). Each donation is screened for hepatitis B (HBsAg), human immunodeficiency virus (HIV) (anti-HIV-1, anti-HIV-2 antibodies and HIV nucleic acid testing), hepatitis C (anti-HCV antibodies and HCV nucleic acid testing), human T-cell lymphotropic virus (anti-HTLV 1 and 2 antibodies) and syphilis (antibody test). Ill and preterm babies born to mothers lacking cytomegalovirus (CMV) antibodies also face a significant risk of neonatal CMV infection if given CMV-seropositive blood. Malaria and other blood-borne parasites pose a significant risk in areas where these are endemic.

Whole blood donations (~470 ml) are collected into 63 ml of citrate phosphate dextrose anti-coagulant. They are then filtered to remove leucocytes. Such leucodepleted blood contains $<1 \times 10^6$ leucocytes per pack and carries a lower risk of vCJD transmission, as well as causing fewer febrile transfusion reactions and alloimmunisation. The main product now provided for clinical use is a 230 ml concentrate with a haematocrit of 55–75% made from this by removing most of the plasma and replacing it with 100 ml of saline, adenine, glucose and mannitol additive solution (SAG-M). Not only are these packs leucodepleted, but they also contain virtually no functional platelets. These packs can be stored for 5 weeks, but ideally, blood <7 days old should be supplied for neonatal use because the potassium and acid load are less and there will be fewer microaggregates. In addition, the oxygen-carrying capacity will be greater (the concentration of 2,3-diphosphoglycerate in the red cells falls with time). Most clotting factors remain relatively stable during storage, but factor V and factor VIII levels fall by 75% within 10 days. Blood for intrauterine and exchange transfusion is plasma reduced to a haematocrit of ~70% and prepared from CMV-negative CPD-A blood. It is also irradiated if the baby is having, or has had, an intrauterine transfusion.

When a 'top-up' transfusion proves necessary, a red cell suspension (usually in SAG-M) is issued. Such suspensions, which contain no clotting factors, increasingly come in 40–45 ml 'paedipacks' (one unit of donor blood usually being used to prepare four to six such packs). Such products can be used for up to 5 weeks after preparation. Such suspensions should **never** be used for an exchange transfusion.

Matching

The laboratory needs to check the recipient's ABO, and Rh D blood group, and to test for the existence of any irregular antibodies before donor blood is released. Maternal blood is still used for detailed matching in some districts, as long as the mother's and baby's ABO groups are compatible, because infants <4 months old rarely make antibodies to red cells, and any neonatal IgG antibody will usually be derived from the mother. If unmatched group O Rh D-negative blood ever needs to be used in an emergency, an attempt should be made to discuss this with a consultant haematologist first.

Adverse reactions

Allergic urticarial reactions are rare in the neonatal period. Symptomatic treatment with 1 mg of chlorphenamine maleate intramuscularly (previously known as chlorpheniramine maleate) may be appropriate. Intravascular haemolysis due to ABO incompatibility is rare but potentially fatal. Immediate signs include flushing, dyspnoea, fever, hypotension and oliguria, with haemoglobinaemia and haemoglobinuria. Stop the transfusion at once, take specimens for laboratory analysis, and watch for renal failure, hyperkalaemia and coagulopathy. Rhesus, Kell, Kidd (Jk^a) and Duffy (Fy) antibodies may cause late reticuloendothelial haemolysis with jaundice and anaemia.

Clinical factors

Intravascular blood volume almost always falls significantly during the first few hours of life as plasma leaves the intravascular compartment but soon stabilises at 80–90 ml/kg with a haematocrit that reflects the extent and direction of any placental transfusion at delivery. Umbilical vein obstruction (as from a tight nuchal cord) can leave a baby hypovolaemic at birth. Replicate

Continued on p. 108

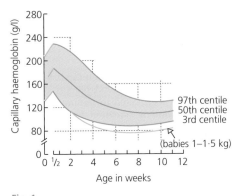

Fig. 1

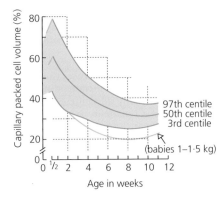

Fig. 2

laboratory haemoglobin estimates from capillary samples can vary by 6 g/l, so apparent changes of 10 g/l may merely reflect sampling error. A capillary haemoglobin may also exceed the venous haemoglobin by 10 g/l. Packed cell volume (PCV) measurements using a centrifuge provide a more rapid and satisfactory way of screening for anaemia in the neonatal period. They are more reproducible, require less blood and provide an immediate sideward answer.

Capillary haemoglobin and PCV ('haematocrit') values for term babies are shown in Figures 1 and 2. Babies born >8 weeks early have values that are about 5% lower than these at birth, and the lower limit of the normal range 4–12 weeks after birth is also lower than in term babies (giving a minimum PCV of 20% instead of 25%). Capillary values exceed venous values by at least 2% (and often by 4–8% in the first few days of life). Such differences can be minimised if free-flowing blood is collected from a warm, well-perfused heel. Micro-centrifuge measurement methods always exceed particle counting estimates by 1–2%.

Indications for transfusion

Symptomatic babies with a venous haematocrit of <40% at birth merit transfusion once a sample of blood has been collected from both the baby and the mother for diagnostic purposes. Watch for the hypovolaemic baby with a normal haematocrit immediately after birth; haematocrit values normally rise in the first 12 hours of life, but in such babies, there will be a fall. Such babies may have lost a quarter to a half of all their blood (20–40 ml/kg). Acute loss is best managed by a prompt rapid transfusion, but chronic anaemia at birth is better managed by exchange transfusion. Since it is the fall in plasma volume rather than the fall in haemoglobin that poses the immediate threat after acute blood loss, 0.9% sodium chloride can be given while waiting for blood to arrive if the patient's condition is critical.

Up to 80% of preterm babies who weighed <1500 g at birth will receive at least one blood transfusion during their neonatal 'career'. Indications for transfusion in this group have largely been based on the haemoglobin concentration combined with the cardiorespiratory status of the baby (e.g. oxygen requirement or respiratory support) and factors such as weight gain; however, the evidence base for such a strategy is, at best, weak. The British Committee for Standards in Haematology (BCSH) Transfusion Guidelines for Neonates and Older Children suggest the transfusion thresholds summarised below:

Postnatal age	Suggested transfusion threshold Hb (g/l)		
	Ventilated	On O$_2$ or CPAP	Off oxygen
First 24 hours	<120	<120	<100
1–7 days old	<120	<100	<100
8–14 days old	<100	<95	<75–85 depending on clinical situation
≥15 days old		<85	

Continued on p. 109

Administration

Treat anaemia with 20–25 ml/kg of blood over 3–4 hours. Multiple small transfusions from different donors are wasteful, and put the patient at increased risk. It is **not** usually necessary to calculate a specific replacement volume or give a 'covering' diuretic. Give blood through a fresh giving set with a 170–200 μm filter into a line previously set up and primed with 0.9% sodium chloride. Terminal co-infusion into a line containing glucose is also safe and does not cause measurable haemolysis, so it is better to do this than terminate the glucose infusion and precipitate reactive hypoglycaemia when it is not practicable to erect a separate intravenous line. Check the crossmatch particulars and the patient's name, and record all the details in the case notes.

Supply

Crossmatched blood stored at 4 °C is available from the local blood bank. Group O rhesus-negative, CMV-negative, plasma-reduced blood is available for emergency use. Use within 4 hours of removal from the fridge. Use a 'paedipack' containing about 40–45 ml of red cell concentrate where possible, particularly if more than one transfusion is likely to be needed within the next 7 days, to conserve stocks and minimise the risk of exposure to several donors.

References   (See also the relevant Cochrane reviews and UK guideline **DHUK**)

Balegar VKK, Kluckow M. Furosemide for packed red cell transfusion in preterm infants: a randomized controlled trial. *J Pediatr* 2011;**159**:913–8.e1. [RCT]

Brotanek JM, Fosz J, Weitzman M, *et al.* Secular trends in the prevalence of iron deficiency among US toddlers, 1976–2002. *Arch Pediatr Adolesc Med* 2008;**162**:374–81.

Doctor A, Spinella P. Effect of processing and storage on red blood cell function in vivo. *Semin Perinatol* 2012;**36**:248–59.

Fergusson DA, Hébert P, Hogan DL, *et al.* Effect of fresh red blood cell transfusions on clinical outcomes in premature, very low-birth-weight infants: the ARIPI randomized trial. *JAMA* 2012;**308**:1443–51.

Hosono S, Mugishima H, Fujita H, *et al.* Umbilical cord milking reduces the need for red cell transfusions and improves neonatal adaptation in infants born less than 29 weeks' gestation: a randomised controlled trial. *Arch Dis Child Fetal Neonatal Ed* 2008;**93**:F14–9. [RCT] (See also pp. F2–3.)

Jankov RP, Roy RND. Minimal haemolysis in blood co-infused with amino acid and dextrose solutions in vitro. *J Paediatr Child Health* 1997;**33**:250–2.

Lacroix J, Hébert PC, Hutchison JS, *et al.* Transfusion strategies for patients in pediatric intensive care units. *N Engl J Med* 2007;**356**:1609–19. [RCT]

Murray NA, Roberts IAG. Neonatal transfusion practice. *Arch Dis Child Fetal Neonatal Ed* 2004;**89**:F101–7.

Norfolk D, ed. *Handbook of transfusion medicine*, 5th edn. London: The Stationary Office, 2013.

van Rheenen PF, Brabin BJ. A practical approach to timing cord clamping in resource poor settings. *Br Med J* 2006;**333**:954–8. [SR]

Venkatesh V, Khan R, Curley A, *et al.* How we decide when a neonate needs a transfusion. *Br J Haematol* 2013;**160**:421–33.

Venkatesh V, Khan R, Curley A, *et al.* The safety and efficacy of red cell transfusions in neonates: a systematic review of randomized controlled trials. *Br J Haematol* 2012;**158**:370–85. [SR]

von Lindern JS, Brand A. The use of blood products in perinatal medicine. *Semin Fetal Neonatal Med* 2008;**13**:271–81.

Use

Bosentan is an oral dual endothelin-1 receptor antagonist that has been used to treat primary pulmonary hypertension in adults and older children. The first clinical trial of this type of drug in humans was published in 1995, and since then, endothelin-1 receptor antagonists have been tested in clinical trials involving heart failure, pulmonary arterial hypertension, resistant arterial hypertension, stroke and subarachnoid haemorrhage and various forms of cancer. The results of most of these trials – except those for pulmonary arterial hypertension and scleroderma-related digital ulcers – were either negative or neutral. This is reflected in the licensed use of bosentan in adults. The manufacturer has yet to endorse use in children or in neonates.

Sporadic reports of use of bosentan to treat neonatal pulmonary hypertension, either with or without congenital heart disease, first appeared in 2008 when it was used in infants who were failing to respond to other, more widely used agents such as nitric oxide (q.v.), epoprostenol (q.v.) and sildenafil (q.v.). In some cases, bosentan is used along with the other agent. To date, only one small randomised placebo-controlled trial has been undertaken using bosentan as an adjuvant therapy.

Pharmacology

Bosentan is a competitive antagonist of endothelin-1 at the endothelin-A (ET-A) and endothelin-B (ET-B) receptors. Endothelin-1 is a 21-amino-acid protein that is one of the most potent vasoconstrictors in the pulmonary vasculature, and pulmonary hypertension is associated with an increased expression of endothelin-1 in vascular endothelial cells.

Maximum plasma concentrations of bosentan are achieved within 3–5 hours after an oral dose. Bioavailability is ~50% and is not affected by food. It is highly protein bound (>98%). In adults, the elimination half-life is 5 hours. Bosentan undergoes hepatic metabolism via CYP2C9 and CYP3A4 (which it also induces) to three metabolites which are cleared by biliary excretion. The pharmacokinetic profile of bosentan in older children appears to be similar to that in adults, although pharmacokinetics in a neonatal population have yet to be studied. Bosentan can cause liver damage, fluid retention and anaemia. Liver enzymes should be monitored before starting therapy and monthly thereafter. If liver enzymes are elevated, therapy may need to be temporarily halted. Fluid retention may be a sign of worsening pulmonary hypertension or a side effect of bosentan and requires a full cardiac assessment.

Bosentan is contraindicated during pregnancy with reports of higher fetal demise and teratogenic effects. Because of induction of hepatic enzymes, hormonal contraceptives are unreliable. Although the high protein binding should mean drug levels in milk are low, the potential for side effects is such that breastfeeding is contraindicated.

Drug interactions

Bosentan interacts with clarithromycin, fluconazole, rifampicin, sildenafil and warfarin.

Treatment

The starting dose in most neonatal studies is 1–2 mg/kg twice a day, increasing to 2–4 mg/kg after 4 weeks.

Supply

Bosentan is available as 62.5 mg tablets costing £27 each. These may be split with a pill cutter and are stable for up to 4 weeks if stored in the original manufacturer's bottle. For children unable to swallow tablets or who require smaller doses, the tablet can be placed in 5–25 ml of water and allowed to disintegrate. The resulting suspension can be used to prepare an aliquot providing the correct dose. The suspension is stable at room temperature for up to 24 hours.

References
See also the relevant Cochrane reviews

Barst RJ, Ivy D, Dingemanse J, *et al*. Pharmacokinetics, safety, and efficacy of bosentan in pediatric patients with pulmonary arterial hypertension. *Clin Pharmacol Ther* 2003;**73**:372–82.

Carter NJ, Keating GM. Bosentan: in pediatric patients with pulmonary arterial hypertension. *Paediatr Drugs* 2010;**12**:63–73.

Goissen C, Ghyselen L, Tourneux P, *et al*. Persistent pulmonary hypertension of the newborn with transposition of the great arteries: successful treatment with bosentan. *Eur J Pediatr* 2008;**167**:437–40.

Continued on p. 111

Haworth SG. The management of pulmonary hypertension in children. *Arch Dis Child* 2008;**93**:620–5.

Mohamed WA, Ismail M. A randomized, double-blind, placebo-controlled, prospective study of bosentan for the treatment of persistent pulmonary hypertension of the newborn. *J Perinatol* 2012;**32**:608–13. [RCT]

Nakwan N, Choksuchat D, Saksawad R, *et al.* Successful treatment of persistent pulmonary hypertension of the newborn with bosentan. *Acta Paediatr* 2009;**98**:1683–5.

Radicioni M, Bruni A, Camerini P. Combination therapy for life-threatening pulmonary hypertension in a premature infant: first report on bosentan use. *Eur J Pediatr* 2011;**170**:1075–8.

Wardle AJ, Wardle R, Luyt K, *et al.* The utility of sildenafil in pulmonary hypertension: a focus on broncho-pulmonary dysplasia. *Arch Dis Child* 2013;**98**:613–7.

Use

Powdered and more recently liquid products have become available for modifying the nutritional content of human breast milk when this is used to feed the very preterm baby. However, the benefits have been modest to date, and the variability of expressed breast milk (EBM) does not make 'tailored' supplementation any easier. They are manufactured from processed cows' milk protein with additional nutritional supplements.

Immunological factors

Human milk is the ideal food for almost every baby. Although the various artificial products (q.v.) available seem to meet all the key nutritional needs of the term and preterm baby, feeding with unpasteurised human milk still confers a number of unique, if poorly understood, immunological advantages. While it is now recommended that all 'donor' milk should be pasteurised before use, mother's own milk is best used without pasteurisation. Milk collected in the home is safe for 8 days if kept at 4 °C and is best given unfrozen.

In a hospital setting, EBM should be stored in accordance with local policy. EBM should only be stored within a suitable fridge for up to 48 hours and, if not used, discarded. If there is any reason why it may not be used within that time, it should be frozen directly after expressing. If EBM has been fortified, it should only be stored in a suitable fridge for 24 hours. Use thawed milk at once.

Cells are damaged by storage and by freezing, but the immunoprotective constituents remain stable when stored at 0–4 °C for 3 days, when frozen at −20 °C for 12 months or when pasteurised at 56 °C for 30 minutes.

Table 1 Composition (per 100 ml) of preterm human milk before and after fortification.

	Protein (g)	Fat (g)	Carbohydrate (g)	Energy (kcal)	Na (mg)	Ca (mg)	P (mg)	Zn (mg)	Vit D (µg)	Vit K (µg)
Preterm human breast milk Tsang *et al.* 2005	1.5	3.5	6.9	65	28.5	25.4	14.2	0.3	0.18	0.83
Cow & Gate (C&G) *Nutriprem fortifier*® Two sachets (4.4 g) per 100 ml	2.6	3.5	9.6	80	63.5	91.4	52.2	0.9	5.18	7.23
SMA *Breast milk fortifier*® Two sachets (4 g) per 100 ml	2.8	4.16	9.4	84.6	48	112	60	0.66	>7.6	>11
Abbott *Similac*® *Human Milk Fortifier* Four sachets (3.6 g) per 100 ml	2.5	3.9	8.7	79	43.5	142	81	1.3	3.2	9.1
Mead Johnson *Enfamil*® *Human Milk Fortifier (powder)* Four sachets (2.8 g) per 100 ml	2.4	5.2	7.8	84	43	113	64	1.07	3.9	6.3
Mead Johnson *Enfamil*® *Human Milk Fortifier Acidified Liquid* Two sachets (4 g) per 100 ml	3.8	5.8	7.9	97	55	141	78	1.33	5	7.7

Nutritional factors

All these products are designed to enhance the nutritional value of human milk. Don't insist on an arbitrary upper limit to oral intake – some preterm babies grow very well on a daily intake of 220 ml/kg when 2 or 3 weeks old. The milk of a mother delivering a preterm baby usually has a relatively high protein content in the first couple of weeks of life, and too high a protein intake could, theoretically, be hazardous. Fortification is probably best not started, therefore, until about 2 weeks after delivery. It seldom needs to be continued once breastfeeding is established or the baby weighs 2 kg. All the products listed in the table in this monograph enhance the protein, calorie and mineral content of the milk.

Continued on p. 113

Supplementation

Human milk contains relatively little protein and a plasma urea lower than 1.6mmol/l may be a sign of suboptimal protein intake. Very preterm babies fed on fortified breast milk will benefit from additional sodium in the first few weeks of life, until their obligatory renal sodium loss decreases. Breastfed babies also almost certainly need additional vitamin K (q.v.) to prevent late vitamin K deficiency bleeding once fortification ceases, unless they have been given a total 'depot' supply of 1 mg IM at birth, irrespective of their weight at delivery, and it is probably easier to start such supplementation early. From about a month of age, all preterm breastfed babies benefit from sustained supplementation with oral iron (q.v.), and a few need zinc (q.v.). Whether it helps to give further vitamin A (q.v.) by mouth is still unclear.

Supply

Enfamil and Similac are widely used in the United States and other countries, but are not commercially available in the United Kingdom. While the SMA product is not on general release, it is available in boxes containing 50×2g sachets to neonatal units stocking and using SMA Gold Prem® low birthweight formula milk. C&G Nutriprem fortifier is supplied in boxes containing 50×2.2g sachets costing £44. The powder is best added just before the baby is fed.

Do not use any of these products to further fortify artificial formula milks.

References

(See also the relevant Cochrane reviews)

Breast Feeding Network (BfN). *Expressing and storing breast milk*. 2009. Downloadable leaflet available at http://www.breastfeedingnetwork.org.uk/pdfs/BFNExpressing_and_Storing.pdf

Geddes D, Hartmann P, Jones E. Preterm birth: strategies for establishing adequate milk production and successful lactation. *Semin Fetal Neonatal Med* 2013;**18**:155–9.

Hands A. Safe storage of expressed breast milk in the home. *MIDIRS Midwifery Digest* 2003;**13**:278–85.

Jones E, King C, eds. *Feeding and nutrition in the preterm infant*. Edinburgh: Elsevier Churchill Livingstone, 2005.

Schanler RJ. Outcomes of human milk-fed premature infants. *Semin Perinatol* 2011;**35**:29–33.

Tsang RC, Uauy R, Koletzko B, *et al.*, eds. *Nutrition of the preterm infant: scientific basis and practical guidelines*, 2nd edn. Cincinnati, OH: Digital Educational Publishing, 2005.

Use

Inhaled steroids, like budesonide, are central to the management of asthma and useful in the management of croup. Prophylactic use has little impact on the incidence of ventilator-induced chronic lung disease.

Pharmacology

Budesonide (patented in 1975) and beclometasone dipropionate (beclomethasone dipropionate = USAN) are steroids of almost equivalent potency with strong glucocorticoid and negligible mineralocorticoid activity. Fluticasone propionate is a related compound which is about twice as potent on a weight-for-weight basis. They are widely used topically on the skin or by inhalation into the lung (as in asthma) and have little systemic effect unless high-dose treatment is employed. There is no contraindication to their use during pregnancy and lactation: indeed, it is particularly important to keep asthma under stable control during pregnancy. Administration is generally from an aerosol or dry powder inhaler. Suspensions of budesonide and fluticasone can also be nebulised, but there seems to be no comparable preparation of beclometasone.

Intra-tracheal steroid use in the preterm baby

Early prophylactic use: A number of trials have demonstrated no benefit for inhaled steroids in reducing the incidence of neonatal chronic lung disease. A major confounding factor is the drug delivery and deposition in the lungs. Numerous factors affect drug delivery and deposition; the number of particles in the respirable range, the delivery technique and the presence of an endotracheal tube and studies have shown the amount of aerosol actually delivered varies from 0.4 to 14% depending on the technique used. Steroid-induced cataracts have been reported after nebuliser use, and significant adrenal suppression is known to occur in some infants treated in this manner. Routine use of prophylactic inhaled steroids is, therefore, not recommended in VLBW infants.

One small study suggests that direct intra-tracheal co-instillation of liquid budesonide with surfactant may be a more effective way of delivering steroids to the lungs, but this method is restricted to the intubated baby.

Treatment of established disease: A recent overview of trial information suggests that while aerosolised or nebulised budesonide or beclometasone can be of some help in weaning babies from ventilator support, they are not as effective as systemic steroids. Use may, however, help to reduce or abolish the need for systemic treatment with dexamethasone in a few babies with chronic lung disease.

Inhaled steroid use in croup

Croup (the sudden onset of hoarseness, a barking cough and distressing inspiratory stridor) is common in young children. It is mainly viral in origin, though atopy plays a part in some children. Symptoms often settle almost as fast as they arise. Brief steroid use can reduce admission, and only 1% of those admitted require intubation (once cases of bacterial epiglottitis are recognised for what they are).

Treatment

Managing ventilator-induced chronic lung disease: 200 (or 500) micrograms of budesonide inhaled twice a day may occasionally aid extubation but is of no other demonstrable long-term benefit. The drug has usually been given from a metered-dose aerosol inhaler into a rigid 'aerochamber' during hand ventilation. Mask administration using a jet nebuliser after extubation can reduce the child's 'symptom score', but trials have failed to show any more general clinical benefit. It may be wise to protect the eyes during mask administration. Only a 10th of the administered dose reaches the baby.

Use in croup: Giving a single 2 mg dose (or two 1 mg doses 30 minutes apart) of nebulised budesonide can reduce the need for hospital admission as effectively as a single 0.6 mg/kg oral (or intramuscular) dose of dexamethasone (q.v.). The dose may be repeated 12 hours later.

Supply and administration

500 micrograms (2 ml) Respules® of budesonide, designed for nebulisation, costs £1.30 each. 500 micrograms (2 ml) Nebules® of fluticasone propionate is also available (costing 90p) for nebulisation.

Continued on p. 115

References

(See also relevant Cochrane reviews)

Berger WE, Qaqundah PY, Blake K, *et al.* Safety of budesonide inhalation suspension in infants aged six to twelve months with mild to moderate persistent asthma or recurrent wheeze. *J Pediatr* 2005;**146**:91–5. [RCT]

Kuo HT, Lin HC, Tsai CH, *et al.* A follow-up study of preterm infants given budesonide using surfactant as a vehicle to prevent chronic lung disease in preterm infants. *J Pediatr* 2010;**156**:537–41. [RCT]

Ozkiraz S, Gokmen Z, Borazan M, *et al.* Bilateral posterior subcapsular cataracts after inhaled budesonide therapy for bronchopulmonary dysplasia. *J Matern Fetal Neonatal Med* 2009;**22**:368–70.

Wilson TT, Waters L, Patterson CC, *et al.* Neurodevelopmental and respiratory follow-up results at 7 years for children from the United Kingdom and Ireland enrolled into a randomized trial of early and late postnatal corticosteroid treatment, systematic and inhaled (the Open Study of Early Corticosteroid Treatment). *Pediatrics* 2006;**117**:2196–205. [RCT]

Yeh TF, Lin HC, Chang CH, *et al.* Early intratracheal instillation of budesonide using surfactant as a vehicle to prevent chronic lung disease in preterm infants: a pilot study. *Pediatrics* 2008;**121**:e1310–8. [RCT]

Use

Bupivacaine is a widely used local anaesthetic. It takes rather longer than lidocaine (q.v.) to become effective and is much more toxic, but the pain relief it provides lasts four times as long.

Pharmacology

Bupivacaine is an amide local anaesthetic, like lidocaine, that blocks the conduction of nerve impulses by decreasing the nerve membrane's permeability to sodium ions. It was first developed in 1957. Sensory nerves are more readily affected than motor nerves. A small amount (~6%) is excreted unchanged in the urine, but most is metabolised by the liver, the neonatal half-life being about 8 hours (at least twice as long as in adults). Tissue levels exceed plasma levels (neonatal steady state V_D ~4 l/kg). All local anaesthetic drugs are potentially toxic. Most are more toxic to the brain than the heart, causing tremor, restlessness, apnoea and fits before they cause an arrhythmia, but the reverse is true of bupivacaine. Check the maximum dose for the baby and do not put more than this in the syringe. Have an intravenous (IV) line in place. Accidental injection into a blood vessel can be particularly dangerous, so aspirate before injecting. Epidural bupivacaine (with or without an opioid) provides lumbar block before surgery and during childbirth. Tissue infiltration can provide local sensory block.

Lidocaine becomes fully effective in adults within 2–4 minutes and blocks all local sensation for about an hour. Bupivacaine, in contrast, takes up to half an hour to become fully effective after infiltration but then blocks all sensation for 2–8 hours (and probably longer than this in the neonate). Anaesthetists have used intra-operative bupivacaine nerve blocks and wound infiltration (in a dose not exceeding 2 mg/kg) to reduce post-operative pain. Epidural bupivacaine has been used during abdominal surgery to avoid the need for morphine in young children, with its attendant risk of respiratory depression. Low epidural blocks have been used, in the same way, during the surgical treatment of inguinal hernia in the preterm baby, obviating the need for a general anaesthetic. The subcutaneous infusion of up to 400 micrograms/kg of bupivacaine an hour post-operatively for up to 3 days into the region of any major incision can also deliver significant pain relief.

Ropivacaine, a related aminoamide anaesthetic first introduced in 1997, has now started to be used to provide caudal and lumbar epidural block in children. Early experience suggests that it is less toxic but also produces less motor block for a given degree of sensory block. The dose used in infancy is 1 ml/kg of a 0.2% solution, followed by a continuous infusion of 200 micrograms/kg/hour (or 400 micrograms/kg/hour in infants more than 6 months old) continued for not more than 72 hours.

Maternal bupivacaine is systemically absorbed after epidural administration, crosses the placenta readily and is detectable in the cord blood in a dose that is high enough to interfere transiently with auditory brainstem evoked responses, but not high enough to induce any significant neurobehavioral changes. The same probably goes for ropivacaine. The amount excreted in human milk is negligible.

Pain relief

Infiltrative local anaesthesia: Do not exceed a dose of 2 mg/kg (0.8 ml/kg of 0.25% bupivacaine), and do not repeat this dose for 8 hours. Use a pulse oximeter (and/or ECG monitor) to detect any early adverse cardiorespiratory effect. *It is essential to avoid accidental injection into a blood vessel*.

Epidural block: Give up to 0.8 ml/kg of 0.25% bupivacaine slowly into the caudal epidural space over 1–2 minutes, aspirating intermittently to check for the presence of blood or CSF. This should produce adequate anaesthesia for inguinal or perineal surgery after about 15 minutes.

Toxicity

Apnoea or a change in heart rate is usually the first sign that too much drug has entered the circulation. Immediate ventilatory support can minimise acidosis (which further augments the drug's toxicity). Hypotension may respond to dobutamine (q.v.). Thiopental sodium (q.v.) may be needed if fits interfere with ventilation. Complete recovery can be anticipated unless an arrhythmia develops that is resistant to these measures and to a 10 micrograms/kg bolus of clonidine.

Continued on p. 117

Supply

10 ml ampoules containing 25 mg of plain bupivacaine hydrochloride (i.e., 0.25% bupivacaine) cost 88p. Note that more concentrated ampoules (0.5%) are also marketed. In addition, bupivacaine is also available in ampoules that contain other drugs: 5 mg/ml bupivacaine with 80 mg/ml glucose is marketed as Marcain Heavy®, bupivacaine (both 2.5 and 5 mg/ml) with 1 in 200,000 (5 micrograms/ml) adrenaline is available in non-proprietary formulations and two strengths of bupivacaine with 2 micrograms/ml of fentanyl for epidural use are marketed as Bufyl®. Care should be taken to ensure that the correct formulation is used.

References

Bösenberg AT, Thomas J, Cronje L, *et al*. Pharmacokinetics and efficacy of ropivacaine for continuous epidural infusion in neonates and infants. *Pediatr Anaesth* 2005;**15**:739–49.

de La Coiussaye JE, Bassoul B, Brugada J, *et al*. Reversal of electrophysiological and haemodynamic effects induced by high dose bupivacaine by the combination of clonidine and dobutamine in anesthetised dogs. *Anesth Analg* 1992;**74**:703–11.

Gallagher TM. Regional anaesthesia for surgical treatment of inguinal hernia in preterm babies. *Arch Dis Child* 1993;**69**:623–4.

Rapp HJ, Molnár V, Austin S, *et al*. Ropivacaine in neonates and infants – a population pharmacokinetic evaluation following single caudal block. *Paediatr Anaesth* 2004;**14**:724–32.

Tirotta CF, Munro HM, Salvaggio J, *et al*. Continuous incisional infusion of local anesthetic in pediatric patients following open heart surgery. *Paediatr Anaesth* 2009;**19**:571–6. [RCT]

Wolf AR, Hughes D. Pain relief for infants undergoing abdominal surgery: comparison of infusions of IV morphine and extra-dural bupivacaine. *Br J Anaesth* 1993;**70**:10–6.

Use
Bromocriptine, cabergoline and quinagolide are three dopamine receptor agonists that are used to treat hyperprolactinaemic amenorrhoea and galactorrhoea. Due to a better side effect profile, cabergoline is preferred to bromocriptine (see web archive) if it is necessary (or justified) to suppress lactation after childbirth. Quinagolide has not been used for this purpose.

Pharmacology
Cabergoline is an ergot derivative with selective inhibitory activity on prolactin secretion by binding to dopamine receptors. It is well absorbed when given by mouth, metabolised in the liver with a half-life of 2–4 days and excreted largely in the bile. A single dose twice a week will restore ovulation in most women with hyperprolactinaemic amenorrhoea. The manufacturers recommend that treatment is stopped before women try to conceive; in reality, this is sometimes not practical; there is a real possibility that withdrawal could prevent ovulation or result in a vision-threatening increase in size if the tumour is already large. First trimester use in humans is not associated with teratogenicity in humans. While high-dose treatment can cause fibrotic heart valve changes, such changes seem rare with low-dose treatment (although a constrictive pericarditis has been reported).

Effect on lactation
Milk formation during late pregnancy occurs under the combined stimulus of oestrogens, prolactin (placental lactogen) and progesterone. Insulin and cortisol may also have a role. Oestrogens antagonise the effects of prolactin, and lactation is stimulated when oestrogen levels fall after delivery.

Oestrogens were once used widely to suppress lactation in the puerperium, but they were found to be relatively ineffective and to increase the risk of potentially life-threatening thromboembolism. Trials undertaken between 1972 and 1984 showed 2.5 mg of bromocriptine twice a week for 2 weeks to be a more effective alternative. However, most drug trials only looked at the immediate effect of drug treatment, and there is some evidence that although bromocriptine reduces pain, engorgement and milk production 1 week after delivery more than a breast binder, the situation is reversed 2 weeks later.

Over the next 10 years, reports started to appear of mothers having seizures, strokes, heart attacks and sudden severe hypertension while taking bromocriptine to suppress lactation. While it is difficult to know whether these symptoms were caused by bromocriptine, problems were reported with sufficient frequency for the manufacturers to stop recommending its use to suppress lactation in 1994. Since discomfort is only a transient problem, there can seldom be a case for using *any* drug to suppress lactation in most mothers, but drug use can still be justified in certain situations. Continued milk production may cause additional anguish to some mothers coping with a stillbirth or early neonatal death.

The dose to completely suppress physiological lactation is given in this monograph. In women with prolactinoma who wish to breastfeed, it is possible to reduce the dose to a level that controls prolactin levels but is still high enough to maintain lactation. On a weight-related basis, the breastfed infant receives less than 1% of the maternal dose. It is also often possible to stop treatment during pregnancy and during lactation because prolactinomas usually only grow slowly at this time.

Use to suppress lactation
A single 1 mg dose of cabergoline by mouth is usually enough to suppress lactation immediately after delivery. If lactation has already been established, give 250 micrograms in four doses at 12 hourly intervals.

Supply
500 microgram scored tablets of cabergoline are available (costing £4 each).

References
(See also the relevant Cochrane reviews)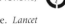

Bhattacharyya S, Shapira A, Mikhailidis DP, *et al.* Drug-induced fibrotic valvular heart disease. *Lancet* 2009;**374**:577–85. [SR]

Caballero GA, Caballero DJL. Caberbolina: Nuevo dopaminérgico a dosis única en la inhibición de la lactación. *Acta Ginecológica* 1996;**53**:172–9. [RCT]

Continued on p. 119

Caballero-Gordo A, Lopez-Nazareno N, Calderay M, *et al.* Single-dose inhibition of puerperal lactation. *J Reprod Med* 1991;**36**:717–21.

Colao A, Abs R, Barcena DG, *et al.* Pregnancy outcomes following cabergoline treatment: extended results from a 12 year observational study. *Clin Endocrinol (Oxf)* 2008;**68**:66–71.

dos Santos Nunes V, El Dib R, Boguszewski CL, *et al.* Cabergoline versus bromocriptine in the treatment of hyperprolactinemia: a systematic review of randomized controlled trials and meta-analysis. Pituitary 2011; **14**:259–65. [SR]

Dutt S, Wong F, Spurway JH. Fatal myocardial infarction associated with bromocriptine for postpartum lactation suppression. *Aust NZ J Obstet Gynaecol* 1998;**38**:116–9.

European Multicentre Study Group for Cabergoline in Lactation Inhibition. Single dose cabergoline versus bromocriptine in inhibition of peurperal lactation: randomised, double-blind, multicentre study. *Br Med J* 1991;**302**:1367–71. [RCT]

Löndahl M, Nilsson A, Lindgren H, *et al.* A case of constrictive pericarditis during cabergoline treatment for hyperprolactinaemia. *Eur J Endocrinol* 2008;**158**:583–5.

Martin NM, Tan T, Meeran K. Dopamine agonists and hyperprolactinaemia. *Br Med J* 2009;**338**:b381.

Rains CP, Bryson HM, Fitton A. Cabergoline. *Drugs* 1995;**49**:255–79. [SR]

Stalldecker G, Mallea-Gil MS, Guitelman M, *et al.* Effects of cabergoline on pregnancy and embryo-fetal development: retrospective study on 103 pregnancies and a review of the literature. *Pituitary* 2010;**13**: 345–50.

Webster J. A comparative review of the tolerability profiles of dopamine agonists in the treatment of hyperprolactinaemia and inhibition of lactation. *Drug Saf* 1996;**14**:228–38.

Use

Caffeine reduces apnoea and speeds extubation, so decreasing the time very preterm babies spend ventilated and in supplemental oxygen. Use also seems to decrease the number of survivors with disability.

Pharmacology

Caffeine is a general stimulant which increases metabolic rate, central chemoreceptor sensitivity to CO_2 and inspiratory drive. It crosses the placenta easily, and a daily intake greater than 300 mg (equivalent to eight cups of tea or three cups of strong coffee) probably increases the risk of miscarriage and stillbirth (see web commentary). The amount in the breast milk of mothers on a normal diet is of no clinical significance, even though the neonatal half-life (60–140 hours) is 16 times as long as it is in adults. Caffeine is well absorbed orally, and intravenous (IV) treatment is seldom necessary. It is mostly excreted, unchanged, in the urine in the first month of life, but clearance rises and approaches the rate found in adults in infants over 4 months old. Use marginally reduces weight gain for a few weeks and does not increase the risk of necrotising enterocolitis. Benefit is most marked in the ventilator-dependent baby started on treatment within 3 days of birth. Tachycardia and agitation are the first signs of toxicity, while a 10-fold overdose may cause hyperglycaemia, hypertonia and heart failure.

Managing neonatal apnoea

Caffeine is preferred to theophylline (q.v.) when managing apnoea, once sepsis, hypoglycaemia, seizures and respiratory exhaustion have been excluded, but medication is no substitute for a sensible nursing strategy. Doxapram (q.v.) may on occasion be useful, but stimulants seldom help when obstructive apnoea is due to reflex glottic closure, or sleep-associated pharyngeal hypotonia, and caffeine can make reflux worse. Continuous positive airway pressure (CPAP) or high flow oxygen may help especially in those babies whose apnoea has an obstructive component.

Serious apnoea is most common in the very preterm baby and becomes more troublesome a few days after birth. It is uncommon in babies with a post-menstrual age of more than 33 weeks, so treatment can usually be stopped 2 weeks before discharge and any monitor removed a week after treatment ceases. Developmental delay is more common when serious apnoea persists longer than this.

Drug equivalence

There is 1 mg of caffeine **base** in 2 mg of caffeine *citrate*. Most neonatologists worldwide have, for the last 25 years, quoted the amount of caffeine citrate used when prescribing this drug, but until recently, the UK drug regulator said that prescribers should state the amount of caffeine base to be given. Fortunately, this advice has been reversed and any prescription should now be written as *caffeine citrate*.

Treatment

Neonatal apnoea: Give a loading dose of 20 mg/kg of caffeine citrate IV or by mouth, followed by a maintenance dose of 5 mg/kg (or *very* occasionally 10 mg/kg) IV or by mouth once every 24 hours. In the few babies who merit treatment at a post-menstrual age of more than 52 weeks, it is sometimes necessary to give a maintenance dose of 5 mg/kg of caffeine citrate four times a day.
Facilitating extubation: The dose used to control neonatal apnoea (see earlier) will usually suffice. A higher loading dose of 80 mg/kg IV followed by 20 mg/kg once a day may further speed tracheal extubation in a few babies of less than 30 weeks gestation, but it often causes quite significant tachycardia (170–190 bpm).

Blood levels

Measurement seldom influences management. While the usual target plasma level is 10–20 mg/l, a few babies respond better to a level of 25–35 mg/l. Signs of toxicity only occur when the level exceeds 50 mg/l (1 mg/l = 5.14 μmol/l). Samples do not need to be collected at any set time.

Supply

IV products: 1 ml non-proprietary vials containing 10 mg of caffeine citrate that cost £4.90 are available. Care must be taken to avoid confusion as there are also 1 ml vials of proprietary caffeine citrate (Peyona®) containing 20 mg (costing £17).

Continued on p. 121

Oral products: Both IV preparations may be given orally. Non-proprietary 5 ml vials containing 50 mg of caffeine citrate (10 mg/ml) and costing £24 are available. Many centres in America, and some in the United Kingdom, continue to make a more easily used (and cheaper) sugar-free preparation 'in-house' with a 1-year shelf life that is useable for a month once opened.

References

(See also the relevant Cochrane reviews)

Brent RL, Christian MS, Diener RM. Evaluation of the reproductive and developmental risks of caffeine. *Birth Defects Res (Part B)* 2011;**92**:152–87.

Doyle LW, Cheong J, Hunt RW, *et al*. Caffeine and brain development in very preterm infants. *Ann Neurol* 2010;**68**:734–52.

Gray PH, Flenady VJ, Charles BG, *et al*. Caffeine citrate for very preterm infants: effects on development, temperament, and behaviour. *J Paediatr Child Health* 2011;**47**:167–72. [RCT]

Pillekamp F, Hermann C, Keller T, *et al*. Factors influencing apnea and bradycardia of prematurity – implications for neurodevelopment. *Neonatology* 2007;**91**:155–61.

Schmidt B, Roberts RS, Davis P, *et al*. Caffeine therapy for apnea of prematurity *N Engl J Med* 2006;**354**:2112–21. [RCT]

Schmidt B, Roberts RS, Davis P, *et al*. The long-term effects of caffeine therapy for apnea of prematurity. *N Engl J Med* 2007;**357**:1893–1902. [RCT] (See also pp. 1967–8.)

Steer P, Flenady V, Shearman A, *et al*. High dose caffeine citrate for extubation of preterm infants: a randomised controlled trial. *Arch Dis Child Fetal Neonatal Ed* 2004;**89**:F499–503. [RCT]

Use

Calcium gluconate can be given orally or intravenously (IV) to control symptomatic neonatal hypocalcaemia, but intramuscular (IM) magnesium sulfate (q.v.) may be preferable in babies presenting 4–10 days after birth.

Pharmacology

Calcium increases myocardial contractility and ventricular excitability. It can also be used to control cardiac hyperexcitability in severe neonatal hyperkalaemia (as outlined in the monograph on the polystyrene sulfonate resins). Dietary supplementation during pregnancy has been shown to reduce the risk of maternal hypertension and pre-eclampsia in high-risk women. Calcium is no longer routinely used during the management of cardiopulmonary resuscitation and is not required for the mild transient hypocalcaemia caused by citrate administration during exchange transfusion.

A degree of 'physiological' hypocalcaemia is common in the first 2 days of life with apathy and hypotonia especially if there is intrapartum asphyxia or respiratory distress. Late hypocalcaemia on the other hand is usually associated with increased tone, jitteriness and multifocal seizures 4–10 days after birth in an otherwise well child. Seizures are usually associated with a serum calcium <1.7 mmol/l (and more specifically an ionised calcium <0.64 mmol/l). Hypomagnesaemia is also often present (<0.68 mmol/l). Most such babies have a QTc of >0.2 seconds on their ECG.

There is no evidence that hypocalcaemia causes permanent neurological damage, and there is little evidence that an asymptomatic baby with transient hypocalcaemia requires any treatment. Calcium gluconate is probably the treatment of choice for early symptomatic hypocalcaemia, but extravasation can cause severe permanent tissue damage with IV administration and has even made partial limb amputation necessary on occasion. A strategy for the early treatment of tissue extravasation is described in the monograph on hyaluronidase (q.v.).

IM magnesium sulfate (q.v.) may be preferable in the first-line management of transient late neonatal hypocalcaemia. Calcium gluconate can also be given orally, but calcium glubionate and lactobionate (Calcium-Sandoz®) is a cheaper and more convenient formulation for sustained oral use. Phenobarbital (q.v.) is effective in controlling seizures but should not be allowed to mask symptoms in the rare baby in whom hypocalcaemia does not resolve within 48 hours. Look for evidence of parathyroid disturbance in mother and/or baby, or maternal vitamin D deficiency, if problems persist.

Correcting hypocalcaemia

Urgent IV correction: Correct serious hypocalcaemia by giving 2 ml/kg (0.46 mmol/kg) of 10% calcium gluconate slowly IV over 5–10 minutes if oral correction does not seem appropriate. This is more than the dose recommended in most British texts but conforms to practice in North America. Watch for arrhythmia and extravasation, and *avoid* intra-arterial and IM administration.
Routine IV supplementation: 2.5 ml/kg of 10% calcium gluconate can be given IV each day for the next 2–3 days, either as a continuous infusion or as four slow bolus doses, while investigations continue into the cause of any persisting abnormality if oral administration is not possible.
Rapid oral correction: Give 4 ml/kg of Calcium-Sandoz syrup (~2 mmol/kg of calcium) a day in divided doses. This more than doubles the calcium intake provided by most artificial infant milks.
Routine oral supplementation: Give 0.5 ml/kg of the Calcium-Sandoz syrup (~250 micromol/kg of calcium) four times a day.

Compatibility

Do not add calcium to any solution containing bicarbonate, sulphate or phosphate, and do not let any IV fluid containing calcium come into even brief contact with any other IV administered drug. An insoluble salt precipitates out on contact with ceftriaxone, and the same may be true of some other drugs.

Supply

One 10 ml ampoule of 10% calcium gluconate contains 1 g of calcium gluconate (or 89 mg of calcium) and costs 60p. This stock preparation, designed primarily for intravenous use, contains 225 micromol (0.46 mEq) of calcium per millilitre. The product should not be used to supplement the calcium content of parenteral nutrition because of its high aluminium content.

Continued on p. 123

An orange-flavoured oral syrup (Calcium-Sandoz) contains calcium glubionate and calcium lactobionate in sucrose (containing 22 mg [0.54 mmol] of calcium per millilitre) is available (cost £4.10 for 300 ml). This product should be avoided in patients with galactosaemia, because the glubionate is hydrolyzed by lactase in the small intestine into galactose and gluconic acid.

References

(See also relevant Cochrane reviews)

Hofmeyr GJ, Duley L, Atallah A. Dietary calcium supplementation for prevention of pre-eclampsia and related problems: a systematic review. *BJOG* 2007;**114**:933–43. [SR]

Hsu SC, Levine MA. Perinatal calcium metabolism: physiology and pathophysiology. *Semin Neonatol* 2004;**9**:23–36.

Mimouni F, Tsang RC. Neonatal hypocalcaemia: to treat or not to treat? *J Am Coll Nutr* 1994;**13**:408–15.

Porcelli PJ, Oh W. Effects of single dose calcium gluconate infusion in hypocalcaemic preterm infants. *J Perinatol* 1995;**12**:18–21.

Srinivasan V, Morris MC, Helfaer MA, *et al.* Calcium use during in-hospital pediatric cardiopulmonary resuscitation: a report from the national registry of cardiopulmonary resuscitation. *Pediatrics* 2008;**121**:e1144–51.

Thomas TC, Smith JM, White PC, *et al.* Transient neonatal hypocalcemia: presentation and outcomes. *Pediatrics* 2012;**129**:e1461–7.

Use

Captopril may be used in the management of babies with congestive cardiac failure. It is also used to control hypertension in older children, but intravenous (IV) labetalol followed by oral nifedipine (q.v.) offers a more reliable strategy for controlling serious hypertension in infancy. Captopril is also used to reduce proteinuria in nephrotic syndrome.

Pharmacology

A range of drugs used to treat heart failure and hypertension work by inhibiting the angiotensin-converting enzyme (ACE) responsible for converting angiotensin I to the potent vasoconstrictor, angiotensin II. These drugs, and the related angiotensin II receptor antagonist group of drugs which share many properties, are fetotoxic in pregnancy causing, in some cases, irreversible renal impairment. This may not be apparent until after the development of oligohydramnios. They are, however, generally safe during breastfeeding since the baby only gets about 0.1% of the maternal dose (on a weight-for-weight basis).

Hyperkalaemia is a hazard in patients co-treated with potassium-sparing diuretics (like spironolactone) or on potassium supplements. The half-life of captopril is only 1–2 hours, but the clinical effect persists much longer than this, possibly because of reconversion of inactive metabolites back to active drug. The half-life of the related ACE inhibitor enalaprilat (and its prodrug enalapril) is 1–2 days.

Because the neonatal response to treatment with an ACE inhibitor is very variable, and some babies become profoundly hypotensive with even a small dose, it is essential first to give a small test dose and then increase the dose cautiously. This seems particularly true in babies under a month old. Reversible adverse effects (including apnoea, seizures and renal failure as well as severe unpredictable hypotension) have been unacceptably common when these drugs were used to control hypertension in the first few months of life. What is more worrying, such episodes have sometimes occurred unpredictably in small babies on maintenance treatment. ACE inhibitors may, however, be of help in infants with chronic congestive failure by decreasing the afterload on the heart, although babies with a left-to-right shunt seldom seem to benefit.

Treatment

Neonatal use: In preterm infants (<37 weeks), start by giving a 'test' dose of 10 micrograms/kg of captopril by mouth and monitor blood pressure carefully. If there are no adverse effects, give 10 micrograms/kg of captopril every 8 hours. This dose can then be increased progressively, as necessary, to no more than 100 micrograms/kg once every 8 hours.

In term neonates, the initial ('test') dose is 10–50 micrograms/kg. The same dose is given 8–12 hourly in the absence of adverse effects and can be increased, if required, to a maximum of 2 mg/kg/day.

Older infants: Start by giving a 100 microgram/kg test dose and monitor blood pressure every 15 minutes for at least 2 hours. Start treatment by giving this dose once every 8–12 hours, and increase the dose cautiously to a total daily dose of no more than 4 mg/kg/day.

Use of enalapril

Enalapril maleate is an alternative oral prodrug which is hydrolyzed in the liver to the even more potent ACE inhibitor enalaprilat (enalaprilat itself being available as an IV preparation in North America, but not in the United Kingdom). The oral bioavailability of enalapril is approximately 60% in adults but variably less than this in neonates. The neonatal response is *very* variable, as is the duration of action. As a result, the starting dose in neonates is 10 micrograms/kg once a day, whereas a starting dose of 100 micrograms/kg is probably safe in older children. Oral doses as high as 1 mg/kg once a day are occasionally used later during the first year of life. The dose should be titrated up slowly as required, watching for possible signs of early renal failure. The drug's main advantage over captopril is the longer half-life and the availability of an IV formulation. The manufacturers have not endorsed the use of this drug in children. Liver failure is a rare hazard.

Supply and administration

Captopril is available as both 5 mg/5 ml and 25 mg/5 ml oral solutions from Martindale Pharma and costs £95 for 100 ml. Captopril and enalapril both come in tablet form (and are only stable when so formulated). Various strengths are available, some costing as little as 5p each. The

Continued on p. 125

tablets dissolve easily in water so a 25 mg tablet dissolved in 25 ml of tap water gives a 1 mg/ml sugar-free solution that is stable for 24 hours.

References

Bullo M, Tschumi S, Bucher BS, *et al*. Pregnancy outcome following exposure to angiotensin-converting enzyme inhibitors or angiotensin receptor antagonists: a systematic review. *Hypertension* 2012;**60**:444–50. [SR]

Bult Y, van den Anker J. Hypertension in a preterm infant treated with enalapril. *J Pediatr Pharm Pract* 1997;**2**:229–31.

Gantenbein MH, Bauersfeld U, Baenziger O, *et al*. Side effects of angiotensin converting enzyme inhibitor (captopril) in newborns and young infants. *J Perinat Med* 2008;**36**:448–52.

Hanssens M, Keirse MJ, Vankelecom F, *et al*. Fetal and neonatal effects of treatment with angiotensin-converting enzyme inhibitors in pregnancy. *Obstet Gynecol* 1991;**78**:128–35. [SR]

Leversha AM, Wilson NJ, Clarkson PM, *et al*. Efficacy and dosage of enalapril in congenital and acquired heart disease. *Arch Dis Child* 1994;**70**:35–9.

Mulla H, Tofeig M, Bu'Lock F, *et al*. Variations in captopril formulations used to treat children with heart failure: a survey in the United Kingdom. *Arch Dis Child* 2007;**92**:409–11.

O'Dea RF, Mirkin BL, Alward CT, *et al*. Treatment of neonatal hypertension with captopril. *J Pediatr* 1988;**113**:403–6.

Perlman JM, Volpe JJ. Neurologic complications of captopril treatment of neonatal hypertension. *Pediatrics* 1989;**83**:47–52.

Tack ED, Perlman JM. Renal failure in sick hypertensive premature infants receiving captopril therapy. *J Pediatr* 1988;**112**:805–10.

Use

Carbamazepine has been in use for generalised tonic–clonic (grand mal) and partial (focal) epilepsy since 1963. It is a valuable first-line drug in the sustained, long-term control of epilepsy in infancy and later childhood. It can only be given by mouth or per rectum.

Pharmacology

Carbamazepine is well but slowly absorbed from the digestive tract and extensively metabolised in the liver before being excreted in the urine along with carbamazepine-10,11-epoxide (one of its primary active metabolites). Peak absorption is delayed when the drug is given as a tablet rather than as a liquid or chew tab. The amount offered should also be increased to 25% when the drug is given into the rectum because of incomplete absorption. Drug clearance is low at birth (half-life 24 hours) but higher in infancy (3–15 hours) than in adult life. The volume of distribution in neonates is 1.5 l/kg.

Start by giving a low dose and increase this gradually. Use should probably be avoided in children with cardiac conduction defects, and caution is appropriate in children with a history of cardiac, hepatic or renal disease. Use frequently exacerbates myoclonic and absence seizures. Side effects are rare but include leucopenia, dystonia and hyponatraemia, and an overdose can cause drowsiness, respiratory depression and convulsions. Babies may also manifest vomiting, urinary retention, tachycardia and dilated pupils. It is not widely used in neonates; limitations include low activity of cytochrome CYP3A4 at birth (activity increases ~20% of adult values at 1 month) and of epoxide hydrolase enzymes as well as reduced renal elimination.

Maternal use during pregnancy is associated with a slightly increased risk of microcephaly and spina bifida. Women are advised to take a folic acid supplement (5 mg daily) prior to, and for 12 weeks after, conception. Serious malformation is otherwise uncommon, and although some mild dysmorphic features are often detectable, there is no evidence that exposure before birth has any impact on the child's later cognitive development. The baby may be hypoprothrombinaemic at birth, but this bleeding tendency is corrected by giving the baby at least 100 micrograms/kg (usually 1 mg) of intramuscular vitamin K (q.v.) at birth. Small amounts of the drug appear in breast milk, but maternal treatment is not a contraindication to breastfeeding because the baby will only receive 5% of the maternal dose on a weight-for-weight basis.

Drug interactions

Concurrent treatment with erythromycin, isoniazid, lamotrigine or valproate (q.v.) causes a rise in the serum level of carbamazepine. The use of two anticonvulsants always increases the risk of drug toxicity.

Treatment

Experience in neonates is limited. Give 5 mg/kg every 12 hours. A larger dose may be necessary in babies over 2 weeks old (maximum intake 15 mg/kg every 12 hours), but larger doses should be introduced slowly. Where oral treatment is not possible, a slightly larger dose of the oral suspension can be given into the rectum after dilution with an equal volume of water to minimise the laxative effect of the standard suspension's high osmolarity (a dose that can probably be repeated if the baby passes a stool within 2 hours of administration).

Blood levels

The optimum anticonvulsant plasma concentration is 4–12 mg/l (1 mg/l=4.23 micromol/l). Levels should be taken shortly before treatment was due. It is, however, important to realise that the drug level in a young baby can take a week to stabilise. Levels above 30 mg/l cause severe toxicity.

Supply

100 ml of a 20 mg/ml caramel-flavoured, sugar-free carbamazepine suspension costs £2 (it also contains 25 mg/ml of propylene glycol). 125 mg suppositories (equivalent to 100 mg orally) cost £1.60 each.

Continued on p. 127

References
(see also the Cochrane review on common antiepileptic drugs in pregnancy)

Gaily E, Kantola-Sorsa E, Hiilesmaa V, *et al.* Normal intelligence in children with prenatal exposure to carbamazepine. *Neurology* 2004;**62**:28–32.

Jentink J, Dolk H, Loane MA, *et al.* Intrauterine exposure to carbamazepine and specific congenital malformations: systematic review and case-control study. *Br Med J* 2010;**341**:c6581.

Kini U, Adab N, Vinten J, *et al.* Dysmorphic features: an important clue to the diagnosis and severity of fetal anticonvulsant syndromes. *Arch Dis Child Fetal Neonatal Ed* 2006;**91**:F80–5.

Korinthenberg R, Haug C, Hannak D. The metabolism of carbamazepine to CBZ-10,11-epoxide in children from the newborn age to adolescence. *Neuropediatrics* 1994;**25**:214–6.

Miles ME, Lawless ST, Tennison MB, *et al.* Rapid loading of critically ill patients with carbamazepine suspension. *Pediatrics* 1990;**86**:263–6.

Morrow J, Russell A, Guthrie E, *et al.* Malformation risks of antiepileptic drugs in pregnancy: a prospective study from the UK Epilepsy and Pregnancy Register. *J Neurol Neurosurg Psychiatry* 2006;**77**:193–8.

Morselli PL, Franco-Morselli R, Bossi L. Clinical pharmacokinetics in newborns and infants: age related differences and therapeutic implications. *Clin Pharmacokinet* 1980;**5**:485–527. (See particularly p. 507.)

Singh B, Singh P, al Hifze I, *et al.* Treatment of neonatal seizures with carbamazepine. *J Child Neurol* 1996;**11**:378–82.

Tulloch JK, Carr RR, Ensom MH. A systematic review of the pharmacokinetics of antiepileptic drugs in neonates with refractory seizures. *J Pediatr Pharmacol Ther* 2012;**17**:31–44.

Veuvonen PJ, Tokola O. Bioavailability of rectally administered carbamazepine mixture. *Br J Pharmacol* 1987;**24**:839–40.

Use

Carglumic acid is primarily used to treat N-acetylglutamate synthase (NAGS) deficiency, a rare urea cycle disorder. It may also reduce ammonia in some patients with branched-chain organic acidaemias.

Biochemistry

N-Acetylglutamate is the natural activator of carbamoyl phosphate synthetase (CPS I), which is the first step in the urea cycle. Patients with NAGS deficiency present with hyperammonaemia in the neonatal period or later in life. Carglumic acid (N-carbamoyl-L-glutamic acid or N-carbamylglutamate) is a synthetic analogue of N-acetylglutamate and has been used since the early 1980s to control hyperammonaemia in patients with NAGS deficiency. After starting carglumic acid, most patients with this disorder tolerate a normal protein intake when they are well, although other measures may be needed, particularly when they are ill. A few patients with partial CPS I deficiency may also respond to carglumic acid.

In branched-chain organic (methylmalonic, propionic and isovaleric) acidaemias, hyperammonaemia is thought to result, at least partly, from inhibition of NAGS, and carglumic acid reduces the ammonia concentration in some, but not all, children with one of these disorders.

Investigating neonatal hyperammonaemia

Plasma ammonia levels do not normally exceed 150 μmol/l, and levels above 200 μmol/l strongly suggest the presence of an inborn error of metabolism. Further investigations should include analysis of plasma amino acids, urine organic acids and urine orotic acid. NAGS is a rare cause of hyperammonaemia and is hard to distinguish from CPS deficiency. A rapid response to carglumic acid strongly suggests the diagnosis: if the drug is available, it can be given while other forms of treatment are being set up.

Specialist advice

Specialist advice on a range of inborn errors of metabolism is available from the British Inherited Metabolic Disease Group (BIMDG) via their website (www.bimdg.org.uk).

> **Note: Treatment with this product should only be initiated after consultation with a specialist centre.**

Treatment

Trial of responsiveness: A trial dose of 200 mg/kg (oral or nasogastric) has been recommended in patients with hyperammonaemia, followed by monitoring of the plasma ammonia concentration every 2 hours; further doses may be given if there is a partial response. It is, however, important not to delay other treatment of hyperammonaemia by promptly administering sodium benzoate, sodium phenylbutyrate and arginine (q.v.) and, in severe cases, beginning haemodialysis.

Long-term management of NAGS deficiency: The total daily dose is usually between 10 and 100 mg/kg a day. It should be given in divided doses two to four times a day before food. During illness, it may be helpful to double the dose; no intravenous preparation is available.

Monitoring

Plasma ammonia and amino acids should be monitored, as in other urea cycle disorders, aiming to keep the plasma ammonia concentration below 60 μmol/l and the plasma glutamine level below 800 μmol/l while maintaining a normal essential amino acid profile.

Supply and administration

Supplies of carglumic acid (Carbaglu®) are available from Orphan Europe. This product was awarded EU marketing authorisation in 2003 and was also identified by the FDA in America for 'fast track' approval as an orphan drug in 2007. The product is currently only available in 200 mg tablet form and in packs of 5 or 60 tablets. The tablets currently cost £60 each.

Continued on p. 129

References

Guffon N, Schiff M, Cheillan D, *et al*. Neonatal hyperammonaemia: the *N*-Carbamoyl-L-glutamic acid test. *J Pediatr* 2005;**147**: 260–2.

Häberle J. Role of carglumic acid in the treatment of acute hyperammonemia due to N-acetylglutamate synthase deficiency. *Ther Clin Risk Manag* 2011;**7**:327–32.

Jones S, Reed CA, Vijay S, *et al*. N-carbamylglutamate for neonatal hyperammonaemia in propionic acidaemia. *J Inherit Metab Dis* 2008;**31** suppl 2:S219–22.

Kasapkara CS, Ezgu FS, Okur I, *et al*. N-carbamylglutamate treatment for acute neonatal hyperammonemia in isovaleric acidemia. *Eur J Pediatr* 2011;**170**:799–801.

Kuchler G, Raboier D, Poggi-Travert F, *et al*. Therapeutic use of carbamylglutamate in the case of carbamoyl-phosphate synthetase deficiency. *J Inherit Metab Dis* 1996;**19**: 220–2.

Wijburg FA, Nassogne M-C. Disorders of the urea cycle and related enzymes. In: Saudubray J-M, van den Berghe G, Walter JH, eds. *Inborn metabolic diseases. Diagnosis and treatment*, 5th ed. Berlin: Springer-Verlag, 2012: pp 263–72.

Use

L-Carnitine is a naturally occurring substance that is required for the transport of fatty acids into mitochondria. It is used in the management of a range of inborn errors of metabolism associated with carnitine deficiency.

Nutritional factors

Carnitine (β-hydroxy-γ-trimethylaminobutyric acid) is a small water-soluble molecule. Most of the body's carnitine is found in skeletal and cardiac muscle. It may be synthesised in the body from lysine and methionine, although synthetic pathways are relatively immature at birth. Most is usually provided by dietary red meat and dairy produce. Human milk and whey-based formula milks all contain l-carnitine; soya-based preparations are usually, but not always, supplemented. Dialysis and defects of renal tubular reabsorption (Fanconi syndrome) may cause secondary deficiency.

Pharmacology

Primary systemic carnitine transporter deficiency is a rare autosomal recessive condition resulting from a defect in the uptake of carnitine across cell membranes. It usually presents with hypoketotic hypoglycaemia, cardiomyopathy or myopathy and is generally associated with a total plasma carnitine level of less than $10\,\mu mol/l$. In countries with expanding newborn screening, it may be diagnosed by tandem mass spectrometry.

Secondary systemic carnitine deficiency occurs in organic acidaemias and fatty oxidation defects. In these conditions, carnitine binds to accumulating intermediate metabolites and is excreted with them in the urine. Organic acidaemias usually present with encephalopathy, often within a few days of birth. Fatty acid oxidation (FAO) defects present in the neonatal period or later with hypoglycaemic encephalopathy or with a cardiac or skeletal myopathy. All these conditions are recessively inherited, and their management should, wherever possible, be guided by a consultant experienced in the management of metabolic disease.

Carnitine is of proven value in primary carnitine deficiency. Use also forms part of the standard strategy for managing organic acidaemias (such as isovaleric, methylmalonic and propionic acidaemias and glutaric aciduria type I). Use in FAO defects is more controversial, although it is often used in the decompensated patient to detoxify acyl-CoA intermediates and replenish the intramitochondrial carnitine pool; long-term supplementation has been questioned in long-chain FAO defects due to accumulation of long-chain fatty acylcarnitines that may cause cardiac arrhythmias. Reports of supplementation in patients on dialysis, on valproate (q.v.) or with Fanconi syndrome have suggested only variable or equivocal benefit. Treatment should always be with the naturally occurring L isomer and not the racemic (DL) mixture. The main dose-related adverse effects of oral treatment are nausea, vomiting, abdominal cramp, diarrhoea and a fish-like smell. Controlled trials in preterm babies (either orally or parenterally fed) have failed to show that routine supplementation reduces apnoea, makes episodic hypoglycaemia less common or improves growth. Women requiring carnitine supplementation should not stop treatment during pregnancy or lactation.

Treatment

Urgent intravenous (IV) treatment: Give 4 mg/kg/hour (0.2 ml/hour of the solution made up as described in 'Supply and administration') as a continuous IV infusion during acute metabolic decompensation. An initial loading dose is no longer generally considered necessary, but if required could be given by infusing 5 ml of the same solution over 30 minutes.

Oral treatment: The usual dose is 25 mg/kg four times a day.

Compatibility

While formal compatibility tests do not seem to have been undertaken, problems have not been encountered when carnitine is terminally co-infused with arginine, sodium benzoate and sodium phenylbutyrate.

Supply and administration

A cherry-flavoured oral paediatric solution dispensed in single-dose bottles of 20 ml (containing 300 mg/ml of L-carnitine) is available commercially costing £21 per bottle. It contains sorbitol and sucrose. A sugar-free oral solution is available in some countries. For IV use, 5 ml ampoules containing 1 g (200 mg/ml) of L-carnitine, which costs £12 each, are available. Take 1 ml of this

Continued on p. 131

preparation for each kilogram that the baby weighs, dilute to 10 ml with 0.9% sodium chloride and infuse at a rate of 0.2 ml/hour. The product is stable at room temperature for 24 hours after reconstitution in this way.

References

(See also the relevant Cochrane reviews)

Kölker S, Christensen E, Leonard JV, *et al.* Diagnosis and management of glutaric aciduria type I – revised recommendations. *J Inherit Metab Dis* 2011;**34**:677–94.

Lee NC, Tang NL, Chien YH, *et al.* Diagnoses of newborns and mothers with carnitine uptake defects through newborn screening. *Mol Genet Metab* 2010;**100**:46–50.

Morris AAM, Spiekerkoetter U. Disorders of mitochondrial fatty acid oxidation and related metabolic pathways. In: Saudubray J-M, van den Berghe G, Walter JH, eds. *Inborn metabolic diseases. Diagnosis and treatment*, 5th ed. Berlin: Springer-Verlag, 2012: pp. 201–16.

Rector RS, Ibdah JA. Fatty acid oxidation disorders: maternal health and neonatal outcomes. *Semin Fetal Neonatal Med* 2010;**15**:122–8.

Scaglia F, Longo N. Primary and secondary alterations of neonatal carnitine metabolism. *Semin Perinatol* 1999;**23**:152–61.

Whitfield J, Smith T, Solluhub H, *et al.* Clinical effects of L-carnitine supplementation on apnea and growth in very low birth weight infants. *Pediatrics* 2003;**111**:477–82. [RCT]

Wilcken B. Fatty acid oxidation disorders: outcome and long-term prognosis. *J Inherit Metab Dis* 2010;**33**:501–6.

Zelnik N, Isler N, Goez H, *et al.* Vigabatrin, lamotrigine, topiramate and serum carnitine levels. *Pediatr Neurol* 2008;**39**:18–21.

Use

Caspofungin is expensive, but it is sometimes the antifungal drug of choice when systemic infection with a *Candida* organism is resistant to fluconazole (q.v.) and when *Aspergillus* infection is resistant to high-dose amphotericin B (q.v.).

Pharmacology

Caspofungin was first licensed for clinical use in 2001 and was the first of a new class of antifungals called echinocandins. Since then, two other members, micafungin (q.v.) and anidulafungin, of the class have emerged. Caspofungin works by inhibiting the synthesis of β-(1,3)-D-glucan, an integral component of fungal cell walls. It demonstrates *in vitro* and *in vivo* activity against *Aspergillus* and a range of *Candida* species, including *C. albicans*, *C. parapsilosis*, *C. tropicalis* and *C. glabrata*, and in a controlled trial published in 2002, adults with invasive candidiasis responded to caspofungin better than they did to amphotericin. There were also fewer side effects. It is not effective in cryptococcal infection.

There are, however, very few published reports as yet of this drug's use in very young children, and the manufacturer is not yet ready to recommend use in children less than 3 months old. Caspofungin was found to be embryotoxic and to interfere with fetal bone formation at standard doses in pregnant rodents, but nothing, understandably, is yet known about the effect of its use in women during pregnancy or lactation (although poor oral bioavailability should limit exposure in the breastfed infant).

Caspofungin blood levels decline in a polyphasic manner, the brief α-phase in adults being followed by a 9–11 hour β-phase and a 40–50 hour γ-phase as widespread tissue redistribution is followed by slow hydrolysis, acetylation and chemical degradation before the resultant metabolites are finally excreted in the urine and faeces. Little pharmacokinetic data in neonates has yet been published, but the volume of distribution in infancy would seem to be even higher than it is in adult life while the β-phase half-life is shorter, making a rather higher dose necessary. Penetration of caspofungin into the CSF is poor in children and adults, but adequate levels in neonatal CSF have been reported when used to eradicate shunt-associated *Candida* meningitis.

Drug interactions

Patients taking any of the hepatic enzyme-inducing drugs, such as carbamazepine, dexamethasone, nelfinavir, nevirapine, phenytoin and rifampicin, probably need to be given a rather higher daily dose because of enhanced drug elimination.

Treatment

Relatively little is known about treatment in the first year of life and even less in the neonatal period. The most appropriate dose in the neonate and infant less than 3 months is probably 25 mg/m² once daily as an infusion made up as described under 'Supply and administration' and given over 1 hour. The dose is increased to 50 mg/m² once daily in infants between 3 and 12 months.

Treatment was continued for 2–3 weeks in most reports published to date with fungal clearance from blood being seen within the first few days of treatment. The dose given does not normally need to be reduced in patients in renal failure, but it is probably not wise to continue giving high-dose treatment to patients showing signs of liver failure.

Supply and administration

Caspofungin comes as a powder ready for reconstitution in 50 mg vials that cost £330 each. Vials are stored at 4°C but brought to room temperature before use. The powder is dissolved in 10.5 ml of 0.9% sodium chloride. For accurate low-dose administration, further dilute the resultant solution to 25 ml with more 0.9% sodium chloride to obtain a solution containing 2 mg/ml of caspofungin, and use this within 24 hours. Caspofungin is incompatible with glucose and has to be given into a line that only contains 0.9% sodium chloride or compound sodium lactate.

References

Belet N, Ciftçi E, Ince E, *et al*. Caspofungin treatment of two infants with persistent fungaemia due to *Candida lipolytica*. *Scand J Infect Dis* 2006;**38**:559–62.

Dodds AES, Lewis ES, Lewis LJS. Pharmacology of systematic antifungal agents. *Clin Infect Dis* 2006;**43**:S29–39.

Continued on p. 133

Fisher BT, Zaoutis T. Caspofungin for the treatment of pediatric fungal infections. *Pediatr Infect Dis J.* 2008;**27**:1099–101.

Gamock-Jones KP, Keam SJ. Caspofungin: in pediatric patients with fungal infections. *Pediatr Drugs* 2009;**11**:259–69.

Jans J, Brüggemann RJ, Christmann V, *et al.* Favorable outcome of neonatal cerebrospinal fluid shunt-associated *Candida meningitis* with caspofungin. *Antimicrob Agents Chemother* 2013;**57**:2391–3.

Manzar S, Kamat M, Pyati S. Caspofungin for refractory candidemia in neonates. *Pediatr Infect Dis J* 2006;**25**:282–3.

Natarajan G, Lulic BM, Rongkavilit C, *et al.* Experience with caspofungin in the treatment of persistent fungemia in neonates. *J Perinatol* 2005;**25**:770–7.

Odio CM, Araya R, Pinto LE, *et al.* Caspofungin therapy in neonates with invasive candidiasis. *Pediatr Infect Dis J* 2004;**23**:1093–7.

Saez-Lorens X, Macias M, Maiya P, *et al.* Pharmacokinetics and safety of caspofungin in neonates and infants less than 3 months of age. *Antiomicrob Agents Chemother* 2009;**53**:869–75.

Smith PB, Steinbach WJ, Cotton CM, *et al.* Caspofungin for the treatment of azole resistant candidemia in a premature infant. *J Perinatol* 2007;**27**:127–9.

Yalaz M, Akisu M, Hilmioglu S, *et al.* Successful caspofungin treatment of multi-drug resistant Candida parapsilosis septicaemia in an extremely low birth weight neonate. *Mycoses* 2006;**49**:242–5.

Use

Cefalexin is one of the few cephalosporin antibiotics that can be given orally. It should only be used in the neonatal period when the sensitivity of the organism under treatment is known. Cefuroxime (q.v.) is a closely related antibiotic with slightly different sensitivities suitable for intravenous (IV) or intramuscular (IM) use.

History

Stimulated by the discovery of penicillin, many other moulds were soon studied to see if they had antimicrobial properties. This soon led Giuseppe Brotzu, Professor of Hygiene at the University of Cagliari, to discover *Acremonium chrysogenum* (formerly called *Cephalosporium acremonium*) in 1948 in a sewage outlet in Sardinia. Extracts of the fungus were soon shown to be active against a range of Gram-negative, as well as Gram-positive, bacteria. However, it took 12 years of further work before the team working with Howard Florey in Oxford had a product (called cephalosporin C, because it had been isolated as a pure crystalline sodium salt) that was ready for clinical use. Its structure was similar to that of penicillin, but it was *not* destroyed by β-lactamase-producing bacteria. Plans to market cephalosporin C were thwarted when Beechams brought methicillin onto the market in 1960, but a wide range of semi-synthetic analogues were developed over the next 20 years.

Cefalexin was one of the first cephalosporins that appeared in 1967. Various 'second-generation' products, including cefoxitin and cefuroxime (q.v.) with a wider spectrum of antibiotic activity, arrived 5 years later, and a third generation of very broad-spectrum cephalosporins, including cefotaxime, ceftazidime and ceftriaxone (q.v.), followed between 1976 and 1979. Fourth-generation cephalosporins are now being used in adults but have yet to find much of a role in neonates.

Pharmacology

Cefalexin is reasonably active against nearly all Gram-positive cocci (including group B streptococci) and most Gram-negative cocci other than enterococci. Gram-positive rods are relatively resistant. While the drug is relatively resistant to staphylococcal β-lactamase, it has no useful activity against methicillin-resistant strains. It should not be used for infections in which *Haemophilus influenzae* is, or is likely to be, implicated or used as an alternative to penicillin for syphilis. Although most *Bacteroides* species are susceptible to cefalexin, this is not true of *Bacteroides fragilis*. Cefalexin has no useful activity against *Listeria*, *Citrobacter* and *Enterobacter* or against *Serratia* and *Pseudomonas* species, and it only penetrates CSF poorly.

Cefalexin, unlike most cephalosporins, is acid resistant and well absorbed when taken by mouth, although absorption is delayed and incomplete when the drug is taken on a full stomach. The dose recommended here takes this into account. Oral treatment usually only has a modest effect on the balance of other bacteria in the gut. Cefalexin is actively excreted by the kidney, the plasma half-life falling from 5 hours at birth to about 2½ hours at 4 weeks. Children more than a year old clear cefuroxime from their plasma almost as fast as adults ($t\frac{1}{2} = 0.9$ hours). Dosage intervals should be extended in babies with severe renal failure.

Problems associated with treatment are uncommon but the same as for all cephalosporins, as discussed in the monograph on ceftazidime (q.v.). Only modest amounts cross the placenta, and there is no evidence of teratogenicity. The baby ingests less than 1% of the weight-related maternal dose when the mother takes this drug while breastfeeding.

Treatment

Give 25 mg/kg by mouth once every 12 hours in the first week of life, every 8 hours in babies 1–3 weeks old and every 6 hours in babies older than this.

Supply

Cefalexin is available as a 25 mg/ml oral suspension. Reconstitute the granules or powder with water and use the resultant suspension within 10 days. 100 ml of the sugar-free non-proprietary product costs £1.40. There are no parenteral formulations available.

References

Boothman R, Kerr MM, Marshall MJ, *et al.* Absorption and excretion of cephalexin in the newborn infant. *Arch Dis Child* 1973;**48**:147–50.

Chen AE, Carroll KC, Diener-West M, *et al.* Randomized controlled trial of cephalexin versus clindamycin for uncomplicated pediatric skin infections. *Pediatrics* 2011;**127**:e573–80. [RCT]

Continued on p. 135

Creatsas G, Pavlatos M, Lolis D, *et al*. A study of the kinetics of cephalosporin and cephalexin in pregnancy. *Curr Med Res Opin* 1980;**7**:43–7.

Disney FA, Dillon H, Blumer JL, *et al*. Cephalexin and penicillin in the treatment of group A beta-hemolytic streptococcal sore throat. *Am J Dis Child* 1992;**146**:1324–9. [RCT]

Kefetzis D, Siafas C, Georgakopoulos P, *et al*. Passage of cephalosporins and amoxicillin into the breast milk. *Acta Paediatr Scand* 1981;**70**:285–8.

McCracken GH Jr, Ginsburg CM, Clahsen JC, *et al*. Pharmacologic evaluation of orally administered antibiotics in infants and children: effect of feeding on bioavailability. *Pediatrics* 1978;**62**:738–43.

Tetzlaff TR, McCracken GH Jr, Thomas, ML. Bioavailability of cephalexin in children: relationship to drug formulations and meals. *J Pediatr* 1978;**92**:292–4.

Use

Cefotaxime is a broad-spectrum cephalosporin largely reserved for empirical use in the management of meningitis and sepsis. It should not be used on its own if *Listeria* or *Pseudomonas* infection is a possibility.

Pharmacology

Cefotaxime is a bactericidal antibiotic introduced into clinical use in 1976 with the same range of activity against Gram-positive organisms as most other third-generation cephalosporins and exceptional activity against most Gram-negative organisms. It is not active against *Listeria monocytogenes*, enterococci or *Pseudomonas*. Tissue penetration is good, and CSF penetration is usually more than adequate when there is meningeal inflammation. Maternal use presents no problem during pregnancy. Use during lactation exposes the baby to considerably less than 1% of the weight-adjusted maternal dose. The neonatal half-life (2–6 hours) varies with gestation and with postnatal age. The drug's primary metabolite, desacetylcefotaxime, which also displays antibiotic activity, has a neonatal half-life twice as long as this. Most of the drug is renally excreted.

Cefotaxime is widely considered to be the antibiotic of choice in the management of most cases of Gram-negative neonatal meningitis at present although, for most infections, there is probably little to choose between cefotaxime and ceftazidime (q.v.). Ceftriaxone (q.v.) is sometimes used in this situation when there is no risk of jaundice because it only has to be given once a day. There is some evidence to suggest that the neurological outcome in proven bacterial meningitis other than that caused by *Neisseria meningitidis may* be improved by the simultaneous early administration of dexamethasone (q.v.).

Neonatal use of the third-generation cephalosporins such as cefotaxime and ceftazidime should probably be limited to the management of proven Gram-negative septicaemia and meningitis because several units have reported the emergence of resistant strains of *Enterobacter cloacae* when cefotaxime is used regularly in the first-line management of possible neonatal sepsis (including coagulase-negative staphylococcal infection). The same potential exists with other organisms (e.g. *Serratia* and *Pseudomonas* species) where inducible β-lactamase production is a possibility.

Diagnosing meningitis

The signs of meningitis are seldom as clear cut in the neonatal period as they are in later childhood and (since babies with meningitis do not always have a positive blood culture) the organism may be missed if a lumbar puncture (LP) is not done when blood is obtained for culture. Even if it is delayed until the baby has been stabilised, an LP should still be done (and done within 2 hours of initiating antibiotic treatment to be sure of isolating the organism), since diagnosis will often influence decisions regarding treatment. Flex the hips and knees, but do not bend the neck to limit respiratory embarrassment. A Gram stain will usually reveal meningitis, but the cell count seen in normal babies overlaps with that seen in babies with early meningitis. The same is true of CSF protein and glucose levels. A combination of benzylpenicillin and an aminoglycoside is widely used in early-onset meningitis of uncertain origin, but cefotaxime should replace benzylpenicillin if Gram-negative organisms are seen (ceftazidime being more appropriate if *Pseudomonas* infection is suspected). Meropenem (q.v.) should be held in reserve for use when a β-lactamase-resistant organism is suspected. Penicillin can replace ampicillin in group B streptococcal infection. Vancomycin should be reserved for proven staphylococcal infection. Viral culture should always be undertaken if no bacteria are seen. Confirm sterility with a second LP after 24–48 hours if the response is uncertain. Meningitis (whatever its cause) remains a notifiable condition in the United Kingdom.

Treatment

Severe neonatal infection should be treated with 50 mg/kg slowly intravenous (IV) (or intramuscular (IM)) once every 12 hours in the first week of life, every 8 hours in babies 1–3 weeks old and once every 6 hours in babies older than this. The dosage interval should be increased in babies with severe renal failure. A single 100 mg/kg IV or IM dose can be used (instead of ceftriaxone) to treat neonatal gonococcal eye infection.

Supply

Stock 500 mg vials, which should be protected from light, cost £2.25. The dry powder should be reconstituted with 2.3 ml of water for injection to give a solution containing 200 mg/ml.

Continued on p. 137

References

Clark RH, Bloom BT, Spitzer AR, *et al.* Empiric use of ampicillin and cefotaxime, compared to ampicillin and gentamicin, for neonates at risk for sepsis is associated with an increased risk of neonatal death. *Pediatrics* 2006;**117**:67–74.

de Man P, Verhoeven BAN, Verbrugh HA, *et al.* An antibiotic policy to prevent emergence of resistant bacilli. *Lancet* 2000;**355**:973–8.

Heath PT, Nik Yusoff NK, Baker CJ. Neonatal meningitis. *Arch Dis Child Fetal Neonatal Ed* 2003;**88**:F173–8. (See also pp. F179–84.)

Kafetzis DA, Brater DC, Kapiki AN, *et al.* Treatment of severe neonatal infections with cefotaxime: efficacy and pharmacokinetics. *J Pediatr* 1982;**100**:438–9.

Kearns GL, Jacobs RF, Thomas BR, *et al.* Cefotaxime and desacetylcefotaxime pharmacokinetics in very low birth weight neonates. *J Pediatr* 1989;**114**:461–7.

Muller-Pebody B, Johnson AP, Heath PT, *et al.* Empirical treatment of neonatal sepsis: are the current guidelines adequate? *Arch Dis Child Fetal Neonatal Ed* 2011;**96**:F4–8.

Trang JM, Jacobs RF, Kearns GL, *et al.* Cefotaxime and desacetylcefotaxime pharmacokinetics in infants and children with meningitis. *Antimicrob Agents Chemother* 1985;**28**:791–5.

Use

Ceftazidime is used in the management of Gram-negative (including *Pseudomonas aeruginosa*) infection, although cefotaxime (q.v.) is more often used for Gram-negative meningitis. The frequent use of any third-generation cephalosporin may rapidly lead to many babies becoming colonised by resistant organisms and can also increase the risk of invasive candidiasis in babies weighing less than 1 kg at birth.

Pharmacology

Ceftazidime is a valuable third-generation bactericidal cephalosporin first patented in 1979. It is resistant to most β-lactamase enzymes and has good *in vitro* activity against a wide range of Gram-negative bacteria, including *P. aeruginosa*. It is reasonably active against group A and group B streptococci and against *Streptococcus pneumoniae* but only has limited efficacy with most other Gram-positive organisms. Ceftazidime is not effective against enterococci, *Listeria, Helicobacter* or *Bacteroides fragilis*. The widespread regular use of this (or any other) cephalosporin can result in an increasing proportion of babies becoming colonised with enterococci and with other potentially dangerous organisms. Generalised fungal infection is also a potential hazard. Ceftazidime should not, therefore, be used on its own in the management of neonatal infection due to an unidentified organism. Ceftazidime is widely distributed in most body tissues including respiratory secretions, ascitic fluid and cerebrospinal fluid (CSF), although CSF penetration is rather variable unless the meninges are inflamed. There is no clear evidence that aminoglycosides are synergistic.

Ceftazidime crosses the placenta freely, but there is no evidence of teratogenicity. Treatment during lactation is equally acceptable since this exposes the baby to less than 1% of the maternal dose on a weight-adjusted basis. The drug is not absorbed when taken by mouth and is excreted unchanged in the urine. The half-life is 4–10 hours at birth, but half this in babies more than a week old.

Adverse effects are not common with *any* of the cephalosporin antibiotics in the neonatal period but can occur. Hypersensitivity reactions are occasionally seen in older patients (sometimes overlapping with hypersensitivity to penicillin). Rashes, phlebitis and leucopenia have all been reported. Diarrhoea can progress to pseudomembranous colitis, due to an overgrowth of antibiotic-resistant bowel organisms, such as *Clostridium difficile*, and if this is not recognised and treated with metronidazole (q.v.), this could prove fatal. A very high blood level, usually because of a failure to reduce dose frequency when the patient is in renal failure, can cause CNS toxicity and fits (as is true of all the β-lactam antibiotics). Bleeding due to hypoproteinaemia (easily reversed by giving vitamin K) has been associated with the prolonged use of cephalosporins in malnourished patients. Ceftriaxone is, on theoretical grounds, the cephalosporin most likely to cause such a problem of the products listed in this compendium.

Some 5% of patients given a cephalosporin develop a transient positive Coombs test (and this can interfere with the crossmatching of blood), but frank haemolytic anaemia is extremely uncommon. Tests may wrongly suggest that there is glucose in the urine because of interference with the alkaline copper reduction test, and interference with the Jaffé reaction may affect the measurement of creatinine (giving a false high reading that can be particularly misleading when renal failure is a concern).

Treatment

Give 25 mg/kg of ceftazidime intravenous (IV) or deep intramuscular (IM) once a day in the first week of life, once every 12 hours in babies 1–3 weeks old and once every 8 hours in babies older than this. Doses of 50 mg/kg should be used in the treatment of suspected or proven meningitis. The dosage interval should be increased in babies with renal failure.

Supply and administration

Ceftazidime is supplied as a powder in 500 mg vials under reduced pressure costing £4.40 each. For IM administration, add 1.6 ml of water to provide a solution containing 250 mg/ml. The bubbles of carbon dioxide will disappear after 1–2 minutes. Reconstitute for IV use with 4.6 ml of water for injection to produce a solution containing 100 mg/ml. Ceftazidime should not be put in the same syringe, or administered in a giving set at the same time, as vancomycin or an aminoglycoside.

Continued on p. 139

References

Bégué P, Michel B, Chasalette JP, *et al.* Etude clinique multicentrique et pharmacocinétique de la ceftazidime chez l'enfant et le nouveau-né. *Pathol Biol* 1996;**34**:525–9.

Cotton CM, McDobald S, Stoll B, *et al.* The association of third-generation cephalosporin use and invasive candidiasis in extremely low birth-weight infants. *Pediatrics* 2006;**118**:717–22.

de Louvois J, Dagan R, Tessin I. A comparison of ceftazidime and aminoglycoside based regimens as empirical treatment of 1316 cases of suspected sepsis in the newborn. *Eur J Pediatr* 1991;**151**:876–84.

Soyer OU, Ozen C, Tiras U, *et al.* Anaphylaxis in a neonate caused by ceftazidime. *Allergy* 2010;**65**:1486–7.

Tessin I, Trollfors B, Thringer K, *et al.* Concentrations of ceftazidime, tobramycin and ampicillin in the cerebrospinal fluid of newborn infants. *Eur J Pediatr* 1989;**148**:678–81.

van den Anker JN, Hop WCJ, Schoemaker RC, *et al.* Ceftazidime pharmacokinetics in preterm infants: effect of postnatal age and postnatal exposure to indomethacin. *Br J Clin Pharmacol* 1995;**40**:439–43.

van den Anker JN, Schoemaker RC, Hop WCJ, *et al.* Ceftazidime pharmacokinetics in preterm infants: effects of renal function and gestational age. *Clin Pharmacol Ther* 1995;**58**:650–9.

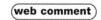

Use

Ceftriaxone is a versatile and useful 'third-generation' cephalosporin that only needs to be given once a day. It should only be given with great caution to any baby with a high unconjugated bilirubin level.

Pharmacology

Ceftriaxone is a β-lactamase-resistant cephalosporin first patented in 1979 that is active, like cefotaxime and ceftazidime (q.v.), against some important Gram-positive and most Gram-negative bacteria. Because of good CSF penetration, even when the meninges are not inflamed, it is now often used as a simpler alternative to cefotaxime in the treatment of meningitis due to organisms other than *Listeria monocytogenes* and faecal streptococci (enterococci). It is also used to treat *Salmonella typhi* infection in countries where this organism is becoming resistant to chloramphenicol (q.v.) and to treat gonorrhoea (*Neisseria gonorrhoeae* infection).

The drug is excreted unaltered almost equally in the bile and urine, so treatment does not normally require adjustment unless there are both renal and hepatic failures. It has a longer half-life than other cephalosporins; the plasma half-life falls from 15 hours at birth to a value only a little in excess of that found in adults (7 hours) over some 2–4 weeks. It crosses the placenta and also appears in amniotic fluid. There is no evidence of teratogenicity in animals, but only limited information regarding its safety during human pregnancy. Very little appears in breast milk: the baby of any mother treated during lactation would be exposed to less than 1% of the maternal dose on a weight-adjusted basis, and little of this would be absorbed.

Ceftriaxone can displace bilirubin from its plasma albumin binding sites, thereby increasing the amount of free unconjugated bilirubin. This initially made many clinicians reluctant to recommend its use in babies less than 6 weeks old, and the drug should only be used in babies at risk of developing unconjugated hyperbilirubinaemia if a lower than usual threshold is adopted for starting phototherapy. High doses often cause a transient precipitate to form in the biliary tract, and small asymptomatic renal stones occasionally form with sustained use. Ceftriaxone has very occasionally caused severe neonatal erythroderma ('red baby' syndrome). Severe, potentially lethal haemolysis is another very rare complication. Other problems are very uncommon but the same as for all cephalosporins, as discussed in the monograph on ceftazidime.

Gonorrhoea

The incidence of this sexually transmitted disease, which can cause vaginal discharge, dysuria and heavy or inter-menstrual bleeding, varies greatly in different parts of the world, and a single 250 mg intramuscular (IM) dose of ceftriaxone is now widely used to treat maternal infection. If it is not possible to test for possible co-infection with *Chlamydia*, it may be appropriate to give a single 1 g dose of azithromycin (q.v.) as well by mouth. There is also a high risk of reinfection unless sexual partners are also seen and treated. Babies run a 30–50% risk of becoming infected at birth and a 4% chance of developing of serious eye infection in the absence of prompt prophylaxis. The presence of intracellular Gram-negative diplococci on a conjunctival Gram stain is virtually diagnostic. The eyes become increasingly purulent and inflamed, and sight can be put at risk if treatment is not started promptly. Untreated discharge from the eye can also cause cross infection. Generalised septicaemia can occur, and this can cause a destructive septic arthritis if early signs are not sought with diligence.

Drug interactions

Never give ceftriaxone intravenous (IV) to any child who is being, or who has recently been, given any IV fluid (such as TPN or Ringer lactate) that contains calcium – precipitation could be potentially lethal. Use cefotaxime instead.

Treatment

Neonatal gonococcal eye infection: A single 125 mg IM dose was shown to be a simple and very effective treatment strategy in one African trial (use 40 mg/kg in any low birthweight baby). Consider giving oral azithromycin or erythromycin (q.v.) as well if there is a possibility of chlamydial co-infection.

Other sepsis: Give 50 mg/kg IM or, preferably, IV once a day for 7 days. Use with great caution in young babies with unconjugated jaundice. Use a 75 mg/kg dose for meningitis in babies over 4 weeks old.

Continued on p. 141

Supply and administration

250 mg vials cost £2.40. They contain 0.9 mmol of sodium. Dissolve the powder in this vial in 4.8 ml of water for injection to obtain a 50 mg/ml solution for IV administration. Infuse this slowly over an hour if the infant is jaundiced; otherwise, it may be given by injection over 2–4 minutes. To make the IM (but *not* IV) injection less painful, dissolve the 250 mg of powder with 0.9 ml of plain 1% lidocaine hydrochloride to make a 250 mg/ml solution.

References

(see the Cochrane review of gonococcal infection in pregnancy)

Duke T, Michael A, Mokela D, *et al*. Chloramphenicol or ceftriaxone, or both, as treatment for meningitis in developing countries? *Arch Dis Child* 2003;**88**:536–9.

Laga M, Naamara W, Brunham RC, *et al*. Single-dose therapy of gonococcal ophthalmia neonatorum with ceftriaxone. *N Engl J Med* 1986;**315**:1382–5. [RCT]

Lamb HM, Ormrod D, Scott LJ, *et al*. Ceftriaxone. *Drugs* 2002;**62**:1041–89. [SR]

Nathan N, Borel T, Djibo A, *et al*. Ceftriaxone as effective as long-acting chloramphenicol in short-course treatment of meningococcal meningitis during epidemics: a randomised non-inferiority study. *Lancet* 2005;**366**:308–13. [RCT]

Steadman E, Raisch DW, Bennett CL, *et al*. Evaluation of a potential clinical interaction between ceftriaxone and calcium. *Antimicrob Agents Chemother* 2010;**54**:1534–40.

Wadsworth SJ, Suh B. In vitro displacement of bilirubin by antibiotics and 2-hydroxybenzoylglycine in newborns. *Antimicrob Agents Chemother* 1988;**32**:1571–5.

Use

This non-toxic broad-spectrum cephalosporin is one of the few available in both parenteral and oral forms.

Pharmacology

Cefuroxime is a β-lactamase-resistant 'second-generation' cephalosporin first patented in 1973. It is active against most Gram-positive organisms (including group B streptococci and penicillin-resistant staphylococci) and a wide range of Gram-negative organisms. It is reasonably active against *Haemophilus influenzae* and *Neisseria gonorrhoeae* but inactive against *Listeria*, enterococci, *Bacteroides* and *Pseudomonas* species. It has sometimes been used prophylactically in neonates undergoing abdominal surgery. It penetrates the CSF only poorly, and coagulase-negative staphylococci are increasingly resistant to this antibiotic. It was once advocated for use (on its own) in asymptomatic babies at birth who were thought to be at risk as a result of prolonged rupture of membranes, maternal pyrexia or meconium aspiration because of its broad spectrum and low potential toxicity for some years. However, controlled trial evidence to support this strategy does not yet exist, and such use has declined in recent years.

Standard cefuroxime is ineffective when given by mouth (<1% is recovered in the urine), but about a third of the administered dose is absorbed when the drug is given as the lipophilic ace-toxyethyl ester, cefuroxime axetil. This prodrug is hydrolysed releasing cefuroxime. There are no published reports of the use of this formulation in children less than 3 months old, but it has been widely used to treat otitis media and other respiratory infections in older children. It is just as effective as treatment with co-amoxiclav (q.v.) and less likely to cause troublesome loose stools. Alternative oral cephalosporins include cefalexin (q.v.) and cefixime.

Cefuroxime is largely excreted by the kidney. Little crosses the placenta and only negligible amounts are found in breast milk. On a weight-for-weight basis, the baby will be exposed to less than 1% of the maternal dose. The plasma half-life falls from 6 hours at birth to about 3 hours at 2 weeks. Babies more than a month old clear cefuroxime from their plasma almost as fast as adults (half-life of 1 hour), but dosage intervals should be extended in babies with severe renal failure. Toxic adverse effects are rare, but oral treatment does sometimes cause nausea and vomiting and a change in stool frequency, and pseudomembranous colitis has occasionally been reported. Other problems, as with cephalosporin in general, are uncommon.

Lyme disease

Lyme disease is caused by a spirochete (*Borrelia burgdorferi*), and human infection is caused by the bite of an infected animal tick. Illness is rare in the United Kingdom, but not uncommon in much of Europe and North America. While a migrating annular skin lesion (erythema migrans) is the classic presentation, symptoms are very variable. Fetal infection was first recognised in 1985, and it is now realised that the risk to the fetus is comparable to that from congenital syphilis. Amoxicillin and cefuroxime axetil are the antibacterials of choice for early Lyme disease in young children (a macrolide may be used if the patient is allergic to penicillin). Intravenous ceftriaxone, cefotaxime or benzylpenicillin is recommended if there are cardiac or neurological complications. The duration of treatment is usually 2–4 weeks.

Treatment

Systemic: Give 25 mg/kg intramuscular (IM) or intravenous (IV) once every 12 hours in the first week of life, every 8 hours in babies 1–3 weeks old and every 6 hours in babies older than this. Double this dose when treating Lyme disease in a baby less than 4 weeks old. The dosage interval needs to be increased if there is serious renal failure.
Oral: Give 15 mg/kg of cefuroxime axetil by mouth once every 12 hours for severe infection. There is no experience of use in babies under 3 months old.

Supply

250 mg vials of the dry powder (costing 94p) should be reconstituted by adding 2.4 ml of sterile water for injection to the vial to get a solution containing 100 mg/ml. A 25 mg/ml oral suspension of cefuroxime axetil containing sucrose is available as a powder for reconstitution with water; 70 ml costs £5.20.

Continued on p. 143

References

Donn KH, James NC, Powell JR. Bioavailability of cefuroxime axetil formulations. *J Pharm Sci* 1994;**83**:842–4.

Eppes SC, Childs JA. Comparative study of cefuroxime axetil versus amoxicillin in children with early Lyme disease. *Pediatrics* 2002;**109**:1173–9. [RCT]

Gooch WM, Blair E, Puopolo A, *et al.* Effectiveness of five days of therapy with cefuroxime axetil suspension for treatment of acute otitis media. *Pediatr Infect Dis J* 1996;**15**:157–64. [RCT]

Scott LJ, Ormrod D, Goa KL. Cefuroxime axetil: an updated review of its use in the management of bacterial infections. *Drugs* 2001;**61**:1455–500.

Smith J, Finn A. Antimicrobial prophylaxis. *Arch Dis Child* 1999;**80**:388–92.

Stanek G, Strle F. Lyme borreliosis. *Lancet* 2003;**362**:1639–47. (See also 2004;**363**:901.)

Wright WF, Riedel DJ, Talwani R, *et al.* Diagnosis and management of Lyme disease. *Am Fam Physician* 2012;**85**:1086–93.

Use

Chloral hydrate has been widely used as a short-term sedative and hypnotic drug for more than a century. It is of no use in controlling pain. The web commentary reviews strategies for safe use in the first year of life.

Pharmacology

Chloral hydrate was synthesised in 1832 and first used as a hypnotic in 1869. Its chemical resemblance to chloroform led early workers to believe that it might work by liberating chloroform in the bloodstream. It is rapidly and effectively absorbed from the stomach and then metabolised by liver enzymes to trichloroacetic acid and the active hypnotic metabolite trichloroethanol (TCE). Further conjugation results in the eventual excretion in the urine as a glucuronide. The half-life of TCE shows wide variability and is at least three times as long in early infancy (10–50 hours) as it is in toddlers and in adult life. It is even longer in the preterm baby and in babies with hepatic or renal disease, making drug accumulation a potential hazard with repeated administration. Hypotension and respiratory depression have been described, and even a low dose may increase the frequency of brief, self-correcting bradycardia.

Chloral hydrate may be used, along with other drugs, to help with symptoms in neonatal abstinence syndrome; however, long-term use has, on occasion, been thought to cause jaundice and worsening of a metabolic acidosis in the neonate. The main adverse effects of oral administration (nausea, vomiting and gastric irritation) can be minimised by giving the drug with a small amount of milk or fruit juice, and this also serves to disguise the drug's unpleasant taste. An overdose can cause coma and a potentially dangerous arrhythmia, probably best controlled using propranolol (q.v.).

Adult insomnia

Chloral hydrate is a good short-term nocturnal sedative for adult patients who find it difficult to sleep while in hospital, and it seems less potentially addictive than benzodiazepines. Long-term use is strongly discouraged. Chloral hydrate is not known to be teratogenic, and while it passes into breast milk, published studies show the breastfed baby ingests only approximately 5% of the weight-related maternal dose.

Infant sedation

Single-dose treatment: A 45 mg/kg oral dose of chloral hydrate usually produces about 1 hour's deep sleep after about 45 minutes. In term babies, a 75 mg/kg dose is occasionally used prior to CT or MRI scanning, echocardiography, etc., but such babies should be monitored because this dose can produce mild hypoxaemia. Rectal administration is sometimes used. A single 100 mg/kg dose is probably safe in infants more than a month old, but only if a pulse oximeter is employed and the child is kept under close surveillance. Staff must also be aware that it can take a *very* variable time for the sedative effect to wear off.

Sustained sedation: 30 mg/kg oral dose of chloral hydrate given once every 6 hours for 1–2 days has been used as an alternative to 400 micrograms/kg of diazepam once every 6 hours in the management of babies with cerebral irritation. It has also been used in some centres to sedate babies requiring respiratory support, but drug accumulation is known to occur especially with repeated use in ill and preterm babies.

Antidote

Flumazenil (as described in the monograph on midazolam) may be of some value in the management of an overdose, but propranolol may be needed to control any arrhythmia.

Supply

An oral elixir of chloral hydrate (Welldorm®) containing just under 30 mg/ml (143.3 mg in 5 ml) is available and costs approximately 6 p/ml. Stocks may be stored at room temperature (5–25 °C). 25, 50, 100 and 200 mg suppositories of chloral hydrate can be obtained from 'special-order' manufacturers or specialist importing companies.

References

(see also the UK guideline on the safe care of any sedated child **DHUK**)

Allegaert K, Daniels H, Naulaers G, *et al*. Pharmacodynamics of chloral hydrate in former preterm infants. *Eur J Pediatr* 2005;**164**:403–7.

American Academy of Pediatrics Committee on Drugs and Committee on Environmental Health. Use of chloral hydrate for sedation in children. *Pediatrics* 1993;**92**:471–3.

Continued on p. 145

Donovan KL, Fisher DJ. Reversal of chloral hydrate overdose with flumazenil. *Br Med J* 1989;**298**:1253.

Esmaeili A, Keinhorst AK, Schuster T, *et al.* Treatment of neonatal abstinence syndrome with clonidine and chloral hydrate. *Acta Paediatr* 2010;**99**:209–14.

Jacqz-Aigrain E, Burtin P. Clinical pharmacokinetics of sedatives in neonates. *Clin Pharmacokinet* 1996;**31**:423–43.

Litman RS, Soin K, Salam A. Chloral hydrate sedation in term and preterm infants: an analysis of efficacy and complications. *Anesth Analg* 2010;**110**:739–46.

Mason KP, Sanborn P, Zurakowski D, *et al.* Superiority of pentobarbital versus chloral hydrate for sedation in infants during imaging. *Radiology* 2004;**230**:537–42.

Napoli KL, Ingrall CG, Martin GR. Safety and efficacy of chloral hydrate sedation in children undergoing echocardiography. *J Pediatr* 1996;**129**:287–91.

Pershad J, Palmisano P, Nichols M. Chloral hydrate: the good and the bad. *Pediatr Emerg Care* 1999;**15**:432–5.

Sury MRJ, Hatch DJ, Deeley T, *et al.* Development of a nurse-led sedation service for paediatric magnetic resonance imaging. *Lancet* 1999;**353**:1667–71.

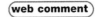
Use

Chloramphenicol is used for typhoid and paratyphoid fever and occasionally used to control meningitis and ventriculitis (because of good CSF penetration). It is also used for sepsis and pneumonia in some countries because oral absorption is good and most alternatives remain expensive.

History

Chloramphenicol came into widespread neonatal use in 1949. Then, in 1959, came a report describing three babies who suffered a 'fatal cardiovascular collapse' (so-called grey baby syndrome). It was not, however, until the result of a prospective controlled trial was published in December 1959 that the potential toxicity of treatment with 100–150 mg/kg/day (the dose then normally recommended) was generally accepted. That most babies had only been given antibiotics to *prevent* infection only added to the anguish. Sadly, the potential toxicity of this drug seems to be a lesson that each new generation of clinicians had to learn afresh, because more deaths from dosing errors were reported in 1983.

Pharmacology

Chloramphenicol kills *Haemophilus influenzae* and *Neisseria* spp. and stops the growth of rickettsiae and most bacteria. It penetrates all body tissues well: the CSF concentration averages 60% of the serum level, while brain levels are said to be nine times higher because of high lipid solubility. Despite this, cefotaxime (q.v.) has now become the drug of choice in the management of suspected or proven Gram-negative meningitis (partly because 2–5% of all strains of *H. influenzae* are now resistant to chloramphenicol). The parenteral drug (chloramphenicol succinate) only becomes biologically active after hydrolysis, and because this can be delayed in the neonate, levels of the active antibiotic can be *very* unpredictable.

The oral drug (chloramphenicol palmitate) also requires prior hydrolysis by pancreatic enzymes that makes it unwise to give the drug by mouth when first starting treatment in early infancy. Much of the inactive ester is excreted by the renal tubules (especially in children), and most of the active drug is first metabolised to the inactive glucuronide, so the dose does not usually need to be modified in renal failure. Excretion and metabolic inactivation are, however, influenced by postnatal age. The half-life decreases from a mean of 27 hours in the first week of life to 8 hours by 2–4 weeks and 4 hours in children over 4 months old.

Maternal treatment does not seem to pose a hazard to the baby at any stage of pregnancy. The breastfed baby receives only approximately 5% of the weight-related maternal dose, so the only reason to discourage breastfeeding is the small (~1:40,000) risk of aplastic anaemia – something that applies to the mother at least as much as it does to the baby. There are a few reports of haemolysis in patients with G6PD deficiency.

Drug interactions

Co-treatment with phenobarbital or rifampicin tends to lower the plasma chloramphenicol level. The effect of phenytoin is more variable, but chloramphenicol can slow the elimination of phenytoin.

Treatment

Neonatal treatment: Give a loading dose of 20 mg/kg intravenous (IV) and then 12 mg/kg orally or IV once every 12 hours in babies less than a week old. Babies 1–4 weeks old should have further doses every 8 hours in the absence of renal failure or liver damage. *Check the dose given carefully: an overdose can be fatal.*

Older children: Children over 4 weeks old can usually be started on 25 mg/kg every 8 hours. The first doses should be given IV or IM in any child who is ill, but further treatment can then be given by mouth.

Eye drops: See the eye drop monograph (q.v.).

Blood levels

Levels should be monitored where facilities exist when this drug is used in babies less than 4 weeks old. Aim for a peak serum concentration of 15–25 mg/l (1 mg/l = 3.1 µmol/l). Levels over 35 mg/l may cause transient marrow suppression. Levels over 50 mg/l can cause cardiovascular collapse.

Continued on p. 147

Supply

1 g vials of chloramphenicol succinate cost £1.40. Add 9.2 ml of water for injection to give a solution containing 10 mg in 0.1 ml. Oral suspensions of the palmitate salt are no longer commercially available in the United Kingdom, but a sugar-free suspension with a 4-week shelf life can be obtained from 'special-order' manufacturers or specialist importing companies.

References

Duke T, Poka H, Dale F, *et al*. Chloramphenicol versus benzylpenicillin and gentamicin for the treatment of severe pneumonia in children in Papua New Guinea: a randomized trial. *Lancet* 2002;**359**:474–80. [RCT]

Mulhall A, de Louvois J, Hurley R. Chloramphenicol toxicity in neonates: its incidence and prevention. *Br Med J* 1983;**2**:1424–7.

Rojchgot P, Prober CG, Soldin S, *et al*. Initiation of chloramphenicol therapy in the newborn infant. *J Pediatr* 1982;**101**:1018–21.

Smith AL, Weber A. Pharmacology of chloramphenicol. *Pediatr Clin North Am* 1983;**30**:209–36.

Weber MW, Gatchalian SR, Ogunlesi O, *et al*. Chloramphenicol pharmacokinetics in infants less than three months of age in the Philippines and The Gambia. *Pediatr Infect Dis J* 1999;**18**:896–901.

Use

Chloroquine was, for a long time, the world's most widely used antimalarial drug, but the most common and virulent parasite, *Plasmodium falciparum*, is now increasingly resistant. Chloroquine can still be used, however, when *P. ovale* and *P. malariae* infection needs treatment, and *P. vivax* is also usually still sensitive.

Pharmacology

Chloroquine (a 4-aminoquinoline developed during World War II) is well absorbed, widely distributed in body tissues, slowly metabolised by the liver and only very slowly cleared from the body. There is no evidence that standard-dose treatment during pregnancy is hazardous, and there is good evidence that weekly prophylaxis is not just safe but also advisable where disease is endemic. Use during lactation exposes the baby to less than 5% of the weight-adjusted maternal dose, which is probably not enough to protect the baby from infection.

Malaria

In 2010, there were an estimated 219 million cases of malaria resulting in 660,000 deaths. Most cases (approximately two-thirds) occur in children. In sub-Saharan Africa, maternal malaria is associated with up to 200,000 estimated infant deaths yearly. Although the incidence of malaria has declined in recent years – largely as a result of the widespread use of insecticide-treated nets and artemisinin-based combination therapies – it remains a significant global problem.

Residents in endemic areas develop considerable immunity over time, but pregnancy makes women more vulnerable, and infection during pregnancy increases the risk of anaemia, miscarriage, stillbirth and prematurity. Transplacental spread is uncommon, but infection sometimes occurs during delivery, although florid symptoms (including fever, jaundice, an enlarged liver and spleen and low platelet count) usually only manifest themselves 2–8 weeks later. Diagnosis of infection, however acquired, depends on recognising the intracellular parasite in a thick smear of stained blood on a microscope slide. Infection is considered severe if there is shock, acidosis, hypoglycaemia or cerebral symptoms or more than 5% of red cells are involved. In *P. vivax* and *P. ovale* infections, treatment with chloroquine can leave some organisms dormant in the liver unless primaquine is given as well (see following text). There are a few areas where even *P. vivax* has now become resistant to chloroquine, and here, it can still be appropriate to treat overt infection with mefloquine (15 mg/kg by mouth followed, after 12 hours, by a second 10 mg/kg dose) or artemether (q.v.) where this is available.

Drug resistance

Chloroquine prophylaxis is still appropriate in the Middle East and Central America. The UK advice on prophylaxis can be obtained from the Public Health England Malaria Reference Laboratory (www.malaria-reference.co.uk), and the WHO advice on travel and the prevalence of drug resistance can be found at http://www.who.int/topics/malaria/en/index.html. Go to http://www.cdc.gov/malaria/ for up-to-date advice from the CDC in America.

Treatment

Prevention in visitors: Offer children 5 mg/kg of chloroquine *base* by mouth once a week in areas where sensitive parasites are endemic. Start 1 week before entering the area and stop 4 weeks after leaving. Consider giving proguanil (q.v.) as well.

Cure: Give a 10 mg/kg loading dose of chloroquine *base* intravenous (IV) or by mouth and then three 5 mg/kg doses (given at 24 hour intervals) starting 6 hours after the loading dose was given. In *P. vivax* or *P. ovale* infections, there may be a case for giving primaquine after this to eliminate any dormant liver parasites.

Eradicating liver organisms

Giving 300 micrograms/kg of primaquine once a day by mouth for 2 weeks will usually kill residual organisms. A higher dose may occasionally be necessary but increases the risk of haemolysis in those with the Mediterranean and Asian variants of G6PD deficiency. Use in young children has not been well studied.

Toxicity

Excess chloroquine is toxic to the heart and the CNS. Prompt high-dose diazepam (2 mg/kg daily) and ventilation seem beneficial. Gastric lavage may be appropriate once the airway has been protected, and activated charcoal may reduce gut absorption. IV adrenaline helps control

Continued on p. 149

hypotension. Correct any acidosis. Phenytoin or a beta-blocker can be used to treat arrhythmia. Dialysis is not helpful.

Supply

Chloroquine base: There are two formulations: a 10 mg/ml syrup containing 13.6 mg/ml of chloroquine sulphate costing £4.60 for 100 ml and a 10 mg/ml syrup containing 16 mg/ml of chloroquine phosphate costing £11 for 75 ml.

Primaquine base: 7.5 and 15 mg tablets are available from specialist importing companies and cost about 70 p each. A 3 mg/ml suspension can be prepared which retains its potency for a week if stored at 4 °C.

References (see also the relevant Cochrane reviews)

Hill DR, Baird JK, Parise ME, *et al.* Primaquine: report from the CDC expert meeting on malaria chemoprophylaxis I. *Am J Trop Med Hyg* 2006;**75**:402–15.

Laufer MK, Thesing PC, Eddington ND, *et al.* Return of chloroquine efficacy in Malawi. *N Engl J Med* 2006;**355**:1959–66. [RCT] (See also pp. 1956–7.)

Law I, Ilett KF, Hackett LP, *et al.* Transfer of chloroquine and desethylchloroquine across the placenta and into milk in Melanesian mothers. *Br J Clin Pharmacol* 2008;**65**:674–9.

Leslie T, Mayan MI Hasan MA, *et al.* Sulfadoxine-pyrimethamine, chlorproguanil-dapsone, or chloroquine for the treatment of *Plasmodium vivax* malaria in Afghanistan and Pakistan: a randomized controlled trial. *JAMA* 2007;**297**:2201–9. [RCT]

Obua C, Hellgren U, Ntale M, *et al.* Population pharmacokinetics of chloroquine and sulfadoxine and treatment response in children with malaria: suggestions for an improved dose regimen. *Br J Clin Pharmacol* 2008;**65**:493–501.

Osadchy A, Ratnapalan T, Koren G. Ocular toxicity in children exposed in utero to antimalarial drugs: review of the literature. *J Rheumatol* 2011;**38**:2504–8.

Parke AL. Antimalarial drugs, pregnancy and lactation. *Lupus* 1993;**2**(suppl 1):S21–3.

Wilby KJ, Ensom MH. Pharmacokinetics of antimalarials in pregnancy: a systematic review. *Clin Pharmacokinet* 2011;**50**:705–23.

Wolfe MS, Cordero JF. Safety of chloroquine in chemosuppression of malaria during pregnancy. *Br Med J* 1985;**290**:1466–7.

Use

Chlorothiazide is a thiazide diuretic used to treat the pulmonary oedema seen in preterm babies with chronic ventilator-induced lung disease. It is also used in the control of fluid retention in congestive heart failure, usually in combination with spironolactone (q.v.). Furosemide (q.v.) is a useful short-term alternative in both conditions when either oral treatment is not possible or a rapid response is required.

Pharmacology

Chlorothiazide was first developed commercially in 1957. It crosses the placenta but shows no definite evidence of teratogenicity, although there is one study suggesting some increased risk associated with use in the first trimester of pregnancy. Diuretic use is, nevertheless, generally considered unwise in pregnancy, except in women with heart disease, because it may further decrease placental perfusion in pre-eclampsia.

Chlorothiazide is moderately well absorbed when taken by mouth and is excreted unchanged into the lumen of the proximal straight tubule where it acts by inhibiting the absorption of sodium and chloride from the urine in the distal tubule, doubling the excretion of potassium and causing a fivefold increase in sodium excretion. The plasma half-life (about 5 hours in the pre-term baby) is much shorter than the functional half-life. It increases when there is renal failure, making drug accumulation possible. Kernicterus is a theoretical possibility in the very jaundiced baby because the drug competes with bilirubin for the available plasma albumin binding sites.

Hydrochlorothiazide is an alternative, closely related, thiazide. It is only available in combinations for use in adults and through specialist importing companies. Both chlorothiazide and hydrochlorothiazide pass into breast milk, but the baby receives less than 2% of the maternal dose on a weight-for-weight basis. Reports that use during lactation can cause thrombocytopenia are unsubstantiated, as are suggestions that thiazide diuretics suppress lactation.

Diuretics are routinely used in patients with heart failure. They can also improve lung compliance in babies with chronic lung damage and pulmonary oedema, but further studies are needed to confirm whether sustained thiazide treatment really reduces the need for supplemental oxygen (as suggested by one small trial). Diuretics often stimulate increased aldosterone secretion, and the addition of spironolactone, which counteracts the sodium-retaining and potassium-excreting effect of aldosterone on the distal tubule, is thought to enhance the response to thiazide use. Combined treatment with spironolactone does, however, cause urinary calcium loss of a magnitude similar to that incurred by furosemide use, and this can cause serious bone demineralisation in the preterm baby. It can also cause nephrocalcinosis detectable on ultrasound (but not, usually, on X-ray); however, this appears to resolve without any sequelae in later infancy when treatment is stopped.

Due to its effect on glucose metabolism (thiazides are known to impair glucose tolerance in adults), chlorothiazide may be used in conjunction with diazoxide (q.v.) to treat severe persistent hyperinsulinism, although its main role is to counter the fluid retention that diazoxide causes.

Treatment

Heart failure: Give 10 mg/kg of chlorothiazide and 1 mg/kg of spironolactone twice a day by mouth. Babies that fail to respond to a standard dose sometimes respond to twice this dose. Potassium supplements are not usually necessary with such combined treatment.

Chronic lung disease: Babies with chronic ventilator-induced lung damage may benefit from a similar dose of chlorothiazide. Whether they should also receive spironolactone requires further study.

Persistent hyperinsulinism: Give 4 mg/kg of chlorothiazide two to three times a day by mouth to minimise the fluid retention caused by diazoxide (q.v.).

Supply

Chlorothiazide is available commercially, to special order, as a suspension containing 50 mg/ml (costing about £12 for 100 ml), but this formulation has to be imported from America at present. This formulation contains sucrose and saccharin. A sugar-free suspension could also be prepared from powder on request, but this suspension is known to have a reduced shelf life. A similar oral suspension of hydrochlorothiazide could be prepared if required.

Continued on p. 151

References

(see also the relevant Cochrane reviews)

Albersheim SG, Solimano AJ, Sharma EK, *et al.* Randomised double blind trial of long term diuretic therapy for bronchopulmonary dysplasia. *J Pediatr* 1989;**115**:615–29. [RCT]

Atkinson SA, Shah JK, McGee G, *et al.* Mineral excretion in premature infants receiving various diuretic therapies. *J Pediatr* 1988;**113**:540–5.

Engelhardt B, Blalock A, DanLevy S, *et al.* Effect of spironolactone-hydrochlorothiazide on lung function in infants with chronic bronchopulmonary dysplasia. *J Pediatr* 1989;**114**:619–24. [RCT]

Fafoula O, Alkhayyat H, Hussain K. Prolonged hyperinsulinaemic hypoglycaemia in newborns with intrauterine growth retardation. *Arch Dis Child Fetal Neonatal Ed* 2006;**91**:F467.

Hussain K, Aynsley-Green A. Hyperinsulinaemic hypoglycaemia in preterm neonates. *Arch Dis Child Fetal Neonatal Ed* 2004;**89**:F65–7.

Kao LC, Durand DJ, McCrea RC, *et al.* Randomised trial of long-term diuretic therapy for infants with oxygen-dependent bronchopulmonary dysplasia. *J Pediatr* 1994;**124**:772–81. [RCT]

Wells TG. The pharmacology and therapeutics of diuretics in the pediatric patient. *Pediatr Clin North Am* 1990;**37**:463–504.

Use

Chlorphenamine is a first-generation histamine H1 receptor antagonist used in allergy, allergic reactions and anaphylaxis. It also features in a number of over-the-counter antihistamine and decongestant or antitussive combinations available for purchase without prescription. Chlorphenamine has also been used to overcome the resistance to treatment encountered with some antimalarials and is sometimes used to ameliorate the symptoms of itch in children with eczema and with chickenpox (varicella) rash.

Pharmacology

Chlorphenamine maleate, first used in 1951, is one of a number of stable, lipid-soluble amines that all have the ethylamine side chain of histamine. Like most other first-generation antihistamines, it causes sedative, anti-emetic and anticholinergic effects that are exploited in a number of conditions. It is, nonetheless, reported to cause less sedation than most first-generation antihistamines.

Chlorphenamine is well absorbed after oral administration, but because of a relatively high degree of metabolism in the intestinal mucosa and the liver, only 25–60% of the drug is available to the systemic circulation. Chlorphenamine and its two metabolites (monodesmethyl- and didesmethyl-chlorphenamine) are excreted by the kidneys. The elimination half-life is approximately 14–25 hours in adults, but is shorter in children (~10 hours). However, the duration of action is only 4–6 hours. Chlorphenamine has, to date, not been implicated in the causation of any fetal malformations, and while it does cross the blood–brain barrier, it is not known whether chlorphenamine crosses the placenta. Like other antihistamines, it passes into breast milk but is probably compatible with breastfeeding although the manufacturers advise against use during lactation. Despite its long history of use, little, if any, published information is available on chlorphenamine pharmacokinetics in neonates, and the manufacturers have yet to endorse its use in children under the age of 12 months.

Chlorphenamine significantly restores the antimalarial efficacy of chloroquine in a setting of almost universal chloroquine resistance. Exactly how it does this is not yet known but may be linked to inhibition of the malarial parasite calmodulin functions.

Uses

Relief of allergic symptoms and pruritus: Oral treatment with chlorphenamine may be used to bring about relief from the symptoms of hay fever, urticaria, food allergy and drug reactions as well as the relief of itch associated with chickenpox and eczema.

Severe allergic reactions and anaphylaxis: Although high-quality evidence for its use in this situation is sparse, chlorphenamine is given by intravenous (IV) (or occasionally IM) injection in cases of severe allergic reactions and anaphylaxis. Administration should only take place after the initial resuscitation. While such reactions are rare in neonates, the manufacturer has not endorsed use of the parenteral preparation in this age group.

Treatment

Oral: A dose of 1 mg may be given twice daily to relieve the symptoms of allergy and itch.
Parenteral: 250 micrograms/kg (or 250 mg if the child is older than 6 months) is given either by slow IV injection (over 1 minute) or by IM injection after the immediate resuscitation in a severe allergic reaction or anaphylaxis. Up to four further doses may be given in a 24 hour period.

Supply and administration

100 ml of a sugar-free oral suspension containing 2 mg/5 ml of chlorphenamine maleate costs £1.70. The prescriber must specify 'sugar-free' in the prescription.

A 1 ml ampoule containing 10 mg of chlorphenamine maleate costs £2.80. Further dilution to 10 ml with 0.9% sodium chloride to a solution containing 1 mg/ml will facilitate administration of small doses. This dilute solution should be used immediately.

References   (see also the Cochrane review and guidelines for the management of anaphylaxis)

Das BP, Joshi M, Pant CR. An overview of over the counter drugs in pregnancy and lactation. *Kathmandu Univ Med J (KUMJ)* 2006;**4**:545–51.
Keleş N. Treatment of allergic rhinitis during pregnancy. *Am J Rhinol* 2004;**18**:23–8.

Continued on p. 153

Munday J, Bloomfield R, Goldman M, *et al.* Chlorpheniramine is no more effective than placebo in relieving the symptoms of childhood atopic dermatitis with a nocturnal itching and scratching component. *Dermatology* 2002;**205**:40–5.

Nelson MM, Forfar JO. Associations between drugs administered during pregnancy and congenital abnormalities of the fetus. *Br Med J* 1971;**1**(5748):523–7.

Simons KJ, Simons FE, Luciuk GH, *et al.* Urinary excretion of chlorpheniramine and its metabolites in children. *J Pharm Sci* 1984;**73**:595–9.

Soar J, Pumphrey R, Cant A, *et al.* Emergency treatment of anaphylactic reactions—Guidelines for healthcare providers. *Resuscitation* 2008;**77**:157–69.

Sowunmi A, Adedeji AA, Gbotosho GO, *et al.* Effects of pyrimethamine sulfadoxine, chloroquine plus chlorpheniramine, and amodiaquine plus pyrimethamine-sulfadoxine on gametocytes during and after treatment of acute, uncomplicated malaria in children. *Mem Inst Oswaldo Cruz* 2006; **101**:887–93.

Swan KE, Fitzsimons R, Boardman A, *et al.* The prevention and management of anaphylaxis. *Paediatr Child Health* 2012; **22**:264–71.

Use

Chlorpromazine hydrochloride is a widely used antipsychotic or 'neuroleptic' drug. It was first used in 1952 in the treatment of schizophrenia but has also been widely used in the short-term management of severe anxiety. It is still used as a short-term tranquilliser in patients of all ages.

Pharmacology

Chlorpromazine is a phenothiazine used to reduce agitation without causing respiratory depression. Phenothiazines have an antihistaminic effect and are sometimes used to combat nausea. They have also been used to reduce peripheral and pulmonary vascular resistance. For this reason, they were used for a few years in the 1980s in the management of neonatal respiratory distress. While chlorpromazine was initially widely offered to psychiatric patients, it soon became even more widely used in the 1950s as an adjunct in preoperative medication and as a joint agent in sedation/anaesthesia because of the way it potentiates the hypnotic, narcotic and analgesic effects of other drugs. Such use has now diminished.

Chlorpromazine is well absorbed orally (although this can occasionally be unpredictable). Deep intramuscular (IM) injection is generally considered preferable to intravenous administration though this is sometimes painful. It is metabolised by the liver into a wide number of different breakdown products with a half-life of about 30 hours in adults and a half-life twice as long as this at birth. Attempts to correlate plasma levels with the clinical effects of treatment have been largely unsuccessful probably because tissue drug levels greatly exceed those in plasma (V_D >8 l/kg).

Chlorpromazine crosses the placenta, and while unpredictable maternal hypotension has been reported following use during labour, there is no evidence of teratogenicity. Extrapyramidal signs have occasionally been suspected for a few days after delivery in babies born to mothers on long-term high-dose antenatal treatment. The breastfed baby only receives approximately 3% of the weight-related maternal dose, and there is a single report of this making the baby drowsy.

Use in babies less than 1 year old has not yet been endorsed by the manufacturer, and very few reports have been published relating to use in the neonatal period. It is, however, sometimes used in the management of babies born to non-opioid drug-abusing mothers. It is also very good at sedating babies with chronic respiratory problems who become seriously agitated and distressed after weeks of care on a ventilator. There is one unconfirmed report of naloxone (q.v.) being an effective antidote after an overdose.

Neonatal abstinence syndrome

Many drugs provoke withdrawal symptoms in the baby after birth. Restlessness, irritability and excessive wakefulness are the most common problems seen. Autonomic dysfunction can include sneezing, yawning, sweating and temperature instability. Feeding can prove difficult. Symptoms can be very unpleasant and occasionally, if particularly severe, dangerous. Those that persist after feeding, swaddling and the use of a dummy or pacifier should be managed with a tapering dose of methadone or morphine (q.v.) if the mother has been taking a narcotic (opioid) drug, but chlorpromazine is an understudied alternative that may achieve weaning faster than a tapering dose of morphine. Using phenobarbital (q.v.) as well may sometimes help where there is a mixed dependency. With amfetamine and most opiate abuse, serious symptoms usually present within 1–2 days, peak early and subside fairly rapidly, because these drugs have a fairly short half-life. Symptoms present more insidiously with other drugs, such as diazepam and the barbiturates, with a longer half-life. Some illicit drugs, such as marijuana (cannabis), seldom cause symptoms. For a fuller discussion, see the methadone website commentary.

Treatment

Start by offering 1 mg/kg by mouth every 8 hours. Most authorities suggest that the *total* daily dose should not exceed 6 mg/kg.

Supply

An oral syrup containing 5 mg/ml of chlorpromazine hydrochloride (costing £2.35 for 150 ml) is available. It can be diluted 10-fold for accurate administration by the pharmacy on request, but the diluted preparation only has a 2-week shelf life. A 1 ml ampoule containing 25 mg of chlorpromazine hydrochloride (costing 60 p) is available for IM use.

Continued on p. 155

References

(see also relevant Cochrane reviews)

Chasnoff IA, ed. Chemical dependency in pregnancy. *Clin Neonatol* 1991;**18**:1–191.

Johnson K. Withdrawal from drugs of addiction in newborn infants. In: David TJ, ed. *Recent advances in paediatrics 22*. London: RSM Press, 2005: pp. 73–83.

Mazurier E, Gambonie G, Barbotte E, *et al*. Comparison of chlorpromazine versus morphine hydrochloride for treatment of neonatal abstinence syndrome. *Acta Paediatr* 2008;**97**:1358–61. (See also pp. 1321–3.)

McElhatton PR. The use of phenothiazines during pregnancy and lactation. *Reprod Toxicol* 1992;**6**:475–90.

Nielsen HC, Wiriyathian S, Rosenfeld CR, *et al*. Chlorpromazine excretion by the neonate following chronic *in utero* exposure. *Pediatr Pharmacol* 1983;**3**:1–5.

Theis JGW, Selby P, Ikizler Y, *et al*. Current management of neonatal abstinence syndrome: a critical analysis of the evidence. *Biol Neonate* 1997;**71**:345–66.

Yoshida K, Smith B, Craggs M, *et al*. Neuroleptic drugs in breast-milk: a study of pharmacokinetics and of possible adverse effects in breast-fed infants. *Psychol Med* 1998;**28**:81–91.

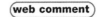
Use

Ciprofloxacin is a broad-spectrum bactericidal antibiotic with activity against a wide range of infectious organisms that can be given by mouth. A single 20 mg/kg dose can be used to treat cholera. Ciprofloxacin is now the first-choice antibiotic for protection after contact with a case of meningococcal infection.

Pharmacology

Ciprofloxacin is a fluoroquinolone, first patented in 1982, with broad-spectrum activity against many Gram-positive and Gram-negative bacteria and against other organisms such as *Chlamydia* and rickettsiae (although gonococci are becoming progressively more resistant). It is particularly useful in the management of enterobacter and other infections resistant to all cephalosporins and all the widely used aminoglycosides. Because it can be given by mouth (oral bioavailability 70%), it is particularly useful in the treatment of pulmonary infection with *Pseudomonas aeruginosa* and *Salmonella*. Intravenous (IV) administration can be painful and cause local erythema and phlebitis unless infused slowly. Ciprofloxacin crosses the placenta and diffuses into most body fluids well, including CSF (adequate levels, >1.0 mg/l, have been documented in the CSF of infants with ventriculitis). It is partly metabolised in the liver but largely excreted unchanged in the urine (where crystalluria may occur if fluid intake is not maintained). The steady-state half-life does not seem to have been studied in babies less than a month old, but the half-life in children and adults is not dissimilar (3–4 hours). Dosage only requires review where there is serious renal or liver dysfunction.

Although the use of this drug was initially discouraged in children because studies had shown lasting damage to the cartilage of weight-bearing joints during growth in animals, no reports of any such complication have appeared following its use in childhood, although transient arthralgia and other musculoskeletal events may occur in about 1.5%. There is one isolated report which suggested that the drug may stain the primary dentition green. Nevertheless, while the drug should not be used in the neonatal period where other alternative treatment strategies are available, use has sometimes proved extremely effective in the treatment of severe septicaemia or meningitis, and *P. aeruginosa* infection, even though the manufacturers have never formally recommended its use children less than 6 years old.

The only pharmacokinetic study performed in septic preterm neonates concluded that a dose of 20 mg/kg/day in two divided doses would be effective for common Gram-negative infections except for *P. aeruginosa* infections. There is some suggestion that the drug can cause seizures in patients with an underlying epileptic tendency and some risk of haemolytic anaemia in babies with G6PD deficiency. Maternal treatment only exposes the breastfed baby to about 3% of the maternal weight-related dose.

Drug interactions

Ciprofloxacin treatment increases the half-life of theophylline and (to a lesser extent) caffeine. Ciprofloxacin can cause prolongation of the QT interval and should be avoided in those with congenital long QT syndrome.

Treatment

Dose: Give 10 mg/kg IV over 30–60 minutes when treating severe infection. A higher dose (15 mg/kg) allows continuation of treatment. Use 20 mg/kg when treating *P. aeruginosa* infection.
Timing: Give one dose every 12 hours in the first month of life and every 8 hours in babies older than this (unless the plasma creatinine is over twice the normal value). Treatment is usually continued for 10–14 days.
Meningococcal prophylaxis: Give a single dose of 30 mg/kg (up to a maximum of 125 mg) orally.

Supply

Ciprofloxacin lactate for IV use is available in 50 ml bottles (cost £7.60) containing 100 mg of ciprofloxacin. A 10 mg/kg dose contains 0.76 mmol/kg of sodium. Bottles must be discarded promptly after they have been opened; capped syringes can be prepared for IV use by the pharmacy on request to minimise drug wastage. 100 ml of sugar-free oral suspension of ciprofloxacin hydrochloride containing 50 mg/ml costs £19.80.

Continued on p. 157

References

Adefurin A, Sammons H, Jacqz-Aigrain E, *et al*. Ciprofloxacin safety in paediatrics: a systematic review. *Arch Dis Child* 2011;**96**:874–80. [SR]

Aggarwal P, Dutta S, Garg SK, *et al*. Multiple dose pharmacokinetics of ciprofloxacin in preterm babies. *Indian Pediatr* 2004;**41**:1001–7.

Bradley JS, Jackson MA; Committee on Infectious Diseases; American Academy of Pediatrics. The use of systemic and topical fluoroquinolones. Pediatrics 2011;**128**:e1034–45.

Chalumeau M, Tonnelier S, d'Athis P, *et al*. Fluoroquinolone safety in pediatric patients: a prospective, multicenter, comparative cohort study in France. *Pediatrics* 2003;**111**:e714–9.

Gendrel D, Chalumeau M, Moulin F, *et al*. Fluoroquinolones in paediatrics: a risk for the patient or for the community? [Review] *Lancet Infect Dis* 2003;**3**:537–46.

Kaguelidou F, Turner MA, Choonara I, *et al*. Ciprofloxacin use in neonates: a systematic review of the literature. *Pediatr Infect Dis J* 2011;**30**:e29–37. [SR]

Lipman J, Gous AGS, Mathivha LR, *et al*. Ciprofloxacin pharmacokinetic profiles in paediatric sepsis: how much ciprofloxacin is enough? *Intensive Care Med* 2002;**28**:493–500.

van den Oever HLA, Verteegh FGA, Theweesen EAPM, *et al*. Ciprofloxacin in preterm neonates: case report and review of the literature. *Eur J Pediatr* 1998;**157**:843–5.

Saha D, Khan WA, Karim MM, *et al*. Single-dose ciprofloxacin versus 12-dose erythromycin for childhood cholera: a randomized controlled trial. *Lancet* 2005;**366**:1085–93. [RCT] (See also pp. 1054–5.)

Use

L-Citrulline may be used instead of L-arginine (q.v.) as an essential nutritional supplement for patients with proximal urea cycle disorders, carbamoyl phosphate synthetase (CPS) deficiency and ornithine carbamoyl transferase (OTC) deficiency, and also in the treatment of deficiency of the ornithine translocase transporter protein. Citrulline is more palatable, but more expensive, than arginine, and facilitates nitrogen excretion (which is the aim of the treatment of urea cycle disorders), together with sodium phenylbutyrate and sodium benzoate (q.v.). It is also used in lysinuric protein intolerance which presents with a secondary urea cycle derangement due to impaired transport of cationic amino acids.

Biochemistry

CPS deficiency is a rare autosomal recessive disorder. It has two distinct clinical phenotypes: neonatal onset (usually severe) and late onset. The time of presentation is dependent on the levels of enzymatic activity which can itself vary within the same family.

OTC deficiency is an X-linked disorder that may occur in males and females. It may occur as a severe neonatal-onset disease in males and as a late-onset disease in both genders. The timing of presentation relates to the level of enzyme activity. Many heterozygous females remain asymptomatic throughout life, but others have problems of variable severity, depending on the X-inactivation pattern as well as the mutation.

Ornithine translocase deficiency (also called hyperornithinaemia–hyperammonaemia–homocitrullinuria or HHH syndrome) is a rare autosomal recessive urea cycle disorder where there is an absence of a transporter protein rather than an enzyme. It results in diminished ornithine transport into the mitochondria.

Lysinuric protein intolerance is a rare autosomal recessive disorder caused by defective cationic amino acid transport which mainly affects intestinal absorption and renal reabsorption.

A high-protein diet or period of catabolic stress can result in the release of amino acids which are then broken down releasing nitrogen which circulates in the body as ammonia. Ammonia is converted into urea via the urea cycle and excreted in the urine. Any enzymatic block of the urea cycle results in the accumulation of excess ammonia which has toxic effects. Citrulline is a naturally occurring amino acid but it is non-structural (i.e. it is not incorporated into proteins). Like arginine, it is normally formed in the urea cycle but this is prevented in the proximal urea cycle disorders. This allows the therapeutic use of L-citrulline in these disorders as a substitute for arginine, and because citrulline occurs in the urea cycle before aspartate is incorporated, it allows the excretion of nitrogen from this amino acid. This does not happen with arginine treatment; thus it can be a significant advantage in severely affected patients. Treatment with L-citrulline needs to be combined with a low-protein diet and supervised by a consultant and dietitian experienced in the management of metabolic disease. Treatment with oral sodium phenylbutyrate and/or sodium benzoate is also usually necessary.

Specialist advice

Specialist advice on a range of inborn errors of metabolism is available from the British Inherited Metabolic Disease Group (BIMDG), and detailed guidance on the management of hyperammonaemia is available on this group's website (www.bimdg.org.uk). Start by clicking on the red box to access a range of emergency protocols.

Treatment

> **NOTE: Treatment with L-citrulline should only be initiated after consultation with a specialist metabolic diseases centre.**

CPS, OTC and ornithine translocase deficiencies: Begin with 150 mg/kg daily in three to four divided doses when the child is able to tolerate enteral feeds. Adjust the dose according to response.
Lysinuric protein intolerance: 100 mg/kg daily (or less) in three to four divided doses. Aim to keep the plasma citrulline levels in the normal range.

Continued on p. 159

Supply and administration

Powdered L-citrulline (100 g) is available from The Specials Laboratory with a 90 day expiry date.

References

Alfadhel M, Al-Thihli K, Moubayed H, *et al*. Drug treatment of inborn errors of metabolism: a systematic review. *Arch Dis Child* 2013;**98**:454–61.

Häberle J, Boddaert N, Burlina A, *et al*. Suggested guidelines for the diagnosis and management of urea cycle disorders. *Orphanet J Rare Dis* 2012;**7**:32.

Lanpher BC, Gropman A, Chapman KA, *et al*. Urea Cycle Disorders Overview. 2003 Apr 29 [Updated 2011 Sep 1]. In: Pagon RA, Adam MP, Bird TD, *et al*., editors. GeneReviews™ [Internet]. Seattle (WA): University of Washington, Seattle; 1993–2013. Available from: http://www.ncbi.nlm.nih.gov/books/NBK1217/. Accessed 14 May 2014.

Martínez AI, Pérez-Arellano I, Pekkala S, *et al*. Genetic, structural and biochemical basis of carbamoyl phosphate synthetase 1 deficiency. *Mol Genet Metab* 2010;**101**:311–23.

Ogier de Baulny H, Schiff M, Dionisi-Vici C. Lysinuric protein intolerance (LPI): a multi organ disease by far more complex than a classic urea cycle disorder. *Mol Genet Metab* 2012;**106**:12–7.

Palmieri F. Diseases caused by defects of mitochondrial carriers: a review. *Biochim Biophys Acta* 2008;**1777**:564–78.

Wraith JE. Ornithine carbamoyltransferase deficiency. *Arch Dis Child* 2001;**84**:84–8.

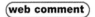
Use

Clarithromycin, like erythromycin and azithromycin (q.v.), can be used to treat neonatal *Chlamydia, Mycoplasma* and *Ureaplasma* infections. It is used widely in upper and lower respiratory tract, ear and skin infections in infants. It is also used as prophylaxis in 'at-risk' individuals who are exposed to pertussis.

Pharmacology

This broad-spectrum macrolide antibiotic was the result of research directed towards development of macrolide antibiotics with increased stability in gastric acid and, consequently, better oral absorption and an improved side effect profile. The antibacterial spectrum is the same as erythromycin, but clarithromycin is also active against *Mycobacterium avium* complex (MAC), *M. leprae* and other atypical mycobacteria. There is a rapid first-pass hepatic metabolism, but the main metabolite, 14-hydroxyclarithromycin, is almost twice as active and has a half-life of 7 hours compared to 5 hours for clarithromycin. The drug and metabolite are extensively distributed throughout the body with tissue concentrations well above peak serum values.

Clarithromycin is used in combination therapy with a proton pump inhibitor and amoxicillin (q.v.) to treat *Helicobacter pylori* in older children and adults. Clarithromycin crosses the placenta in greater amounts than other macrolides, but there do not appear to be any teratogenic effects. It also enters breast milk, reaching levels of up to 75% of maternal concentrations, but seems safe with few reported neonatal effects.

Like other macrolides, clarithromycin has been used to eradicate *Ureaplasma urealyticum* in infants at risk from chronic lung disease (CLD), and in one single centre study to reduce CLD, when started in the first 3 days of life, in preterm infants with *U. urealyticum* isolated from nasopharyngeal swabs.

The manufacturer has yet to endorse **intravenous (IV)** treatment in children less than 12 years.

Prevention of pertussis

When a diagnosis of pertussis has been made and there is a vulnerable individual (i.e. an unimmunised or partially immunised child under 1 year of age) in close contact with the index case, the family and the 'at-risk' child should be given clarithromycin. Unfortunately, the immunity imparted by childhood pertussis immunisation wanes within 10 years, and staff working in neonatal units may pose a risk to a large cohort of unimmunised neonates. See web commentary for full details.

Drug interactions

Clarithromycin is a potent inhibitor of the hepatic cytochrome, CYP3A4, and increases the half-life of a number of drugs such as midazolam, theophylline and carbamazepine producing potential toxicity. It also prolongs the QT interval, and this effect can be dangerously potentiated by interaction with other drugs.

Treatment

Pertussis prophylaxis: In neonates and young infants, give 7.5 mg/kg orally twice a day. Once the child reaches 8 kg, give 62.5 mg twice daily, until they reach 11 kg when the dose is 125 mg twice a day. Give the antibiotic for 7 days.

Treatment of infection: In neonates and young infants, give 7.5 mg/kg orally twice a day. Once the child reaches 8 kg, give 62.5 mg twice daily, until they reach 11 kg when the dose is 125 mg twice a day. Treatment is normally for 7 days but may be extended to 14 days. In severe infections or where oral dosing is not possible, clarithromycin 7.5 mg/kg (made up as described below) may be given intravenously every 12 hours into central or large proximal veins.

Supply and administration

70 ml of the oral suspension of clarithromycin (25 mg/ml) costs £5 and can be kept for up to 2 weeks after being reconstituted from the dry powder. This solution contains 2.4 g of sucrose per 5 ml. Clarithromycin lactobionate for IV injection is available in 500 mg vials (cost £9.50). Vials should first be reconstituted with 10 ml water for injection, before further dilution with 5% glucose or 0.9% sodium chloride to a concentration of 2 mg/ml. The required dose should be infused over 1 hour into a central or large proximal vein.

Continued on p. 161

References

See also the relevant Cochrane reviews

Haiduven DJ, Hench CP, Simpkins SM, *et al.* Standardized management of patients and employees exposed to pertussis. *Infect Control Hosp Epidemiol* 1998;**19**:861–4.

Koletzko S, Jones NL, Goodman KJ, *et al.* Evidence-based guidelines from ESPGHAN and NASPGHAN for *Helicobacter pylori* Infection in children. *J Pediatr Gastroenterol Nutr* 2011;**53**:230–43.

Maltezou HC, Ftika L, Theodoridou M. Nosocomial pertussis in neonatal units. *J Hosp Infect* 2013;**85**:243–8.

Ozdemir R, Erdeve O, Dizdar EA, *et al.* Clarithromycin in preventing bronchopulmonary dysplasia in *Ureaplasma urealyticum*-positive preterm infants. *Pediatrics* 2011;**128**:e1496–501.

Viscardi RM. Ureaplasma species: role in neonatal morbidities and outcomes. *Arch Dis Child Fetal Neonatal Ed* 2014;**99**:F87–92.

Use

Clindamycin hydrochloride is a lincosamide antibiotic related to lincomycin and is used in the prophylaxis and treatment of anaerobic infections. It can also be used to protect against bacterial endocarditis in penicillin allergic individuals, and neonatal group B streptococcal infection if the mother is allergic to penicillin.

Pharmacology

Clindamycin has a mainly bacteriostatic effect on Gram-positive aerobes and a wide range of anaerobic bacteria. It acts by inhibiting protein synthesis in much the same way as erythromycin. Lincomycin was originally isolated from the bacterium *Streptomyces lincolnensis*, found in a soil sample, but was later superseded by clindamycin which was first synthesised in 1967. It is rapidly absorbed when given by mouth and penetrates most tissues well, although CSF penetration is poor.

Clindamycin is metabolised by the liver with a half-life in adults of 2–3 hours. The dose given does not normally need to be changed when there is renal failure because only a little is excreted unmetabolised in the urine. The half-life is long and extremely variable 3–15 hours in the preterm baby, falling to adult values by 2 months, and the manufacturers do not recommend intravenous (IV) use in babies less than 4 weeks old. The risk of diarrhoea, and of occasionally fatal antibiotic-related pseudomembranous colitis (characterised by bloody diarrhoea and abdominal pain), has limited the neonatal use of this antibiotic. Treatment must be stopped at once if this adverse reaction is suspected. Oral vancomycin (15 mg/kg every 8 hours) and parenteral nutrition are often used to treat this colitis which seems to be due to *Clostridium difficile* toxin. Other adverse effects include skin rashes and other hypersensitivity reactions, blood dyscrasias and disturbances of hepatic function. The drug is still sometimes used as an alternative to sodium fusidate (q.v.) in the management of resistant staphylococcal osteomyelitis and to control the anaerobic sepsis associated with necrotising enterocolitis (although the only controlled trial raised the possibility that clindamycin might increase the risk of late stricture formation). Clindamycin is occasionally used in the management of protozoal infection (including malaria and toxoplasmosis). It is now also being increasingly used to treat overt bacterial vaginosis, and some also advocate screening for asymptomatic vaginosis in early pregnancy if vaginal pH exceeds 4.5. There is no evidence of teratogenicity, and treatment during lactation only exposes the baby to about 3% of the maternal dose on a weight-for-weight basis. There is just one anecdotal report of a baby who passed two bloody stools while being breastfed by such a mother.

Prophylaxis

Bacterial vaginosis: Clindamycin (5 g of the 2% vaginal cream once a day for 7 days or 300 mg twice daily by mouth for 5 days) reduced the risk of very preterm birth in two trials when given to women with a clearly abnormal vaginal flora or frank bacterial vaginosis in *early* pregnancy (before 20 weeks).

Maternal group B streptococcal carriage: Clindamycin (900 mg IV once every 8 hours) can be used, like penicillin (q.v.) or erythromycin, to reduce the risk of the baby becoming infected during delivery.

In children with heart defects: Short courses of clindamycin are still sometimes given during surgery involving a site where infection is suspected to reduce the risk of endocarditis in patients who are allergic to penicillin. Give 20 mg/kg of clindamycin by mouth 1 hour before the procedure is due.

Treatment

Neonates (age under 14 days): Give 5 mg/kg by mouth or (slowly) IV once every 8 hours for 7–10 days to manage severe staphylococcal infection or the septicaemia associated with necrotising enterocolitis.

Infants (more than 2 weeks old): Give 5 mg/kg by mouth or (slowly) IV once every 6 hours.

Supply and administration

300 mg (2 ml) ampoules of clindamycin phosphate (containing 0.9% w/v benzyl alcohol) cost £6.20. To obtain a solution containing 5 mg/ml for accurate administration, first dilute the contents of the 300 mg ampoule to 15 ml with 5% glucose, and then take 0.25 ml (5 mg) of this solution for each kilogram that the baby weighs, dilute this with 0.75 ml/kg of 5% glucose, and infuse over at least 10 minutes. Clindamycin palmitate could also be made available as an oral suspension. This is stable for 2 weeks at room temperature after reconstitution. A 40 g pack of the 2% vaginal cream costs £10.86.

Continued on p. 163

> **Note: Very immature babies may be at risk from the effects of benzyl alcohol, which is an excipient of the IV product.**

References

See also the relevant Cochrane reviews

Bell MJ, Shackelford P, Smith R, *et al*. Pharmacokinetics of clindamycin phosphate in the first year of life. *J Pediatr* 1984;**105**:482–6.

Deajani AS, Taubert KA, Wilson W, *et al*. Prevention of bacterial endocarditis: recommendations by the American Heart Association. *JAMA* 1997;**277**:1794–801.

Faix RG, Polley TZ, Grasela TH. A randomised, controlled trial of parenteral clindamycin in neonatal necrotising enterocolitis. *J Pediatr* 1988;**112**:271–9. [RCT]

Hall CM, Milligan DWA, Berrington J. Probable adverse reaction to a pharmaceutical excipient. *Arch Dis Child Fetal Neonatal Ed* 2004;**89**:F184.

Koren G, Zarfin Y, Maresky D, *et al*. Pharmacokinetics of intravenous clindamycin in newborn infants. *Pediatr Pharmacol* 1986;**5**:187–92.

Larsson P-G, Fåhraeus L, Carlsson B, *et al*. Late miscarriage and preterm birth after treatment with clindamycin: a randomised consent design study according to Zelen. *Br J Obstet Gynecol* 2006;**113**:629–37. [RCT] (See also pp. 1483–4.)

Ugwamadu A, Manyonda I, Reid F, *et al*. Effect of early oral clindamycin on late miscarriage and preterm delivery in asymptomatic women with abnormal vaginal flora and bacterial vaginosis: a randomised controlled trial. *Lancet* 2003;**361**:983–8. [RCT]

Use

Clonazepam, like lorazepam (q.v.), is sometimes used in the neonatal period to control severe continuous seizure activity resistant to routine anticonvulsant treatment, despite increasing concern that its sedative effect may sometimes mask the fact that cortical seizure activity has not been suppressed.

Pharmacology

Clonazepam is a benzodiazepine which is completely and readily absorbed from the gastrointestinal tract, peak plasma levels occurring after 60–90 minutes. Steady-state tissue levels exceed plasma levels (V_D~3 l/kg). Clonazepam is extensively metabolised to inactive compounds, but the neonatal half-life is 24–48 hours. It may be given by intravenous (IV) injection if rapid onset of action is required.

Clonazepam has been used since the mid-1970s as an anticonvulsant in various types of epilepsy but is now mostly used in the management of panic attacks and some movement disorders, including hyperekplexia ('exaggerated surprise'), and in the treatment of myoclonic and absence seizures. It crosses the placenta but no adverse fetal effects have been noted. It has also been used in late pregnancy without causing any obvious sedation of the infant after birth. It appears in breast milk like other benzodiazepines. Breastfed babies need to be monitored for drowsiness, and apnoea is a theoretical possibility.

Clonazepam has often been given as a slow, continuous IV infusion in the neonatal period, but this approach is of no particular benefit since clonazepam is only slowly cleared from the brain (unlike diazepam). In addition, its onset of action will be seriously delayed if an initial loading dose is not given. There is no good controlled trial data on the use of clonazepam in the control of neonatal seizures. Drug tolerance becomes a problem if treatment is continued for any extended period, and increasing seizure activity may occur if the serum level exceeds 125 micrograms/l.

> Clonazepam pharmacokinetics during therapeutic hypothermia have not been established, but as the drug is metabolised extensively by hepatic cytochrome P450 enzymes, the already long half-life is likely to be extended further in cooled infants.

Major adverse effects are drowsiness, ataxia and behavioural changes. Bronchial hypersecretion and salivation are said to be a problem in infancy, particularly if there is neurological dysfunction with impaired swallowing. As with all benzodiazepine anticonvulsants, withdrawal of clonazepam should be gradual – over at least 6 weeks if medication has been used for any length of time – in order to reduce the risk of withdrawal (rebound) seizures.

Drug interactions

Concurrent treatment with phenytoin or carbamazepine reduces the half-life of clonazepam.

Treatment

Neonates: Give 100 micrograms/kg IV as a slow bolus injection once every 24 hours for 2–3 days in seizures resistant to routine anticonvulsant medication.

Infants (1–12 months): In status epilepticus, give 50 micrograms/kg repeat after 10 minutes if necessary.

Antidote

Flumazenil is a specific antidote (as described in the monograph on midazolam).

Blood levels

Plasma levels are usually 30–100 micrograms/l (1 micrograms/l = 3.16 nmol/l), but levels do not always correlate with clinical efficacy.

Supply and administration

Stock ampoules containing 1 mg of clonazepam in 1 ml of solvent (cost 63p) are supplied with a further 1 ml ampoule of water for injection. The content of *both* ampoules should be drawn into a syringe *immediately* before use and then diluted to 10 ml with 10% glucose saline to give a

Continued on p. 165

solution that contains 100 micrograms/ml suitable for slow bolus IV administration. Such a solution should *not* be used to give a continuous IV infusion. Each 1 ml ampoule contains 30 mg of benzyl alcohol and a significant (but otherwise unspecified) amount of propylene glycol.

References

André M, Boutroy MJ, Bianchetti G, *et al.* Clonazepam in neonatal seizures: dose regimes and therapeutic efficiency. *Eur J Clin Pharmacol* 1991;**40**:193–5.

André M, Boutroy MJ, Dubrruc C, *et al.* Clonazepam pharmacokinetics and therapeutic efficacy in neonatal seizures. *Eur J Clin Pharmacol* 1986;**30**:585–9.

Boylan GB, Rennie JM, Chorley G, *et al.* Second-line anticonvulsant treatment of neonatal seizures: a video-EEG study. *Neurology* 2004;**62**:486–8. [RCT]

Dhahar E, Raviv R. Sporadic major hyperekplexia in neonates and infants: clinical manifestations and outcome. *Pediatr Neurol* 2004;**31**:30–4.

Rivera S, Villega F, de Saint-Martin A, *et al.* Congenital hyperekplexia: five sporadic cases. *Eur J Pediatr* 2006;**165**:104–7.

Slaughter LA, Patel AD, Slaughter JL. Pharmacological treatment of neonatal seizures: a systematic review. *J Child Neurol* 2013;**28**:351–64.

van Rooij LG, van den Broek MP, Rademaker CM, *et al.* Clinical management of seizures in newborns: diagnosis and treatment. *Paediatr Drugs* 2013;**15**:9–18.

Use

Co-amoxiclav was developed in response to the increasing numbers of β-lactamase-producing bacteria that were formerly treated with amoxicillin (q.v.). It is a combination of the sodium salt of amoxicillin and potassium salt of clavulanic acid in various ratios. These ratios are expressed in the form X/Y where 'X' and 'Y' are the strengths in milligrams of amoxicillin and clavulanic acid, respectively.

Pharmacology

Discovered in 1974, clavulanic acid is produced naturally by the Gram-positive bacterium *Streptomyces clavuligerus*. It was found to have almost no antimicrobial activity, despite sharing the β-lactam ring characteristic of β-lactam antibiotics. Instead, the similarity in its chemical structure allows it to covalently interact with and then inactivate the β-lactamase molecule. This, in turn, renders the bacteria susceptible to β-lactam antibiotics. The pharmacokinetics of clavulanic acid and amoxicillin are very similar. Both are rapidly absorbed after oral administration and have similar half-life of 1–1.5 hours in older children. Both are excreted by the kidney.

Both the amoxicillin and clavulanic acid components cross the human placenta, but use has not been associated with teratogenicity in either animal or human studies. Its use in women with preterm prolonged rupture of membranes may increase the risk of necrotising enterocolitis, and for this reason, it is no longer widely used in the later stages of pregnancy. Other than allergic reactions, the main concern with co-amoxiclav is its association with cholestatic jaundice that can occur either during or shortly afterwards. The risk of acute liver toxicity is about six times greater with co-amoxiclav than with amoxicillin alone; however, these reactions are very rare in children and if they do occur are usually self-limiting and rarely fatal.

Indications

Co-amoxiclav is rarely used in a neonatal intensive care setting; group B streptococcus remains susceptible to penicillin, making this (with or without gentamicin) the first-line treatment for early-onset sepsis. Co-amoxiclav is widely used in the primary and secondary care settings for the treatment of infants and children with infections, particularly of the respiratory tract and middle ear (acute otitis media) where amoxicillin alone is not appropriate.

Controversy continues about how best to manage acute otitis media, not all children require antibiotics, but the prevalence of β-lactamase-producing strains of *Haemophilus influenzae* and *Moraxella catarrhalis* in middle ear fluid isolates means that co-amoxiclav remains a useful choice. Many children respond to simple analgesia only.

Treatment

Intravenous (IV) therapy: Give 30 mg/kg (0.5 ml/kg of a solution made up as described in the section 'Supply and administration') of co-amoxiclav by slow intravenous injection over 3–4 minutes) twice daily in neonates and infants up to the age of 3 months. For infants of 3–12 months, give co-amoxiclav 8 hourly. Alternatively, it may be infused over 30 minutes.
Oral therapy: Co-amoxiclav sugar-free oral suspension is available in a number of different combinations of amoxicillin and clavulanic acid; any prescription needs to specify the amount of co-amoxiclav (in 5 ml of the suspension) as well as the volume per dose.

Oral suspension strength	125/31 in 5 ml	400/57 in 5 ml
Neonate	0.15 ml/kg three times a day	Not recommended
1 month–1 year	0.25 ml/kg three times a day	—
2 months–2 years	—	0.15 ml/kg twice daily

Continued on p. 167

Supply and administration

Vials containing co-amoxiclav 500/100 (amoxicillin 500 mg as sodium salt and clavulanic acid 100 mg as potassium salt) powder for reconstitution cost £1.20. Add 10 ml of water for injection to give a solution containing 60 mg/ml. Give 0.5 ml of this for every kilogram the infant weighs.

Various strengths of oral suspension are available and are not interchangeable. Sugar-free co-amoxiclav 125/31 (costing £2.10 per 100 ml) contains 125 mg of amoxicillin and 31 mg of potassium clavulanate in 5 ml. Sugar-free co-amoxiclav 400/57 (costing £4.10 for 35 ml) contains 400 mg of amoxicillin and 57 mg of potassium clavulanate in 5 ml. The reconstituted suspension should be stored in a refrigerator (at 2–8 °C) and used within 7 days.

References

(See the relevant Cochrane reviews)

Al-Sabbagh A, Moss S, Subhedar N. Neonatal necrotising enterocolitis and perinatal exposure to co-amoxyclav. *Arch Dis Child Fetal Neonatal Ed* 2004;**89**:F187.

Hita EO, García JA, Gonzalez JC, *et al.* Amoxicillin-clavulanic acid hepatotoxicity in children. *J Pediatr Gastroenterol Nutr* 2012;**55**:663–7.

Kenyon S, Boulvain M, Neilson J. Antibiotics for preterm rupture of the membranes: a systematic review. *Obstet Gynecol* 2004;**104**:1051–7.

Kenyon SL, Taylor DJ, Tarnow-Mordi W; ORACLE Collaborative Group. Broad-spectrum antibiotics for preterm, prelabour rupture of fetal membranes: the ORACLE I randomised trial. ORACLE Collaborative Group. *Lancet* 2001;**357**:979–88.

Reading C, Cole M. Clavulanic acid: a beta-lactamase-inhibiting beta-lactam from *Streptomyces clavuligerus*. *Antimicrob Agents Chemother* 1977;**11**:852–7.

Tähtinen PA., Laine MK., Huovinen P, *et al.* A placebo-controlled trial of antimicrobial treatment for acute otitis media. *N Engl J Med* 2011;**364**:116–26.

Use

Codeine is an opioid analgesic frequently given by mouth to adults together with aspirin or paracetamol. Use in adults is being discouraged because of evidence that it is becoming a drug of addiction. In Europe, but not North America, paediatric codeine use is restricted to its use in acute pain relief in children over the age of 12 years. Paracetamol or ibuprofen (q.v.) is used to provide oral analgesia in young children.

Pharmacology

Codeine was first isolated from the opioid juices left over after morphine had been extracted from poppy juice in 1832. The name chosen came from the Greek word *codeia*, meaning a poppy capsule. Codeine is only a mild narcotic but it is probably as effective an antitussive (cough suppressant) as morphine. When given by mouth, its analgesic effect starts to become apparent after 30 minutes and peaks at 2 hours. Absorption is as rapid but less complete after rectal administration, making a larger dose necessary.

Few pharmacokinetic studies have yet been done in early infancy. Tissue levels exceed plasma levels (V_D ~3 l/kg). The drug is partly metabolised by the liver (morphine being one of the metabolites), and it is increasingly thought that metabolism to morphine probably explains much of the drug's analgesic effect. The extent to which this occurs depends on which genetic variant of the CYP2D6 cytochrome P450 enzyme the individual has inherited, making the exact analgesic effect of any given dose hard to predict. People can be classified as *poor, intermediate, extensive* or *ultra-rapid* metabolisers. Poor metabolisers convert very little codeine into morphine and therefore obtain little or no pain relief with codeine; in contrast, ultra-rapid or extensive metabolisers may quickly produce excessive amounts of morphine, which can lead to severe side effects due to its effects on the brain and on respiration.

Codeine causes as much nausea, vomiting, constipation and ileus as a dose of morphine of similar analgesic potency. It also causes as much respiratory depression and hypotension (due to histamine release). Much is finally excreted after conjugation with glucuronic acid in the urine, making repeated, or high-dose, administration hazardous where there is renal or liver failure. Little has been published relating to the use of codeine in babies less than 3 months old.

Codeine is also an ingredient of many of the compound analgesic preparations routinely available (including a range of preparations that are available 'over the counter') even though it is a schedule 2 controlled drug – a fact that those travelling abroad need to bear in mind. Codeine crosses the placenta, but there is no evidence of teratogenicity. Tolerance develops with repeated use, and withdrawal symptoms have been documented, even in infancy. Heavy maternal usage in the period immediately before delivery can even, occasionally, cause neonatal symptoms of opiate withdrawal 1–2 days after delivery.

Codeine and its active metabolite, morphine, are excreted into breast milk. While the highest blood level usually achieved is less than a third of the lowest therapeutic blood level, a minority of babies inherit a gene that results in their metabolising very much more of the codeine into morphine, and there is one recent report where this may have caused death from opiate toxicity. In the United Kingdom and Europe, codeine is now contraindicated during breastfeeding. Some other countries still allow use, and the breastfed baby of any mother taking codeine for more than 1–2 days **must**, therefore, be monitored for lethargy and somnolence.

Antidote

Overdose causes drowsiness, pinpoint pupils and hypotension and can cause dangerous respiratory depression. Naloxone (q.v.) is a specific antidote for all the opiate drugs.

Treatment

Because it is contraindicated in children less than 12 years, no dosing is given here.

Supply

Staff caring for mothers should be aware that some tablets of co-codamol, still widely used as an analgesic after childbirth, contain as much as 30 mg of codeine as well as 500 mg of paracetamol.

Continued on p. 169

References

Broussard CS, Rasmussen SA, Reefhuis J, *et al*. Maternal treatment with opioid analgesics and risk for birth defects. *Am J Obstet Gynecol* 2011;**204**:314.e1–11.

Koren G, Cairns J, Chitayat D, *et al*. Pharmacogenetics of morphine poisoning in a breast fed neonate of a codeine-prescribed mother. *Lancet* 2006;**368**:704. (See also *Lancet* 2008;**372**;606–7 and 625–6.)

Magnani B, Evans R. Codeine intoxication in the neonate. *Pediatrics* 1999;**104**:e75.

McEwan A, Sigston PE, Andrews KA, *et al*. A comparison of rectal and intramuscular codeine phosphate in children following neurosurgery. *Paediatr Anaesth* 2000;**10**:189–93. [RCT]

Meny RG, Naumburg EG, Alger LS, *et al*. Codeine and the breast fed neonate. *J Hum Lactation* 1993; **9**: 237–40.

Sistonen J, Madadi P, Ross CJ, *et al*. Prediction of codeine toxicity in infants and their mothers using a novel combination of maternal genetic markers. *Clin Pharmacol Ther* 2012;**91**:692–9.

Williams DG, Hatch CJ, Howard RF. Codeine phosphate in paediatric medicine. *Br J Anaesth* 2001;**86**:413–21.

Williams DG, Patel A, Howard RF. Pharmacogenetics of codeine metabolism in an urban population of children and its implications for analgesic reliability. *Br J Anaesth* 2002;**89**:839–45.

Zhang WY, Li Wan Po A. Analgesic efficacy of paracetamol and its combination with codeine and caffeine in surgical pain – a meta-analysis. *J Clin Pharm Ther* 1996;**21**:261–82. [SR]

Use

Co-trimoxazole is used to treat cholera (*Vibrio cholerae* infection) and to prevent and treat *Pneumocystis jiroveci* (formerly *carinii*) infection. It is an effective treatment for two important protozoan intestinal infections (isosporiasis and cyclosporiasis). It has also been used to treat uncomplicated falciparum malaria and is sometimes used in the management of neonatal meningitis because of good tissue and CSF penetration.

Pharmacology

Co-trimoxazole is a 5:1 mixture of two different antibiotics that inhibit folic acid synthesis in protozoa and bacteria (and, to a lesser degree, in man). It was first marketed in 1969. The bacteriostatic effect of the long-acting sulphonamide (sulfamethoxazole) is augmented by the synergistic effect of trimethoprim (q.v.). The two drugs in combination are active against most common pathogens except *Pseudomonas* and *Mycobacterium tuberculosis*. Both drugs are well absorbed by mouth and actively excreted by the kidney with half-lives of about 12 hours. They also cross the placenta with ease. CSF levels approach half those in the plasma, while levels in the urine and in bronchial and vaginal secretions exceed those in plasma. Use during lactation only exposes the baby to about 3% of the weight-adjusted maternal dose.

Because both drugs are folate antagonists, the manufacturers still caution against their use during pregnancy, but teratogenicity has only been encountered in folate-deficient animals, and the drug has now been in widespread clinical use for more than 30 years. The manufacturers have also declined to recommend use in babies less than 6 weeks old, but there is no specific reason for this caution other than the risk of haemolytic anaemia in babies with G6PD deficiency and the risk of kernicterus (although sulfamethoxazole competes for the protein binding sites usually available to bilirubin in babies with jaundice less than most of the other sulphonamide antibiotics). Caution is understandable however given the unnecessary deaths caused by the prophylactic use of sulphonamide drugs in the early 1950s (as outlined in the monograph on sulfadiazine).

Rapid intravenous (IV) administration can cause an allergic reaction or anaphylaxis. Other adverse effects, which can be fatal, are usually only seen in elderly patients or following high-dose treatment in patients with AIDS. Nevertheless, since the problems (including rashes, erythema multiforme and marrow depression) are almost certainly due to the sulphonamide component, trimethoprim is now increasingly prescribed on its own.

Drug interactions

Treatment with co-trimoxazole increases the plasma half-life of phenytoin.

Prescribing

Specify the *total* amount of active drug in milligrams. Thus, 20 mg/kg of sulfamethoxazole and 4 mg/kg of trimethoprim are prescribed as 24 mg/kg of active drug.

Prophylaxis

Immunodeficiency: Give a single dose as detailed in the table by mouth once a day **3 days a week** to babies with possible combined immunodeficiency, or HIV, to reduce the risk of bacterial infection and of *P. jiroveci* pneumonia.

Measles: Complications in a resource-poor country can be reduced by giving co-trimoxazole for 7 days.

Surface area (m²)	Dose (mg)
<0.25	120
0.25–0.39	240
0.4–0.49	360
0.5–0.75	480
0.76–1	720
>1	960

Continued on p. 171

Treatment

Dose: Treat severe systemic infection with 24 mg/kg of active drug by mouth (or IV, if oral treatment is impracticable). Avoid in babies with limited renal function, unless the plasma sulfamethoxazole trough level is kept below 120 mg/l (1 mg/l = 3.95 mmol/l), and in babies with serious unconjugated jaundice.

Timing: Give once a day in the first week of life and once every 12 hours after that. Treat *Pneumocystis* once every 6 hours in babies over 4 weeks old, even if the blood level exceeds 120 mg/l.

Supply and administration

A sugar-free paediatric oral suspension containing 48 mg of active drug per ml (240 mg/5 ml) costs £1.10 per 100 ml. 5 ml ampoules for IV use containing 96 mg/ml (costing £1.60 per ampoule) are also available: to give the standard neonatal dose (24 mg/kg), dilute 0.25 ml/kg of the contents of the ampoule into at least 15 times the same volume of 10% glucose in 0.18% sodium chloride and then infuse this over 2 hours. The IV preparation contains 45% w/v propylene glycol. Avoid IM use in small children. More concentrated solutions have been given using a central line.

References (See also the relevant Cochrane reviews)

Chintu C, Bhat GJ, Walker AS, *et al.* Co-trimoxazole as prophylaxis against opportunistic infections in HIV-infected Zambian children (CHAP): a double-blind randomised placebo-controlled trial. *Lancet* 2004;**364**:1865–71. [RCT] (See also 2005;**365**:749–50.)

Escobedo AA, Almirall P, Alfonso M, *et al.* Treatment of intestinal protozoan infections in children. *Arch Dis Child* 2009;**94**:478–82.

Fehintola FA, Adedeji AA, Tambo E, *et al.* Cotrimoxazole in the treatment of acute uncomplicated falciparum malaria in Nigerian children: a controlled clinical trial. *Clin Drug Invest* 2004;**24**:149–55. [RCT]

Garly M-L, Balé C, Martins CL, *et al.* Prophylactic antibiotics to prevent pneumonia and other complications after measles: community based randomised double blind placebo controlled trial in Guinea-Bissau. *Br Med J* 2006;**333**:1245–7. [RCT]

Graham SM. Prophylaxis against *Pneumocystis carinii* pneumonia for HIV-exposed infants in Africa. *Lancet* 2002;**360**:1966–8.

Use

Dalteparin sodium is a fractionated, low molecular weight derivative of heparin (q.v.) with most of the properties similar to the parent drug, but with a longer duration of action, and is given subcutaneously rather than by intravenous (IV) injection.

Pharmacology

Dalteparin is prepared by nitrous acid degradation of unfractionated heparin from porcine intestinal mucosa. It is composed of strongly acidic sulphated polysaccharide chains with an average molecular weight of 5000 and about 90% of the material within the range of 2000–9000. As with all other LMWHs, it has a more predictable response, a greater bioavailability and a longer anti-Xa half-life than unfractionated heparin. Dalteparin is eliminated through the kidneys, and the half-life of 3–5 hours after subcutaneous injection is substantially extended in patients with renal impairment.

Dalteparin can also be safely used in most pregnant women. Like other LMWHs and unfractionated heparin, it does not cross the placenta. If required during lactation, the molecular weight makes significant transfer into breast milk very unlikely, and in any case, drug entering the milk would be inactivated in the baby's gut before absorption. Reports of use in children and infants are rare (most experience of LMWHs in this age group has been with enoxaparin).

Maternal thromboembolism

Prophylaxis: High-risk obstetric patients with thrombophilia, immobility, obesity, pre-eclampsia or a past history of deep vein thrombosis should be assessed for their risk factors and considered for prophylactic LMWH. The daily dose depends on the patient's weight (see table). Doses of 7500 units or higher may be given as two smaller doses, but otherwise, once daily dosing is appropriate.

Weight (kg) at booking	Total daily dose of dalteparin
<50 kg	2500 units
50–90 kg	5000 units
91–130 kg	7500 units
131–170 kg	10,000 units
>170 kg	75 units/kg

Experience indicates that monitoring of anti-Xa levels is not required during thromboprophylaxis with LMWH. Stop 24 hours prior to any planned operative (or epidural) delivery until 4 hours after the procedure is over. Women receiving antenatal LMWH should be advised that, if they have any vaginal bleeding or once labour begins, they should not inject any further LMWH. There is no need to monitor platelets routinely unless there has been exposure to unfractionated heparin.

Treatment: Give a 100 unit/kg dose of dalteparin by subcutaneous injection once every 12 hours. Start treatment promptly, as soon as a clot or embolus is seriously suspected, after first taking blood for a full thrombophilia screen and confirm that renal and liver function are normal. Routine measurement of peak anti-Xa activity is not usually indicated unless the woman weighs less than 50 kg or more than 90 kg. As with prophylaxis, LMWH should be stopped at the onset of labour or 24 hours before any planned operative delivery or an epidural.

Neonatal treatment (including infants up to 12 months)

Bear in mind that experience is extremely limited.
Prophylaxis: 100 units/kg once every 24 hours.
Treatment: 100 units/kg every 12 hours. Adjust the dose according to the peak anti-Xa level.

Dose monitoring

Take blood 3–4 hours after subcutaneous injection to assess the peak anti-Xa level, and adjust the dose to achieve a level of 0.6–1.0 units/ml during treatment and 0.35–0.7 units/ml during prophylaxis. Activated partial thromboplastin time (APTT) or thrombin time should not be used

Continued on p. 173

because these tests are relatively insensitive to the activity of dalteparin. Increasing the dose of dalteparin in an attempt to prolong APTT may result in bleeding.

Antidote

Protamine sulphate will usually stop overt haemorrhage as summarised in the monograph on heparin.

Supply and administration

The drug is available in a range of pre-filled syringes (0.2–0.72 ml) containing 12,500 units/ml of dalteparin sodium; syringes cost from £1.90 to £10 each. Avoid the use of the 4 ml multi-dose vial (contains 100,000 units) which contains benzyl alcohol. To make a more dilute 1250 unit/ml preparation for accurate neonatal use, draw 0.1 ml into a 1 ml syringe and make up to 1 ml with water for injection just before use.

References   (See also the UK guideline on thromboprophylaxis in pregnancy)

Merli GJ, Groce JB. Pharmacological and clinical differences between low-molecular-weight heparins: implications for prescribing practice and therapeutic interchange. *P T* 2010;**35**:95–105.

Nohe N, Flemmer A, Rümler R, *et al.* The low molecular weight heparin dalteparin for prophylaxis and therapy of thrombosis in childhood: a report on 48 cases. *Eur J Pediatr* 1999;**158**(suppl 3):S134–9.

Rey E, Garneau P, David M, *et al.* Dalteparin for the prevention of recurrence of placental-mediated complications of pregnancy in women without thrombophilia: a pilot randomized controlled trial. *J Thromb Haemost* 2009;**7**:58–64.

Use

The use of a single 2-day course of dexamethasone or, preferably, betamethasone (q.v.) to accelerate surfactant production in the fetal lung *before* birth is known to be safe, but the safety of sustained high-dose use in the weeks *after* birth remains extremely uncertain.

Pharmacology in pregnancy

Dexamethasone, a potent glucocorticoid that is well absorbed by mouth, was developed in 1958. It crosses the placenta and has a half-life of about 3 hours. It appears as effective as betamethasone in accelerating surfactant production by the preterm fetal lung, reducing the risk of death from respiratory distress. Maternal treatment alters fetal heart rate and its variability and marginally enhances renal maturation. Treatment can control virilisation in fetuses with congenital adrenal hyperplasia, and 4 mg a day may improve the outcome if maternal lupus erythematosus causes fetal heart block (with salbutamol if the heart rate is <55 bpm). Dexamethasone is excreted into breast milk, but it would require prolonged courses of high doses to produce effects in the breastfed infant.

Pharmacology in the neonate

Dexamethasone can speed extubation in a minority of babies with laryngeal oedema. It can also reduce the amount of time that preterm babies with acute lung injury due to some combination of mechanical ventilation, low-grade infection and oxidative stress (so-called bronchopulmonary dysplasia or BPD) need to spend in oxygen before being discharged home. Steroids should not be given lightly, however, because their use is associated with a 50% increase in the risk of secondary infection, while protein catabolism also affects growth. The associated rise in blood pressure and blood glucose rarely calls for intervention, and the hypertrophy of the ventricular myocardium seen in a minority is reversible, but steroid use increases the risk of nephrocalcinosis in babies on diuretics. Gastrointestinal haemorrhage and perforation can occur, while continuous treatment for over 10 days can also cause adrenal suppression for 2–4 weeks. If steroids are going to be beneficial, some improvement will almost always be seen within 48 hours.

Increased survival rather than time in oxygen is, however, what matters. Improved survival free from evidence of chronic lung disease at 36 weeks postmenstrual age has only been seen when treatment is limited to babies who are still ventilator dependent and in substantial oxygen 7–14 days after birth. Intervention outside this 'time window' seems to have no measurable impact on survival. Even more worryingly, the combined results from 11 trials involving 1388 children followed after discharge show more disability among the steroid-treated children (although frequent 'open-label' steroid use in controls in some studies complicates meaningful analysis). Perhaps, as with all drugs, dexamethasone has the potential to do good and do harm.

Unfortunately, despite two decades of widespread use, we still know little about the best dose to use or the optimum length of treatment. Inhaled steroids have not proved as effective as was hoped, as the monograph on budesonide makes clear. Neither have short, 3-day 'pulses' of treatment proved an advance. However, Durand's low-dose regimen (see the section on 'Treating chronic lung disease') has been shown to improve pulmonary function in the first week of treatment as effectively as the regimen used in the past while reducing corticosteroid exposure by two-thirds, and the short-term outcome of the Australian DART trial which had to close early for lack of support (see web commentary) has now confirmed this. In the end, however, any *short*-term benefit seen may only be worth having if the *long*-term outcome is equally reassuring – an issue still unaddressed by any large study. In so far as use reduces BPD, it may achieve this largely by facilitating earlier extubation.

One study has suggested that treating established BPD with a tapering 3-week course of hydrocortisone (75 mg/kg in total) may be as effective as standard high-dose dexamethasone treatment (6 mg/kg in total) and generate fewer adverse effects. Many will take this as evidence that the use of a different corticosteroid is worth more study; others that this just shows that the early studies used too high a dose of dexamethasone, even though one recent meta-analysis has suggested that a high dose might be better.

Drug equivalence

Each 1 mg dose of dexamethasone **base** is equivalent to 1.2 mg of dexamethasone phosphate or 5 mg of dexamethasone sodium phosphate. Minimise confusion by prescribing the amount of **base** to be given.

Continued on p. 175

Prophylaxis

Congenital adrenal hyperplasia: Giving the mother 7 micrograms/kg of dexamethasone *base* once every 8 hours, preferably before the eighth week of pregnancy, reduces virilisation in the affected female fetus but may have some impact on working memory in children treated unnecessarily. Reduce the dose in the third trimester to minimise side effects. Hydrocortisone (q.v.) is used once diagnosis is confirmed after birth.

Fetal lung maturation: Give 12 mg of dexamethasone *base* by intramuscular (IM) injection to the mother and repeat once after 24 hours if there is a risk of preterm delivery. Oral treatment (four 6 mg doses once every 12 hours) is sometimes preferred, although one small trial has suggested that the outcome is marginally less satisfactory. One important observational study suggests that betamethasone (q.v.) may be better.

Early BPD: Early postnatal steroid use can no longer be justified except as part of a formal controlled trial.

Meningitis: 150 micrograms/kg of dexamethasone *base* given six hourly by intravascular (IV) injection, IM or by mouth for 2 days started *early* can reduce the risk of subsequent deafness in young children with early *Haemophilus* or pneumococcal meningitis (possibly by moderating toxins from rapid bacterial lysis caused by treatment with cefotaxime).

Treating chronic lung disease

Ventilated preterm babies who are still seriously oxygen dependent 7–10 days after birth are at serious risk of developing chronic lung disease. While parents may understandably want treatment with dexamethasone tried if it is starting to look as though progressive lung disease may jeopardise survival, it remains uncertain which – if any – of the following treatment strategies is best. Low-dose strategies are now favoured.

DART trial regimen: 60 micrograms/kg of dexamethasone *base* twice a day IV (or orally) on days 1–3, 40 micrograms/kg twice a day on days 4–6, 20 micrograms/kg twice a day on days 7–8 and 8 micrograms/kg twice a day on days 9–10 (a total of 712 micrograms/kg over 10 days). Repeat once if necessary.

Durand trial regimen: 100 micrograms/kg of dexamethasone *base* IV twice a day for 3 days and then 50 micrograms/kg twice a day for 4 days (a total of 1 mg/kg over 7 days).

Traditional regimen: 250 micrograms/kg of dexamethasone *base* orally or IV twice a day for 7 days was, until about 10 years ago, the most widely used regimen. Some babies were also offered a second course.

Treating other conditions

Hypotension: One 100 micrograms/kg dose followed, if necessary, by 50 micrograms/kg IV twice a day for 1–2 days often 'cures' inotrope-resistant neonatal hypotension. Low-dose hydrocortisone is also effective.

Facilitating extubation in the preterm baby: Even if the DART regimen (see preceding text) does not reduce chronic lung damage, it *does* facilitate extubation, and less than half this dose seemed to help in one small study. The Minidex study used a dose of microgram per kilograms per day for 10 days followed by alternate-day doses for 6 days. The effects of this very low dose have not yet been reported in a randomised trial.

Treatment for post-intubation laryngeal oedema: Three 200 micrograms/kg doses of dexamethasone *base* orally or IV at 8 hourly intervals (started at least 4 and preferably 12 hours before the endotracheal tube is removed) may aid extubation in babies and in older children with an oedematous or traumatised larynx.

Croup: Viral croup responds to a single 150 micrograms/kg dose of oral dexamethasone *base* as well as it does to an IM dose. Effects are seen within 30 minutes of administration. The dose can be repeated after 12 hours if necessary. Inhaled budesonide and oral prednisolone (q.v.) are alternatives with comparable efficacy.

Surgical stress: To cover possible adrenal suppression, babies on dexamethasone or who last completed a course of dexamethasone lasting more than 1 week less than 4 weeks ago should receive 1 mg/kg of hydrocortisone IV prior to surgery and then every 6 hours IV or IM for 24–48 hours.

Supply and administration

Several products exist and care must be taken to avoid the confusion caused by different labelling. 1 ml vials are available containing either 3.3 mg dexamethasone base or 4 mg of dexamethasone phosphate (depending on the supplier – these are equal amounts of the drug).

Continued on p. 176

Vials cost 91 p–£1.10. *Avoid products with a sulphite preservative* (for reasons outlined in the website commentary). Draw 0.3 ml of fluid from the vial into a syringe and dilute to 10 ml with 5% glucose to get a solution containing 100 micrograms/ml of base for IV or oral use. Scored 500 micrograms tablets are available (costing 2p each). So is a sugar-free 0·4 mg/ml oral solution (costing £42.30 for 150 ml) with a 3-month shelf-life which can be further diluted if necessary just before use (although this contains propylene glycol).

References

(See also the relevant Cochrane reviews)

Ausejo M, Saenz A, Pham B, *et al*. The effectiveness of glucocorticoids in treating croup: meta-analysis. *Br Med J* 1999;**319**:595–600. [SR]

Bjornson CL, Klassen TP, Williamson J, *et al*. A randomized trial of a single dose of oral dexamethasone for mild croup. *N Engl J Med* 2004;**351**:1306–13. [RCT] (See also pp. 1283–4.)

Brook CGD. Antenatal treatment of a mother bearing a fetus with congenital adrenal hyperplasia. *Arch Dis Child Fetal Neonatal Ed* 2000;**82**:F176–8. (See also associated commentaries pp. 178–81.)

Dobrovoljac M, Geelhoed GC. How fast does oral dexamethasone work in mild to moderately severe croup? A randomized double-blinded clinical trial. *Emerg Med Australas* 2012;**24**:79–85. [RCT]

Doyle LW, Davis PG, Morley CJ, *et al*. Low-dose dexamethasone facilitates extubation among chronically ventilator-dependent infants: a multicenter, international, randomized, controlled trial. *Pediatrics* 2006;**117**:75–83. [RCT] (See also 2007;**119**:716–21.)

Doyle LW, Halliday HL, Ehrenkranz RA, *et al*. Impact of postnatal systematic corticosteroids on mortality and cerebral palsy in preterm infants: effect modification by risk for chronic lung disease. *Pediatrics* 2005; **115**:655–61. (See also p. 794.) [SR]

Gaissmaier RE, Pohlandt F. Single-dose dexamethasone treatment of hypotension in preterm infants. *J Pediatr* 1999;**134**:701–5. [RCT]

Jaeggi ET, Fouron J-C, Silverman ED, *et al*. Transplacental fetal treatment improves the outcome of prenatally diagnosed complete atrioventricular heart block without structural heart disease. *Circulation* 2004;**110**: 1542–8.

Lukkassen IMA, Hassing MBF, Markhirst DG. Dexamethasone reduces reintubation rate due to postextubation stridor in a high-risk paediatric population. *Acta Paediatr* 2006;**95**:74–6.

New MI, Abraham M, Yuen T, *et al*. An update on prenatal diagnosis and treatment of congenital adrenal hyperplasia. *Semin Reprod Med* 2012;**30**:396–9.

Noori S, Siassi B, Durand M, *et al*. Cardiovascular effects of low-dose dexamethasone in very low birth weight neonates with refractory hypotension. *Biol Neonate* 2006;**89**:82–7.

Onland W, Offringa M De Jaegere AP, *et al*. Finding the optimal postnatal dexamethasone regimen for preterm infants at risk of bronchopulmonary dysplasia: a systematic review of placebo-controlled trials. *Pediatrics* 2009;**123**:367–77. [SR]

Tanney K, Davis JW, Halliday H, *et al*. Extremely low-dose dexamethasone to facilitate extubation in mechanically ventilated preterm babies. *Neonatology* 2011;**100**:285–9.

van der Heide-Jalving M, Kamphuis PJGH, van der Laan MJ, *et al*. Short- and long-term effects of neonatal glucocorticoid therapy: is hydrocortisone an alternative to dexamethasone? *Acta Paediatr* 2003;**92**:827–35.

Yates HL, Newell SJ. Minidex: very low dose dexamethasone (0.05 mg/kg/day) in chronic lung disease. *Arch Dis Child Fetal Neonatal Ed* 2011;**96**:F190–4.

Yeh TF, Lin YJ, Lin HC, *et al*. Outcomes at school age after postnatal dexamethasone for lung disease of prematurity. *N Engl J Med* 2004;**350**:1304–13. [RCT] (See also pp. 1349–51.)

Use

Diamorphine has been used to control neonatal pain, but morphine (q.v.), which has been more fully evaluated in neonates, is equally effective.

Pharmacology

Diamorphine hydrochloride is a potent semi-synthetic opioid analgesic. Because it is all converted, within minutes, to morphine and 6-monoacetylmorphine in the body, almost all the drug's properties and adverse effects, including reduced peristalsis, urinary retention and respiratory depression, are essentially the same as for morphine. It is well absorbed by mouth, but bioavailability is reduced by rapid first-pass liver metabolism. Some enters the CNS after bolus intravenous (IV) administration causing intense euphoria, and it is this that probably makes the drug so addictive. Clearance is very variable, inversely related to gestational age and essentially the same as for morphine. High solubility is the drug's only clinical advantage, because this makes it possible to give a large intramuscular dose in a small-volume injection, but this is of no relevance to its use in infancy.

There are *no* good pharmacological reasons for using diamorphine rather than morphine in young children, and parents can be very disconcerted to discover, possibly by chance, that their child is 'on heroin'. It was first manufactured on a commercial basis in 1898 but eventually banned in America in 1924 after its full addictive potential became apparent. Many other countries have since introduced similar bans. Placental transfer is rapid, but there is no reason why a mother given diamorphine in labour should not breastfeed, although the baby may be too drowsy to suckle vigorously for several hours, unless offered naloxone (q.v.).

Maternal addiction

While there have been suggestions that diamorphine could be teratogenic, the malformations reported conform to no discernible pattern, and all the mothers in the studies reported had been taking heroin of uncertain purity as well as other drugs during pregnancy. Fetal growth is often reduced, and there may be an increased risk of fetal death. Most mothers in the United Kingdom admitting to opiate addiction are now placed on methadone (q.v.) during pregnancy to minimise these problems. Even so, babies exposed to *any* opiate drug in pregnancy, including methadone, show slight (but significant) developmental delay when 2–3 years old.

While morphine is still widely used to control any symptoms of withdrawal that appear in the baby after delivery, methadone may be used as an alternative. Some babies seem to benefit from being given phenobarbital (q.v.) as well, and there is a belief that chlorpromazine (q.v.) can be helpful if an opiate is not the only illicit drug that the mother is taking. The use of paregoric (a variable cocktail of opium, glycerine, alcohol and benzoic acid) lacks rational justification. Some assessment scales have the perverse effect of suggesting that an increasingly sedated baby is improving, but the main aim of treatment must be to improve the baby's ability to feed normally as well as sleep normally, and an unnecessarily complex weaning strategy merely serves to delay discharge. Mothers are sometimes discouraged from breastfeeding, but lactation can be used as part of a controlled weaning strategy as long as the mother is not also taking other serious drugs of abuse, since the baby only receives, on a weight-for-weight basis, about 5–10% of the maternal dose.

Pain relief

Give ventilated babies in serious pain a loading dose of 180 micrograms/kg IV followed by a maintenance infusion of 15 micrograms/kg/hour (or 6 ml/hour *for 1 hour* followed by 0.5 ml/hour of a solution made up as described under 'Supply and administration') accepting that this can depress any respiratory activity that may allow the baby to 'trigger' the ventilator. Sedation only requires 9 micrograms/kg/hour IV (0.3 ml/hour). Intra-nasal administration gives good relief after approximately 20 minutes.

Antidote

Naloxone is a specific antidote for all the opioid drugs.

Supply and administration

10 mg ampoules of diamorphine cost £3.10. The ampoule should be reconstituted with 1 ml of water to give a solution containing 10 mg/ml. To set up a continuous infusion, dilute this reconstituted liquid to 10 ml with 0.9% sodium chloride; place 1.5 ml of this diluted preparation for

Continued on p. 178

each kilogram the baby weighs in a syringe, dilute to 50 ml with 10% glucose saline, and infuse at a rate of 0.5 ml/hour in order to provide a continuous infusion of 15 micrograms/kg/hour. The drug is stable in solution, so it is not necessary to change the infusate daily.

References
(See also the relevant Cochrane reviews)

Barker DP, Simpson J, Barrett DA, *et al*. Randomised double blind trial of two loading dose regimens of diamorphine in ventilated newborn infants. *Arch Dis Child Fetal Neonatal Ed* 1995; **73**:F22–6. [RCT]

Barrett DA, Barker DP, Rutter N, *et al*. Morphine, morphine-6-glucuronide and morphine-3-glucuronide pharmacokinetics in newborn infants receiving diamorphine infusions. *Br J Clin Pharmacol* 1996;**41**:531–7.

Hunt RW, Tzioumi D, Collins E, *et al*. Adverse neurodevelopmental outcome of infants exposed to opiate in-utero. *Early Hum Dev* 2008;**84**:29–35. [SR]

Kidd S, Brennan S, Stephen R, *et al*. Comparison of morphine concentration-time profiles following intravenous and intranasal diamorphine in children. *Arch Dis Child* 2009;**94**:974–8.

O'Grady MJ, Hopewell J, White MJ. Management of neonatal abstinence syndrome: a national survey and review of practice. *Arch Dis Child Fetal Neonatal Ed* 2009;**94**:F249–52.

Use
Diazepam is a sedative and anxiolytic. Its effect as a muscle relaxant is used in the management of neonatal tetanus. Seizures are better controlled using other benzodiazepines such as lorazepam or midazolam (q.v.).

Pharmacology
Diazepam, first marketed in 1963, has also been used to control status epilepticus. It has a long half-life (20–60 hours), and both the parent drug and its pharmacologically active metabolite N-desmethyl diazepam both accumulate in maternal and fetal tissues ($V_D \sim 1.3 \, l/kg$). The neonatal half-life is even longer, and a maternal dose of 30 mg or more in the 15 hours before delivery (once commonly used to manage toxaemia) can cause severe hypotonia, respiratory depression, temperature instability and feeding difficulty particularly in babies of short gestation. Some (but not all) reports suggest that high-dose exposure in early pregnancy could be teratogenic. Withdrawal symptoms with jitteriness and hypertonia are common in babies born to women using this drug in an addictive way during pregnancy. Use during lactation only exposes the baby to a tenth of the maternal dose (on a weight-for-weight basis), but there are reports of sedation and poor weight gain, particularly in babies who had also been exposed to diazepam before delivery.

Neonatal tetanus
Tetanus (lockjaw), due to infection with *Clostridium tetani*, was recently estimated by WHO to be causing the death of up to 6% of all newborn babies in some parts of the world. This anaerobic, spore-forming, Gram-positive bacillus typically gains access to the body through a wound or area of damaged tissue contaminated by dirt or faecal material, giving off a neurotoxin with an effect similar to strychnine that last several weeks. Ear drops, if contaminated, can cause tetanus in young children with chronic otitis media. Umbilical infection must be suspected *immediately* in any baby starting to develop increasingly frequent, stimulus-triggered muscle spasms and sympathetic overactivity 4–14 days after birth. Start high-dose metronidazole (q.v.) or, if that is unavailable, intravenous (IV) or intramuscular (IM) penicillin, and debride any gangrenous tissue. Give a 150 mg/kg IM dose of human (or equine) tetanus immunoglobulin at once to neutralise systemic toxins, and consider one intrathecal dose (1000 units of the preservative-free IV product diluted to 2 ml with sterile water) in patients presenting early. Give 0.5 ml of tetanus toxoid into a different limb. Minimal handling, care in a quiet dark room, tube feeding and sedation, followed by regular oral (or IV) diazepam, can minimise the painful spasms. A continuous IV infusion of magnesium sulfate (q.v.) reduced the need for other medication in one recent trial in adult patients. Some babies need respiratory support. Prior maternal immunisation (two 0.5 ml doses of vaccine a month apart) and appropriate cord care could completely eliminate this painful, costly illness.

Treatment
Tetanic muscle spasm: A titration of 0.5 mg/kg/hour IV will usually control spasm, but a few need double this dose. Switch to oral (or rectal) treatment and then reduce the dose used over 2–4 weeks. Depression of the swallowing reflex can render oral secretions hazardous. Monitor respiration.
Seizures: A 300 micrograms/kg dose IV will stop most seizures for several hours. A 500 micrograms/kg rectal dose is usually, but not always, equally effective. Other anticonvulsants, such as lorazepam or midazolam, provide more sustained control.

Antidote
Flumazenil is a specific antidote (as described in the monograph on midazolam).

Supply and administration
Diazepam: Use the emulsified IV preparation (Diazemuls®) for the neonate; 2 ml (10 mg) ampoules cost 91p. Dilute any continuous infusion in 10% glucose, and use within 6 hours. Other IV formulations contain potentially toxic benzyl alcohol (15–55% w/v), and some also contain 40% w/v propylene glycol. A 1 mg/ml oral solution is available in some countries. A rapidly absorbed rectal preparation (Stesolid®) is also available in 2.5 ml tubes containing 2.5, 5 or 10 mg of diazepam per tube (costing £1.13–£1.37 each). Avoid the IM route – it is painful, and absorption is slow and incomplete.

Continued on p. 180

Tetanus immunoglobulin: Human anti-tetanus immunoglobulin (HTIG) is available for IM use in 250 unit ampoules. It is available from Bio Products Laboratory Limited, Elstree, Herts. Store at 4 °C.

Tetanus vaccine: Five doses of tetanus vaccine are sufficient to provide lifelong protection; these are currently provided by the three infant immunisations, the preschool booster and a final booster before leaving school. Unimmunised individuals should be given three doses of the combined adsorbed diphtheria, tetanus and inactivated poliomyelitis vaccine.

References

(See also the relevant Cochrane reviews and the UK Guideline on tetanus immunisation **DHUK**)

Ahmadsyah I, Salim A. Treatment of tetanus: an open study to compare the efficacy of procaine penicillin and metronidazole. *Br Med J* 1985;**291**:648–50.

Khoo BH, Less EL, Lam KL. Neonatal tetanus treated with high dose diazepam. *Arch Dis Child* 1978;**53**:737–9.

Miranda-Filho Dde B, Ximenes RA, Barone AA, *et al.* Randomised controlled trial of tetanus treatment with antitetanus immunoglobulin by the intrathecal or intramuscular route. *Br Med J* 2004;**328**:615–7. [RCT]

Ogatu BR, Newton CRJC, Crawley J, *et al.* Pharmacokinetics and anticonvulsant effects of diazepam in children with severe falciparum malaria and convulsions. *Br J Clin Pharmacol* 2002;**53**:49–75.

Tullu MS, Deshmukh CT, Kamat JR. Experience of pediatric tetanus. Cases from Mumbai. *Indian Pediatr* 2000;**37**:765–71.

Use

Diazoxide is used to treat intractable hypoglycaemia in the neonate when this is being caused by persisting excessive insulin production (hyperinsulinism).

Pharmacology

Diazoxide was once quite widely used to control hypertension in pregnancy, but high-dose (75 mg) bolus use can cause dangerous hypotension, while use during labour can affect uterine tone and delay labour unless oxytocin is prescribed as well. Use in labour can also have a transient impact on neonatal glucose homeostasis. Use during lactation has not been studied, but because of the drug's low molecular weight, it probably appears in breast milk. Diazoxide is now most commonly used to control the hypoglycaemia caused by hyperinsulinism. Insulin secretion by pancreatic beta cells is controlled by ATP-sensitive potassium (K_{ATP}) channels. In the presence of glucose, the channels close, leading to depolarisation of the cell membrane, an influx of calcium ions and insulin secretion. Diazoxide inhibits insulin secretion by opening these channels.

Neonatal hyperinsulinism sometimes resolves within 1–2 days of birth (as it does in infants of diabetic mothers) making drug treatment quite unnecessary. In other babies, hyperinsulinism can persist for some weeks (usually following intrauterine growth retardation or perinatal asphyxia), and diazoxide can be helpful in these patients. More persistent hyperinsulinaemic hypoglycaemia ('nesidioblastosis') is a heterogeneous condition, but most cases appear to result from genetic defects and many cases respond to treatment with diazoxide. However, an IV line for giving glucose ***must*** remain in place until a management regimen has been established that eliminates all risk of damaging symptomatic hypoglycaemia. If this proves difficult, there must be no delay in arranging prompt tertiary referral. Some severe cases require partial pancreatectomy (for focal adenomatous islet cell hyperplasia) or subtotal pancreatectomy (for diffuse beta cell hyperfunction).

Diazoxide is well absorbed by mouth and has a long half-life (10–20 hours), so it can usually be given by mouth. In patients only thought to have transient hyperinsulinism, fasting tolerance should be monitored for about 5 days after diazoxide is withdrawn, to ensure that there is no longer a risk of hypoglycaemia. Complete resolution is less likely in cases of hyperinsulinism persisting beyond the neonatal period, but the severity of the problem decreases with time, and in most children, it is possible to withdraw treatment after 5–6 years. Excessive hair growth is almost inevitable if treatment is continued for more than a few months, and leucopenia and eosinophilia are also seen on occasion. Although diazoxide is a thiazide derivative, it has an *anti*diuretic effect: giving chlorothiazide (q.v.) prevents fluid and salt retention and helps to raise glucose concentrations. A few patients who do not have the K_{ATP} channel defect benefit (for reasons that are not very clear) from being given 100–800 micrograms/kg of oral nifedipine (q.v.) once every 8 hours. The management of children who cannot be stabilised with diazoxide is outlined in the monograph on octreotide (q.v.).

Diagnosis

Any baby who is persistently found to need more than 9 mg/kg of IV glucose a minute to maintain a normal blood glucose level is almost certainly displaying at least transient evidence of hyperinsulinism.

Treatment

Diazoxide: Start by giving 5 mg/kg once every 8 hours (orally rather than IV where possible) as soon as it is clear that there is hyperinsulinaemia. Doses higher than this are seldom necessary, but a few babies derive optimum benefit when given 20 mg/kg a day. If the baby is going to respond, some benefit will be seen within 48 hours. The dose can then be reduced gradually once normoglycaemia has been achieved, but care *must* be taken not to let the blood glucose level fall below 3.5 mmol/l. Treatment can usually be stopped once a child only seems to need a 1.5 mg/kg dose, but 'weaning' should only be attempted in a hospital setting.

Managing episodes of hypoglycaemia

Hypoglycaemia is particularly dangerous when caused by a high insulin level because, in this situation, fatty acid and ketone body formation is reduced. Give 0.5–1 mg of glucagon IM (q.v.) if IV access is not immediately available, but get IV glucose started after this to counteract the rebound in insulin this will cause.

Continued on p. 182

Supply

Ampoules of diazoxide (300 mg in 20 ml) cost £30 each. Protect from light. A sugar-free oral suspension that is stable for a week can be made from a powder provided by Idis World Medicine, and a 50 mg/ml oral suspension (Proglycem®) containing 7.25% alcohol is available in America.

References

Arnoux JB, Verkarre V, Saint-Martin C, *et al*. Congenital hyperinsulinism: current trends in diagnosis and therapy. *Orphanet J Rare Dis* 2011;**6**:63.

Hoe FM, Thornton PS, Wanner LA, *et al*. Clinical features and insulin regulation in infants with a syndrome of prolonged neonatal hyperinsulinism. *J Pediatr* 2006;**148**:207–12.

Kapoor RR, Flanagan SE, James C, *et al*. Hyperinsulinaemic hypoglycaemia. *Arch Dis Child* 2009;**94**:450–7.

Lindley KJ, Dunne MJ. Contemporary strategies in the diagnosis and management of neonatal hyperinsulinaemic hypoglycaemia. *Early Hum Dev* 2005;**81**:61–72.

Michael CA. Intravenous labetalol and intravenous diazoxide in severe hypertension compromising pregnancy. *Aus N J Obstet Gynaecol* 1986;**26**:26–9. [RCT]

Mohnike K, Blankenstein O, Pfluetzner A, *et al*. Long-term non-surgical therapy of severe persistent congenital hyperinsulinism with glucagon. *Horm Res* 2008;**70**:59–64.

Palladino AA, Stanley CA. A specialized team approach to diagnosis and medical versus surgical treatment of infants with congenital hyperinsulinism. *Semin Pediatr Surg* 2011;**20**:32–7.

Use

Dichloroacetate has been used to reduce lactic acid levels in congenital lactic acidaemias; however, it has not been shown to improve long-term outcomes. It is generally well tolerated, but continued administration is associated with an increased frequency of peripheral neuropathy.

Biochemistry

Lactic acidosis can occur in many different circumstances; the most common is a secondary lactic acidosis due to hypoxia, hypoperfusion and shock which can be seen in a number of disease states. It is important to exclude and treat these before considering a metabolic cause for the lactic acidosis. Lactic acidosis may also be seen in other metabolic disorders as a secondary complication of the metabolic disease (e.g., propionic acidaemia, methylmalonic acidaemia, fatty acid oxidation defects, etc.) particularly during periods of acute illness.

Congenital lactic acidaemias are a group of inherited disorders that have variable clinical features such as progressive neuromuscular deterioration and in which there is accumulation of lactate in blood, urine and cerebrospinal fluid. In most patients, there are defects of the mitochondrial respiratory chain or the pyruvate dehydrogenase complex (PDH). The prognosis for these conditions is largely poor. Various approaches have been used to provide alternate dietary substrate fuels and/or vitamins and other cofactors that might stimulate residual enzyme activity or circumvent the enzyme defect.

Dichloroacetate indirectly stimulates the activity of PDH. This catalyses the conversion of pyruvate to acetyl-CoA and CO_2, thus determining whether glucose is metabolised oxidatively or is converted into lactate. Randomised study showed that the blood lactate levels were lowered in treated individuals, regardless of the underlying defect, but treatment with dichloroacetate, even in patients where PDH activity is increased by treatment, had little effect on actual disease progression.

Specialist advice

Specialist advice on a range of inborn errors of metabolism is available from the British Inherited Metabolic Disease Group (BIMDG) via their website (www.bimdg.org.uk).

Treatment

> **Note: Treatment with dichloroacetate should only be initiated after consultation with a specialist metabolic diseases centre.**

Neonate: Begin with 12.5 mg/kg in four divided doses. The dose should be adjusted according to response (up to 200 mg/kg daily has been used).
Infant >28 days: Begin with 12.5 mg/kg in four divided doses. The dose should be adjusted according to response (up to 200 mg/kg daily may be required).

Supply and administration

Sodium dichloroacetate is available as powder from Special Products Ltd. which when reconstituted with water provides 200 ml of a solution containing 50 mg/ml.

References

Kaufmann P, Engelstad K, Wei Y, *et al*. Dichloroacetate causes toxic neuropathy in MELAS: a randomized, controlled clinical trial. *Neurology* 2006;**66**:324–30. [RCT]

Stacpoole P, Barnes C, Hurbanis M, *et al*. Treatment of congenital lactic acidosis with dichloroacetate. *Arch Dis Child* 1997;**77**:535–41.

Stacpoole PW, Kerr DS, Barnes C, *et al*. Controlled clinical trial of dichloroacetate for treatment of congenital lactic acidosis in children. *Pediatrics* 2006;**117**:1519–31. [RCT]

Stacpoole PW, Wright EC, Baumgartner TG, *et al*. A controlled clinical trial of dichloroacetate for treatment of lactic acidosis in adults. The Dichloroacetate-Lactic Acidosis Study Group. *N Engl J Med* 1992;**327**:1564–9. [RCT]

Use

Digoxin immune fragmented antibodies (Fab) are indicated for the treatment of patients with life-threatening or potentially life-threatening digoxin toxicity or overdose associated with either ventricular arrhythmias or bradyarrhythmias that are unresponsive to atropine and when measures beyond the withdrawal of digoxin and correction of any electrolyte abnormalities are considered necessary. The original commercially available digoxin immune fragmented antibody preparation (Digibind®) was discontinued in the United Kingdom in 2011; it has been replaced by a similar preparation (DigiFab®) which has been used in North America since 2002.

Digoxin toxicity

The most common symptoms of digoxin toxicity in adults and older children are cardiac arrhythmias (e.g., ventricular extrasystoles, ventricular fibrillation, AV blockade, sinus brady-cardia). Extra-cardiac symptoms can occur, and gastrointestinal (GI) symptoms (nausea, vomiting, diarrhoea and abdominal pain) are the most predominant and frequently observed in infants. ECG signs may appear when the neonatal serum level exceeds 2 nanograms/ml; *clinical* symptoms (with partial AV block or a PR interval of >0.16 seconds) only appear when the level exceeds 3 nanograms/ml. Serum levels are not the best way to define toxicity as hypokalaemia can potentiate the toxic effects.

Pharmacology

Digoxin immune Fab are monovalent immunoglobulin fragments obtained from the blood of healthy sheep given a digoxin analogue, digoxin dicarboxymethoxylamine, which contains the functionally essential cyclopentaperhydrophenanthrene:lactone ring. The antibody fragments have a higher affinity for digoxin than the drug has for its sodium pump receptor. As a result, the antibody fragments reduce free digoxin levels and reduce the receptor binding and the cardio-toxic effects. Antibody–digoxin complexes are then cleared by the kidney and reticuloendothelial system. The half-life of the digoxin immune Fab in adults is 15–20 hours (prolonged in renal failure). No data exist for neonates.

Maternal use

The safety of digoxin immune Fab in pregnancy has not been established; however, use of such an antidote and the health of the mother are likely to take precedence. Use during lactation is unlikely to result in any adverse effects as the antibody fragments, even if they are excreted in the mother's milk, are likely to be digested in the breastfed infant's GI tract.

Management of digoxin toxicity

Treat any hyperkalaemia with salbutamol (q.v.). Give atropine for AV block. Give lidocaine (q.v.) or, if this fails, phenytoin (q.v.) for tachyarrhythmia. Severe bradycardia or block may require transvenous pacing. Ventricular fibrillation will only respond to a DC shock.

Consider intravenous (IV) digoxin immune Fab in severe toxicity. Improvement in signs and symptoms should occur 2–30 minutes following IV infusion of digoxin immune Fab.

Treatment

Acute ingestion of known amount: First, calculate the **body load of digoxin** by multiplying the amount of digoxin ingested (in mg) by 0.8, and then for each mg body load of digoxin, give 20 mg of digoxin-specific antibody fragments as described under 'Supply and administration'.

Based on steady-state digoxin level: Multiply the babies weight (in kg) by the serum digoxin level (in nanograms/ml). Further multiply this by 0.4 to give the dose of digoxin-specific antibody fragments (in mg) to be given.

Supply and administration

Vials containing 40 mg of lyophilised digoxin-specific antibody fragments (DigiFab) cost £750. Vials should be stored at 2–8 °C. Reconstitute the contents of the vial with 4 ml sterile water for injection to give a 10 mg/ml solution. This reconstituted solution is best further diluted for ease of administration in small infants to a 1 mg/ml solution using 0.9% saline. Administer by IV infusion over 30 minutes. If an infusion-related reaction occurs, stop the infusion and restart at a slower rate.

Continued on p. 185

References

Hastreiter AR, van der Horst RL, Chow-Tung E. Digitalis toxicity in infants and children. *Pediatr Cardiol* 1984;**5**:131–48.

Husby P, Farstad M, Brock-Utne JG, *et al*. Immediate control of life-threatening digoxin intoxication in a child by use of digoxin-specific antibody fragments (Fab). *Paediatr Anaesth* 2003;**13**:541–9.

Johnson GL, Desai NS, Pauly TH, *et al*. Complications associated with digoxin therapy in low-birth weight infants. *Pediatrics* 1982;**69**:463–5.

Nybo M, Damkier P. Gastrointestinal symptoms as an important sign in premature newborns with severely increased S-digoxin. *Basic Clin Pharmacol Toxicol* 2005;**96**:465–8.

Presti S, Friedman D, Saslow J, *et al*. Digoxin toxicity in a premature infant: treatment with Fab fragments of digoxin-specific antibodies. *Pediatr Cardiol* 1985;**6**:91–3.

Ward SB, Sjostrom L, Ujhelyi MR. Comparison of the pharmacokinetics and in vivo bioaffinity of DigiTAb versus Digibind. *Ther Drug Monit* 2000;**22**:599–607.

Use
Digoxin is still sometimes used to manage supraventricular tachycardia (SVT) and occasionally heart failure.

Pharmacology
William Withering's 1785 description of the foxglove leaf as a herbal remedy for 'dropsy' (or cardiac failure) is well known. The active ingredient, digoxin, is still sometimes given to women (250 micrograms, three times a day) to control fetal tachycardia, because placental transfer is relatively brisk after maternal digitalisation. Aim for a level at the top of the therapeutic range. It is by no means universally effective, especially in the hydropic fetus, and flecainide (q.v.) is considered a better option. Quinidine sulfate (starting with 200 mg every 6–8 hours) has occasionally been of benefit in fetuses with atrial flutter after prior digitalisation. Adenosine (q.v.) is the most appropriate first-line treatment for SVT after birth.

Digoxin is present in breast milk, but this excretion can be ignored when considering clinical management. Digoxin is largely eliminated by the kidney without prior degradation (clearance exceeding GFR). Marked tissue binding occurs, the myocardial levels being linearly related to (and some 20 times) the serum concentration and twice as high in infancy as in adults, while the neonatal serum half-life (55–90 hours) is nearly three times as long as in adults ($V_D \sim 9\,l/kg$). Clearance is unaffected by the serum level, so doubling the dose will double the serum concentration.

Drug interactions
Patients on amiodarone will need, and those on indometacin *may* need, a lower dose. Occasionally, the same is true with erythromycin. Arrhythmias have been reported when digitalised patients are given pancuronium or suxamethonium.

Treatment
The conventional starting dose in microgram per kilogram is:

Weight	Total slow IV loading dose	Total oral loading dose	Daily oral maintenance dose
<1.5 kg	20	25	5
1.5–2.5 kg	30	35	7.5
>2.5 kg	35	45	10

Seek consultant advice. Give half the total loading dose immediately, and a quarter of the total dose after 8 and 16 hours. Digoxin is rather erratically absorbed intramuscularly and bioavailability when given by mouth only 80% of that achieved by intravenous (IV) administration (as reflected above). Use a reduced dose in babies with renal failure and monitor the blood level. *Check each dose carefully*. Overdose can cause serious arrhythmia and a life-threatening reduction in cardiac output without warning.

Toxicity
While ECG signs may appear when the neonatal serum level exceeds 2 nanograms/ml, *clinical* symptoms (with partial AV block or a PR interval of >0.16 seconds) only appear when the level exceeds 3 nanograms/ml. Serum levels are not the best way to define toxicity. Control hyperkalaemia with salbutamol (q.v.). Give atropine for AV block. Give lidocaine (q.v.) or, if this fails, phenytoin (q.v.) for tachyarrhythmia. Severe bradycardia or block may require transvenous pacing. Ventricular fibrillation will only respond to a DC shock. Control severe toxicity with IV digoxin immune Fab antibody fragments (q.v.).

Blood levels
Levels can take 10 days to stabilise because of the 2–4 day half-life. Collect at least 0.2 ml of serum or plasma six or more hours after the last dose was administered. The therapeutic range of digoxin is 0.9–2 nanograms/ml (1 nanogram/ml = 1.28 nmol/l).

Continued on p. 187

Supply

1 ml (100 micrograms) ampoules cost 70p. The oral syrup (Lanoxin PG®) containing 50 micrograms/ml costs £5.35 for 60 ml. Both products contain 10% v/v ethanol; the ampoules contain 43% and the syrup 5% v/v propylene glycol. Do not give digoxin intramuscularly.

References

(See also the relevant Cochrane reviews)

Balaguer Gargallo M, Jordán García I, Caritg Bosch J, *et al*. Taquicardia paroxistica supraventricular en el niño y el lactante. *Ann Pediatr (Barc)* 2007;**67**:133–8.

Hastreiter AR, John EG, van der Horst RL. Digitalis, digitalis antibodies, digitalis-like immunoreactive substances, and sodium homeostasis: a review. *Clin Perinatol* 1988;**15**:491–522.

Husby P, Farstad M, Brock-Utne JG, *et al*. Immediate control of life-threatening digoxin intoxication in a child by use of digoxin-specific antibody fragments (Fab). *Paediatr Anaesth* 2003;**13**:541–6.

Skinner JR, Sharland G. Detection and management of life threatening arrhythmias in the perinatal period. *Early Hum Dev* 2008;**84**:161–72.

Yukawa E, Akiyama K, Suematsu F, *et al*. Population pharmacokinetic investigation of digoxin in Japanese neonates. *J Clin Pharmacol Ther* 2007;**32**:381–6.

Use

Deciding to use an inotrope and then choosing the right inotrope requires an understanding not only of the physiological and pathological processes occurring in the baby but also of how various inotropes work. While dopamine (q.v.) appears to result in a better blood pressure, dobutamine seems to be better at improving systemic blood flow, and there is a growing consensus that although it is harder to measure, cardiac output and systemic tissue perfusion usually matter more than blood pressure. Milrinone (q.v.) could be tried if dobutamine proves ineffective, although there also may be an argument for using adrenaline (q.v.) or noradrenaline (q.v.).

Neonatal hypotension

Neonatal hypotension is defined as a clinical condition of abnormally low arterial blood pressure affecting perfusion. While few would disagree that inadequate perfusion should be treated, defining neonatal hypotension itself is difficult; there is no single accepted value that defines low blood pressure, and while imminently measurable, blood pressure on its own is only part of the equation. Different gestational norms, different pathophysiologies and the transition from fetal to *ex utero* circulation all compound the difficulties in making an informed choice about which inotrope to use (or, in some cases, whether one is required in the first place). See the website commentary for a detailed discussion of this topic.

Common misconceptions in neonatology are that normal blood pressure, however this is defined, equates to normal systemic blood flow and that improving blood pressure means that blood flow must also improve. Unfortunately, simply treating a low blood pressure without consideration for which inotrope best suits the situation to use might worsen both systemic blood flow and tissue perfusion.

Pharmacology

Dobutamine hydrochloride is a synthetic inotropic catecholamine developed in 1973 by the systemic alteration of isoprenaline with a view to reducing some of the latter's unwanted adrenergic effects (i.e. chronotropism, arrhythmias, vascular constriction). It has to be given intravenously because of rapid first-pass metabolism. Dobutamine is a $\beta1$ agonist like dopamine, but in high doses, its $\beta2$ effects can decrease rather than increase peripheral resistance. For a brief summary of how drug receptors act, see the monograph on noradrenaline. It is about four times as potent as dopamine in stimulating myocardial contractility in low concentration, and of proven value in increasing left ventricular output in the hypotensive preterm neonate, but has less effect than dopamine on blood pressure because it has little effect on systemic vascular resistance. The right dose to use needs to be *individually assessed* because clearance is very variable in children; the drug's short half-life means that this assessment can be made as soon as 10–15 minutes. Tachycardia may occur, and increased pulmonary blood pressure leading to pulmonary oedema has been reported. In general, however, side effects are rare as long as the dose does not exceed 15 micrograms/kg/minute. Extravasation seldom causes the sort of tissue damage seen with dopamine. Note that manufacturers have still not formally endorsed the use of dobutamine in children.

Treatment

Start with 5 micrograms/kg/minute (0.5 ml/hour of a solution made up as described under 'Supply and administration'). Adjust this dose if necessary after approximately 20 minutes because of the drug's variable half-life accepting that a few babies need twice as much as this. Prepare a fresh solution every 24 hours.

Compatibility

Compatible with noradrenaline and the same drugs as dopamine (q.v.). Do not mix with sodium bicarbonate.

Supply and administration

20 ml vials of dobutamine hydrochloride costing £5.20 each contain 12.5 mg/ml of dobutamine. To give 10 micrograms/kg of dobutamine per minute, place 2.4 ml (30 mg) of this solution for each kilogram that the baby weighs in a syringe, dilute to 50 ml with 10% glucose or glucose saline, and infuse at a rate of 1 ml/hour. Less concentrated solutions of glucose or glucose saline can be employed.

Continued on p. 189

References

(See also relevant Cochrane reviews)

Dempsey EM, Al Hazzani F, Barrington KJ. Permissive hypotension in the extremely low birthweight infant with signs of good perfusion. *Arch Dis Child Fetal Neonatal Ed* 2009;**94**:F241–4.

Martinez AM, Padbury JF, Thio S. Dobutamine pharmacokinetics and cardiovascular responses in critically ill neonates. *Pediatrics* 1992;**89**:47–51.

Osborn D, Evans N, Kluckow M. Randomised trial of dobutamine versus dopamine in preterm infants with low systemic blood flow. *J Pediatr* 2002;**140**:183–91. [RCT]

Robel-Tillig E, Knüpfer M, Pulzer F, *et al*. Cardiovascular impact of dobutamine in neonates with myocardial dysfunction. *Early Hum Dev* 2007;**83**:307–12.

Steinberg C, Notterman, DA. Pharmacokinetics of cardiovascular drugs in children: inotropes and vasopressors. *Clin Pharmacokinet* 1994;**27**:345–67.

Use
This drug is, at present, quite widely used across Europe to treat children with gastro-oesophageal reflux, although there is little evidence of efficacy and some evidence that it could increase the risk of arrhythmia. It has sometimes been used to manage post-operative gastrointestinal stasis although, in infancy, erythromycin (q.v.) is a better studied alternative. Severe nausea and vomiting is best treated with ondansetron (q.v.).

Pharmacology
Domperidone is a dopamine D_2-receptor antagonist used to relieve nausea and vomiting. It stimulates gastric and upper intestinal motility and also acts on the chemoreceptor trigger zone. Like metoclopramide (q.v.), it seems to *increase* gastro-oesophageal, and *decrease* pyloric, sphincter tone. It first came into clinical use in 1978 largely as a potent anti-emetic.

Because of its effect on prolactin excretion, it has sometimes been used as a galactogogue to stimulate lactation although the manufacturers have never endorsed its use for this purpose. Several studies have suggested that use can augment (without altering the composition of) the milk supply of some mothers who were expressing their milk following the birth of a preterm baby. Use in pregnancy is little studied, but the drug is not teratogenic in animals. Maternal use during breastfeeding is not contraindicated because the baby will receive less than 1% of the maternal dose when intake is calculated on a weight-for-weight basis.

Dystonic and extrapyramidal reactions can occur but are much rarer than with metoclopramide, probably because only a little of the drug crosses the blood–brain barrier. Domperidone is rapidly metabolised by the liver after absorption into the portal vein following oral administration, and because of this 'first-pass' metabolism, systemic bioavailability is quite low (15%). Rectal bioavailability is much the same, but the blood level only peaks after an hour (rather than 30 minutes) when the drug is given rectally. The volume of distribution in adults is high ($V_D \sim 5.5\,l/kg$), and the elimination half-life about 7 hours, most of the drug being excreted in the bile and the urine, mainly as inactive metabolites. The only intravenous formulation was withdrawn after high-dose use was occasionally found to cause arrhythmia and even sudden death, and a serious oral overdose could, conceivably, be equally dangerous. Very few pharmacokinetic studies seem to have been undertaken into the drug's use in infancy or childhood. Sustained use for more than 12 weeks is not recommended even in adults, and the manufacturers have not, as yet, made any recommendation as to use in children, except to control the nausea and vomiting caused by cytotoxic drugs and by radiotherapy. Although the drug has a licence for use in Canada, it has not been approved for use in the United States, and the US authorities have previously taken steps to try and stop its illegal importation and unapproved use.

Very few formal studies have been undertaken into the use of domperidone in children, and the only trials done to date suggest that domperidone does little for babies with gastro-oesophageal reflux. Since it has now been shown to interfere with cardiac conduction, causing QT prolongation, this risk should be assessed in any infant so treated because cisapride was eventually withdrawn from sale in Europe and North America after it was found to cause similar problems.

Treatment
Mother: A 10 mg (or 20 mg) dose three times a day for 1–2 weeks may help initiate lactation in the mothers of babies too premature to be put to the breast. Use for longer than this has not yet been studied.

Baby: The usual dose is 200–400 micrograms/kg by mouth, repeatable every 4–8 hours as necessary. There is relatively little experience of sustained use, and no published data on the drug's use in babies less than 1 month old. It is probably wise to do a paired ECG test to see if treatment significantly prolongs the QT time.

Supply
Domperidone is available as a 1 mg/ml sugar-free suspension (100 ml costs £6.30). Small quantities (packs containing not more than twenty 10 mg doses) are available 'over the counter' in the United Kingdom to treat flatulence, epigastric discomfort and heart burn in adults, but it has never been licensed for use in the United States.

Continued on p. 191

References

Bines JE, Quinlan J-E, Treves S, *et al*. Efficacy of domperidone in infants and children with gastroesophageal reflux. *J Pediatr Gastroenterol Nutr* 1992;**14**:400–5. [RCT]

Campbell-Yeo ML, Allen AC, Joseph KS, *et al*. Effect of domperidone on the composition of preterm human breast milk. *Pediatrics* 2010;**125**:e107–14.

da Silva OP, Knoppert DC, Angelini MM, *et al*. Effect of domperidone on milk production in mothers of premature newborns: a randomized, double-blind, placebo-controlled trial *Can Med Assoc J* 2001;**164**:17–21. [RCT]

Djeddi D, Kongolo G, Lefiax C, *et al*. Effect of domperidone on QT interval in neonates. *J Pediatr* 2008;**153**:663–6. (See also pp. 596–8.)

Ingram J, Taylor H, Churchill C, *et al*. Metoclopramide or domperidone for increasing maternal breast milk output: a randomised controlled trial. *Arch Dis Child Fetal Neonatal Ed* 2012;**97**:F241–5. [RCT]

O'Meara A, Grill BB, Hillemeier AC, *et al*. Effects of domperidone therapy on symptoms and upper gastrointestinal motility in infants with gastroesophageal reflux. *J Pediatr* 1985;**106**:311–6.

Pritchard DS, Baber N, Stephenson T. Should domperidone be used for the treatment of gastro-oesophageal reflux in children? Systematic review of randomised controlled trials in children aged 1 month to 11 years old. *Br J Clin Pharmacol* 2005;**59**:725–9. [SR]

Wan EW-X, Davey K, Page-Sharp M, *et al*. Dose-effect study of domperidone as a galactogogue in preterm mothers with insufficient milk supply, and its transfer into milk. *Br J Clin Pharmacol* 2008;**62**:283–9. [RCT]

Use

Dopamine is widely used to treat neonatal hypotension, but it has a variable, unpredictable dose-dependent impact on vascular tone, and use too often fails to recognise that adequate tissue perfusion, rather than supply pressure *per se*, should be the aim of treatment. Hydrocortisone (q.v.) may work better, and a dobutamine (q.v.) or adrenaline infusion (q.v.) is a more logical strategy if low cardiac output is the primary problem.

Physiology

Hypotension is currently over-diagnosed (see web commentary), and the 'rule of thumb' that so classifies any baby with a mean arterial pressure (in mmHg) that is less than gestation (in weeks) can often result in a quarter of all day-old babies being classed as hypotensive. In addition, an apparent response to treatment may simply reflect the rise in pressure that normally occurs anyway during the first 2 days of life.

Pharmacology

Dopamine hydrochloride is a naturally occurring catecholamine precursor of noradrenaline (q.v.) that was first synthesised in 1910 and shown to be a neurohormone in 1959. *Low*-dose infusion (2 micrograms/kg/minute) normally causes dopaminergic coronary, renal and mesenteric vasodilatation, but there is little evidence that this is clinically beneficial, and there is good controlled trial evidence that such treatment does *not* protect renal function, although it does cause some increase in urine output. *High* doses cause vasoconstriction, increase systemic vascular resistance and eventually decrease renal blood flow. While a moderate dose increases myocardial contractility and cardiac output in adults and older children, a dose of more than 10 micrograms/kg/minute can cause an increase in systemic resistance, a fall in gut blood flow and a *reduction* in cardiac output in the neonate especially in the first few days of life.

Correct any acidosis first, and look to see if there is a reason why the baby is hypotensive rather than just treating the symptom alone. Use high-dose treatment with caution after cardiac surgery or where there is coexisting neonatal pulmonary hypertension, because the drug can cause a detrimental change in the balance between pulmonary and systemic vascular resistance. High doses can also cause tachycardia and arrhythmia in adults. Lack of response may suggest vasopressin exhaustion (q.v.). Side effects are easily controlled by stopping the infusion because the half-life is only 5–10 minutes. There are no known teratogenic effects. Dopamine causes suppression of serum TSH, T4 and prolactin levels in VLBW infants, which reverses after cessation of treatment; however, it is not known if this short-term iatrogenic pituitary suppression has any longer-term consequences.

Drug interactions

There are reports of phenytoin and tolazoline causing severe hypotension in patients on dopamine.

Treatment

Start by giving 3 micrograms/kg/minute (or 0.3 ml/hour of a solution made up as described under 'Supply and administration'), and increase this every half an hour as necessary because the response (like the drug's blood level) is known to vary greatly. Always use ultrasound to check the haemodynamic response when using a dose of more than 10 micrograms/kg/minute. Prepare a fresh infusion daily, and stop high-dose treatment slowly.

Compatibility

Dopamine is inactivated by alkali but can be added (terminally) to a line containing fentanyl, lignocaine, midazolam, milrinone, morphine or standard TPN (with or without lipid).

Supply and administration

Supply: One stock 5 ml (200 mg) ampoule (pH 2.5–4.5) costs £3.90. To give an infusion of 10 micrograms/kg/minute of dopamine, place 0.75 ml (30 mg) of the concentrate for each kilogram the baby weighs in a syringe, dilute to 50 ml immediately before use with 10% glucose or glucose saline, and infuse at a rate of 1 ml/hour (a less concentrated solution of glucose or glucose saline can be used where necessary).

Administration: Extravasation can cause serious tissue damage, and the management of this is discussed in the monograph on hyaluronidase. Indeed, serious blanching along the line of the

Continued on p. 193

vein can, in itself, be enough to cause tissue ischaemia. Any dopamine infusion is always best given through an umbilical venous catheter or percutaneous 'long line'.

References

(See also relevant Cochrane reviews)

Batton B, Zhu X, Fanaroff J, *et al.* Blood pressure, anti-hypotensive therapy, and neurodevelopment in extremely preterm infants. *J Pediatr* 2009;**154**:351–7.

Dempsey EM, Al Kazzani F, Barrington KJ. Permissive hypotension in the extremely low birthweight infants with signs of good perfusion. *Arch Dis Child Fetal Neonatal Ed* 2009;**94**:F241–4.

Dempsey EM, Barrington KJ. Evaluation and treatment of hypotension in the preterm infant. *Clin Perinatol* 2009;**36**:75–85.

Filippi L, Pezzati M, Poggi C, *et al.* Dopamine versus dobutamine in very low birthweight infants: endocrine effects. *Arch Dis Child Fetal Neonatal Ed* 2007;**92**:F367–71. [RCT]

Laughon M, Bose C, Allred E, *et al.* Factors associated with treatment for hypotension in extremely low gestational age newborns during the first postnatal week. *Pediatrics* 2007;**119**:273–80.

Limperopoulos C, Bassan H, Kalish LA, *et al.* Current definitions of hypotension do not predict abnormal cranial ultrasound findings in preterm infants. *Pediatrics* 2007;**120**:966–77.

Shah DM, Condò M, Bowen J, *et al.* Blood pressure or blood flow: which is important in the preterm infant? A case report of twins. *J Paediatr Child Health* 2012;**48**:E144–6.

Use

Oral or intravenous (IV) doxapram can sometimes be useful in preterm babies who continue to have troublesome apnoea despite treatment with caffeine citrate (q.v.). The effects of caffeine and doxapram appear to be additive.

Pharmacology

Doxapram (first developed commercially in 1964) stimulates all levels of the cerebrospinal axis, and respiration appears to be stimulated at doses that cause little general excitation. A plasma concentration of 2 mg/l doubles minute volume in healthy adults, but there is no evidence of any additive benefit from raising the plasma level above 1 mg/l in babies. High doses cause convulsions, and subconvulsive doses can still cause tachycardia, hypertension, hyperpyrexia, jitteriness, laryngospasm and vomiting.

Oral caffeine is usually considered the drug of choice in the management of idiopathic neonatal apnoea, but adding doxapram can sometimes bring additional benefit. The drug is usually given as a continuous infusion, but oral treatment is often very effective as long as the dose is doubled to compensate for poor absorption. Developmental delay is not uncommon in survivors, and while severe apnoea may merely be the first sign of some existing cerebral dysfunction that later manifests as developmental delay, a drug-related effect cannot be ruled out until an appropriately designed trial is done. Nasal continuous positive airway pressure (CPAP) or high flow oxygen may make tracheal intubation and ventilation unnecessary.

Doxapram is metabolised by the liver, the half-life in babies (about 7 hours) being double that seen in adults. It is longer still in the first week of life. Significant tissue accumulation occurs ($V_D \sim 6$ l/kg), and some of the metabolic breakdown products are also potentially metabolically active. The optimum respiratory response is usually seen with a plasma level of 2–4 nanograms/ml, but the dose needed to achieve this plasma level varies.

Adverse effects are increasingly common when the level exceeds 5 nanograms/ml. The dose recommended in certain neonatal texts (2.5 mg/kg/hour) is almost certainly potentially toxic in some babies (especially if there is evidence of a parenchymal cerebral bleed or an existing seizure disorder). Watch for adverse effects (including hyperexcitability, AV heart block, hypokalaemia and a rise in blood pressure if more than 1 mg/kg/hour has to be infused for more than 36–48 hours). Use of doxapram in children has not yet been endorsed by the manufacturers.

Treatment

IV administration: Start with 2.5 mg/kg as a loading dose over at least 5–10 minutes followed by a maintenance infusion 300 micrograms/kg/hour (0.3 ml/hour of a solution made up as described under 'Supply and administration'), and increase the dose cautiously as required. Babies over a week old sometimes only respond to a continuous infusion of 1 or even 1.5 mg/kg/hour. Tissue extravasation can cause skin damage.

Oral administration: Babies who respond to IV doxapram can usually be transferred onto oral maintenance treatment. Take half the total daily dose found effective IV and give this once every 6 hours by mouth diluted in a little 5% glucose. High-dose oral treatment sometimes slows gastric emptying. Such problems can usually be resolved by reverting to IV treatment.

Post-anaesthetic use: A single 1 mg/kg IV bolus will sometimes rouse the post-operative preterm baby.

Compatibility

Doxapram can probably be added (terminally) into a line containing standard TPN (but not lipid) when absolutely necessary.

Supply and administration

5 ml (100 mg) ampoules cost £3. To give an infusion of 1 mg/kg/hour of doxapram, place 2.5 ml of the concentrate for each kilogram the baby weighs in a syringe, dilute to 50 ml with 10% glucose or glucose saline, and infuse at 1 ml/hour (a less concentrated solution of glucose or glucose saline can be used where necessary). Doxapram is stable in solution, so IV lines do not require changing daily. Nor does IV material made available for oral use. The US formulation contains 0.9% benzyl alcohol.

Continued on p. 195

References

(See also the relevant Cochrane reviews)

Barbé F, Hansen C, Badonnel Y, *et al*. Severe side effects and drug plasma concentrations in preterm infants treated with doxapram. *Ther Drug Monit* 1999;**21**:547–52.

Dani C, Bertini G, Pezzati M, *et al*. Brain hemodynamic effects of doxapram in preterm infants. *Biol Neonate* 2006;**89**:69–74.

De Villiers GS, Walele A, Van der Merwe P-L, *et al*. Second-degree atrioventricular heart block after doxapram administration. *J Pediatr* 1998;**133**:149–50.

Fischer C, Ferdynus C, Gouyon JB, *et al*. Doxapram and hypokalaemia in very preterm infants. *Arch Dis Child Fetal Neonatal Ed* 2013;**98**:F416–8.

Huon C, Rey E, Mussat P, *et al*. Low-dose doxapram for treatment of apnoea following early weaning in very low birthweight infants: a randomised double-blind study. *Acta Paediatr* 1998;**87**:1180–4. [RCT]

Malliard C, Boutroy M, Fresson J, *et al*. QT interval lengthening in premature infants treated with doxapram. *Clin Pharmacol Ther* 2001;**70**:540–5.

Poets CF, Darraj S, Bohnhorst B. Effect of doxapram on episodes of apnoea, bradycardia and hypoxaemia in preterm infants. *Biol Neonate* 1999;**76**:207–13.

Sreenan C, Etches PC, Demianczuk N, *et al*. Isolated developmental delay in very low birth weight infants: association with prolonged doxapram therapy of apnea. *J Pediatr* 2001;**139**:832–7. (See also 2002;**141**:296–7.)

Use

A Gastrografin® enema can be both diagnostic and therapeutic in a baby with low intestinal obstruction. Macrogols (polyethylene glycols), which act by enhancing the water content of stool in the colon, are the best way to relieve and to control constipation in later infancy.

Pathophysiology

Once X-rays and clinical examination have rendered a diagnosis of atresia, volvulus or an obstructing hernia unlikely and the possibility that the failure to pass stool is an iatrogenic complication of opiate sedation has been ruled out, a range of other diagnostic possibilities require consideration.

Meconium plug syndrome: All that may be required to relieve a 'plug' of hard dried gelatinous meconium in the distal colon in the term baby after birth is a 1 mg glycerin suppository plus, on occasion, a rectal washout. Similar problems in the absence of an obvious 'plug' are not uncommon in the preterm baby.

Meconium ileus: Obstruction in the terminal ileum makes meconium ileus a more likely possibility. A dis-impacting Gastrografin enema may be all that is needed to deal with the sticky viscid meconium, but a minority require the resection of 20–40 cm of the small bowel and a primary re-anastomosis. Many of these children will be found to have cystic fibrosis, requiring treatment with pancreatin (q.v.) and access to long-term, high-quality care to try and minimise the inevitable complications of this recessively inherited condition.

Milk curd obstruction: Early milk feeding can sometimes result in undigested milk curds reaching the far end of the small bowel and impacting there. A Gastrografin enema carried out skilfully can be both diagnostic and therapeutic, but some cases come to surgery especially if there has been a focal perforation. The problem, if recognised promptly, should have no long-term consequences and can be distinguished from necrotising enterocolitis (NEC) because there is no intramural gas on X-ray and histology fails to reveal any bacterial invasion of the gut wall.

Faecal constipation: Serious constipation is rare in infancy. When it does occur, it is probably best treated (once Hirschsprung's disease has been excluded), as in older children, by using an osmotic agent to increase the water content of the stool. There is good evidence that the best approach is to use a macrogol (polyethylene glycol) first to dis-impact the rectum and then, in a lower dose, for a sustained period until bowel tone returns to normal. Delay can cause behavioural problems to develop, and the longer the problem is left unaddressed, the longer it will take for function to recover. Chronic idiopathic pseudo-obstruction is an extremely rare cause of very severe intestinal dysmotility due to an as yet poorly understood disorder of the enteric neuromusculature that can present with intractable constipation from a very early age.

Treatment

Bowel impaction in the neonate: A Gastrografin enema, administered under fluoroscopic control, has been widely used to disimpact the lower bowel in babies without resort to surgery ever since Helen Noblett first described this approach in 1969. A rectal biopsy to exclude Hirschsprung's disease is called for if the stool pattern does not become normal after this.

Constipation in later infancy: Give 600 mg/kg of macrogol once a day by mouth. More may sometimes be needed, especially at first. Manufacturers have not recommended use in children less than 1 year old.

Supply and administration

Macrogols: Non-absorbed polymers of high molecular weight (such as polyethylene glycol 3350) are usually used. Movicol® Paediatric Plain (which contains supplementary electrolytes) is the commercial product most often used in Europe. Dissolve one 6.5 g sachet of powder (costing 15p) in 65 ml of water immediately before use to obtain a 100 mg/ml solution. An identical generic product is available in America, but here, an electrolyte-free product (MiraLAX®) in 17 g packs is most commonly used to treat constipation.

Gastrografin: 100 ml of this iodinated monomeric contrast medium (sodium and meglumine amidotrizoate) costs £14.70. It should be diluted 15–30 ml with five times as much 0.9% sodium chloride and then given slowly into the rectum using a plain 8 FG catheter while screening the enema's progress into the colon.

Glycerol: Pre-moistened 1 g suppositories (costing 7p each) are often given to preterm babies.

Continued on p. 197

References

Burke MS, Ragi JM, Karamanoukian HL, *et al.* New strategies for nonoperative management of meconium ileus. *J Pediatr Surg* 2002;**37**:760–4.

Candy D, Belsey J. Macrogol (polyethylene glycol) laxatives in children with functional constipation and faecal impaction: a systematic review. *Arch Dis Child* 2009;**94**:156–60. [SR]

Hajivassiliou CA. Intestinal obstruction in neonatal pediatric surgery. *Semin Pediatr Surg* 2003;**12**:241–53.

Heneyke S, Smith VV, Spitz L, *et al.* Chronic intestinal pseudo-obstruction: treatment and long term follow up of 44 patients. *Arch Dis Child* 1999;**81**:21–7.

Keckler SJ, St Peter SD, Spilde TL, *et al.* Current significance of meconium plug syndrome. *J Pediatr Surg* 2008;**43**:896–8.

Noblett HR. Treatment of uncomplicated meconium ileus by gastrografin enema: a preliminary report. *J Pediatr Surg* 1969;**4**:190–7.

Pijpers MAM, Tabbers MM, Benninga MA, *et al.* Currently recommended treatments of childhood constipation are not evidence based: a systematic literature review on the effect of laxative treatment and dietary measures. *Arch Dis Child* 2009;**94**:117–31. [SR]

Emil S, Nguyen T, Sills J, *et al.* Meconium obstruction in extremely low-birth-weight neonates: guidelines for diagnosis and management. *J Pediatr Surg* 2004;**39**:731–7.

Use

Enoxaparin is a low molecular weight derivative of heparin (q.v.) with most of the same properties as the parent compound but with a longer duration of action and given subcutaneously rather than by intravenous (IV) injection.

Pharmacology

Enoxaparin was first prepared by the depolymerisation of porcine heparin in 1981. A range of other low molecular weight heparins (LMWHs) are now available, including certoparin, dalteparin sodium (q.v.), reviparin sodium and tinzaparin sodium. All have very similar properties, although the recommended dose of the various products can vary. Enoxaparin has been the most widely studied of LMWHs in pregnancy and the neonatal period, although the manufacturers have yet to recommend use in children in the United Kingdom or in the United States.

LMWHs have a longer half-life, cause less osteoporosis and thrombocytopenia and have a more predictable pharmacodynamic (anticoagulant) effect than heparin. Despite this, the effective dose varies widely and needs to be individually titrated. Neonates also generally need a high dose (as with heparin). Administration by subcutaneous rather than IV injection makes treatment much easier but also makes an overdose less easily treatable. There is no evidence of teratogenicity and placenta transfer does not occur. Lactation during treatment is also safe; the molecular weight makes significant transfer into breast milk very unlikely, and any drug entering the milk would be inactivated in the gut before absorption.

Maternal thromboembolism

Prophylaxis: High-risk obstetric patients with thrombophilia, immobility, obesity, pre-eclampsia or a past history of deep vein thrombosis should be assessed for their risk factors and considered for prophylactic LMWH. The daily dose depends on the patient's weight (see table). Doses of 60 mg or higher may be given as two smaller doses, but otherwise, once daily dosing is appropriate.

Weight (kg) at booking (kg)	Total daily dose of enoxaparin
<50	20 mg (2000 units)
50–90	40 mg (4000 units)
91–130	60 mg (6000 units)
131–170	80 mg (8000 units)
>170	0.6 mg/kg (600 units/kg)

Experience indicates that monitoring of anti-Xa levels is not required during thromboprophylaxis with LMWH. Stop 24 hours prior to any planned operative (or epidural) delivery until 4 hours after the procedure is over. Women receiving antenatal LMWH should be advised that, if they have any vaginal bleeding or once labour begins, they should not inject any further LMWH. There is no need to monitor platelets routinely unless there has been exposure to unfractionated heparin.

Treatment: Give a 1 mg/kg subcutaneous injection once every 12 hours. Start treatment promptly, as soon as a clot or embolus is seriously suspected, after first taking blood for a full thrombophilia screen and confirming that renal and liver functions are normal. Then adjust treatment for maintenance purposes to optimise the peak anti-Xa level. As with prophylaxis, treatment should be withheld at the start of labour or 24 hours before any planned operative delivery or epidural.

Neonatal treatment

Prophylaxis: Experience is extremely limited. Try 750 micrograms/kg once every 12 hours (or 500 micrograms/kg in babies over 2 months old).

Treatment: A subcutaneous dose of 1.5–2 mg/kg once every 12 hours normally produces an anti-Xa level of 0.5–1.0 units/ml, but all treatment needs to be individualised. Preterm babies sometimes need over 2 mg/kg, while babies over 2 months old usually only need about 1 mg/kg every 12 hours.

Continued on p. 199

Dose monitoring

Take blood 3–4 hours after subcutaneous injection to assess the peak anti-Xa level, and adjust the dose to achieve a level of 0.6–1.0 units/ml during treatment and 0.35–0.7 units/ml during prophylaxis.

Antidote

Protamine sulphate will usually stop overt haemorrhage as summarised in the monograph on heparin.

Supply and administration

The drug is available in a range of pre-filled syringes (0.2–1.0 ml) containing 100 mg/ml (10,000 units/ml) of enoxaparin; syringes cost from £2.30 to £8 each. Avoid the use in neonates of the 300 mg (0.3 ml) ampoules which contain benzyl alcohol. To make a more dilute 10 mg/ml preparation for accurate neonatal use, draw 0.1 ml into a 1 ml syringe and make up to 1 ml with water for injection just before use.

References   (See also the UK guideline on thromboprophylaxis in pregnancy **DHUK**)

Guillonneau M, de Crepy A, Aufrant C, *et al.* Breast-feeding is possible in case of maternal treatment with enoxaparin. *Arch Pediatr* 1996;**3**:513–4.

Lim W, Eikelboom JW, Ginsberg JS. Inherited thrombophilia and pregnancy associated venous thromboembolism. [Review] *Br Med J* 2007;**334**:1318–21.

Malowany JI, Managle P, Knoppert DC, *et al.* Enoxaparin for neonatal thrombosis: a call for a higher dose in neonates. *Thromb Res* 2008;**122**:826–30.

McLintock C, McCowan LME, North RA. Maternal complications and pregnancy outcomes in women with mechanical prosthetic heart valves treated with enoxaparin. *BJOG* 2009;**116**:1585–92.

Meneveau N. Safety evaluation of enoxaparin in currently approved indications. *Expert Opin Drug Saf* 2009;**8**:745–54.

Michaels LA, Gurian M, Hegyi T, *et al.* Low molecular weight heparin in the treatment of venous and arterial thromboses in the premature infant. *Pediatrics* 2004;**114**:703–7.

Paidas MJ, Ku D-HW, Arkel YS. Screening and management of inherited thrombophilias in the setting of adverse pregnancy outcome. *Clin Perinatol* 2004;**31**:783–805.

Streif W, Goebel G, Chan AKC, *et al.* Use of low molecular mass heparin (enoxaparin) in newborn infants: a prospective cohort study of 62 patients. *Arch Dis Child Fetal Neonatal Ed* 2003;**88**:F365–70.

Use

Enzyme replacement therapy (ERT) using recombinant DNA technology allows treatment of an increasing number of conditions that are caused by a specific congenital enzyme deficiency. While treatment, which may need to be lifelong unless stem cell transplantation is an option, is both burdensome and expensive, use can be justified for some seriously disabling conditions. There is now more evidence about early treatment, and while not all conditions are suitable for early use, a few are. If the diagnosis is made at birth (or antenatally), treatment may be started in the neonatal period as earlier treatment tends to give a better prognosis. Newborn screening programmes for some conditions are beginning to appear.

Pharmacology

A variety of animal, transformed human and even plant cell lines are now genetically engineered to secrete the missing enzyme which is then given intravenous (IV) infusion every 1–2 weeks after careful purification. All ERTs can cause an antibody response that in some patients means premedication may be required for transfusion reactions.

Congenital enzyme deficiencies

Gaucher's disease: In this autosomal recessively inherited lysosomal storage disorder (LSD), sphingolipid accumulation occurs because of acid β-glucosidase deficiency. Manifestations are highly variable, and the diagnosis is seldom obvious at birth. It presents with anaemia, thrombocytopenia and a bleeding tendency, noticeable hepatosplenomegaly and progressive skeletal problems. There is extensive experience of using **imiglucerase** in type I disease (where there is no neurological involvement). Treatment, if sustained, can render patients almost symptom-free. However, because the enzyme does not cross the blood–brain barrier, this is of little help to the minority with early progressive neurological involvement (type II disease). Treatment should not be stopped during pregnancy or lactation. **Velaglucerase alfa** is a newer ERT with an identical amino acid sequence to the naturally occurring enzyme (imiglucerase has a single amino acid substitution) that is equally effective but with, it seems, fewer hypersensitivity reactions and fewer antibodies than imiglucerase. Many patients, including infants and younger children in whom there is increasing experience, were switched to velaglucerase alfa during shortage of imiglucerase, but there does not appear to be any evidence to support superiority of one product over the other. A further ERT, taliglucerase, has been approved as a treatment for adult Gaucher's disease by the FDA in the United States, but this is not available in Europe due to a 10-year market exclusivity that had been granted by the EMEA for velaglucerase alfa.

Hurler's syndrome (MPS type I): A recessively inherited deficiency of α-L-iduronidase causes the accumulation of mucopolysaccharides in this condition. Patients with severe symptoms are classed as having Hurler's syndrome, and those with only minor symptoms as having Scheie disease. **Laronidase** can contain symptoms, but because it does not cross the blood–brain barrier, stem cell transplantation is usually offered to younger patients, despite the risk involved, once a match is found.

Hunter's syndrome (MPS type II): An X-linked deficiency of iduronate-2-sulphatase leads to the accumulation of heparan and dermatan sulphates. Although the mean age at diagnosis is 3–4 years, symptoms begin during the first year of life but may not be immediately recognised as due to Hunter's syndrome. Eventually, distinctive coarse facial features appear and multi-organ involvement (particularly the heart, lungs, airway and skeletal and nervous system) follows. **Idursulfase** may be used to prevent or treat non-CNS manifestations, but because the enzyme does not cross the blood–brain barrier, this is of little benefit to those with neurological manifestations.

Maroteaux–Lamy syndrome (MPS type VI): This recessively inherited LSD is caused by deficiency of the enzyme N-acetylgalactosamine-4-sulphatase. As with other mucopolysaccharidoses, most individuals are normal at birth, and symptoms and signs of short stature, hepatosplenomegaly, dysostosis multiplex, corneal clouding, cardiac abnormalities and facial dysmorphism appear as glycosaminoglycans accumulate; however, there is usually no CNS involvement. **Galsulfase** may be used to prevent manifestations and treatment is usually lifelong (stem cell transplantation is now rare in MPS VI).

Pompe's disease: In this LSD, a recessively inherited α-glucosidase enzyme deficiency causes excess glycogen to accumulate in muscle. Expression is variable. In the infantile form, cardiomyopathy and profound myopathy used to cause death within 18 months. **Alglucosidase alfa** has been successful when started early, although some skeletal myopathy may remain.

Continued on p. 201

Treatment

> Note: Treatment with any of these products should only be initiated after consultation with a specialist centre.
>
> Most treatment schedules were designed with older children and adults in mind and may not be suitable for neonates and young infants. The following rates and infusions are suitable for infants greater than 6 months; for neonates and infants less than 6 months, seek additional advice from the specialist centre. Prematurity is not usually a contraindication to treatment. Infusions are usually started at a low rate which is then increased as the infusion progresses.

Imiglucerase: Give 60 units/kg IV slowly over 1–2 hours once every two weeks. Dose is adjusted according to response, and in some children, doses of 30 units/kg every 2 weeks may be effective.

Velaglucerase alfa: Give 60 units/kg IV slowly through a 0.2 µm filter over 1–2 hours once every 2 weeks. Dose is adjusted according to response. In some children, doses of 30 units/kg may be effective.

Laronidase: Give 100 units/kg (0.58 mg/kg) as a slow IV infusion through a 0.2 µm filter over 4 hours once a week.

Idursulfase: Give 500 micrograms/kg as a slow IV infusion over 3 hours once a week.

Galsulfase: Give 1 mg/kg as a slow IV infusion through a 0.2 µm filter over 4 hours once a week.

Alglucosidase alfa: Give 20 mg/kg as a slow IV infusion through a 0.2 µm line filter over approximately 4 hours once every 2 weeks.

Supply and administration

Keep all vials at 2–8 °C, but let these come to room temperature for 20 minutes before reconstitution.

Imiglucerase: 200 unit vials cost £535; 400 unit vials cost £1070. Reconstitute the powder with water for injection (5.1 ml of water for the 200 unit vial, 10.2 ml for the 400 unit vial) to obtain a 40 units/ml solution. Take 1.5 ml/kg (60 units/kg) of the reconstituted imiglucerase and dilute this with 0.9% sodium chloride to a total volume of 100–200 ml. Slowly infuse this solution at a rate not exceeding 0.5 units/kg/minute (for the initial dose only, subsequent doses may be given at a rate up to 1 unit/kg/minute) within 3 hours of reconstitution.

Velaglucerase alfa: 400 unit vials cost £1400. Reconstitute the powder with 4.3 ml water for injection to obtain a 100 units/ml solution. Take 0.6 ml/kg (60 units/kg) of the reconstituted velaglucerase and dilute this with 0.9% sodium chloride to a total volume of 100 ml. Infuse this solution over 1 hour.

Laronidase: 500 unit (5 ml) vials cost £460. Take 1 ml/kg and dilute this with 0.9% sodium chloride to a total volume of 100 ml. Infuse initially at a rate of 2 units/kg/hour, and then increase gradually every 15 minutes to max. 43 units/kg/hour.

Idursulfase: 6 mg (2 mg/ml) vials cost £1985. Take 0.25 ml/kg and dilute this with 0.9% sodium chloride to a total volume of 100 ml. Infuse this solution over 3 hours. Subsequently, the infusion duration can be gradually reduced to 1 hour if there are no transfusion reactions.

Galsulfase: 5 mg (1 mg/ml) vials cost £980. Take 1 ml/kg and dilute this with 0.9% sodium chloride to a total volume of 100 ml. Infuse this over at least 4 hours.

Alglucosidase alfa: 50 mg vials cost £360. Reconstitute the powder by allowing 10.3 ml of water for injection to run slowly down the side of the vial to obtain a 5 mg/mL solution. Check that this solution is colourless and clear (a few colourless strands may persist). Draw 4 ml/kg into large syringe, and add enough 0.9% sodium chloride to achieve a concentration of 0.5–4 mg/ml. Infuse this at an initial rate of 1 mg/kg/hour, increasing by 2 mg/kg/hour every 30 minutes to a maximum of 7 mg/kg/hour.

References

Anderson H, Kaplan P, Kacena K, *et al.* Eight-year clinical outcomes of long-term replacement therapy for 884 children with Gaucher disease type I. *Pediatrics* 2008;**122**:1182–90.

Continued on p. 202

Burrow TA, Grabowski GA. Velaglucerase alfa in the treatment of Gaucher disease type 1. *Clin Investig (Lond)* 2011;**1**:285–93.

Chakrapani A, Vellodi A, Robinson P, *et al.* Treatment of infantile Pompe disease with alglucosidase alpha: the UK experience. *J Inherit Metab Dis* 2010;**33**:747–50.

Chien Y-H, Lee N-C, Thurberg BL, *et al.* Pompe disease in infants: improving the prognosis by newborn screening and early treatment. *Pediatrics* 2009;**124**:e1116–25.

Clarke LA, Wraith JE, Beck M, *et al.* Long-term efficacy and safety of laronidase in the treatment of muco-polysaccharidosis I. *Pediatrics* 2009;123;**123**:229–40.

Coman DJ, Hayes IM, Collins V, *et al.* Enzyme replacement therapy for mucopolysaccharidoses: opinions of patients and families. *J Pediatr* 2008;**152**:723–7.

Elstein Y, Eisenberg V, Granbovsky-Grisaru S, *et al.* Pregnancies in Gaucher disease: a 5-year study. *Am J Obstet Gynecol* 2004;**190**:435–41.

Grabowski GA, Kacena K, Cole JA, *et al.* Dose-response relationships for enzyme replacement therapy with imiglucerase/alglucerase in patients with Gaucher disease type I. *Genet Med* 2009;**11**:90–100.

Harmatz PR, Garcia P, Guffon N, *et al.* Galsulfase (Naglazyme®) therapy in infants with mucopolysaccharidosis VI. *J Inherit Metab Dis* 2014;**37**:277–87.

Morris JL. Velaglucerase alfa for the management of type 1 Gaucher disease. *Clin Ther* 2012;**34**:259–71.

Sohn YB, Cho SY, Park SW, *et al.* Phase I/II clinical trial of enzyme replacement therapy with idursulfase beta in patients with mucopolysaccharidosis II (Hunter syndrome). *Orphanet J Rare Dis* 2013;**8**:42.

Tylki-Szymanska A, Jurecka A, Zuber Z, *et al.* Enzyme replacement therapy for mucopolysaccharidosis II from 3 months of age: a 3-year follow-up. *Acta Paediatr* 2012;**101**:e42–7.

Vanier MT, Caillaud C. Disorders of sphingolipid metabolism and neuronal ceroid-lipofuscinoses. In: Saudubray J-M, van den Berghe G, Walter JH. eds. *Inborn metabolic diseases. Diagnosis and treatment*, 5th ed. Berlin: Springer-Verlag, 2012: pp. 555–78.

Vellodi A, Tylski SA, Davies EH, *et al.* Management of neuropathic Gaucher disease: revised recommendations. *J Inherit Metab Dis* 2009;**32**:660–4.

Wraith JE. Mucopolysaccharidoses and oligosaccharidoses In: Saudubray J-M, van den Berghe G, Walter JH, eds. *Inborn metabolic diseases. Diagnosis and treatment*, 5th ed. Berlin: Springer-Verlag, 2012: pp. 579–90.

Wynn RF, Mercer J, Page J, *et al.* Use of enzyme replacement therapy (laronidase) before hematopoietic stem cell transplantation for mucopolysaccharidosis I: experience in 18 patients. *J Pediatr* 2009;**154**:135–9. (See also pp. 609–11.)

Use

Epoprostenol (PGI$_2$) is used in the treatment of adults and children with severe, sustained pulmonary arterial hypertension. Treatment, involving continuous intravenous (IV) infusion, is expensive and 'high maintenance', demanding an ongoing commitment by the parents/carers and co-operation of the child. There have been a few reports of IV (or nebulised) administration improving oxygenation in the term baby even when treatment with nitric oxide (q.v.) has proved ineffective.

Pharmacology

Epoprostenol is a prostaglandin-like substance first discovered in 1976. It is an extremely powerful inhibitor of platelet aggregation sometimes used during renal dialysis and in the management of haemorrhagic meningococcal purpura. Epoprostenol produces rapid dose-related decreases in pulmonary arterial pressure and pulmonary vascular resistance and came to be used experimentally, therefore, in the management of babies with persistent pulmonary hypertension or cyanosis due to a persisting transitional circulation. The drug is not metabolised during passage through the lung, but only has a 3 minute half-life, making continuous infusion necessary. The drug's rapid action makes efficacy easy to judge but can also leave the baby very drug dependent. Systemic hypotension can also be a serious problem because of marked systemic vasodilatation.

More recently, there have been reports where aerosolised prostacyclin improved oxygenation *without* affecting systemic blood pressure. A reduction in intrapulmonary shunting seemed to account for much of the improvement. **Iloprost** is a synthetic analogue of prostacyclin that has been approved for inhalation but not IV use. Concerns exist, however, due to airway irritation and damage of mechanical ventilator valves from the alkaline nature of the solution, condensation and loss of medication and alteration of mechanical ventilation characteristics due to added gas flow during nebulisation.

Treatment

Intravenous epoprostenol: Begin the infusion at a rate of 2 nanograms/kg/minute and adjust according to response up to a maximum of 20 nanograms/kg/minute (may be increased up to 40 nanograms/kg/minute).
Inhaled iloprost: The inhaled dose has not been established in neonates. Studies report starting at 1 micrograms/kg every 2 hours and titrating according to response.

Supply and administration

Vials containing 500 micrograms of epoprostenol powder (costing £22), with 50 ml of glycine diluent buffer for reconstitution, are available. Vials and diluent must be stored at 2–8 °C, protected from light and discarded promptly after use. To prepare epoprostenol for use, draw 10 ml of sterile diluent (pH 10.5) into a syringe, inject into the epoprostenol vial, and dissolve the contents completely. Draw the epoprostenol back into the syringe and reunite the contents of the syringe with the residue of the original 50 ml of diluent (giving a solution of 10 micrograms/ml). Then choose which instructions to follow according to the baby's weight:

Weight <2 kg: Take **15 ml (150 micrograms)** of the reconstituted solution for every kilogram the baby weighs and dilute to a final volume of 50 ml with 0.9% saline. An infusion rate of 0.1 ml/hour provides a dose of **5 nanograms/kg/minute.**

Weight ≥2 kg: Take **6 ml (60 micrograms)** of the reconstituted solution for every kilogram the baby weighs and dilute to a final volume of 50 ml with 0.9% saline. An infusion rate of 0.1 ml/hour provides a dose of **2 nanograms/kg/minute.**

Make up a fresh supply once every 24 hours (the manufacturer recommends once every 12 hours, but potency only falls 5% in this time). Watch for tissue extravasation, and tail off any infusion over a number of hours. Iloprost is available in 1 ml vials containing 10 micrograms (cost £13).

Continued on p. 204

References

Bindl I, Fahrenstick H, Peukert U. Aerosolised prostacyclin for pulmonary hypertension in neonates. *Arch Dis Child Fetal Neonatal Ed* 1994;**71**:F214–6.

Eronen M, Pohjavouri M, Andersson S, *et al*. Prostacyclin treatment for persistent pulmonary hypertension of the newborn. *Pediatr Cardiol* 1997;**18**:3–7.

Gokce I, Kahveci H, Turkyilmaz Z, *et al*. Inhaled iloprost in the treatment of pulmonary hypertension in very low birth weight infants: a report of two cases. *J Pak Med Assoc* 2012;**62**:388–91.

Kaapa P, Koivisto M, Ylikorkala O, *et al*. Prostacyclin in the treatment of neonatal pulmonary hypertension. *J Pediatr* 1985;**107**:951–3.

Kelly LK, Porta NFM, Goodman DM, *et al*. Inhaled prostacyclin for term infants with persistent pulmonary hypertension refractory to inhaled nitric oxide. *J Pediatr* 2002;**141**:830–2.

Lammers AE, Hislop AA, Flynn Y, *et al*. Epoprostenol treatment in children with severe pulmonary hypertension. *Heart* 2007;**93**:739–43.

Lock JE, Olley PM, Coceani F, *et al*. Use of prostacyclin in persistent fetal circulation. *Lancet* 1979;**1**:1343.

Olmsted K, Oluola O, Parthiban A, *et al*. Can inhaled prostacyclin stimulate surfactant in ELBW infants? *J Perinatol* 2007;**27**:724–6.

Pappert D, Busch T, Gerlach H, *et al*. Aerosolized prostacyclin *versus* inhaled nitric oxide in children with severe acute respiratory distress syndrome. *Anesthesiology* 1995;**82**:1507–11.

Piastra M, De Luca D, De Carolis MP, *et al*. Nebulized iloprost and noninvasive respiratory support for impending hypoxaemic respiratory failure in formerly preterm infants: a case series. *Pediatr Pulmonol* 2012;**47**:757–62.

Soditt V, Aring C, Gronceck P. Improvement in oxygenation in a preterm infant with persistent pulmonary hypertension of the newborn. *Intensive Care Med* 1997;**23**:1275–8.

Use

Erythromycin, like azithromycin (q.v.), is used to treat neonatal *Chlamydia*, *Mycoplasma* and *Ureaplasma* infections. Azithromycin is now more widely used to reduce whooping cough cross infection. Erythromycin marginally, but usefully, delays delivery in a few women with preterm pre-labour rupture of membranes (pPROM) and helps some babies with gut motility problems.

Pharmacology

This broad-spectrum macrolide antibiotic, first isolated in 1952, does not enter the CSF. Only small amounts cross the placenta, and the amount ingested in breast milk exposes the baby (weight for weight) to only 2% of the maternal dose. There is no evidence of teratogenicity. Erythromycin may be given in labour to mothers allergic to penicillin where there is a risk of group B streptococcal infection. Giving mothers with pPROM 250 mg by mouth four times a day reduced delivery within 48 hours by 15% in the ORACLE trial but delivered no long-term benefit and only delivered a significant reduction in neonatal problems in singleton pregnancy (which was not a pre-specified trial outcome). More significantly, pre-delivery use in preterm labour *not* associated with pre-labour membrane rupture was associated with a greater risk of cerebral palsy.

Erythromycin is well absorbed orally and intravenous (IV) treatment is seldom necessary. The oral preparation (erythromycin ethylsuccinate) has to be hydrolysed to the active base after absorption, and the ester occasionally causes reversible liver toxicity. Sudden arrhythmia has occurred with rapid IV administration, and vomiting and diarrhoea (occasionally caused by pseudomembranous colitis) have been reported in older children, but the drug is, in most respects, one of the more innocuous antibiotics in current use. The serum half-life is short (2–4 hours), is unaffected by renal function and changes little during the neonatal period. Some of the drug appears in the bile and urine, but most is unaccounted for. Erythromycin is a motilin receptor agonist; its value in speeding up full enteral feeding and reduction of TPN-associated cholestasis must be balanced against a knowledge that pyloric stenosis can occur after high-dose use. Low-dose regimes (3 mg/kg per dose) seem to be effective, and high-dose (12.5 mg/kg per dose) regimes are best reserved for 'rescue' treatment.

Chlamydia infection

Chlamydiae are small intracellular bacteria that need living cells to multiply. Genitourinary infection is particularly common among young women who have had a new sexual partner in the last 12 months if they are not using barrier contraception. Some 5% of women of child-bearing age are infected (two-thirds are asymptomatic) and at risk of tubal infertility and tubal pregnancy. Screening should be offered to all women requesting termination of pregnancy and to all under 25 booking for antenatal care. Babies often develop conjunctivitis at delivery, and a few develop an afebrile pneumonitis. Failure to recognise that this is due to *Chlamydia*, and to refer as appropriate, exposes the mother to all the risks associated with progressive unchecked pelvic inflammatory disease. Chronic eye infection (trachoma) causes progressive damage to the upper eyelid, and the resultant corneal scaring is the most common cause of preventable blindness in many countries.

Drug interactions

Erythromycin increases the half-life of midazolam, theophylline and carbamazepine producing potential toxicity. It also prolongs the QT interval and this effect can be dangerously potentiated by interaction with other drugs. Increased oral bioavailability can also cause toxicity in a minority of patients on digoxin. Erythromycin also seems to potentiate the anticoagulant effect of warfarin.

Treatment

Systemic infection: Give 12.5 mg/kg every 6 hours by mouth, or infuse 10–12.5 mg IV over 1 hour (to avoid the risk of arrhythmia) as described under 'Supply and administration'. There is no satisfactory intramuscular preparation.

Conjunctivitis: See the monograph on eye drops (q.v.), but where chlamydia is suspected, the most effective choice is almost certainly a single 20 mg/kg oral dose of azithromycin (q.v.).

Gut dysmotility: Try 3 mg/kg by mouth once every 6 hours (12.5 mg/kg if TPN-associated cholestasis is a concern).

Continued on p. 206

Supply and administration

The IV (lactobionate) salt is available in 1 g vials (cost £11). When made up with 20 ml of water for injection (not saline), the resultant stock solution contains 50 mg/ml. Individual doses containing 5 mg/ml can be prepared by drawing 5 ml of the stock solution into a syringe and diluting this to 50 ml with non-buffered 0.9% saline (or with buffered glucose previously prepared by adding 5 ml of 8.4% sodium bicarbonate to a 500 ml bag of 10% glucose or glucose saline). Give IV doses within 8 hours of preparation. 100 ml of the sugar-free oral suspension of erythromycin ethylsuccinate (25 mg/ml) costs £2.50 and can be kept for up to 2 weeks after being reconstituted from the dry powder if stored at 4 °C.

References 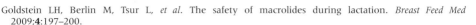 (See also the relevant Cochrane reviews)

Goldstein LH, Berlin M, Tsur L, *et al*. The safety of macrolides during lactation. *Breast Feed Med* 2009;**4**:197–200.

Kenyon S, Pike K, Jones DR, *et al*. Childhood outcomes after prescription of antibiotics to pregnant women with spontaneous preterm labour: 7 year follow-up of the ORACLE II trial. *Lancet* 2008;**372**:1319–27. [RCT] (See also pp. 1310–8.)

Lam HS, Ng PC. Use of prokinetics in the preterm infant. *Curr Opin Pediatr* 2011;**23**:156–60.

Maheshwai N. Are young infants treated with erythromycin at risk for developing hypertrophic pyloric stenosis? *Arch Dis Child* 2007;**92**:271–3.

Ng PC, Lee CH, Wong SPS, *et al*. High-dose oral erythromycin decreased the incidence of parenteral nutrition-associated cholestasis in preterm Infants. *Gastroenterology* 2007;**132**:1726–39. [RCT]

Use

Erythropoietin stimulates red blood cell production but has little impact on the need for blood transfusion if blood sampling is kept to a minimum, and use within a week or so of birth seems to increase the risk of serious retinopathy of prematurity (ROP). High-dose use also increases mortality in adults in renal failure.

Recombinant EPO (r-EPO) has a variety of glycosylation patterns giving rise to alfa, beta, delta, theta and omega forms. In addition, **darbepoetin alfa**, a long-acting analogue, is available which has two additional glycosylation sites. This modification gives a longer half-life and thereby enables less frequent dosing.

Pharmacology

Erythropoietin is a natural glycoprotein produced primarily in the kidneys which stimulates red blood cell production, particularly when there is relative tissue anoxia. During fetal life, it is mostly produced in the liver. Two commercial versions (epoetin alfa and epoetin beta), synthesised using recombinant DNA technology, became available in 1986. They have identical amino acid sequences but different glycosylation patterns. Since then, further versions have become available. The prescriber must specify which of these biosimilar products is to be given. Epoetin beta is the only product the manufacturer has been authorised to recommend for use in treatment of anaemia of prematurity in Europe. Progressive hypertension and severe red cell aplasia are the most serious adverse effects seen in adults, but they have not been reported in neonates to date. The platelet count may rise. Erythropoietin does not seem to cross the human placenta, and the amount absorbed from breast milk is not enough to effect haemopoiesis (although it could enhance gut maturity), so women should not be denied treatment just because they are pregnant or breastfeeding.

Numerous randomised and blinded, or placebo-controlled, trials have now shown that early and sustained treatment with erythropoietin can stimulate red cell production in the very preterm baby, as long as supplemental iron is also given. Perhaps among the most important findings of the first randomised controlled trials of r-EPO was that implementing standard criteria for RBC transfusion alone safely reduced the number of transfusions administered, even for patients in the control group.

However, large doses have to be given because clearance and the volume of distribution are both three to four times as high as in adult life. Treatment certainly has a place in the early care of vulnerable babies born to families who are reluctant to sanction blood transfusion on religious grounds. Nevertheless, although early treatment reduces the need for replacement transfusion, especially in the smallest babies, it seldom eliminates it, and no response to treatment is generally seen for 1–2 weeks. The benefits of r-EPO on the need for early transfusion are modest and must be weighed against other benefits (such as a reduction in chronic lung disease, possibly due to anti-inflammatory and antioxidative actions) and disadvantages (an increase in significant ROP and the numbers of infantile haemangiomas). There does appear to be a slighter larger effect of r-EPO on the need for late transfusions, which, given the association between these and the subsequent development of necrotising enterocolitis (NEC), may argue in favour of r-EPO treatment. Darbepoetin alfa has been shown in one randomised trial to be as effective as epoetin in reducing transfusion need, but the manufacturer has yet to endorse use in young children.

Treatment

Epoetin beta: Give 250 units/kg by subcutaneous injection into the thigh three times a week, starting within 3 days of birth and continuing for 6 weeks.
Darbepoetin alfa: Give 10 micrograms/kg by subcutaneous injection once a week, starting within 3 days of birth and continuing for 6 weeks.

Compatibility

Erythropoietin seems equally effective given as a continuous (but not as a bolus) infusion in parenteral nutrition (q.v.), together with 1 mg/kg a day of parenteral iron if oral iron cannot be given.

Supply

500 unit and 2000 unit pre-filled syringes of epoetin beta cost £3.50 and £14, respectively. The large multi-dose vials, which require water for reconstitution, should not be used when treating babies because they contain benzyl alcohol. Supplies should be stored at 4°C. Pre-filled syringes containing 10 micrograms of darbepoetin alfa (25 micrograms/ml) cost £14.70.

Continued on p. 208

References

(See also the relevant Cochrane reviews)

Doege C, Pritsch M, Frühwald MC, *et al.* An association between infantile haemangiomas and erythropoietin treatment in preterm infants. *Arch Dis Child Fetal Neonatal Ed* 2012;**97**:F45–9.

Franz AR, Pohlant F. Red blood cell transfusions in very and extremely low birthweight infants under restrictive transfusion guidelines: is exogenous erythropoietin necessary? *Arch Dis Child Fetal Neonatal Ed* 2001;**84**:F96–100.

Garcia MG, Hutson AD, Christensen RD. Effect of recombinant erythropoietin on "late" transfusions in the neonatal intensive care unit: a meta-analysis. *J Perinatol* 2002;**22**:108–11. [SR]

Kotto-Kome AC, Garcia MG, Calhoun DA, *et al.* Effect of beginning recombinant erythropoietin treatment within the first week of life, among very-low-birth-weight neonates, on "early" and "late" erythrocyte transfusions: a meta-analysis. *J Perinatol* 2004;**24**:24–9. [SR]

Ohls RK. Erythropoietin treatment in extremely low birth weight infants: blood in versus blood out. *J Pediatr* 2002;**141**:3–6.

Ohls RK. Human recombinant erythropoietin in the prevention and treatment of anemia of prematurity. *Paediatr Drugs* 2002;**4**:111–21.

Ohls RK, Christensen RD, Kamath-Rayne BD, *et al.* A randomized, masked, placebo-controlled study of darbepoetin alfa in preterm infants. *Pediatrics* 2013;**132**:e119–27. [RCT]

Phrommintikul A, Haas SJ, Elsik M, *et al.* Mortality and target haemoglobin concentrations in anaemic patients with chronic kidney disease treated with erythropoietin: a meta-analysis. *Lancet* 2007;**369**:381–8. [SR] (See also pp. 346–50.)

Use

Eye drops are necessary to treat a number of neonatal conditions; antibiotic eye drops are used to treat acute infective conjunctivitis, and saline eye drops (or fresh tap water) are used to treat chemical conjunctivitis seen in the early days. Mydriatic eye drops dilate the pupil, while cycloplegics paralyse the ciliary muscle, allowing diagnostic or therapeutic procedures. Proxymetacaine provides surface anaesthesia. Hypromellose eye drops ('artificial tears') are used to moisten the cornea when tear production is inadequate or the baby is paralysed or unconscious. Steroid drops are sometimes prescribed after surgery to the eye.

Pharmacology

Because penetration is limited and rather variable when antibiotics are prescribed topically as drops, a systemic antibiotic should always be given as well if there is deep-seated infection. High doses of mydriatics can cause adverse systemic side effects (including ileus). Many eye drops also contain antimicrobial preservatives; one of the most common is benzalkonium chloride; however, these are best avoided due to their propensity to cause problems with the tear film, cornea and conjunctiva with long-term use (see commentary).

Infections

Conjunctival inflammation during the first month of life (*ophthalmia neonatorum* or neonatal conjunctivitis) occurs in up to a quarter of neonates. The most serious infections are those caused by *Neisseria gonococcus* and *Chlamydia trachomatis*. Chloramphenicol eye drops are still widely used to deal with low-grade conjunctivitis (especially where this seems to be due to staphylococcal or coliform infection). Gonococcal infection is probably best treated with a single large intravenous or intramuscular dose of ceftriaxone or ceftazidime (q.v.), while overt *Chlamydia* infection, which can cause inclusion conjunctivitis (or very rarely, if not treated, trachoma), is best managed with oral azithromycin (q.v.). The mother should always be seen and treated as well when venereally acquired neonatal gonococcal or chlamydial infection is encountered. It may also be important to trace the mother's contacts too. *Pseudomonas* infection, which is potentially very dangerous, should be treated with gentamicin eye drops and appropriate systemic antibiotics under the supervision of a consultant ophthalmologist. Look for keratitis or a corneal ulcer using fluorescein if in any doubt after first anaesthetising the cornea. Herpes conjunctivitis as a first manifestation of generalised neonatal herpes infection requires equally expert management with topical and systemic aciclovir (q.v.). A chronic watery discharge is usually due to congenital nasolacrimal duct obstruction (a very common condition that almost always cures itself and seldom needs treatment unless overt infection supervenes).

Steroids

Steroid eye drops should only be used under the supervision of a consultant ophthalmologist and after the exclusion of herpetic eye disease. They may be used to reduce inflammation after eye surgery, including laser treatment of retinopathy of prematurity.

Fundal examination and screening for retinopathy of prematurity

Various antimuscarinic and sympathomimetic drops are available to bring about mydriasis (dilatation of the pupil) or cycloplegia (paralysis of the ciliary muscle of the eye) making examination easier. Antimuscarinics dilate the pupil and paralyse the ciliary muscle; they vary in potency and duration of action. The action of tropicamide lasts about 4–6 hours, that of cyclopentolate up to 24 hours, and that of atropine up to 7 days. Phenylephrine causes mydriasis that lasts up to 5–7 hours.

Topical anaesthetics

Oxybuprocaine and proxymetacaine are widely used topical local anaesthetics. Proxymetacaine causes less initial stinging. The BNF and BNF for Children continue to assert that use of topical anaesthetics is ill-advised in the preterm baby *because of the immaturity of the enzyme system which metabolises the ester type local anaesthetics in premature babies*. The original statement reflected a theoretical concern, and there is no published evidence that use has actually proved hazardous. Gentle pressure on the duct in the inner corner of the eye may stop the drops draining into the nose and into the blood.

Continued on p. 210

Miscellaneous

Hypromellose and a number of other 'artificial tears' are available and should be considered where the eye does not close. Some formulations, however, contain benzalkonium chloride.

Supply

Anti-infective eye preparations: Azithromycin dihydrate 1.5% single-dose solution in container costs £1.20. It may be used in simple bacterial conjunctivitis but may also be used to treat trachomatous conjunctivitis in conjunction with oral azithromycin (q.v.). Single use (Minims®) **chloramphenicol 0.5%** costs 51p each; 10 ml of **chloramphenicol 0.5%** costs £1.50; both are used in simple mild bacterial conjunctivitis. **Fusidic acid 1%** in gel basis (which liquefies on contact with eye) costing £2.70 for a 5 g tube may be used in simple mild bacterial conjunctivitis but is especially useful in staphylococcal conjunctivitis. This contains benzalkonium chloride. **Gentamicin sulfate 0.3%** drops (suitable for aural or ocular use) are available in 10 ml bottles (cost £2.10) which contain benzalkonium chloride. A stronger 1.5% preparation is available as a manufactured special from Moorfields Eye Hospital. **Aciclovir 3% ointment** (cost £9.30 for 4.5 g) is available to treat herpes infections of the eye (along with systemic aciclovir).

Steroid eye drops: Various preparations are available, and some combined with antibiotics. **Betamethasone sodium phosphate 0.1%** drops costing £2.30 for 10 ml and **prednisolone sodium phosphate 0.5%** drops costing £2 for 10 ml are among those used (both preparations contain benzalkonium chloride). Avoid the stronger prednisolone drops (Pred Forte®).

Cycloplegics and mydriatics: Atropine sulfate 0.5% costs £19 for 10 ml. **Cyclopentolate hydrochloride** (in a solution containing benzalkonium chloride) is available in 0.5% and 1% strengths costing £6.70 for 5 ml. Single use (Minims) **cyclopentolate** 0.5% and 1% drops are preservative-free and cost 48p. **Tropicamide** is available in two strengths: 0.5% costing £1.30 and 1% costing £1.60 for 5 ml (these contain benzalkonium chloride). Single use (Minims) **tropicamide** 0.5% and 1% drops are preservative-free and cost 50p, and Minims of **phenylephrine hydrochloride** 2.5% costs 53p.

Topical anaesthetics: Single use (Minims) of **oxybuprocaine hydrochloride** 0.4% costs 47p, while **proxymetacaine hydrochloride** 0.5% costs 53p per Minims. They provide corneal anaesthesia in half a minute.

Miscellaneous: Hypromellose 0.3% costs £1.10 for 10 ml (some preparations contain benzalkonium chloride). Single use drops are available but vary considerably in price. **Saline** (0·9% sodium chloride) eye drops (as Minims) do not need a prescription. However, they cost 25p each and their use is hard to justify in babies with a mild (probably chemical) conjunctivitis. Such eyes merely need to be bathed periodically with clean fresh tap water.

References   (See also the relevant Cochrane reviews)

Baudouin C, Labbé A, Liang H, *et al*. Preservatives in eyedrops: the good, the bad and the ugly. *Prog Retin Eye Res* 2010;**29**:312–34.

Darling EK, McDonald H. A meta-analysis of the efficacy of ocular prophylactic agents used for the prevention of gonococcal and chlamydial ophthalmia neonatorum. *J Midwifery Womens Health* 2010;**55**:319–27. [SR]

Isenberg SJ, Apt L, Del Signore M, *et al*. A double application approach to ophthalmia neonatorum prophylaxis. *Br J Ophthalmol* 2003;**87**:1449–52.

Isenberg SJ, Apt L, Wood M. A controlled trial of povidone-iodine as prophylaxis against ophthalmia neonatorum. *N Engl J Med* 1995;**332**:562–6. [RCT] (See also pp. 600–1.)

Rose PW, Harden A, Brueggemann AB, *et al*. Chloramphenicol treatment for acute infective conjunctivitis in children in primary care: a randomised double-blind placebo-controlled trial. *Lancet* 2005;**366**:37–43. [RCT] (See also 6–7 and 1431–2.)

Wiholm B-E, Kelly JP, Kaufman D, *et al*. Relation of aplastic anemia to use of chloramphenicol eye drops in two international case-control studies. *Br Med J* 1998;**316**:666. (See also p. 667.)

Use

Fentanyl is used to provide perioperative pain relief. Remifentanil (q.v.) is a very short-acting alternative. A continuous infusion will cause tolerance to develop and exposes babies to symptoms of opiate withdrawal.

Pharmacology

Fentanyl citrate is a synthetic fat-soluble opioid developed as an analogue of pethidine and haloperidol in 1964. It is used to provide rapid short-lived pain relief during surgery and during epidural anaesthesia in childbirth. Administration, particularly if rapid, can sometimes cause muscle rigidity and seizure-like activity. Few haemodynamic effects are seen, and the drug seems to be good at inhibiting the haemodynamic and metabolic effects of surgical stress. It is well absorbed from the gastrointestinal tract, but bioavailability is limited by rapid liver metabolism. Transdermal patches are useful for chronic pain in older children.

While fentanyl is a short-acting narcotic, it has a prolonged elimination half-life. Significant doses rapidly cause respiratory depression. The peak effect occurs within 5 minutes (4–8 times sooner than morphine) but may only last 30–60 minutes due to rapid and cumulative redistribution into fat and muscle (neonatal V_D 6–12 l/kg). Fentanyl is primarily metabolised by cytochrome P450 3A4. Elimination is controlled by N-dealkylation and hydroxylation in the liver and is dose dependent. The half-life, like that of morphine, is very variable in the neonate (6–30 hours) and only slightly influenced by gestation but seems to approach that seen in adult life (2–7 hours) within 2–3 months of birth.

> **Fentanyl pharmacokinetics during therapeutic hypothermia have not been established, but as the drug is metabolised by hepatic cytochrome P450 enzymes, the half-life is likely to be longer in cooled infants. In a hypothermic pig model, there was a 25% increase in plasma fentanyl concentrations during hypothermia that persisted for 6 hours after re-warming.**

Tolerance is more likely if fentanyl is used for more than 3 days, whereas this is seen with morphine after a couple of weeks. Higher plasma levels (and higher doses) become necessary. An unpleasant and potentially alarming withdrawal can then occur, with irritability and hypertonia, unless the drug is gradually withdrawn. Alfentanil might, on theoretical grounds, be a useful alternative, because less tissue accumulation occurs, but muscle rigidity is even more common, and the shorter half-life seen in adults is not replicated in infancy.

Embryotoxic, but not teratogenetic, effects are seen in rodents; however, use in humans has not revealed any malformations. Long-term use during pregnancy (e.g. through transdermal patches) can lead to neonatal abstinence. Short-term maternal analgesic use appears to have no effect on the fetus or newborn infant. Although it rapidly crosses the placenta, fetuses should always be given a 15 micrograms/kg injection (based on estimated fetal weight) if undergoing painful procedures *in utero*. There is some evidence that epidural use (together with bupivacaine) during childbirth may make lactation rather harder to establish, but breastfed babies only ingest about 3% of the maternal dose on a weight-for-weight basis. Even then, the bioavailability is limited by the rapid liver metabolism, and no adverse effects have been reported in breastfed infants.

Pain relief

Short-term use: Smaller doses (1–3 micrograms/kg), given over 30 seconds, may be used to provide analgesia in the spontaneously breathing infant, but a 5 micrograms/kg intravenous dose will abolish respiration while providing good brief analgesia; twice this dose is effective for an hour.

Sustained use: Give 5 micrograms/kg and then infuse at a rate of 1.5 micrograms/kg an hour. Adjust according to response.

Use during therapeutic hypothermia: There are currently insufficient data from hypothermic newborns to recommend any specific dosing schedule; however, it would seem sensible to begin by halving the 'normothermic' doses (i.e. by giving 5 micrograms/kg and then infusing at 0.75 micrograms/kg/hour) and titrating according to the response of the infant.

Continued on p. 212

Premedication for induction

Fentanyl at a dose of 2–3 micrograms/kg is used as premedication for intubation in a number of combinations with suxamethonium (q.v.) and atropine (q.v.) or similar.

Antidote

Bradycardia after excess fentanyl administration may respond to atropine. Muscle rigidity will respond to muscle relaxants. Naloxone (q.v.) is an effective fentanyl antidote.

Compatibility

Fentanyl can be added (terminally) to a line containing midazolam, milrinone or standard TPN (including lipid).

Supply and administration

2 ml and 10 ml ampoules containing 50 micrograms/ml cost 30p and 75p, respectively. Take 0.2 ml (10 micrograms) and dilute to 1 ml with 5% glucose to obtain a solution containing 10 micrograms/ml for accurate low-dose administration.

References

Arnold JH, Truog RD, Scavone JM, *et al*. Changes in the pharmacodynamic response to fentanyl in neonates during continuous infusion. *J Pediatr* 1991;**119**:639–43. (See also pp. 588–9.)

Fahnenstich H, Steffan J, Kau N, *et al*. Fentanyl-induced chest wall rigidity and laryngospasm in preterm and term infants. *Crit Care Med* 2000;**28**:836–9.

Fisk NM, Gitau R, Teixeira JM. Effect of direct fetal opioid analgesia on fetal hormonal and hemodynamic stress response to intrauterine needling. *Anesthesiology* 2001;**95**:828–35.

Frank LS, Vilardi J, Durand D, *et al*. Opioid withdrawal in neonates after continuous infusions or morphine or fentanyl during extracorporeal membrane oxygenation. *Am J Crit Care* 1998;**9**:364–9.

Mattingly JE, D'Alessio J, Ramanathan J. Effects of obstetric analgesics and anesthetics on the neonate: a review. *Paediatr Drugs* 2003;**5**:615–27.

Saarenmaa E, Neuvonen PJ, Fellman V. Gestational age and birth weight effects on plasma clearance of fentanyl in newborn infants. *J Pediatr* 2000;**136**:767–70.

Taddio A. Opioid analgesia for infants in the neonatal period. *Clin Perinatol* 2002;**29**:493–509.

Use

Fibrin sealants (also known as tissue adhesives or glues) are used in a wide range of surgical procedures to rapidly arrest bleeding and assist in wound healing. They can be applied by dripping the solution or by spraying the solution using a pressure regulator onto a bleeding tissue where they form a fibrin clot. They have been used in a few, largely, preterm infants with an intractable pneumothorax in order to achieve pleurodesis.

Product

Fibrin sealants are two-component products made from fibrinogen and thrombin. The thrombin converts the fibrinogen to fibrin within 10–15 seconds depending on the concentration of thrombin employed. While both extrinsic and intrinsic coagulation pathways are bypassed, the sealant mimics the final common coagulation pathway. A variety of preparations are available. The older fibrin sealants were largely of bovine origin, but more recently, human products have become available. They are theoretically better than collagen-, cellulose- and gelatin-based haemostats that relied on intact clotting mechanisms and that may also produce foreign body reactions. The use of products containing human fibrinogen and thrombin brings with it theoretical hazards associated with the use of a non-sterilised human product.

Fibrin sealants must not be injected or allowed to enter a large blood vessel because it could cause extensive, potentially lethal, intravascular clotting. Sprays have been reported to cause life-threatening or fatal air embolism and are best avoided in young children. They can sometimes be used with surgical meshes to fill defects.

Treatment of persistent or recurrent pneumothorax

Pulmonary air leaks usually respond to drainage and expectant management within 2–3 days, but high-frequency ventilation, selective ventilation of a single lung and surgical exploration are occasionally called for. As a last resort, if all else fails, approximately 2 ml of reconstituted thrombin can be instilled into the pleural cavity followed, after 2 minutes, by 2 ml of fibrinogen. The pleural drains need to be clamped for 3–5 minutes during this procedure. Such a strategy should not be adopted without first discussing the case with a paediatric or thoracic surgeon.

Treatment of chylothorax

Congenital chylothorax usually resolves with conservative management but carries a high mortality. Pleurodesis has occasionally been used and octreotide (q.v.) has also been used with apparent success when other measures fail. An intravenous infusion (1–3 micrograms/kg/hour) sustained for several days was used in the 12 reports published to date.

Supply and administration

Various fibrin sealants are available; EVICEL® Fibrin Sealant (Human) contains only human products and is available in a number of different size kits (1, 2 and 5 ml) consisting of one vial each of fibrinogen (55–85 mg/ml) and thrombin (800–1200 IU/ml human thrombin) in frozen solutions. It thaws within 10 minutes at room temperature and is usable within 1 minute. TISSEEL® is available as a freeze-dried kit or as pre-filled frozen syringes (total volumes, 2, 4 and 10 ml). While both the fibrinogen (67–106 mg/ml) and thrombin (400–625 units/ml) are of human origin, the product contains synthetic aprotinin, which delays fibrinolysis but which can cause anaphylaxis even with first time use. ARTISS® Fibrin Sealant (Human) comes as frozen solution and lyophilised powder for solution for topical application. It is used primarily for skin grafts rather than haemostasis; the fibrinogen content (67–106 mg/ml) is the same as TISSEEL®, but the thrombin content is lower (2.5–6.5 units/ml). It also contains aprotinin.

References

Atrah HI. Fibrin glue. Topical use for areas of bleeding large and small. *Br Med J* 1994;**308**:933–4.

Berger JT, Gilhooly J. Fibrin glue treatment of persistent pneumothorax in a premature infant. *J Pediatr* 1993;**122**:958–60.

Brissaud O, Desfrere L, Mohsen R, *et al.* Congenital idiopathic chylothorax in neonates: chemical pleurodesis with povidone-iodine (Betadine). *Arch Dis Child Fetal Neonatal Ed* 2003;**88**:F531–3.

Dhillon S. Fibrin sealant (evicel® [quixil®/crosseal™]): a review of its use as supportive treatment for haemostasis in surgery. *Drugs* 2011;**71**:1893–915.

Dunn CJ, Goa KL. Fibrin sealant. A review of its use in surgery and endoscopy. *Drugs* 1999;**58**:863–86. [SR]

Continued on p. 214

Kuint J, Lubin D, Martinowitz U, *et al.* Fibrin glue treatment for recurrent pneumothorax in a premature infant. *Am J Perinatol* 1996;**13**:245–7.

Moreira Dde A, Santos MM, Tannuri AC, *et al.* Congenital chylous ascites: a report of a case treated with hemostatic cellulose and fibrin glue. *J Pediatr Surg* 2013;**48**:e17–9.

Moront MG, Katz NM, O'Donnell J, *et al.* The use of topical fibrin glue at cannulation sites in neonates. *Surg Gynecol Obstet* 1988;**166**:358–9.

Nishizaki N, Suganuma H, Nagata S, *et al.* Use of fibrin glue in the treatment of pneumothorax in premature infant. *Pediatr Int* 2012;**54**:416–9.

Pratap U, Sklavik Z, Ofoe VD, *et al.* Octreotide to treat postoperative chylothorax after cardiac operations in children. *Ann Thorac Surg* 2001;**72**:1740–2.

Sarkar S, Hussain N, Herson V. Fibrin glue for persistent pneumothorax in neonates. *J Perinatol* 2003;**23**:82–4.

Zeidan S, Delarue A, Rome A, *et al.* Fibrin glue application in the management of refractory chylous ascites in children. *J Pediatr Gastroenterol Nurt* 2008;**46**:478–81.

Use

Flecainide is increasingly replacing digoxin (q.v.) in the control of fetal and neonatal supraventricular arrhythmia. Amiodarone (q.v.) will usually work where flecainide does not. Because the manufacturer has not yet endorsed the use of either of these in children, they should only be used under the direct supervision of a paediatric cardiologist.

Pharmacology

Flecainide is a class I antiarrhythmic agent that functions as a sodium channel blocker. It is a fluorinated derivative of procainamide, first synthesised in 1975. The drug is well absorbed orally. It is extensively metabolised in the liver to a number of inactive metabolites as well as being partly excreted by the kidney. There is one isolated report suggesting that diarrhoeal illness may actually cause blood levels to rise due to altered absorption. The half-life in adults is about 14 hours, and such evidence as there is suggests that the half-life is shorter than this in infancy. Tissue levels greatly exceed plasma levels ($V_D \sim 10 \, l/kg$).

The drug crosses the placenta and can be used to control any fetal supraventricular arrhythmia that does not respond to digitalisation. It is increasingly being used from the outset where there is fetal hydrops. It suppresses most re-entry tachycardias and is also effective in atrial ectopic and His bundle tachycardias.

Most children with tachycardia first manifesting itself in the perinatal period become asymptomatic within a year. Where problems persist or return 5–8 years later, radiofrequency catheter ablation of the offending pathways is becoming a progressively more effective long-term solution.

Teratogenic effects have been reported with high-dose treatment in laboratory animals: the relevance of this to the drug's use in early pregnancy remains to be established. The drug causes slowing of atrial, AV nodal and infra-nodal conduction, increasing the atrial and ventricular muscle's refractory period. The drug exerts little effect on sinus node function, but it increases the PR interval and the duration of the QRS complex. Few extra-cardiac adverse effects have been noted to date. Some caution should be exercised when the drug is used during lactation because the baby will receive 5–10% of the maternal dose when intake is calculated on a weight-for-weight basis. Overdose is rare but sodium bicarbonate may be beneficial in overcoming the sodium channel blockade.

The β-blocker sotalol (q.v.) has sometimes been used as an alternative for controlling supraventricular arrhythmia, but such comparative information as there is suggests that flecainide is probably the better drug to use both before and after birth. Sotalol may, however, be a better drug to use in the management of atrial flutter (a rare, and potentially lethal, fetal arrhythmia with an excellent long-term prognosis if identified in time).

Treatment

Oral treatment: Start by giving 2 mg/kg by mouth once every 8 hours, and monitor the ECG for at least the first 48 hours because, in one child in 20, this will trigger a slower but incessant form of supraventricular tachycardia. A broad P wave, widened QRS and prolonged PR interval provide early signs of toxicity.

Intravenous (IV) treatment: Where other strategies fail, a single 1–2 mg/kg dose given IV over about 10 minutes may successfully arrest a dangerous arrhythmia, but this should only be attempted by someone experienced enough to recognise and deal with any unexpected response. Oral treatment should then be started promptly.

Blood levels

The therapeutic plasma range in children is 0.25–0.75 mg/l, lower than the level needed in adults (1 mg/l of flecainide acetate = 2.10 µmol/l).

Supply

15 ml ampoules containing 10 mg/ml of flecainide acetate cost £4.40 each. An oral liquid containing 5 mg in 1 ml is available for 'named' patients from Penn Pharmaceutical Services. It should *not* be refrigerated.

Continued on p. 216

References

Fenrich AL, Perry JC, Freidman RA. Flecainide and amiodarone: combined therapy for refractory tachyarrhythmias in infancy. *J Am Coll Cardiol* 1995;**25**:1195–8.

Hahurij ND, Blom NA, Lopriore E, *et al*. Perinatal management and long-term cardiac outcome in fetal arrhythmia. *Early Hum Dev* 2011;**87**:83–7.

Jang DH, Hoffman RS, Nelson LS. A case of near-fatal flecainide overdose in a neonate successfully treated with sodium bicarbonate. *J Emerg Med* 2013;**44**:781–3.

O'Sullivan J, Gardiner H, Wren C. Digoxin or flecainide for prophylaxis of infant supraventricular tachycardia. *J Am Coll Cardiol* 1995;**26**:991–4.

Paul T, Bertram H, Bökenkamp R, *et al*. Supraventricular tachycardia in infants, children and adolescents. *Paediatr Drugs* 2000;**2**:171–81.

Perry JC, Garson A Jr. Flecainide acetate for treatment of tachyarrhythmias in children: review of world literature on efficacy, safety, and dosing. *Am Heart J* 1992;**124**:1614–21.

Use

Flucloxacillin is the drug of choice for penicillinase-resistant staphylococcal infection (unless the strain has also become methicillin resistant).

Pharmacology

Flucloxacillin is a non-toxic, semi-synthetic, acid-resistant, isoxazolyl penicillin first developed in 1964. It has a side chain that protects the β-lactam ring from attack by staphylococcal (and some other) penicillinases, giving it properties similar to meticillin (known in the United States as methicillin). Cloxacillin, nafcillin and oxacillin are closely related products, less well absorbed orally but given in the same parenteral dose as flucloxacillin. Cloxacillin is generally available in most parts of the world, but flucloxacillin is the only product available in the United Kingdom. Dicloxacillin (differing from flucloxacillin with the substitution of chlorine for a fluorine atom) is the product available in the United States with virtually identical properties.

Flucloxacillin and dicloxacillin are both well absorbed orally and mostly inactivated within the body, although a third may appear in the urine. Because they are very non-toxic, the dose only needs to be reduced when there is profound renal failure. Bioavailability approaches 50% when the drug is given by mouth both in babies and in adults, although the presence of food in the stomach delays absorption. The half-life is only 1 hour in adults. It is five times longer than this at birth but falls rapidly during the first month of life. Drug penetration into the meninges and into the bone is limited, but because of its lack of toxicity, high-dose treatment can be used safely in these situations. Anaphylaxis (extremely uncommon in the neonatal period) can occur and patients who are allergic to one of the penicillins are often sensitive to others.

Placental transfer is poor and teratogenicity is not seen. Very little drug appears in breast milk (1 mg/l). Transient diarrhoea is quite common with oral flucloxacillin. While severe, delayed and occasionally lethal cholestatic jaundice has occasionally been seen in adults treated with flucloxacillin for more than 2 weeks, no such problem has yet been recognised with neonatal use.

Maternal mastitis

The main problem, especially in the early days, is usually local engorgement. This can be overcome by relieving the obstruction and 'emptying' the breast. Recurrent trouble is almost always due to poor positioning, as is confirmed by the fact that the affected breast is nearly always on the side the mother less instinctively holds her baby. A red, swollen, tender area is *not* always a sign of bacterial infection, even if the temperature and pulse are up or rigors appear, although this possibility always merits treatment if symptoms persist. Since infection is almost always staphylococcal in origin, the most appropriate treatment is oral flucloxacillin (250 mg once every 6 hours by mouth). Cefalexin (q.v.) is a widely used alternative. Antibiotics are, however, no substitute for dealing with the engorgement and reviewing the mother's feeding technique. Never stop feeding just because antibiotics have been started. Instead, advise the mother to feed more often, offering the affected breast first. Ibuprofen (q.v.) may help both the pain and the inflammation. Localised *nipple* pain is usually traumatic but can be due to *Candida* infection (see the monographs on fluconazole and nystatin).

Treatment

Dose: Use a dose of 100 mg/kg by intravenous (IV) or intramuscular (IM) injection when treating staphylococcal osteomyelitis, meningitis or cerebral abscess. Otherwise, a dose of 50 mg/kg is adequate for most other purposes. These doses are higher than those usually recommended. A dose of 25 mg/kg by mouth is more than adequate when managing most minor infections.

Timing: Give one dose every 12 hours in the first week of life, one dose every 8 hours in babies 1–3 weeks old and one dose every 6 hours in babies four or more weeks old. Treatment should be sustained for 2 weeks in proven septicaemia, for at least 3 weeks in babies with infections of the central nervous system and for 4 weeks in babies with osteitis or proven staphylococcal pneumonia. Oral medication can often be used to complete a course of treatment, and the dosage recommended here allows for the fact that treatment may well need to be given to a baby who has recently been fed.

Supply and administration

Stock 250 mg flucloxacillin vials cost £1.20 each. Add 2.3 ml of sterile water for injection to get a solution containing 100 mg/ml. There is no published evidence to suggest that IV doses need to be injected slowly over more than 3–4 minutes. Vials should be discarded after use and never

Continued on p. 218

kept for more than 24 hours after reconstitution. A 100 mg/kg dose contains 0.23 mmol/kg of sodium. Sustained IV treatment can cause a reactive phlebitis. The stock oral suspension (25 mg/ml) costs £21.40 for 100 ml; a 'sugar-free' version may be prescribed.

References

Adrianzen Vargas MR, Danton MH, Javaid SM, *et al*. Pharmacokinetics of intravenous flucloxacillin and amoxicillin in neonatal and infant cardiopulmonary bypass surgery. *Eur J Cardiothorac Surg* 2004; **25**:256–40.

Bergdahl S, Eriksson M, Finkel Y. Plasma concentration following oral administration of di- and flucloxacillin in infants and children. *Pharmacol Toxicol* 1987;**60**:233–4.

Herngren L, Ehrnebo M, Boréus LO. Drug distribution in whole blood of mothers and their newborn infants: studies of cloxacillin and flucloxacillin. *Eur J Clin Pharmacol* 1982;**22**:351–8.

Ladhani S, Garbash M. Staphylococcal skin infections in children: rational drug therapy recommendations. *Pediatr Drugs* 2005;**7**:77–102.

Use

Fluconazole is commonly used both to prevent and to treat invasive neonatal *Candida albicans* infection.

Pharmacology

Fluconazole is a potent, selective, triazole inhibitor of the fungal enzymes involved in ergosterol synthesis. The drug is reasonably effective against most *Candida* species, other than *C. krusei* and *C. glabrata*. It is also of value in the treatment of cryptococcal infection (although treatment needs to be sustained for several weeks). It was first synthesised and patented in 1982. It is water soluble, well absorbed by mouth even in infancy and largely excreted unchanged in the urine. Penetration into the CSF is good. While high-dose systemic exposure (400 mg/day) in the first trimester of pregnancy can produce a constellation of serious fetal abnormalities, there are, as yet, no reports of teratogenicity with a single 150 mg dose in the first trimester or with topical or oral use later in pregnancy. Fluconazole is probably the best antifungal to use when *Candida* infects the mother's milk ducts during lactation, even though the manufacturers have never endorsed such use, because the baby only gets approximately 10% of the weight-adjusted maternal dose.

Fluconazole is increasingly used in the treatment of ***invasive*** (systemic) *C. albicans* infection. Studies suggest that it is less toxic and at least as effective as amphotericin B. Liver function tests sometimes show a mild self-correcting disturbance, and rashes can occur, but serious drug eruptions have only been seen in immunodeficient patients. The half-life is 40–60 hours at birth but doubles within 2 weeks. It is 20 hours throughout infancy and childhood but 30 hours in adults. There is no good reason to give amphotericin B as well as high-dose fluconazole, but there is evidence that effective treatment of all *Candida* species with a minimum inhibitory concentration of ≤8 micrograms/ml requires a higher dose than many reference texts currently quote (Wade *et al.*, 2009). *In vitro* modelling also suggests that high-dose treatment makes the emergence of resistant strains less likely. Oral fluconazole is widely used to treat ***superficial*** (topical) infection in adults and is now starting to be used for this purpose in babies. Prophylactic use has been widely studied in the last ten years (see web commentary), but some prefer to use nystatin (q.v.), which is not systemically absorbed, to minimise the risk of fluconazole-resistant strains proliferating.

Diagnosing systemic candidiasis

Systemic candidiasis is difficult to diagnose, but not rare in colonised ill babies. The isolation of *Candida* from blood should never be ignored. Unfortunately, blood cultures may take days to reveal evidence of infection and can be misleadingly negative. The presence of budding yeasts or hyphae in freshly voided urine should lead to an immediate search for further evidence of infection. A suprapubic tap can be used to collect urine for microscopy and fungal culture to clinch any diagnosis and prove that treatment has been effective. Treatment should not necessarily await the outcome of laboratory studies. Congenital infection from ascending vaginal infection can occur. Tracheal colonisation frequently precedes systemic infection.

Candida infection of the breast

Give the mother a 150–300 mg loading dose by mouth and then 100–200 mg once a day for at least 10 days. Treat the baby as well, and take steps to minimise the risk of reinfection as outlined in the web commentary.

Prophylactic use in the neonate

Age under 2 weeks: Give 6 mg/kg of fluconazole on day 1 and then a further 6 mg/kg every third day.
Age 2–4 weeks: Give 6 mg/kg of fluconazole on day 1 and then a further 6 mg/kg every second day.

Treatment of invasive candidiasis

Age under 2 weeks: Give 6–12 mg/kg of fluconazole every third day.
Age 2–4 weeks: Give 6–12 mg/kg of fluconazole every second day.
Age 4 weeks to 1 year: Give 6–12 mg/kg of fluconazole every 24 hours.
A loading dose of 25 mg/kg has sometimes been recommended and shortens the time to achieving therapeutic levels. Double the dosage interval after the first two doses if there is renal failure.

Continued on p. 220

Supply

25 ml bottles for intravenous use containing 2 mg/ml of fluconazole cost £7.30. A 12 mg/kg dose contains 0.92 mmol/kg of sodium. A powder for oral use which, when reconstituted, provides 35 ml of a 10 mg/ml solution costs £16.60. It contains 5.6 g/ml of sucrose. Do not dilute this further or keep more than 2 weeks after reconstitution. 50, 150 and 200 mg capsules for adult use cost between £2.40 and £9.50 each.

References   (See also the relevant Cochrane reviews)

Driessen M, Ellis JB, Copper PA, *et al.* Fluconazole vs. amphotericin B for the treatment of neonatal fungal septicaemia: a prospective randomised trial. *Pediatr Infect Dis J* 1996;**15**:1107–12. [RCT]

Long SS, Stevenson DK. Reducing *Candida* infections during neonatal intensive care: management choices, infection control, and fluconazole prophylaxis. *J Pediatr* 2005;**147**:135–41.

Manzoni P, Stolfi I, Pugni L, *et al.* A multi-center randomized trial of prophylactic fluconazole in preterm neonates. *N Engl J Med* 2007;**356**:2483–95. [RCT]

Piper L, Smith PB, Hornik CP, *et al.* Fluconazole loading dose pharmacokinetics and safety in infants. *Pediatr Infect Dis J* 2011;**30**:375–8.

Schwarze R, Penk A, Pittrow L. Administration of fluconazole in children below 1 year. *Mycoses* 1998;**42**:3–16. [SR]

Wade KC, Benjamin CK, Kaufman DA, *et al.* Fluconazole dosing for the prevention or treatment of invasive Candidiasis in young infants. *Pediatr Infect Dis J* 2009;**28**:717–23.

Use

Flucytosine has been used, with amphotericin B (q.v.), to treat respiratory and systemic fungal infection. This combination is used to treat aspergillosis, coccidioidomycosis and cryptococcosis and is also often used to treat systemic *Candida* infection, although many now prefer to use fluconazole (q.v.). Nystatin or miconazole (q.v.) is more appropriately used to treat superficial *Candida* infection.

Pharmacology

Flucytosine (previously called 5-fluorocytosine) is a fluorinated pyrimidine first developed in 1957 which acts as a competitive inhibitor of uracil metabolism. The drug is well absorbed by mouth and more than 90% is excreted unchanged in the urine. Renal clearance is about three-quarters that achieved for creatinine. The half-life in the neonatal period is *very* variable but usually about 8 hours. The drug is distributed widely through body tissues including the CSF.

Synergy with amphotericin (q.v.) means they are frequently used together and flucytosine makes up for the lack of CSF penetration by amphotericin. While flucytosine has been used on its own to treat *Candida* renal tract infection, resistant strains have been reported. Co-treatment with either amphotericin or fluconazole is now universally recommended to reduce the emergence of drug resistance. *Candida* species are usually said to be resistant to flucytosine when the minimum inhibitory concentration (MIC) exceeds 60 micrograms/ml, and *Cryptococcus* when this MIC exceeds 12.5 micrograms/ml.

Sustained use can cause leucopenia and thrombocytopenia. Because co-treatment with amphotericin and the underlying fungal infection can both cause renal impairment, monitoring the trough blood level is important if the plasma creatinine level exceeds 40 μmol/l. Vomiting and diarrhoea can occur, and reversible liver function changes have been reported. Flucytosine has been given in pregnancy without seeming to cause any apparent harm to the baby, but the risk of teratogenicity cannot be discounted (in part due to its conversion to 5-fluorouracil). It is not known whether the drug appears in breast milk.

Treatment

Neonatal use: Give 50 mg/kg by mouth or intravenous (IV) injection once every 12 hours for at least 10 days. Start with 50 mg/kg once every 24 hours if there is evidence of renal failure. Any IV infusion is probably best given using a 15 μm in-line filter to trap any possible drug crystals. The manufacturers also recommend slow infusion over at least 20 minutes, although they offer no reason for this recommendation.

Older children: A dose of 50 mg/kg every 6 or 8 hours is normally used in older children. Always check the blood level after 1–2 days if a dose as high as this is used in a young baby.

Blood levels

Marrow toxicity can occur when the blood level exceeds 100 mg/l for any length of time, so it is advisable to check the serum level when the fourth dose is due if renal function could be impaired. Most large hospitals now have access to a laboratory that can measure this, given at least 0.5 ml of whole blood. Peak levels occur a variable time after oral administration in young babies, so it is probably better to monitor the trough level, aiming for a level of 25–40 mg/l (1 mg/l = 7.75 μmol/l) because lower levels are sub-therapeutic.

Supply and administration

250 ml bottles of a 10 mg/ml IV formulation cost £30. This can be infused (terminally) into a line containing glucose or glucose saline. It can also be given by mouth. A 50 mg/kg dose contains 0.69 mmol/kg of sodium. This *must* be kept at room temperature and should be protected from light. Crystals of flucytosine may precipitate out if the temperature falls below 18 °C (these will be trapped by the 15 μm filter if used). If precipitation is suspected, the bottle can be heated to 80 °C for 30 minutes to redissolve the precipitate, but decomposition (and 5-fluorouracil formation) occurs with sustained storage at temperatures over 25 °C.

References

Baddley JW, Pappas PG. Antifungal combination therapy: clinical potential. *Drugs* 2005;**65**:1461–80.
Baley JE, Meyers C, Klegmann RM, *et al*. Pharmacokinetics, outcome of treatment, and toxic effects of amphotericin B and 5-fluorocytosine in neonates. *J Pediatr* 1990;**116**:791–7.

Continued on p. 222

Butler KM, Baker CJ. Candida: an increasingly important pathogen in the nursery. *Pediatr Clin North Am* 1988;**35**:543–63.

Diasio RB, Lakings DE, Bennett JE. Evidence for conversion of 5-fluorocytosine to 5-fluorouracil in humans: possible factor in 5-fluorocytosine clinical toxicity. *Antimicrob Agents Chemother* 1978;**14**:903–8.

Loke HL, Verber I, Szymonowicz W, *et al*. Systemic candidiasis and pneumonia in preterm infants. *Aust Paediatr J* 1988;**24**:138–42.

Pappas PG, Rex JH, Sobel JD, *et al*. Guidelines for treatment of candidiasis. *Clin Infect Dis* 2004;**38**:161–89.

Soltani M, Tobin CM, Bowker KE, *et al*. Evidence of excessive concentrations of 5-flucytosine in children below 12 years: a 12-year review of serum concentrations from a UK clinical assay reference laboratory. *Int J Antimicrob Agents* 2006;**28**:574–7.

Vermes A, Guchelaar H-J, Dankert J. Flucytosine: a review of its pharmacology, clinical indications, pharmacokinetics, toxicity and drug interactions. *J Antimicrob Chemother* 2000;**46**:171–9.

Use

Folic acid is necessary to prevent megaloblastic anaemia. Supplementation prior to conception can also reduce the risk of several fetal defects especially anencephaly or spina bifida. Several uncommon conditions, including primary and secondary cerebral folate deficiency and folinic acid-responsive seizures, result in progressive neurological deterioration.

Nutritional factors

Folic acid was first synthesised in 1945, but it is tetrahydrofolic acid, the metabolically active form, that participates in DNA synthesis and red cell maturation. Peas, beans, green vegetables, yeast extract, Bovril and fortified cereals are all good dietary sources. Excessive intake does not seem to be dangerous. Liver is a rich source of folate, but this should be avoided in pregnancy because of its high vitamin A content.

Serum and red cell folate levels are higher in the newborn infant than the mother; deficiency is only seen if the mother is grossly deficient. Folate is actively excreted in breast milk and well absorbed in the duodenum and jejunum. Human milk contains 3–6 micrograms/100 ml. Term formula milks contain 11–13 micrograms/100 ml and preterm formula milks contain 30–35 micrograms/100 ml. It is often claimed that folate requirements in infancy are as high as 20–50 micrograms/day (4–10 times the adult requirement). This is more than most babies get by mouth for some months after birth. Despite this discrepancy and that both serum and red cell folate levels fall after delivery, especially in LBW babies, symptomatic deficiency has not been observed in the absence of chronic infection, malabsorption (e.g. coeliac disease) or diarrhoea. Supplementary folic acid fails to produce any rise in haemoglobin in the absence of megaloblastic anaemia, even in babies with severe haemolytic disease. Many units still offer a routine supplement of 50 micrograms/day to every preterm baby, but there is no evidence that this is necessary.

Maternal prophylaxis

In countries that have not adopted a policy of food supplementation, women should take 400 micrograms once a day *before* conception and for the first 12 weeks of pregnancy to minimise the risk of neural tube defects. Suitable tablets are available 'over the counter' in the United Kingdom without prescription. Three months of Preconceive® costs £4.50, but the free 'Healthy Start' product (cf. vitamin D monograph) is only available to those already pregnant. Women at high risk (i.e. if there has been a previously affected pregnancy, if either parent is affected, if the mother is taking an anticonvulsant or has coeliac disease) should take 5 mg once a day. Diabetes UK also recommends that women with diabetes should also use this dose.

Treating folate deficiency diseases in infancy

Cerebral folate deficiency: This rare neurological disorder, due to diverse metabolic pathways and unrelated processes, is characterised by decreased CSF but normal serum 5-methyltetrahydrofolate (5-MTHF) levels that affect development after 4–6 months. Further deterioration can be arrested by starting **folinic acid** at a dose of 0.5–1 mg/kg a day. Increase this slowly to no more than 2.5 mg/kg a day under guidance from a paediatric neurologist. Folic acid should **not** be given; this may exacerbate the CSF 5-MTHF deficiency.

Folinic acid-responsive seizures: This condition is due to mutations in the ALDH7A1 (antiquin) gene giving α-aminoadipic semialdehyde dehydrogenase (α-AASA) deficiency and is identical to the major form of pyridoxine-dependent epilepsy. Treatment with 2.5 mg/kg of **folinic acid** twice a day stops the seizures, but developmental delay persists. The optimum maintenance dose has not yet been established. The addition of pyridoxine has been suggested together with a lysine-restricted diet.

Megaloblastic anaemia: In the absence of vitamin B_{12} deficiency, infants are usually treated with 1 mg of folic acid daily by mouth. If this is due to dietary deficiency rather than malabsorption or disorders of folate metabolism, then they should respond rapidly to physiological doses of folic acid (50 micrograms/day). Symptoms develop insidiously during the first months of life, and deficiency can have permanent consequences unless the diagnosis is made before growth has already been affected.

Supply

Folic acid: 150 ml of a 50 micrograms/ml sugar-free oral suspension costs £9. For maternal use, 400 micrograms tablets (which need no prescription) and 5 mg tablets cost approximately 2p each.

Continued on p. 224

Folinic acid: The product usually dispensed is calcium folinate (known as leucovorin in America). 30 mg (10 ml) vials suitable for intravenous, intramuscular or oral administration cost £4.60, and 15 mg tablets cost £4.50. Levofolinic acid, the levo-isomer of folinic acid, is also available but is considerably more expensive (175 mg vials cost £85).

References (See also the relevant Cochrane reviews)

Cheriajn A, Seena S, Bullock RK, *et al.* Incidence of neural tube defects in the least-developed area of India: a population-based study. *Lancet* 2005;**366**:930–1. (See also pp. 871–2.)

De Wals P, Tairou F, Van Allen MI, *et al.* Reduction in neural-tube defects after folic acid fortification in Canada. *N Engl J Med* 2007;**357**:135–42.

Djukic A. Folate-responsive neurological diseases. *Pediatr Neurol* 2007;**37**:387–97.

Gallagher RC, Van Hove JL, *et al.* Folinic acid-responsive seizures are identical to pyridoxine-dependent epilepsy. *Ann Neurol* 2009;**65**:550–6.

Hyland K, Shoffner J, Heales SJ. Cerebral folate deficiency. *J Inherit Metab Dis* 2010;**33**:563–70.

Ramaekers VT, Rothenberg SP, Sequeira JM, *et al.* Autoantibodies to folate receptors in the cerebral folate deficiency syndrome. *N Engl J Med* 2005;**352**:1985–91.

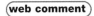

Use

While breastfeeding remains the ideal source of nutrition for babies, a number of those who are formula fed develop symptoms of intolerance or allergy. Specialised infant formula milks with modified protein, carbohydrate or fat content are available to treat a range of conditions. Advice from a paediatric dietitian may ensure the most appropriate feed choice.

Lactose intolerance

Lactose intolerance may be congenital, primary (including congenital) or secondary. Secondary lactose intolerance is usually temporary and due to loss of lactase enzyme expression in the brush border of intestinal villi following inflammatory or structural damage (e.g. after gastroenteritis). Symptoms (flatus, diarrhoea, abdominal distension and discomfort) are due to the osmotic effects of lactose and its fermentation by intestinal bacteria. The similarity to non-IgE-mediated cow's milk protein allergy (CMPA) means that the two may be mistaken for each other. While babies who are receiving breast milk should continue to do so, formula-fed babies who are intolerant of lactose should receive lactose-free formula milk. The enzyme lactase (Colief®) may sometimes be given to breastfed babies to help with their symptoms.

Cow's milk protein allergy

Cow's milk is the most common food allergen in infants. It can be IgE mediated (usually causing urticaria, wheezing, rhinitis, eczema and anaphylaxis) or non-IgE mediated. Non-IgE-mediated CMPA presents with predominantly abdominal symptoms (gastro-oesophageal reflux, repetitive vomiting, with or without diarrhoea, abdominal pain and bloody stools) and develops several hours after ingestion of the offending food. While breast milk and most formula milks contain whole protein, hydrolysed formula milk contains peptide chains or amino acids. The extent of protein hydrolysis and protein source varies between products (see table). Amino acid-based formula milks are required only by 5–10% of babies with the most severe cow's milk protein sensitivity. An extensively hydrolysed milk formula is otherwise suitable for most others with this condition. Soy-based formula milk should be avoided wherever possible in babies <6 months with either CMPA or lactose intolerance due to theoretical risks of phytoestrogens and possible soya sensitisation.

Other uses

Hydrolysed formula milks are sometimes used after gut surgery or trauma and/or in liver disease. They are sometimes used in the absence of the mother's own breast milk (or banked milk) during the initiation of feeds in preterm babies, but they do not meet the long-term nutritional needs of the growing preterm baby. They may also be used, with dietetic input, in some malabsorption states. While they may be effective in infantile colic, they should be used only as a last resort.

Further supplements

These formula milks are not designed for premature infants and do not meet their nutritional requirements. They should only be used when breast milk is not available and the clinical rationale is justified. Most babies can accept an oral intake of over 200 ml/kg a day once feeding is fully established. However, babies with malabsorption are unlikely to tolerate such large volumes. In some babies <2 kg, growth can be enhanced by increasing the concentration of the feed or by supplementation to achieve an adequate protein, energy, sodium, vitamin, mineral and LCP content (see *Formula milks for preterm babies*).

Supply

Lactase (Colief) is available in a 7 ml bottle containing 50,000 units/g (cost £8.40). Four drops should be mixed with expressed breast milk and given to the baby before the feed.

See the monograph on *Formula milks for preterm babies* for information about subsidising of the cost of formula milk supplied to hospitals and risks of infection with pathogenic bacteria such as *Salmonella* and *Enterobacter sakazakii*.

Continued on p. 226

Table 1 Composition (per 100ml) of human milk and 'specialised' formula milks.

	Protein or equivalent (g)	Fat (g)	Carbohydrate (g)	Energy (kcal)	Na (mg)	Ca (mg)	P (mg)	Zn (mg)	Vit D (micrograms)	Vit K (micrograms)	Lactose-free?
Typical mature human breast milk	1.4	4.0	6.6	67	25.3	25	13	0.34	<0.1	0.2	No
Lactose-free formula milks											
Aptamil Lactose Free®	1.3	3.5	7.3	66	17	55	30	0.56	1.2	4.5	Yes
Mead Johnson Enfamil O-Lac®	1.4	3.7	7.2	68	31	78	52	0.68	1.0	10.1	Yes
SMA Lactose Free®	1.5	3.6	7.2	67	24	55	37	0.89	1.8	10	Yes
Amino acid-based formula milks											
Abbott Similac Alimentum®	1.86	3.75	6.62	67.6	30	71	44	0.51	1.01	5.4	Yes
Mead Johnson Nutramigen AA®	1.9	3.5	6.9	67	31.3	63	35	0.7	0.8	5.3	Yes
SHS Neocate LCP®	1.8	3.4	7.2	67	26.1	65.6	47.1	0.73	1.2	5.9	Yes
Hypoallergenic extensively hydrolysed, casein-based formula milks											
Mead Johnson Nutramigen Lipil 1®	1.9	3.4	7.5	68	32	77	53	0.48	1.0	8.8	Yes
Mead Johnson Nutramigen Lipil 2®	1.7	2.9	8.6	68	25	94	50	0.75	1.1	8.8	Yes
Mead Johnson Pregestimil Lipil® with MCT	2.8	5.6	10.2	68	47	94	52	1	0.8	12	Yes
Hydrolysed, whey-based formula milks											
Aptamil Pepti 1®	1.6	3.5	7.1	67	20	47	26	0.5	1.3	4.7	No
Aptamil Pepti 2®	1.6	3.1	8	68	25	63	36	0.5	1.4	5	No
Cow & Gate Pepti-Junior® with MCT	1.8	3.5	6.8	66	18	50	28	0.5	1.3	4.7	Yes

Continued on p. 227

Typical costs are shown below.

	Approximate prices (United Kingdom)
Aptamil *Lactose Free®*	£5 per 400g tin*
Mead Johnson *Enfamil O-Lac®*	£4.50 per 400g tin*
SMA *Lactose Free®*	£5 per 400g tin*
Abbott *Similac Alimentum®*	£9 per 400g tin
Mead *Johnson Nutramigen AA®*	£25 per 400g tin
SHS *Neocate LCP®*	£27.50 per 400g tin
Mead Johnson *Nutramigen Lipil 1®*	£10 per 400g tin
Mead Johnson *Nutramigen Lipil 2®*	£10 per 400g tin
Mead Johnson *Pregestimil Lipil®*	£11 per 400g tin
Aptamil *Pepti 1®*	£9.50 per 400g tin/£21.50 per 900g tin
Aptamil *Pepti 2®*	£20.50 per 900g tin
Cow & Gate *Pepti-Junior®* with MCT	£12 per 450g tin

The cost of lactose-free milks is similar to that of standard formula milks. Thus, it is hard to justify prescribing them.

While some of these milks are available for parents to buy over the counter, most are available in the United Kingdom on prescription and carry Advisory Committee on Borderline Substances (ACBS) approval for treatment of specific conditions. Such prescriptions should be issued in accordance with the Committee's advice and endorsed 'ACBS'. Thus, for example, Neocate LCP should only be prescribed for *proven whole protein intolerance, short bowel syndrome, intractable malabsorption or other gastrointestinal disorders where an elemental diet is indicated.*

References

Agostoni C, Axelsson I, Goulet O, *et al.* Soy protein infant formulae and follow-on formulae: a commentary by the ESPGHAN Committee on Nutrition. *J Pediatr Gastroenterol Nutr* 2006;**42**:352–61.

American Academy of Pediatrics. Committee on Nutrition. Hypoallergenic infant formulas. *Pediatrics* 2000;**106**:346–9.

American Academy of Pediatrics. Committee on Nutrition. Iron fortification of infant formulas. *Pediatrics* 1999;**104**:119–23.

British Dietetic Association. Paediatric group position statement on the use of soya protein for infants. *J Fam Health Care* 2003;**13**:93.

Committee on Toxicity. *Phytoestrogens and health.* Committee on Toxicity of Chemicals in Food, Consumer Products and the Environment. The Food Standards Agency, London, 2003 (available at http://cot.food.gov.uk/pdfs/phytoreport0503).

du Toit G, Meyer R, Shah N, *et al.* Identifying and managing cow's milk protein allergy. *Arch Dis Child Educ Pract Ed* 2010;**95**:134–44.

Elizur A, Cohen M, Goldberg MR, *et al.* Mislabelled cow's milk allergy in infants: a prospective cohort study. *Arch Dis Child* 2013;**98**:408–12.

Fiocchi A, Brozek J, Schünemann H, *et al.* World Allergy Organization (WAO) Diagnosis and Rationale for Action against Cow's Milk Allergy (DRACMA) Guidelines. *World Allergy Organ J* 2010;**3**:57–161.

Lomer MC, Parkes GC, Sanderson JD. Review article: lactose intolerance in clinical practice-myths and realities. *Aliment Pharmacol Ther* 2008;**27**:93–103.

Ludman S, Shah N, Fox AT. Managing cows' milk allergy in children. *Br Med J* 2013;**347**:f5424.

Tsang RC, Uauy R, Koletzko B *et al.* eds. *Nutrition of the preterm baby: scientific basis and practical guidelines*, 2nd ed. Cincinnati, OH: Digital Educational Publishing, 2005.

Vandenplas Y, Koletzko S, Isolauri E, *et al.* Guidelines for the diagnosis and management of cow's milk protein allergy in infants. *Arch Dis Child* 2007;**92**:902–8.

Venter C, Pereira B, Voigt K, *et al.* Prevalence and cumulative incidence of food hypersensitivity in the first 3 years of life. *Allergy* 2008;**63**:354–9.

Use

Artificial milks for healthy term infants (called 'breast milk substitutes' although they cannot hope to achieve anywhere near the short- or long-term beneficial effects that breastfeeding brings) have been commercially available for 40 years. Modified formulae designed for use in preterm babies have been developed more recently. Breast milk fortifiers (q.v.) are available to supplement breast milk when it is used to feed the preterm baby. These should not be mixed with formula milk.

Nutritional factors

Most milk formulae are made from demineralised protein-enriched whey, skimmed milk, vegetable oils and milk fat, glucose, lactose and/or maltodextrin, with mineral and vitamin supplements. While breast milk is the food of choice for almost every baby (including those born prematurely), most will grow very well on 130–150 kcal/kg/day of any formula milk in the neonatal period. Most babies can accept an oral intake of over 200 ml/kg a day once feeding is fully established. In some babies of <2 kg, growth can be enhanced by using a nutrient-enriched preterm formula.

Formula milk for preterm babies can be, somewhat artificially, divided into those used while in hospital (low-birthweight formulae) and those for use after discharge (post-discharge nutrient-enriched formulae). These differ slightly in their nutritional contents and are designed to address the needs of the baby at different stages.

All have a potassium content of between 1.4 and 2.0 mmol/100 ml. With the exceptions of the substances noted in the following paragraphs, formula milks contain adequate quantities of all the nutrients, trace elements and vitamins known to be necessary for growth in the neonatal period. In particular, there is no evidence that babies ever need further supplemental vitamin K (q.v.) once established on an artificial milk formula. Nor do babies need more folic acid (q.v.) than is provided by every one of the artificial infant milk products currently on sale in the United Kingdom, even when born preterm.

Further supplements

Sodium: Most babies of <30 weeks' gestation require further routine sodium with their milk to bring their total intake up to between 4.5 and 6.0 mmol/kg/day. This high requirement is caused by the immature kidney's limited ability to conserve sodium. The extra sodium is best provided by adding a further 2 mmol of sodium chloride to every 100 ml of preterm milk formula or breast milk fed to all babies of <30 weeks' gestation (for details, see the monograph on sodium chloride). Loss should also be monitored intermittently, because some very preterm babies require more supplemental sodium than most, especially in the first 2 weeks of life. If the sodium content of a 'spot' urine sample is high, something is limiting renal tubular reabsorption, unless intake has been abnormally high.

Vitamin D: Babies are known to require 10 micrograms of vitamin D a day irrespective of their weight. The vitamin D content of most artificial milk only averages 1 microgram/100 ml (with an agreed maximum of 5 micrograms/100 ml because of the risk associated with excessive intake). For further details, see the monograph on vitamin D (q.v.).

Iron: All babies have reasonable iron stores at birth even if born prematurely, but dietary iron becomes necessary within 2–3 months of birth to provide the additional iron needed by the child's growing red cell mass. Repeated blood sampling may further reduce available body iron if the blood taken is not replaced by transfusion. All standard artificial UK milk formulae contain enough iron to provide for the needs of babies born at term, being formulated to contain much more iron than breast milk in order to compensate for poor iron absorption. The same is not true in all countries.

The preterm formulae available in the United Kingdom contain similar supplements of iron, but there is no evidence that babies absorb this iron in the first month of life, even when they are offered it, and there are theoretical reasons for limiting early supplementation because this interferes with the antimicrobial activity of lactoferrin in the gut.

Phosphate: Human milk is capable of sustaining excellent bone growth in the full-term baby, but bone growth and increased bone mineralisation are so rapid in the preterm baby that babies weighing <1.3 kg at birth are at serious risk of osteopenia and of spontaneous pathological fractures in the second and third month of life if not offered further supplementation. Both calcium and phosphorus are usually provided, and all artificial preterm milk formulae provide some supplementation. Calcium and phosphorus absorptions are linked and a calcium/phosphorus ratio of between 1.4:1 and 2:1 seems to optimise absorption and minimise the risk of late

Continued on p. 229

Table 1 Composition (per 100 ml) of human milk and formula milks for preterm babies.

	Protein (g)	Fat (g)	Carbohydrate (g)	Energy (kcal)	Na (mg)	Ca (mg)	P (mg)	Zn (mg)	Vit D (micrograms)	Vit K (micrograms)
Typical mature (>2 weeks post-partum) human breast milk	1.4	4.0	6.6	67	25.3	25	13	0.34	<0.1	0.2
Preterm human breast milk (Tsang et al. 2005)	1.5	3.5	6.9	65	28.5	25.4	14.2	0.3	0.18	0.83
Low-birthweight formula milks										
Cow & Gate Nutriprem 1®	2.6	3.9	8.4	80	70	94	62	1.1	3	6
Aptamil for Preterm®	2.6	3.9	8.4	80	70	94	62	1.1	3	6
SMA Gold Prem 1®	2.2	4.4	8.4	82	44	101	61	0.8	3.4	6.3
Post-discharge nutrient-enriched formula milks										
Cow & Gate Nutriprem 2®	2	4	7.5	75	28	87	47	0.9	1.7	5.9
SMA Gold Prem 2®	1.9	3.9	7.5	73	27	73	42	0.73	1.5	6.3

Continued on p. 230

neonatal hypocalcaemia. Phosphorus is well absorbed and its availability seems to limit calcium absorption. It is now thought that optimum phosphorus intake in the growing preterm baby is probably provided by a milk containing between 1.3 and 2.3 mmol of phosphorus per 100 ml. Human milk only contains a third of this and requires regular supplementation (see the monograph on phosphate). Additional calcium is probably not necessary if adequate phosphorus is provided. Most commercial preterm milks contain at least the minimum amount of phosphorus now recommended.

Bicarbonate: Some preterm babies develop a late metabolic acidosis on formula feeds due to the neonatal kidney's limited ability to excrete acid. Oral bicarbonate will relieve this, improving weight gain and nitrogen retention, as described in the monograph on sodium bicarbonate (q.v.).

Supply

Manufacturers are banned from subsidising the cost of formula milk supplied to hospitals or from providing free samples in an attempt to increase their share of the market with newly delivered mothers (the practice has been shown in nine controlled trials to reduce the number of mothers achieving a sustained lactation).

Infant formulae and modular feeds are a food source and therefore an excellent medium for bacterial and microbial proliferation. Powdered infant formula is a non-sterile product, and there is an inherent risk of infection with pathogenic bacteria such as *Salmonella* and *Enterobacter sakazakii* in neonates, preterm, low-birthweight and immunocompromised infants who are most at risk. For this reason, most of the low-birthweight and post-discharge milks are available as ready-made bottles (for use in hospitals), and the post-discharge milks are available as either powder or ready-made in cartons.

References   (See also the relevant Cochrane reviews)

Agostoni C, Buonocore G, Carnielli VP, *et al.* Enteral nutrient supply for preterm infants: commentary from the European Society of Paediatric Gastroenterology, Hepatology and Nutrition Committee on Nutrition. *J Pediatr Gastroenterol Nutr* 2010;**50**:85–91.

American Academy of Pediatrics. Committee on Nutrition. Iron fortification of infant formulas. *Pediatrics* 1999;**104**:119–23.

Edmond K, Bahl R. *Optimal feeding of low-birth-weight infants.* [WHO technical review] Geneva: World Health Organisation, 2006.

ESPGHAN Committee on Nutrition. Medical Position Paper: Feeding Preterm Infants after Hospital Discharge. A Commentary by the ESPGHAN Committee on Nutrition. *J Pediatr Gastroenterol Nutr* 2006;**42**:596–603.

Griffin IJ, Cooke RJ. Nutrition of preterm infants after hospital discharge. *J Pediatr Gastroenterol Nutr* 2007;**45**(suppl 3):S195–203.

McGuire W, Anthony MY. Donor human milk versus formula for preventing necrotising enterocolitis in preterm infants: systematic review. *Arch Dis Child Fetal Neonatal Ed* 2003;**88**:F11–4. [SR]

Radde IC, Chance GW, Bailey K, *et al.* Growth and mineral metabolism 1. Comparison of the effects of two modes of NaHCO₃ treatment of late metabolic acidosis. *Pediatr Res* 1975;**9**:564–8. [RCT]

Steer PA, Lucas A, Sinclair JC. Feeding the low birthweight infant. In: Sinclair JC, Bracken MB, eds. *Effective care of the newborn infant.* Chapter 7. Oxford: Oxford University Press, 1992: pp 94–140. (See also pp. 161–77.) [SR]

Tsang RC, Uauy R, Koletzko B *et al.* eds. *Nutrition of the preterm baby: scientific basis and practical guidelines*, 2nd ed. Cincinnati, OH: Digital Educational Publishing, 2005.

Use
Fresh frozen plasma (FFP) and cryoprecipitate can be used to treat symptomatic vitamin K deficiency, bleeding in disseminated intravascular coagulation (DIC) and coagulation factor deficiency (when specific coagulation factor concentrate is unavailable, e.g. factor V deficiency).

Product
Standard 200–250 ml packs of fresh plasma containing albumin, immunoglobulin and stable clotting factors are prepared and frozen at −30 °C within 6 hours of collection from a single donation of whole blood. Cryoprecipitate, which is the precipitate formed during controlled thawing of fresh pooled frozen plasma, contains an eightfold concentrate of fibrinogen together with a range of other coagulation factors (especially factor VIII) in 20 ml packs. Solvent-/detergent-treated (virally inactivated) packs of FFP are now becoming available that make HIV and hepatitis B and C transmission unlikely, but human parvovirus B19 and hepatitis A virus transmission could still occur – especially as most supplies come from pooled donors. The UK Department of Health now requires that children under 16 years of age requiring FFP should receive pathogen-reduced FFP of non-UK origin to minimise the risks of vCJD.

Assessment and use
Neonatal FFP transfusions should be considered in the clinical context of bleeding (e.g. vitamin K dependent), disseminated intravascular coagulopathy and very rare inherited coagulation factor deficiencies. Abnormalities of standard coagulation tests should not be interpreted in isolation, but alongside reference ranges for gestational age and postnatal age and other haemostatic markers, such as platelet count. There is **no** evidence to support the prophylactic use of FFP to prevent intraventricular haemorrhage, as a volume expander or to manage either sepsis or thrombocytopenia.

Healthy babies have values in the range shown below at birth. The normal prothrombin and activated partial thromboplastin times both decrease by about 10% in the first month of life. While D-dimer levels are usually below 250 micrograms/l, normal babies occasionally have values as high as 1000 micrograms/l.

Coagulation screening tests (95% confidence intervals)

Test	Gestation (weeks) 24–29	30–36	37–41
Prothrombin time (seconds)	12.2–21.0	10.6–16.2	10.1–15.9
International normalised ratio (INR)	–	0.61–1.70	0.53–1.62
Activated partial thromboplastin time (seconds)	43.6–101	27.5–79.4	31.3–54.5
Thrombin clotting time (seconds)	–	19.2–30.4	19.0–28.3
Fibrinogen (g/l)	0.69–4.12	1.50–3.73	1.67–3.99
Platelets (×10⁹/l)	150–350	150–350	150–350

Treatment
Infuse 10–20 ml/kg of blood group compatible FFP over 30–60 minutes. Use material from a group AB rhesus-negative donor or, failing this, blood of the same ABO group as the baby. Each millilitre of undiluted plasma contains 1 IU of each coagulation factor; thus, 10–20 ml/kg of FFP is expected to sufficiently correct a factor-deficient patient by approximately 30%.

Cryoprecipitate may be of more use in the bleeding patient with low fibrinogen levels (<1 g/l) where there are concerns about volume overload.

Supply
Stocks of FFP and cryoprecipitate are held in local blood banks, and some also stock 50–70 ml 'minipacks'. The packs should be thawed by the blood bank staff immediately prior to issue and used within 6 hours. Hold the material at 2–6 °C if there is any unavoidable last-minute delay in administration. A filter is not necessary.

Continued on p. 232

References

(See also the relevant Cochrane reviews and UK guideline **DHUK**)

Buchanan GR. Coagulation disorders in the neonate. *Pediatr Clin North Am* 1986;**33**:203–20.

Cohen H. Avoiding the misuse of fresh frozen plasma. *Br Med J* 1993;**307**:395–6.

Murray N, Roberts I. Neonatal transfusion of blood products. In: David TJ, ed. *Recent advances in paediatrics 23*. London: Royal Society of Medicine, 2006: pp. 139–53.

NNNI Trial Group. Randomised trial of prophylactic early fresh frozen plasma or gelatin or glucose in preterm babies: outcome at 2 years. *Lancet* 1996;**348**:229–32. [RCT]

Norfolk DR, Glaser A, Kinsey S. American fresh frozen plasma for neonates and children. *Arch Dis Child* 2005;**90**:89–91.

Poterjoy BS, Josephson CD. Platelets, frozen plasma, and cryoprecipitate: what is the clinical evidence for their use in the neonatal intensive care unit? *Semin Perinatol* 2009;**33**:66–74.

Seguin JH, Topper WH. Coagulation studies in very low birth weight infants. *Am J Perinatol* 1994;**11**:17–9.

Venkatesh V, Khan R, Curley A, *et al*. How we decide when a neonate needs a transfusion. *Br J Haematol* 2013;**160**:421–33.

Use
Furosemide is a valuable, powerful and rapidly acting diuretic that is particularly useful in the management of acute congestive cardiac failure. Alternatives (such as chlorothiazide with or without spironolactone) are cheaper and preferable for maintenance treatment.

Pharmacology
Furosemide was first marketed in 1962. It is both filtered by the glomerulus and also actively excreted by the proximal renal tubule. It then inhibits active chloride reabsorption and, as a result, passive sodium reabsorption from the ascending limb of the loop of Henle and distal tubule (hence the term 'loop' diuretic). While this can result in a sixfold increase in free water clearance in adults, its efficacy in the preterm baby (and fetus when the drug is given to the mother) remains less clearly quantified.

Furosemide is protein bound in plasma, but does not significantly influence bilirubin binding. Sustained use increases urinary sodium and potassium loss and can cause hypokalaemia. Urinary calcium excretion triples in the preterm baby, causing marked bone mineral loss, and renal and biliary calcium deposition. It crosses the placenta, and while it has been used to treat fetal hydrops, the effects are variable. The response of the fetal kidney appears to be poor and diuresis is not seen. There is no good evidence that it is teratogenic. It is excreted into breast milk, but no adverse effects have been reported.

Furosemide stimulates renal synthesis of prostaglandin E_2, thus enhancing, and modifying, renal blood flow. Early use is associated with some increase in the incidence of symptomatic patent ductus in babies requiring ventilation for respiratory distress, and this might be due to increased prostaglandin production. Furosemide also has a direct effect on lung fluid reabsorption, but does not speed the resolution of transient tachypnoea of the newborn. Aerosol administration can transiently improve lung function, and sustained intravenous (IV) or oral use can improve oxygenation in babies over 3 weeks old with chronic lung disease, but there is no evidence, as yet, of sustained clinical benefit.

The half-life is ~8 hours in the term newborn baby but approaches adult values (2 hours) within a few months. It may be as long as 24 hours in the very preterm baby, making progressive accumulation possible with repeated use, and this may be a factor in the increased risk of serious late-onset deafness seen in neonates exposed to sustained diuretic treatment. The related diuretic **bumetanide** may be less ototoxic, but neonatal use has not yet been fully evaluated; it might also be more effective in renal failure, because entry into the tubular lumen is less dependent on glomerular filtration and clearance less dependent on renal excretion. The dose of bumetanide in neonates is 10–50 micrograms/kg orally, IV or intramuscular (IM) injection once every 24–48 hours in preterm infants, increasing to once every 12–24 hours in term infants.

Drug interactions
Concurrent furosemide use significantly increases the risk of aminoglycoside ototoxicity.

Treatment
Use as a diuretic: Try 1 mg/kg of furosemide IV or IM, or 2 mg/kg by mouth, repeatable after 12–24 hours. Do not give more than once a day to babies with a post-menstrual age <29 weeks. Patients on long-term treatment with furosemide may require 1 mmol/kg/day of oral potassium chloride (q.v.) to prevent hypokalaemia.

Renal failure: Give a single 5 mg/kg dose of furosemide IV as soon as renal failure is suspected to lower the metabolic activity of the chloride pump, minimise the risk of ischaemic tubular damage and reduce the shutdown in glomerular blood flow that follows from this.

Chronic lung disease: 1 mg/kg of the IV preparation of furosemide added to 2 ml of 0.9% sodium chloride and given by nebuliser every six hours may temporarily improve lung compliance in ventilator-dependent babies without affecting renal function.

Supply and administration
Furosemide: 2 ml (20 mg) ampoules cost 35p. Precipitation can occur when mixed with any IV fluid (such as glucose and glucose saline) with a pH <5.6, so it should *always* be separated by a 1 ml 'bolus' of 0.9% sodium chloride when given IV. The IV preparation can be given orally after dilution, but a sugar-free oral solution containing 4 mg/ml is available (150 ml costs £14). Some preparations contain 10% alcohol.

Bumetanide: 4 ml (2 mg) ampoules of bumetanide cost £1.80. An oral liquid containing 200 micrograms/ml costs £128 for 150 ml.

Continued on p. 234

References

(See also the relevant Cochrane reviews)

Borradori C, Fawer C-L, Buclin T, *et al*. Risk factors of sensorineural hearing loss in preterm infants. *Biol Neonate* 1997;**71**:1–10.

Karabayir N, Kavuncuoglu S. Intravenous frusemide for transient tachypnoea of the newborn. *J Paediatr Child Health* 2006;**42**:640–2. [RCT]

Moghal NE, Shenoy M. Furosemide and acute kidney injury in neonates. *Arch Dis Child Fetal Neonatal Ed* 2008;**93**:F313–6.

Pai VB, Nahata MC. Aerosolised furosemide in the treatment of acute respiratory distress and possible bronchopulmonary dysplasia in preterm neonates. *Ann Pharmacother* 2000;**34**:386–92. [SR]

Segar JL. Neonatal diuretic therapy: furosemide, thiazides, and spironolactone. *Clin Perinatol* 2012;**39**:209–20.

Sullivan JE, Witte MK, Yamashita TS, *et al*. Dose-ranging evaluation of bumetanide pharmacodynamics in critically ill infants. *Clin Pharmacol Ther* 1996;**60**:424–34.

Use

Parenteral ganciclovir is used to treat cytomegalovirus (CMV) infection in neonates and AIDS patients when sight is threatened by CMV retinitis. Valganciclovir is an L-valine ester prodrug of ganciclovir that can be given orally.

Pharmacology

Ganciclovir, developed in 1980, is a synthetic nucleoside with properties similar to aciclovir (q.v.). It accumulates after phosphorylation in CMV-infected cells inhibiting virus replication. It is much more toxic than aciclovir, frequently causing neutropenia and thrombocytopenia. Treatment should be suspended (or the dose reduced) if the neutrophil count is $<0.5 \times 10^9/l$. Concurrent treatment with zidovudine (q.v.) increases the drug's toxicity. Both ganciclovir and valganciclovir are rapidly excreted by the kidney with an average half-life of 3 hours. Both drugs may affect fertility, and animal studies suggest that both these drugs are not only fetal teratogens but also potential mutagens and carcinogens. Despite this, limited case reports of use during human pregnancy largely report good outcomes. Breastfeeding is inadvisable due to the marrow toxicity.

Cytomegalovirus infection

Approximately 50% of women of childbearing age have already had an asymptomatic infection before the start of pregnancy (often in early childhood), but primary or reactivated infection is thought to cause congenital or perinatal infection in about 1 in every 300 UK pregnancies. Most babies are asymptomatic, but ~5% develop disseminated cytomegalic inclusion disease with thrombocytopenic petechiae, hepatitis, chorioretinitis, intracranial calcification and/or microcephaly. Severe progressive deafness may sometimes develop in asymptomatic babies especially when infection occurred in the first trimester. Overt cytomegalic inclusion disease may also result from neonatal cross infection or exposure to CMV-infected blood or human milk; such babies often develop pneumonia as well as many of the symptoms listed earlier. Hand washing is important to prevent congenitally infected babies causing iatrogenic cross infection. There is limited evidence that any antiviral agent can alter the course of congenitally acquired infection, but ganciclovir can temporarily eradicate virus excretion and sustained use after birth seems to reduce the risk of later progressive hearing loss. Valaciclovir (a prodrug of aciclovir) given to the mother at a dose of 2 g four times a day may reduce fetal damage. Alternatively, 200 units/kg of hyperimmune globulin may be of benefit. CMV-specific immunoglobulin is available in some countries.

Treatment

Seek expert advice – treatment is only recommended for symptomatic babies. Explain that use seldom eliminates the virus and that the manufacturer has not yet endorsed use in children. Watch for neutropenia, and increase the dosage interval if there is renal impairment. Treatment is usually for 6 weeks, of which the majority should be given intravenously. Monitor progress by measuring the viral load in blood.

Intravenous (IV) treatment: Give 6 mg/kg IV of ganciclovir (5 ml of the solution made up as described under 'Supply and administration') over 1 hour once every 12 hours until oral treatment is possible. Maintain hydration during IV use.

Oral treatment: Start by giving a 16 mg/kg dose of valganciclovir twice a day.

Supply and administration

Undiluted ganciclovir is very caustic (pH ~ 11). Both products are potential teratogens and carcinogens, so gloves and goggles should be used during reconstitution. Wash at once to limit accidental contact with skin.

Ganciclovir: 500 mg vials cost £30 each. The freeze-dried powder must be reconstituted with 9.7 ml of water for injection to give a solution containing 50 mg/ml (water containing a bacteriostatic such as *para*-hydroxybenzoate may cause precipitation). Shake to dissolve, and use promptly. Do not use the vial if there is any particulate matter still present. To give 6 mg/kg of ganciclovir, take 1.2 ml of this solution for each kilogram the baby weighs, dilute to 50 ml with 10% glucose or glucose saline, and infuse 5 ml over 1 hour.

Valganciclovir: 450 mg tablets are available (cost £18 each) as is a powder which, when reconstituted, gives an oral suspension containing 50 mg/ml (cost £230 for 100 ml).

Continued on p. 236

References

Adler SP, Nigro G. Findings and conclusions from CMV hyperimmune globulin treatment trials. *J Clin Virol* 2009;**46**(Suppl):S54–7.

Capretti MG, Lanari M, Lazzarotto T, *et al*. Very low birth weight infants born to cytomegalovirus-seropositive mothers fed with their mother's milk: a prospective study. *J Pediatr* 2009;**154**:842–8.

Coll O, Benoist G, Ville Y, *et al*., for the WAPM Consensus Group. Guidelines on CMV congenital infection. *J Perinat Med* 2009;**37**:433–45.

Evans C, Brooks A, Anumba D, *et al*. Dilemmas regarding the use of CMV-specific immunoglobulin in pregnancy. *J Clin Virol* 2013;**57**:95–7.

Jacquemard F, Yamamoto N, Costa J-M, *et al*. Maternal administration of valaciclovir in symptomatic intrauterine cytomegalovirus infection. *BJOG* 2007;**114**:1113–21.

Kadambari S, Williams EJ, Luck S, *et al*. Evidence based management guidelines for the detection and treatment of congenital CMV. *Early Hum Dev* 2011;**87**:723–8.

Kimberlin DW, Acosta EP, Sánchez PJ, *et al*. Pharmacokinetic and pharmacodynamic assessment of oral valganciclovir in the treatment of symptomatic congenital cytomegalovirus disease. *J Infect Dis* 2008;**197**:836–45.

Kimberlin DW, Lin C-Y, Sanchez PJ, *et al*. Effect of ganciclovir therapy on hearing in symptomatic congenital cytomegalovirus disease involving the central nervous system: a randomized, controlled trial. *J Pediatr* 2003;**143**:16–25. [RCT] (See also pp. 4–6.)

Marshall BC, Koch WC. Antivirals for cytomegalovirus infection in neonates and infants: focus on pharmacokinetics, formulations, dosing and adverse events. *Pediatr Drugs* 2009;**11**:309–21.

Nigro G, Adler SP, La Torre R, *et al*. Passive immunisation during pregnancy for congenital cytomegalovirus infection. *N Engl J Med* 2005;**353**:1350–62.

Puliyanda DP, Silverman NS, Lehman D, *et al*. Successful use of oral ganciclovir for the treatment of intrauterine cytomegalovirus infection in a renal allograft recipient. *Transpl Infect Dis* 2005;**7**:71–4.

Use

Gentamicin is widely used to treat Gram-negative bacterial infection, but it is of variable efficacy (and not the treatment of choice) for known staphylococcal sepsis. It has to be given intravenous (IV) or intramuscular (IM) (or occasionally nebulised).

Pharmacology

Gentamicin is a naturally occurring substance produced by the environmental Gram-positive bacteria *Micromonospora*. It was first isolated in 1963 and is a mixture of related compounds. It crosses the placenta, producing fetal levels that are about half the maternal level, but it has never been known to have caused ototoxicity *in utero*. Absorption from the gut is too limited to disallow maternal use during lactation (although the baby's gut flora could be altered). Gentamicin is passively filtered unchanged by the glomerulus and concentrated in the urine. As a result, in healthy babies, the half-life decreases by more than 50% in the first 7–10 days after birth. Corrected gestational age also affects the half-life to a lesser extent. Renal tubular damage is progressive with time and can even produce a Bartter-like syndrome. Co-treatment with vancomycin can exacerbate these problems, which are usually reversible on cessation of treatment and seldom severe. Cochlear impairment is uncommon in young children, but gentamicin can cause balance problems as well as high-tone deafness, and these can become permanent if early symptoms go unrecognised. Blood levels should always be measured in order to minimise this risk where facilities exist. It is *at least* as important to avoid simultaneous treatment with furosemide and to try to stop treatment after 7–10 days.

Therapeutic strategy

Aminoglycosides are only effective against many bacteria when the serum level is high enough to be potentially toxic. A high peak level (at least eight times the minimum inhibitory dose) enhances the drug's bactericidal effect. Gram-negative organisms stop taking up the drug after an hour and only do so again 2–10 hours later ('adaptive resistance'); therefore, repeat treatment during this time is ineffective. Serious toxicity is predominantly seen with treatment longer than 7–10 days where there are sustained high trough serum levels and/or co-exposure to other oto-toxic drugs. In patients with normal renal function, treatment is optimised, and adverse effects are minimised, by following a once a day ('high peak, low trough') policy. An increasing number of studies have now suggested that this is the right strategy to adopt in babies and children. When aminoglycosides *are* given more than once a day in children, the serum level will remain sub-therapeutic for many hours if an initial loading dose is not given (because of the large V_D).

Treating suspected sepsis

Dose: Give 5 mg/kg IV or IM to babies less than 4 weeks old and 7 mg/kg to children older than this.
Timing: Give a dose once every 36 hours in babies less than 32 weeks gestation in the first week of life. Give all other babies a dose once every 24 hours unless renal function is poor.
Individualised treatment: A strategy to individualise treatment in very immature infants (≤28 weeks gestation) may be followed by measuring the gentamicin level 22 hours after a single dose of 5 mg/kg. The timing of the next dose is then calculated according to the level.

Level at 22 hours	Dosing interval
≤1.2 mg/l	24 hourly
1.3–2.6 mg/l	36 hourly
2.7–3.5 mg/l	48 hourly
≥3.6 mg/l	Withhold the next dose. Repeat level 24 hours later and base dosing interval on the time to achieve a level <2 mg/l

Gentamicin is frequently used in babies undergoing therapeutic hypothermia. These babies typically have renal impairment, close monitoring is mandatory, and dose adjustments are frequently needed. A 4 mg/kg dose and a 36 hourly regime is reported as best for these babies.

Continued on p. 238

Managing ventriculitis

CSF penetration is poor so it can *sometimes* be appropriate to give 1–2 mg of the ***intrathecal*** preparation once every 24–48 hours as a direct intraventricular injection and to monitor the CSF drug level (aim for 5–10 mg/l) when treating chronic ventriculitis, especially when this complicates shunt surgery. Ceftazidime, cefotaxime, co-trimoxazole and chloramphenicol (q.v.) all achieve better CSF penetration than gentamicin when given IV.

Blood levels

Measure trough levels just before the fourth dose (or, preferably, before the third dose in babies <7 days old and in babies with poor renal function) aiming for a level of about 1 mg/l. Extend the dosing interval if this level exceeds 2 mg/l. The peak level only needs to be measured when using a non-standard treatment.

Supply

A 2 ml (20 mg) vial costs £1.40 and a 1 ml (5 mg) intrathecal ampoule costs 74p.

References

(See also the relevant Cochrane reviews)

Alshaikh B, Dersch-Mills D, Taylor R, *et al*. Extended interval dosing of gentamicin in premature neonates ≤28-week gestation. *Acta Paediatr* 2012;**101**:1134–9.

Dersch-Mills D, Akierman A, Alshaikh B, *et al*. Validation of a dosage individualization table for extended-interval gentamicin in neonates. *Ann Pharmacother* 2012;**46**:935–42.

English M, Mohammed S, Ross A, *et al*. A randomised, controlled trial of once daily and multi-dose daily gentamicin in young Kenyan infants. *Arch Dis Child* 2004;**89**:665–9. [RCT]

Frymoyer A, Lee S, Bonifacio SL, *et al*. Every 36-h gentamicin dosing in neonates with hypoxic-ischemic encephalopathy receiving hypothermia. *J Perinatol* 2013;**33**:778–82.

Nestaas E, Bangstad H-J, Sandvik L, *et al*. Aminoglycoside extended interval dosing in neonates is safe and effective: a meta-analysis. *Arch Dis Child Fetal Neonatal Ed* 2005;**90**:F294–300. [SR]

Thingvoll ES, Guillet R, Caserta M, *et al*. Observational trial of a 48-hour gentamicin dosing regimen derived from Monte Carlo simulations in infants born at less than 28 weeks' gestation. *J Pediatr* 2008;**153**:530–4.

Use

Glucagon can be useful in the management of neonatal hypoglycaemia and may be useful in neonates with symptoms of β-blockade after maternal treatment.

Pharmacology

Glucagon is a polypeptide hormone produced by α cells of the pancreatic islets. It has a natural half-life of 5–10 minutes. It was formerly extracted from animal pancreatic islet cell tissue, but a recombinant 29-amino-acid product, identical to human glucagon, is now the main product available. Glucagon mobilises hepatic glycogen and increases hepatic glucose and ketone production, causing increased amino acid uptake and free fatty acid flux. It is also known to stimulate growth hormone release. Glucagon activates the adenyl cyclase system even when the β-adrenoreceptors are blocked, and a continuous infusion is of proven value in the management of unintentional overtreatment with β-blockers such as atenolol, labetalol and propranolol (q.v.). Isoprenaline (q.v.) may be of value if glucagon is not effective.

Glucagon does not appear to cross the placenta. Rodent teratogenicity studies are reassuring. It is not known whether glucagon enters breast milk; however, as a peptide, glucagon will be digested within the GI tract. There is no evidence why glucagon cannot be used for the treatment of severe hypoglycaemia during pregnancy and lactation.

In hypoglycaemia, a single bolus injection of glucagon can sometimes increase the blood glucose level enough to make further treatment unnecessary. It is not clear how this effect is achieved, but glucagon may act by inducing key gluconeogenic enzymes in the period immediately after birth. A subcutaneous or intramuscular (IM) injection is sometimes used to counteract accidental hyperinsulinism in patients with diabetes. An IM injection can also be used as a temporary expedient to reduce the risk of reactive hypoglycaemia in an infusion-dependent baby when an intravenous (IV) drip suddenly 'tissues' and proves difficult to resite. Continuous infusions are not recommended by the manufacturer, but have sometimes been used in growth-restricted babies with persisting neonatal hypoglycaemia despite a substantial infusion of IV glucose (q.v.). They have also been used in the initial short-term management of babies with endogenous hyperinsulinism, sometimes in conjunction with octreotide (as outlined in the monograph on diazoxide), since glucagon can itself stimulate insulin production. High-dose infusion can cause nausea and vomiting.

Treatment

Single-dose treatment: Give 200 micrograms/kg of glucagon subcutaneously, IM or as a bolus IV. This can sometimes raise the blood glucose level permanently out of the hypoglycaemic range in the first few days of life (sometimes even making it unnecessary to erect an IV drip).

Continuous IV infusion: Start with 300 nanograms/kg/minute (0.3 ml/hour of a solution made up as described under 'Supply and administration') and increase this, if necessary, to a dose of not more than 900 nanograms/kg/minute. Prepare a fresh solution if treatment needs to be continued for more than 24 hours.

Supply and administration

Vials containing 1 mg of powder (1 mg = 1 unit), suitable for single-dose administration, are available costing £11.50 each. Reconstitute with the diluent provided to obtain a solution containing 1 mg/ml. To give an infusion of 100 nanograms/kg/minute, take 300 micrograms (0.3 ml) of this reconstituted material for each kilogram the baby weighs, dilute this to 5 ml with further 5% glucose to obtain a solution containing 60 micrograms/kg/ml, and infuse this at a rate of 0.1 ml/hour.

Vials should be stored at 4 °C and reconstituted immediately before use. The fluid has a pH of 2.5–3.0. Avoid co-infusion with any fluid containing calcium (to avoid immediate precipitation), and do not use the reconstituted solution if it is not clear.

References

Arnoux JB, de Lonlay P, Ribeiro MJ, *et al*. Congenital hyperinsulinism. *Early Hum Dev* 2010;**86**:287–94.

Carter PE, Lloyd DJ, Duffty P. Glucagon for hypoglycaemia in infants small for gestational age. *Arch Dis Child* 1988;**63**:1264–5.

Charsha DS, McKinley PS, Whitfield JM. Glucagon infusion for treatment of hypoglycemia: efficacy and safety in sick preterm infants. *Pediatrics* 2003;**111**:220–1.

Hawdon JM, Aynsley Green A, Ward Platt MP. Neonatal blood glucose concentrations: metabolic effects of intravenous glucagon and intragastric medium chain triglyceride. *Arch Dis Child* 1993;**68**:255–61.

Continued on p. 240

Mehta A, Wootton R, Cheng KL, *et al*. Effect of diazoxide or glucagon on hepatic glucose production rate during extreme neonatal hypoglycaemia. *Arch Dis Child* 1987;**62**:924–30.

Miralles RE, Lodha A, Perlman M, *et al*. Experience with intravenous glucagon infusions as a treatment for resistant neonatal hypoglycemia. *Arch Pediatr Adolesc Med* 2002;**156**:999–1004.

Stevens TP, Guillet R. Use of glucagon to treat neonatal low-output congestive heart failure after maternal labetalol therapy. *J Pediatr* 1995;**127**:151–3.

Young J, Anwar A. Diabetic medications in pregnancy. *Curr Diabetes Rev* 2009;**5**:252–8.

Use

Glucose is among the most frequently used (and abused) drugs in the neonatal setting. It is a key component of parenteral nutrition (q.v.).

Pharmacology

Dextrose is the naturally occurring D-isomer of glucose. A 5% solution is isotonic with blood. More concentrated solutions can cause thrombophlebitis due, in part, to the fact that autoclaved solutions have a relatively low pH. A correctly placed 'long line' is the best way to deliver any solution stronger than 10–12.5%.

Hypoglycaemia: Few subjects provoke such controversy as does the measurement of blood glucose in an otherwise healthy newborn baby; the widespread adoption of 2.6 mmol/l as a cut-off for defining 'neonatal hypoglycaemia' has led to many such babies receiving interventions which they did not require. Early blood glucose concentration changes in these babies reflect simply the change from placental to enteral supply of food, a process for which most are well prepared because the brain is protected by a range of alternative fuels. There are, however, groups of babies who are at risk of more profound or prolonged fall in blood glucose or more importantly a failure to mount the normal metabolic responses. To avoid unnecessary treatment, suggested thresholds for intervention in healthy term babies may be adopted (in the following table).

Subsequently, a laboratory whole-blood glucose of <2.5 mmol/l (45 mg/dl) is very unusual in any baby being maintained on a sustained infusion of 9 mg/kg/minute (~130 ml/kg/day) of 10% glucose within 48 hours of birth, and hyperinsulinism should be suspected if this level can only be sustained by giving more than 12 mg/kg/minute.

Suggested blood glucose thresholds for intervention in healthy term babies (from Cornblath *et al.*, 2000).

Clinical picture	Blood glucose
Healthy well baby	Any single value <1.0 mmol/l
Baby with abnormal clinical signs	Any single value <2.5 mmol/l
'At-risk' baby without clinical signs	Any single measurement <2.0 mmol/l and still <2.0 mmol/l at next measurement

Most asymptomatic hypoglycaemia is caused by delayed feeding, compounded by an inadequate (and frequently interrupted) glucose infusion rate. Milk is the best prophylaxis, and the best treatment, for any well baby since it contains 50% more calories than 10% dextrose. Mild asymptomatic hypoglycaemia may respond to oral dextrose gel or intramuscular glucagon (q.v.), making intravenous (IV) glucose unnecessary. Sustained hypoglycaemia due to hyperinsulinism may respond to diazoxide or octreotide (q.v.).

Hyperglycaemia: Although most healthy babies can metabolise at least 14 mg/kg of glucose per minute, babies of <1 kg are often relatively intolerant at first, and all babies may show small amounts of glycosuria for several days especially after any period of stress. Uptake saturation is best dealt with by reducing the rate of glucose infusion by 75% for 6–12 hours. Insulin (q.v.) is seldom needed. Levels measured using any blood specimen taken from a line containing glucose will always be misleadingly high, even if a vigorous attempt was made to clear the 'dead space' first. Sudden hyperglycaemia in a previously stable baby may be caused by pain, infection, necrotising enterocolitis or an intracranial bleed.

Treatment of hypoglycaemia

Feed the otherwise well asymptomatic baby. 200 mg/kg (0.5 ml/kg) of 40% dextrose gel massaged into the buccal mucosa may aid the process and avoid the need for IV dextrose.

Starting a 5 ml/kg/hour (120 ml/kg/day) infusion of 10% glucose will raise the blood sugar level out of the hypoglycaemic range within 10 minutes in 90% of babies. A loading dose of 2.5 ml/kg over 5 minutes will speed the control of hypoglycaemic stupor or fits. The infusion must then be continued at a steady rate and only reduced slowly as the milk intake is increased. Avoid 'bolus' injections of any strength – they only destabilise the body's regulatory mechanisms.

Continued on p. 242

A maintenance infusion containing more than 10% glucose may be necessary where water intake has to be kept below 100 ml/kg/day.

Supply

500 ml bags containing 5, 10 and 15% glucose, 4% glucose in 0.18% sodium chloride and 10% glucose in 0.18% sodium chloride are available as stock and cost 48p to 158p each. The web page associated with this entry shows how to calculate commonly used strength of dextrose if these are not available.

References

Cornblath M, Hawdon JM, Williams AF, *et al.* Controversies regarding definition of neonatal hypoglycemia: suggested operational thresholds. *Pediatrics* 2000;**105**:1141–5.

Coulthard MG, Hey EN. Renal processing of glucose in well and sick neonates. *Arch Dis Child Fetal Neonatal Ed* 1999;**81**:F92–8.

Harris DL, Weston PJ, Signal M *et al.* Dextrose gel for neonatal hypoglycaemia (the Sugar Babies Study): a randomised, double-blind, placebo-controlled trial. *Lancet* 2013;**382**:2077–83. [RCT]

Hawdon JM, Modder J, eds. Glucose control in the perinatal period. *Semin Fetal Neonat Med* 2005;**10**:305–400. [The whole issue.]

Hawdon JM, Ward Platt MP, Aynsley-Green A. Patterns of metabolic adaptation for preterm and term infants in the first neonatal week. *Arch Dis Child* 1992;**67**:357–65.

Lilien LD, Grajwer LA, Pildes RS. Treatment of neonatal hypoglycaemia with continuous intravenous glucose infusions. *J Pediatr* 1977; **91**:779–82. (See also 1980;**97**:295–8.)

Rozance PJ, Hay WW. Hypoglycemia in newborn infants: features associated with adverse outcomes. *Biol Neonat* 2006;**90**:74–86. (See also PP. 87–8.)

Use

The main neonatal use of glyceryl trinitrate (GTN) is in the management of low-output cardiac failure. It may be used topically to counteract tissue ischaemia caused by vasoconstrictive inotropes like dopamine (q.v.).

Pharmacology

The main use of GTN is in the treatment of coronary heart disease. When first used for angina in 1879, it was presumed that it had a direct effect on the coronary arteries, but it is now recognised to have other systemic effects that help to reduce cardiac oxygen requirements:

- *Low* doses (between 0.5 and 3 micrograms/kg/minute) decrease ventricular filling pressure ('preload') by reducing venous tone, thus decreasing pulmonary artery pressure and increasing cardiac output. It also improves coronary artery perfusion and decreases myocardial oxygen consumption making secondary cardiac ischaemia less likely.
- *Moderate* doses (4–6 micrograms/kg/minute) cause pulmonary and systemic arteriolar dilatation.
- *High* doses (7–10 micrograms/kg/minute) cause hypotension and secondary tachycardia.

GTN is taken up avidly by vascular smooth muscle. Nitric oxide (q.v.) is then liberated causing a marked decrease in venous and arterial tone. It is also quickly metabolised (half-life 1–4 minutes) by glutathione-organic nitrate reductase in the liver and must, therefore, be given by continuous infusion. Therapy can be complicated by methaemoglobinaemia (an oxidation by-product of the reaction between nitric oxide and haemoglobin), but this has been described in only one paper where there were prolonged infusions and concomitant use of sodium nitroprusside. It can also produce raised intracranial pressure although this has not been described in the newborn either.

There is no evidence of teratogenicity, and there is growing evidence that it can be used as a safe, rapid onset, short-acting, tocolytic agent (one 100 micrograms 'bolus' IV) to manage placental retention, or fetal entrapment during caesarean section or vaginal twin delivery, or to control uterine tone during external cephalic version. Transdermal patches have recently been used to control preterm labour, but such treatment often causes headache. It is not known if GTN enters breast milk. However, considering the indication, dosing and rapid clearance, infrequent GTN use is unlikely to pose a significant risk to the breastfed infant.

Treatment

Intravenous use: Continuous infusions have been used in the management of patients with systemic or pulmonary venous congestion due to poor ventricular function. Start with a low dose of between 0.5 and 3 micrograms/kg/minute and increase as necessary. It is important to exclude hypovolaemia, and sometimes use an inotrope as well.

Topical use: Serious catheter-related vasospasm can sometimes be corrected by the application of 2% GTN ointment or topical spray. Papaverine (q.v.) may be an equally effective way of controlling vasospasm.

Compatibility

Glyceryl trinitrate can be added (terminally) to an IV line containing atracurium, dobutamine and/or dopamine, midazolam, milrinone or nitroprusside.

Supply and administration

Check the strength of the ampoule carefully before use. Several strengths exist: 1 mg/ml (in 5, 10 and 50 ml ampoules costing £1.80, £5.90 and £15.90 respectively) and 5 mg/ml (in 5 and 10 ml costing £6.49 and £12.98). Most formulations contain some propylene glycol (a maximum of 30% v/v).

To give an infusion of 1 microgram/kg/minute, draw up 15 mg of GTN for each kilogram the baby weighs, dilute to 25 ml with 10% glucose or glucose saline, and infuse at a rate of 0.1 ml/hour (a less concentrated solution of glucose or glucose saline can be used if necessary). Ampoules should be protected from strong light, discarded if the fluid is discoloured and disposed of promptly after use. Glyceryl trinitrate is absorbed by polyvinyl chloride and should only be given using syringes and tubing made of polyethylene. A fresh solution should be prepared every 24 hours.

Continued on p. 244

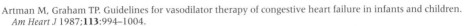

An ointment containing 2% GTN (60 g costing £11) can be obtained on request. Transdermal patches and sprays are used in adults with coronary heart disease.

References

(See also relevant Cochrane reviews)

Artman M, Graham TP. Guidelines for vasodilator therapy of congestive heart failure in infants and children. *Am Heart J* 1987;**113**:994–1004.

Baserga MC, Puri A, Sola A. The use of topical nitroglycerin ointment to treat peripheral tissue ischaemia secondary to arterial line complications in neonates. *J Perinatol* 2002;**22**:416–9.

Black RS, Lees C, Thompson S, *et al.* Maternal and fetal cardiovascular effects of transdermal glyceryl trinitrate and intravenous ritodrine. *Obstet Gynecol* 1999;**94**:572–6.

Kamar R, van Vonderen JJ, Lopriore E, *et al.* Nitroglycerin for severe ischaemic injury after peripheral arterial line in a preterm infant. *Acta Paediatr* 2013;**102**:e144–5.

Keeley SR, Bohn DJ. The use of inotropic and afterload-reducing agents in neonates. *Clin Perinatol* 1988;**15**:467–89.

Smith GN, Walker MC, Ohlsson A, *et al.* Randomized double-blind placebo-controlled trial of transdermal nitroglycerin for preterm labour. *Am J Obstet Gynecol* 2007;**196**:37.e1–8. [RCT]

Tamura M, Kawano T. Effects of intravenous nitroglycerin on hemodynamics in neonates with refractory congestive heart failure or PFC. *Acta Paediatr Jpn* 1990;**32**:291–8.

Williams RS, Mickell JJ, Young ES, *et al.* Methemoglobin levels during prolonged combined nitroglycerin and sodium nitroprusside infusions in infants after cardiac surgery. *J Cardiothorac Vasc Anesth* 1994;**8**:658–62.

Wong AF, McCulloch LM, Sola A. Treatment of peripheral tissue ischaemia with topical nitroglycerin ointment in neonates. *J Pediatr* 1992;**121**:980–3.

Use

Glycine is used in the management of isovaleric acidaemias. This rare, autosomal recessive, inborn error of metabolism is caused by a deficiency of isovaleryl-CoA dehydrogenase, an enzyme on the catabolic pathway of leucine. Treatment is aimed at reducing production of isovaleric and increasing its removal. The patients are treated with a low-protein diet, glycine and L-carnitine (q.v.).

Biochemistry

Glycine is a naturally occurring amino acid. In isovaleric acidaemia, the administration of additional glycine greatly speeds the conversion of isovaleryl-CoA to isovalerylglycine, which is then excreted in the urine. Aspirin should be avoided as it is a competitive substrate for one of the essential metabolic steps involved.

Isovaleric acidaemia

Deficiency of isovaleryl-CoA dehydrogenase causes a range of metabolites, including isovaleric acid, to accumulate. Glycine and carnitine are conjugated to isovaleric acid and then excreted in the urine. Some patients present soon after birth (often within 3–6 days) with poor feeding, vomiting and drowsiness. Tremor, twitching and seizures may be seen before the child lapses into coma and death. Other patients present for the first time when rather older with similar symptoms precipitated by intercurrent illness. Symptoms are often accompanied by acidosis, ketosis and a high blood ammonia level (sometimes >500 μmol/l). There can often be neutropenia, thrombocytopenia and hypo- or hyperglycaemia when the condition first presents in the neonatal period. High isovaleric acid levels may give rise to a characteristic unpleasant odour, which has been likened to that of 'sweaty feet'. Patients present, very occasionally, with progressive generalised developmental delay.

The condition is most easily diagnosed by detecting excess isovalerylglycine (and 3-hydroxy-isovaleric acid) in the urine or abnormal acylcarnitines in the blood. Patients are generally treated with glycine and carnitine, a low-protein diet and measures to minimise catabolism during intercurrent illnesses. The prognosis can be good with early diagnosis, but many patients suffer neurological damage prior to diagnosis. Symptomatic disturbance becomes less common in later childhood, and the condition is compatible with normal adult life (including a normal uneventful pregnancy). There is no reason to think that lactation would be unwise while the mother herself remains well. Carnitine may become depleted in isovaleric acidaemias, and levocarnitine (q.v.) is also given routinely by mouth (or intravenously if a metabolic crisis occurs).

Treatment

Acute illness: Withdraw all protein from the diet, and give IV glucose to minimise catabolism. Start treatment with oral glycine (see under 'Maintenance care'). Haemodialysis, exchange transfusion or the use of sodium benzoate or sodium phenylbutyrate may be indicated if there is severe hyperammonaemia (>500 μmol/l) when the patient first presents.

Maintenance care: The usual maintenance dose is 50 mg/kg of glycine three times a day although, during acute illness, the amount given can be increased to 100 mg/kg six times a day. The normal maintenance dose may need to be modified if there is liver or kidney impairment and stopped if there is anuria. Long-term management involves dietary protein restriction supervised by someone experienced in the management of metabolic disease.

Supply and administration

Glycine is available as a powder from SHS International, and a stable solution containing 50 or 100 mg/ml can be provided on request. 100 g of power costs £5. No IV preparation is available, but glycine can be given by nasogastric tube, and the likelihood of vomiting can be reduced by giving small frequent doses.

References

Cohn RM, Yudkoff M, Rothman R, *et al.* Isovaleric acidemia: use of glycine therapy in neonates. *N Engl J Med* 1978;**299**:996–9.

de Baulny HO, Dionisi-Vici C, Wendel U. Branched-chain organic acidurias/acidemias. In: Saudubray J-M, van den Berghe G, Walter JH. eds. *Inborn metabolic diseases. Diagnosis and treatment*, 5th ed. Berlin: Springer-Verlag, 2012: pp. 297–96.

Continued on p. 246

Dixon MA, Leonard JV. Intercurrent illness in inborn errors of intermediary metabolism. *Arch Dis Child* 1992;**67**:1387–91.

Heimler R, Hennes H, Khayata S, *et al*. Isovaleric acidaemia in a premature infant: diagnosis and treatment. *J Inherit Metab Dis* 1988;**11**:313–4.

Shih VE, Aubry RH, DeGrande G, *et al*. Maternal isovaleric acidemia. *J Pediatr* 1984;**105**:77–8.

Sweetman L, Williams JC. Branched chain organic acidurias. In: Scriver CR, Beaudet AL, Sly WS, *et al*., eds. *The metabolic and molecular bases of inherited disease*, 8th ed. New York: McGraw-Hill, 2001: pp. 2125–63.

Use

Glycopyrronium, like atropine (q.v.), can be used to combat vagal bradycardia and to control salivation and tracheal secretions during general anaesthesia and elective intubation. It is given to control the muscarinic effects of neostigmine (q.v.) when this is used to reverse the effect of a non-depolarising muscle relaxant.

Pharmacology

Glycopyrronium bromide is a quaternary ammonium drug with peripheral antimuscarinic effects similar to those of atropine that is rapidly redistributed into the tissues after intravenous (IV) or intramuscular (IM) injection. It was first introduced into clinical use in 1960. The full effect of IM administration is only seen after 15 minutes, and vagal blockade lasts about 3 hours. The plasma half-life is only 5–10 minutes during childhood and adult life, with almost half the drug being excreted in the urine within 3 hours. The way that babies handle this drug when less than a month old has not yet been studied. Many anaesthetists prefer glycopyrronium to atropine and the other belladonna alkaloids, partly because very little crosses the blood–brain barrier. Transplacental passage is also less than for atropine, and the amount detected in umbilical cord blood following use during caesarean delivery is small. Rapid plasma clearance makes it extremely unlikely that use during lactation would pose any problem. Oral absorption is poor, but a 50 micrograms/kg oral dose has been used with some success to control drooling in older children with severe cerebral palsy.

Glycopyrronium, given with neostigmine, achieves an excellent controlled reversal of the neuromuscular blockade seen with the competitive muscle relaxant drugs such as pancuronium (q.v.), but it may take at least 30 minutes to effect the full reversal of deep blockade. A 1:5 drug ratio seems to minimise any variation in heart rate. The risk of dysrhythmia is lower with glycopyrronium, and the lack of any effect on the central nervous system speeds arousal after general anaesthesia.

Treatment

Premedication: The usual dose is 5 micrograms/kg IV shortly before the induction of anaesthesia. Oral premedication with 50 micrograms/kg 1 hour before surgery is not as effective as a 20 micrograms/kg oral dose of atropine at controlling the bradycardia associated with anaesthetic induction.

Reversing neuromuscular block: 10 micrograms/kg of glycopyrronium and 50 micrograms/kg of neostigmine (0.2 ml/kg of a combined solution made up as described under 'Supply and administration'), given IV, will reverse the muscle relaxing effect of pancuronium (and, where necessary, atracurium, rocuronium and vecuronium).

Drooling: 50 micrograms/kg by mouth two to three times a day may help control drooling in cerebral palsy.

Alternatives

Neuromuscular blockade can be reversed just as effectively with atropine and neostigmine if glycopyrronium is not available. Give 20 micrograms/kg of atropine IV followed by a 40 micrograms/kg dose of IV neostigmine.

Supply and administration

Plain 1 ml ampoules simply containing 200 micrograms of glycopyrronium bromide cost 54p. A combination of neostigmine metilsulfate (2.5 mg) and glycopyrronium bromide (500 micrograms) is available in 1 ml ampoules (cost £1.15). Take the contents of one of these 1 ml ampoules, dilute to 10 ml with 0.9% sodium chloride, and give 0.2 ml/kg of this diluted solution to reverse the neuromuscular block caused by non-depolarising muscle relaxant drugs.

Dispersible 1 and 2 mg tablets for oral use are available on a 'named-patient' basis from specialist importing companies. Alternatively, the injection solution may be given by mouth.

References

(See also relevant Cochrane reviews)

Ali-Melkkilä T, Kaila T, Kanto J, *et al*. Pharmacokinetics of glycopyrronium in parturients. *Anesthesia* 1990;**45**:634–7.

Bachrach SJ, Walter RS, Trzeinski K. Use of glycopyrrolate and other anticholinergic medications for sialorrhea in children with cerebral palsy. *Clin Pediatr* 1998;**37**:485–90.

Continued on p. 248

Cartabuke RS, Davidson PJ, Warner LO. Is premedication with oral glycopyrrolate as effective as oral atropine in attenuating cardiovascular depression in infants receiving halothane for induction of anaesthesia? *Anesth Analg* 1991;**73**:271–4. [RCT]

Goldhill DR, Embree PB, Ali HH, *et al*. Reversal of pancuronium. Neuromuscular and cardiovascular effects of a mixture of neostigmine and glycopyrronium. *Anaesthesia* 1988;**43**:443–6.

Jongerius PH, van den Hoogen FJA, van Limbeek J, *et al*. Effect of botulinum toxin in the treatment of drooling: a controlled clinical trial. *Pediatrics* 2004;**114**:620–7. [RCT]

Mirrkakhur RK, Shepherd WFI, Jones CJ. Ventilation and the oculocardiac reflex. Prevention of oculocardiac reflex during surgery for squints: role of controlled ventilation and anticholinergic drugs. *Anaesthesia* 1986;**41**:825–8. [RCT]

Norman E, Wikström S, Hellström-Westas L, *et al*. Rapid sequence induction is superior to morphine for intubation of preterm infants: a randomized controlled trial. *J Pediatr* 2011;**159**:893–9.

Parr JR, Buswell CA, Banerjee K *et al*. Management of drooling in children: a survey of UK paediatricians' clinical practice. *Child Care Health Dev* 2012;**38**:287–91.

Rautakorpi P, Ali-Melkkila T, Kaila T, *et al*. Pharmacokinetics of glycopyrrolate in children. *J Clin Anesth* 1994;**6**:217–20.

van der Burg JJW, Jongerius PH, van Limbeek J, *et al*. Drooling in children with cerebral palsy: effect of salivary flow reduction on daily living and care. *Dev Med Child Neurol* 2006;**48**:103–7.

Use

Granulocyte colony-stimulating factor (G-CSF) and granulocyte–macrophage colony-stimulating factor (GM-CSF) are naturally occurring proteins involved in proliferation and differentiation of myeloid precursors. Purified recombinant factors are commercially available; **filgrastim** (unglycosylated rhG-CSF) and **lenograstim** (glycosylated rhG-CSF) have similar effects and can promote the production of neutrophils in a variety of neutropenic states. **Sargramostim** (rhGM-CSF) is marketed in the United States, but it is not generally available in the United Kingdom. The current preparations no longer contain EDTA which was reported to be the reason for adverse events that occurred with some of the early formulations.

Physiology

Neutrophils play an essential role in the body's defence against bacteria. After leaving the bone marrow pool, they remain in circulation for ~6 hours before entering other body tissues. Birth causes a transient increase in the number in circulation, especially when this is stressful. Neonatal sepsis can rapidly *decrease* the number in circulation, because production is already close to its peak at birth. This and functional immaturity of the baby's immune system make them vulnerable to infection. Very low birthweight babies often have very low counts soon after birth and again at 2–4 weeks of age when the marrow mounts its first response to the growing post-delivery anaemia.

Pharmacology

Marrow colony-stimulating factors are naturally occurring glycoprotein growth promoters (cytokines) that stimulate the proliferation and differentiation of red and white blood cell bone precursors in bone marrow. A number of these factors, including erythropoietin (q.v.), have been produced by recombinant DNA technology in the last 20 years. Both filgrastim and lenograstim enhance the production and release of neutrophil white blood cells from bone marrow, and filgrastim is widely used to prevent chemotherapy-induced neutropenia and speed neutrophil recovery after bone marrow transplantation.

Subcutaneous rather than intravenous (IV) use doubles the elimination half-life to about 3 hours and is believed to increase therapeutic efficacy while minimising the risk of toxicity associated with high peak blood levels. Adverse effects, including fever, dyspnoea, nausea and vomiting, have been very uncommon with neonatal use. Use during pregnancy is associated with increased fetal death in primates. Use during lactation has not been studied but seems unlikely, on theoretical grounds, to pose any serious risk.

The early postnatal and sepsis-induced neutropenia ($<1.5 \times 10^9$/l) often seen in the preterm baby can frequently be prevented by giving rhG-CSF, but while studies *in vitro* and in animal models and early trials showed encouraging improvements in neutrophil counts, larger trials and systematic reviews have identified no substantial evidence that treatment reduces mortality. Accordingly, the current role of rhG-CSF in neonates does not include prevention of infection or treatment of suspected or proven infection, but does include cases of severe chronic neutropenia, where it can be very helpful or even life-saving.

Treatment

Administer 1 million units/kg (10 micrograms/kg) of filgrastim or lenograstim subcutaneously (or IV over 30 minutes) once a day for 3 days. This equates to 0.1 ml/kg of either of the products made up as described under 'Supply and administration'.

Supply and administration

Almost all the neonatal studies reported to date have used filgrastim, but the related product, lenograstim, comes in low-dose vials that can be more economical to use. The manufacturers have not yet endorsed the use of lenograstim in children <2 years old or the use of filgrastim in neonates.

Filgrastim: Add 2 ml of 5% glucose to the 300 micrograms (30 million unit) 1 ml vials of filgrastim (costing £53) to obtain a preparation containing 100 micrograms/ml. Store all vials at 4°C, and do not keep material more than 24 hours once the vial has been opened, even if it is still stored at 4°C.

Lenograstim: 105 micrograms (13.4 million unit) 1 ml vials cost £40. Dissolve the lyophilisate with 1 ml of water for injection (as supplied). Agitate gently, but do not shake. Vials can be stored at room temperature. Reconstituted material should not be kept for more than 24 hours even if stored at 4°C.

Continued on p. 250

References

 (See also the relevant Cochrane reviews)

Ahmad A, Laborada G, Bussel J, *et al*. Comparison of recombinant granulocyte colony-stimulating factor, recombinant granulocyte-macrophage colony-stimulating factor and placebo for treatment of septic preterm infants. *Pediatr Infect Dis J* 2002;**21**:1061–5. [RCT]

Bernstein HM, Pollock BH, Calhoun DA, *et al*. Administration of recombinant granulocyte colony-stimulating factor to neonates with septicemia: a meta-analysis. *J Pediatr* 2001;**138**:917–20. [SR]

Carr R. The role of colony stimulating factors and immunoglobulin in the prevention and treatment of neonatal infection. *Arch Dis Child Fetal Neonatal Ed* 2013;**98**:F192–4.

Carrison G, Ahlin A, Dahllöf G, *et al*. Efficacy and safety of two different rG-CSF preparations in the treatment of patients with severe congenital neutropenia. *Br J Haematol* 2004;**126**:1327–32.

Kuhn P, Paupe A, Espagne S, *et al*. A multicenter, randomized, placebo-controlled trial of prophylactic recombinant granulocyte-colony stimulating factor in preterm neonates with neutropenia. *J Pediatr* 2009;**155**:324–30. [RCT]

Use

This vaccine, made from protein-conjugated polysaccharides, provides moderately well-sustained protection from *Haemophilus influenzae* type b (Hib) infection. Serious adverse reactions are rare.

Haemophilus infection

H. influenzae can be differentiated into six capsulated serotypes (Hia–Hif) and non-capsulated (ncHi) strains. Before immunisation, serotype b (Hib) accounted for >80% of invasive disease, mainly in children under five, causing meningitis (60%), epiglottitis (15%), septicaemia (10%), septic arthritis, osteomyelitis, cellulitis and pneumonia. Hib vaccination, introduced to the United Kingdom in 1992, resulted in a rapid and sustained reduction in Hib disease.

Hib cases increased between 1999 and 2003, but since the introduction of a routine 12-month Hib booster in 2006, the incidence of Hib disease is very low. Other types of *H. influenzae* are now relatively more common. In 2008, only 20 cases of invasive Hib disease in children were reported, compared with 65 ncHi and 15 non-type b encapsulated *H. influenzae* cases. In the newborn, ncHi infections have a 10-fold higher incidence than Hib. They can be associated with septicaemia in the mother, increased complications during labour and preterm delivery. Invasive ncHi infection usually develops within the first 48 hours of life, follows a fulminant clinical course and is associated with significantly higher case fatality than Hib infections. After the neonatal period, ncHi usually cause non-invasive respiratory tract infections, while invasive ncHi infection occurs mainly in children with significant co-morbidities. All invasive *H. influenzae* infections are notifiable in England and Wales, whereas since 2010 only the Hib organism is notifiable in Scotland.

Indications

All children should be offered immunisation against *Haemophilus* (Hib) as part of their routine immunisations.

Contraindications

Immunisation should be delayed in any child who is acutely unwell and not be offered if a previous dose triggered an anaphylactic reaction. A minor non-febrile infection is no reason to delay immunisation, and the contraindications associated with the use of a live vaccine (cf. measles) do not apply.

Administration

Children under a year old: The Hib vaccine is given as part of the routine childhood immunisations as one of two combined products; the diphtheria toxoid, tetanus toxoid, 5-component acellular pertussis, inactivated polio vaccine and *H. influenzae* type b (DTaP/IPV/Hib) vaccine given at 2, 3 and 4 months; and the Hib/MenC conjugate vaccine given at 12–13 months of age.

Older children: Children between 1 and 10 years of age who have not been immunised or not completed a primary course of diphtheria, tetanus, pertussis or polio vaccination should receive the outstanding doses of DTaP/IPV/Hib vaccination at monthly intervals. Children of the same age but who have completed a primary course of diphtheria, tetanus, pertussis or polio should have Hib/MenC conjugate vaccine.

Anaphylaxis

The management of anaphylaxis (which is very rare) is outlined in the monograph on immunisation.

Supply

Pediacel® manufactured by Sanofi Pasteur MSD, is the currently used product in the United Kingdom for the primary DTaP/IPV/Hib immunisations and Menitorix (Hib/MenC) conjugate vaccine, manufactured by GlaxoSmithKline is used at 12–13 months.

Continued on p. 252

References

(See also the relevant Cochrane reviews and UK guidelines **DHUK**)

Adegbola RA, Secka O, Lahai G, *et al.* Elimination of Haemophilus influenzae type b (Hib) disease from The Gambia after the introduction of routine immunisation with a Hib conjugate vaccine: a prospective study. *Lancet* 2005;**366**:144–50. (See also pp. 101–2.)

Cowgill KD, Ndirity M, Nyiro J, *et al.* Effectiveness of *Haemophilus influenzae* Type b conjugate vaccine introduction into routine childhood immunization in Kenya. *JAMA* 2006;**296**:671–8.

Gessner BD, Sutanto A, Linchan M, *et al.* Incidences of vaccine-preventable *Haemophilus influenzae* type b pneumonia and meningitis in Indonesian children: hamlet-randomised vaccine-probe trial. *Lancet* 2005;**365**:43–52. [RCT] (See also pp. 5–7.)

Heath PT. Booy R, McVernon J, *et al.* Hib vaccination in infants born prematurely. *Arch Dis Child* 2003;**88**:206–10. (See also pp. 379–83.)

Ladhani S, Slack MP, Heys M, *et al.* Fall in *Haemophilus influenzae* serotype B disease following implementation of a booster campaign. *Arch Dis Child* 2008;**93**:665–9.

McVernon J, Trotter CL, Slack MPE, *et al.* Trends in *Haemophilus influenzae* group b infections in adults in England and Wales: surveillance study. *Br Med J* 2004;**329**:655–8.

Peltola H, Salo E, Saxén H. Incidence of *Haemophilus influenzae* type b meningitis during 18 years of vaccine use: observational study using routine hospital data. *Br Med J* 2005;**330**:18–9.

Watt JP, Wolfson LJ, O'Brien KL, *et al.* Burden of disease caused by *Haemophilus influenzae* type b in children younger than 5: global estimates. *Lancet* 2009;**374**:903–11. (See also pp. 854–6.)

Use

Heparin can help maintain catheter patency and is used during and after cardiovascular surgery. Low molecular weight heparins (LMWHs), such as enoxaparin and dalteparin (q.v.), are now generally used to prevent and manage venous thromboembolism, but there is, as yet, little experience of their use in the neonate.

Pharmacology

Heparin is an acid mucopolysaccharide of variable molecular weight (4,000–40,000 Da). It was first obtained from the liver (hence its name) in a form pure enough to make clinical trials possible in 1935. While it has some thrombolytic action, it is mostly used to prevent further blood clot formation rather than to lyse those that have already formed. The higher molecular weight heparins also inhibit platelet activity. It works *in vitro* by activating plasma antithrombin inhibitor, which then deactivates thrombin and factor Xa. It is metabolised by *N*-desulphation after intravenous (IV) administration and then rapidly cleared from the body. The half-life of conventional unfractionated heparin is dose dependent, increasing as the plasma level rises. It averages 90 minutes in adults, but may be less at birth.

LMWHs weigh 4,000–6,000 Da and have a much longer half-life. Unlike unfractionated heparin, they do not cause osteopenia during long-term use, show much greater bioavailability when given subcutaneously and are mostly excreted by the kidneys. All products occasionally cause an immune-mediated thrombocytopenia, most commonly 5-10 days after the start of treatment. Because this can, paradoxically, cause a major thromboembolic event, the platelet count *must* be monitored. Stop treatment at once if thrombocytopenia develops, and do not give platelets. Heparin does not cross the placenta, is not teratogenic and can be given with complete safety during lactation (very small amounts of the LMWHs can appear in breast milk when these are used, but there is no effect on the baby).

Women at high risk of thromboembolism because of immobility, obesity, high parity, previous deep vein thrombosis or an inherited thrombophilia are now increasingly given LMWH during pregnancy and, more particularly, operative delivery and the early puerperium. Warfarin (q.v.) continues to be used to anticoagulate women with pulmonary vascular disease and patients with an artificial heart valve or atrial fibrillation, but time may show that they, too, can be protected with LMWH.

Indications for neonatal use

Although one small study has suggested that full **heparinisation** may reduce the formation of arterial thrombi, the effect of any such approach on the risk of intraventricular haemorrhage remains uncertain. Three observational studies even suggest a correlation between total heparin exposure and the risk of intraventricular haemorrhage in babies of <1500 g in the first week of life. However, this may merely mean that some babies got more heparin because they were already less well. No adequate sized trials have ever been performed, and neonatal use has never been subjected to serious study. However, while adverse effects of heparin are rare, heparinised babies can bleed unpredictably, so it is probably unwise to use heparin in babies with intracranial or gastrointestinal haemorrhage. Uncorrected thrombocytopenia ($<50 \times 10^9$/l) is also a contraindication, and intramuscular injections should not be given to any heparinised patient. Lumbar puncture can also be hazardous. Alteplase and streptokinase (q.v.) are almost certainly better at removing clots that have already formed. Prophylactic **low-dose** use to maintain catheter patency is much better established (see under 'Monitoring lines' – pp. 17–21).

Prophylactic strategies

Monitoring lines: Intravascular catheters are often used to monitor blood pressure and to make blood sampling possible without disturbing the patient. A steady 0.5 or 1.0 ml/hour infusion containing 1–2 units of heparin for each ml of fluid prolongs catheter patency. Glucose shortens the line's life and makes it impossible to monitor blood glucose levels. The use of 0.45% rather than 0.9% sodium chloride reduces the risk of sodium overload. Clear the 1 ml catheter 'dead space' carefully after sampling and consider using water rather than dextrose or saline for this in order to avoid sudden swings in blood glucose and the infusion of further unmeasured quantities of sodium chloride. Any water or saline used to 'flush' the dead space does not need to contain further heparin and should not, when treating a small baby, come from an ampoule containing a bacteriostatic for the reasons outlined in the archived monograph on benzyl alcohol.

Continued on p. 254

'Stopped-off' lines and cannulas: 'Normal' saline containing 10 units/ml of heparin is commonly flushed through and left in 'stopped-off' cannulas after use, but the addition of heparin does little to prolong patency. Central venous long lines are often left primed with a fluid containing 5000 units/ml of heparin, but a solution containing 1 mg/ml of alteplase (q.v.) seems to be a better way of keeping the catheter patent.

Cardiac catheterisation: A 100 unit/kg IV bolus at the start of the procedure greatly reduces the risk of symptomatic thromboembolism.

Intravascular infusions: Neonatal trials have shown that adding heparin to the infusate prolongs the patency, not only of arterial catheters, but also of peripherally inserted central venous lines. The most recent trial in babies with a central venous line in place used a dose of 0.5 unit/kg/hour. Such use caused a fivefold reduction in the number of catheters needing replacement because of blockage, but it did not reduce the number needing replacement because of extravasation or suspected sepsis (an equally common reason for replacement) or the risk of a clot forming close to where the tip of the catheter was (or had been). Only two small trials have yet been done (involving just 200 children) to see whether the use of a heparin-bonded catheter helps to sustain catheter patency.

Full anticoagulation

The indications for this in the neonate remain unclear. There is no good evidence that anticoagulation reduces the risk of an existing clot enlarging, fragmenting and shedding emboli or reforming after lysis. If treatment *is* indicated, start by giving a loading dose of 75 units/kg IV over 10 minutes (a loading dose of 50 units/kg may be safer in babies with a post-menstrual age of <37 weeks). Maintenance requirements vary; start with a continuous IV infusion of 25 units/kg/hour (1 ml/hour of a solution made up as described in the following text) and assess the requirement by measuring the activated partial thromboplastin time (APTT) after 4 hours. Monitor the platelet level weekly.

Dose monitoring

The anticoagulant dose used during extracorporeal membrane oxygenation (ECMO) and to lyse thrombi is one that raises the APTT to 1.8–2.0 times the normal level. Never take blood for this test from an intravascular line that has contained heparin: sufficient heparin will remain to invalidate the result even if the line is flushed through first. Normal neonatal APTT times are given in the monograph on fresh frozen plasma.

Antidote

Protamine sulphate is a basic protein which combines with heparin to produce a stable complex devoid of anticoagulant activity. The effect of heparin can, therefore, be neutralised by giving 1 mg of protamine sulphate IV over about 5 minutes for every 100 units of heparin given in the previous 2 hours. Excess protamine is dangerous because it binds platelets and proteins such as fibrinogen, producing, in itself, a bleeding tendency.

Compatibility

It is known that adrenaline, atracurium, fentanyl, glyceryl trinitrate, insulin, isoprenaline, lidocaine, midazolam, milrinone, morphine, nitroprusside, noradrenaline, propofol, prostaglandin E_1, ranitidine, streptokinase, TPN (the standard formulation with or without lipid) and urokinase can be added (terminally) to a line containing heparin. So can plain amphotericin (but not the liposomal formulation because of concern that this may destabilise the colloid). So, too, can dopamine, but there are reports suggesting that although heparin is compatible with dobutamine when suspended in 0.9% sodium chloride, precipitation may occur (somewhat unpredictably) when the two drugs are mixed, even briefly, in a glucose solution.

Supply and administration

Care should be taken with use of heparin; vials which differ in strength by 100- or even 1000-fold are routinely stocked together, with little or no visible differentiation in packaging.

There are three strengths of standard, unfractionated heparin sodium – 1,000, 5,000 and 25,000 units/ml – and all are available in volumes (vials or ampoules) of 1 and 5 ml. The 1,000 units/ml strength is also available in 10 and 20 ml ampoules, and the 25,000 units/ml strength in a 0.2 ml ampoule. Vials can be stored at room temperature (5–25 °C) for 18 months, but are best not kept more than 28 days once open. These may contain up to 50 mg of benzyl alcohol.

Continued on p. 255

Small 5 ml preservative-free ampoules of Hep-Lock® and Hepsal® flush solution contain 0.75 mmol of sodium and 50 units of unfractionated heparin.

Full anticoagulation: To give 25 units/kg of heparin per hour, draw 1250 units for each kilogram the baby weighs into a syringe, dilute this to 50 ml with 0.9% sodium chloride, and infuse at a rate of 1 ml/hour.

Flush solution: Accurate dilution is best achieved by making any syringe containing 1 unit/ml of heparin 'flush' solution up from a 500 ml bag of 0.9% (or 0.45%) IV sodium chloride freshly prepared by the addition of 500 units of heparin. Heparin is stable in solution, so IV lines do not need to be replaced after some set time on these grounds.

Protamine sulphate: 5 ml ampoules containing 10 mg/ml cost £1.15 each.

References

(See also the relevant Cochrane reviews and UK guideline on thromboembolic disease in pregnancy **DHUK**)

Hecker JF. Potential for extending survival of peripheral intravenous infusions. *Br Med J* 1992;**304**:619–24. [SR]

Horgan MJ, Bartoletti A, Polansky S. Effect of heparin infusates in umbilical arterial catheters on frequency of thrombotic complications. *J Pediatr* 1987;**111**:774–8.

Monagle P, Chalmers E Chan A, *et al.* Antithrombotic therapy in neonates and children: American College of Chest Physicians evidenced-based clinical practice guidelines (8th edition). *Chest* 2008;**133** (Suppl 6):887S–968S.

Monagle P, Studdert DM, Newall F. Infant deaths due to heparin overdose: time for a concerted action on prevention. *J Paediatr Child Health* 2012;**48**:380–1.

Newall F, Barnes C, Igjatovic V, *et al.* Heparin-induced thrombocytopenia in children. *J Paediatr Child Health* 2003;**39**:289–92. [SR]

Newall F, Johnston L, Ignjatovic V, *et al.* Unfractionated heparin therapy in infants and children. *Pediatrics* 2009;**123**:e510–8.

Pierce CM, Wade Amok Q. Heparin-bonded central venous lines reduce thrombotic and infective complications in critically ill children. *Intensive Care Med* 2000;**26**:967–72. [RCT]

Pryce R. Cannula patency: should we use flushes or continuous fluids, or heparin? *Arch Dis Child* 2009;**94**:992–4. [SR]

Randolph AG, Cook DJ, Gonzales CA, *et al.* Benefit of heparin in peripheral venous and arterial catheters: systematic review and meta-analysis of randomised controlled trials. *Br Med J* 1998;**316**:969–75. [SR]

Shah PS, Kalyn A, Satodia P, *et al.* A randomized, controlled trial of heparin versus placebo infusion to prolong the usability of peripherally placed percutaneous central venous catheters (PCVCs) in neonates: the HIP (Heparin Infusion for PCVC) study. *Pediatrics* 2007;**119**:e284–91. [RCT].

Silvers KM, Darlow BA, Winterbourn CC. Pharmacological levels of heparin do not destabilise neonatal parenteral nutrition. *J Parent Ent Nutr* 1998;**22**:311–4.

Use

Hepatitis B vaccine provides active immunity to the hepatitis B virus (HBV); hepatitis B specific immunoglobulin (HBIg) can be used to provide immediate short-lasting passive immunity. Maternal treatment with lamivudine (q.v.) is sometimes used to prevent vertical transmission of this virus.

Hepatitis B

Hepatitis B is a major worldwide problem. Illness starts insidiously and is of variable severity. Infection can result from sexual contact, from contaminated blood or from a blood-contaminated needle. Some 2–10% of the adults so infected become chronic carriers, and nearly a quarter of these eventually develop chronic disease (with possible cirrhosis or hepatocellular carcinoma). Infection can also pass from mother to child. Transplacental passage is rare, but 80% of babies become infected during delivery, and 90% of those so infected become chronic carriers. Universal early immunisation is the policy recommended by WHO, and the approach is now being adopted in most parts of the world. Maternal screening and selective neonatal immunisation remains the approach still being adopted in Scandinavia and the United Kingdom, but this is only going to be effective if robust steps are taken to make sure that the babies so identified do get the treatment they need. The present vaccines contain 10 or 20 micrograms/ml of hepatitis B surface (Australia) antigen (HBsAg) adsorbed on an aluminium hydroxide adjuvant. Hepatitis B, like any form of hepatitis, is a notifiable infection.

Indications

Babies born to mothers with the HBsAg need prompt active immunisation. Babies born to mothers developing hepatitis B during pregnancy or born to mothers who are both surface and hepatitis B core (e) antigen (HBeAg) positive are at particularly **high risk** and need immediate bridging protection with specific HBIg as well. Where the mother's 'e' marker status is unknown or the baby weighs <1.5 kg at birth, the baby should be treated as if it were at high risk. The United Kingdom's current policy of selective immunisation can only be made to work if the policy of universal antenatal screening is fully implemented, and there is a fail-safe callback system so that those identified get all the treatment recommended. Active immunisation is also offered to all healthcare staff and to all children on haemodialysis, requiring frequent or large blood transfusions or repeated factor concentrates.

Contraindications

Side effects of immunisation (other than local soreness) are rare, and contraindications to immunisation almost non-existent (although vaccination should be delayed in the face of intercurrent illness). Vaccination should not be withheld from a high-risk woman because she is pregnant since infection in pregnancy can result in severe illness and chronic infection in the baby.

Administration

Universal vaccination: Doses are usually given at 0–2, 1–4 and 6–18 months. Premature babies given their first dose within a month of birth benefit from a fourth dose. Protection wanes over time.

Selective vaccination: At-risk babies need a first 0.5 ml intramuscular (IM) injection of hepatitis B vaccine within 24 hours of birth and booster injections 1, 2 and 12 months later. A preschool booster is also advised at 4 years. High-risk babies (as defined earlier) also need 200 units of hepatitis B specific immunoglobulin (HBIg) IM into the other thigh within 24 hours of birth (irrespective of birthweight). Breastfeeding can safely continue. This provides 95% protection, but it is prudent to check the baby's surface antigen (HBsAg) status at 12 months.

Supply

Vaccine: Give a 0.5 ml injection irrespective of which product is used. The SmithKline Beecham (Engerix B®) vaccine comes in 0.5 ml (10 micrograms) vials; Aventis Pasteur produces an interchangeable product (HBvaxPRO Paediatric®) in 0.5 ml (5 micrograms) vials. Both cost £9.10 each. Store at 2–8 °C but do not freeze. Shake before use. *Always* record administration in the child's personal health record.

Immunoglobulin: Ampoules containing 200 or 500 units of HBIg prepared by the Bio Products Laboratory are available in the United Kingdom from most Health Protection Agency laboratories. HBIg is expensive and only limited supplies are available. Store all ampoules at 4 °C.

Continued on p. 257

References

(See also full UK website guidelines **DHUK**)

Aggarwal R, Ranjan P. Preventing and treating hepatitis B infection. *Br Med J* 2004;**329**;1080–6. (See also pp. 1059–60.)

Han L, Zhang HW, Xie JX, *et al.* A meta-analysis of lamivudine for interruption of mother-to-child transmission of hepatitis B virus. *World J Gastroenterol* 2011;**17**:4321–33. [SR]

Lee C, Gong Y, Brok J, *et al.* Effect of hepatitis B immunisation in newborn infants of mothers positive for hepatitis B surface antigen: systematic review and meta-analysis. *Br Med J* 2006;**332**:328–31. [SR]

Lin Y-C, Chang M-H, Ni Y-H, *et al.* Long-term immunogenicity and efficacy of universal hepatitis B virus vaccine vaccination in Taiwan. *J Infect Dis* 2003;**187**:134–8.

Petersen KM, Bulkow LR, McMahon BJ, *et al.* Duration of hepatitis B immunity in low risk children receiving hepatitis B vaccinations from birth. *Pediatr Infect Dis J.*2004;**23**:650–5.

Zanetti AR, Mariano A, Romanò L, *et al.* Long-term immunogenicity of hepatitis B vaccination and policy for booster: an Italian multicentre study. *Lancet* 2005;**366**:1379–84. (See also pp. 1337–8.)

Use

Extravasation can cause severe tissue injury when irritant fluid leaks from a vein during infusion, and hyaluronidase can, if started within 2 hours of the injury, potentially limit such damage. It can also be used to aid subcutaneous rehydration ('hypodermoclysis') when venous access proves difficult.

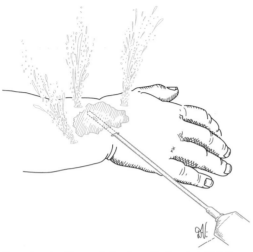

Reproduced with permission from Davies *et al.* (1994).

Pharmacology

Hyaluronidase is a naturally occurring enzyme that has a temporary and reversible depolymerising action on the polysaccharide hyaluronic acid present in the intercellular matrix of connective tissue. It can be used to enhance the permeation of local anaesthetics, subcutaneous infusions and intramuscular injections into the body tissues. It can also aid the resorption of excess tissue fluid. The product widely used since 1980 is a purified extract of sheep semen. The dose recommended here (the dose usually employed in the United Kingdom) is five times the dose generally used in the United States. Hyaluronidase was initially used on its own in an attempt to disperse damaging extravasated fluid, but immediate saline irrigation (with or without prior infiltration with hyaluronidase) with a view to washing away any irritant fluid is probably a much more effective strategy. There is still, regrettably, almost no good controlled trial evidence on which to base the management of extravasation injury.

Treating intravenous extravasation tissue damage

Clean the damaged area of skin and then infiltrate it immediately with a 0.3 ml/kg of 1% lidocaine (q.v.). Bupivacaine (q.v.) could, alternatively, be used to provide a more sustained pain relief although it takes longer to become effective. Then inject 500–1000 units of hyaluronidase into the subcutaneous tissues under the area of damaged skin. The simplest approach is merely to inject some hyaluronidase into the cannula through which extravasation occurred (if this is still in place), but it is said to be better, especially with large lesions, to make three or four small 'incisions' into the skin with a sharp scalpel round the edges of the area to be treated (Davies *et al.*, 1994), insert a blunt Veress needle into each incision in turn, inject the hyaluronidase and then irrigate the damaged tissue with 25–100 ml of 0.9% saline using the needle and three-way tap (i.e. a total of 100–400 ml of irrigating fluid in all, depending on the size of the lesion). Saline should flow freely out of the other incisions. Excess fluid can be massaged out of the incisions by gentle manipulation. The damaged area is probably then best kept reasonably moist. Dressings are a very poorly researched topic. Options include hydrocolloids, silicones or paraffin gauze (tulle gras). These dressings should aid autodebridement.

Extravasation of vasoconstrictive drugs

It has been traditional to manage the dangerous ischaemia and the dermal necrosis that can result from the extravasation of fluid containing vasoconstrictive drugs such as adrenaline, dopamine and noradrenaline (q.v.) by prompt infiltration with not more than 5 mg of phentolamine mesilate in 5 ml 0.9% sodium chloride using a fine needle. There is, however, some evidence that the application of 25 mm (16 mg) of topical 2% glyceryl trinitrate ointment (q.v.) may prove a simpler and equally effective strategy. Peripherally administered infusions of dopamine in particular seem capable of causing ischaemic tissue damage even when there has been no visible extravasation. It may be necessary to stop the infusion if there is blanching along the side of the vein.

Continued on p. 259

Emergency rehydration when venous access is difficult

A similar initial dose of hyaluronidase can be used to speed the subcutaneous delivery of any isotonic fluid.

Supply

Hyaluronidase: Ampoules containing 1500 units of hyaluronidase cost £7.60 each. Dissolve the contents in 3 ml of water for injection to give a solution containing 500 units per ml just before use.

Phentolamine mesilate: 1 ml ampoules containing 10 mg of phentolamine mesilate are available from 'special-order' manufacturers or specialist importing companies.

Needles: Veress needles are widely used to insufflate air during laparoscopy. They are available through NHS supplies from a number of supply companies.

References

(See also the relevant Cochrane reviews **DHUK**)

Allen CH, Etzwiler LS, Miller MK, *et al.* Recombinant human hyaluronidase-enabled subcutaneous pediatric rehydration. *Pediatrics* 2009;**124**:e858–67.

Casanova D, Bardot J, Magalon G. Emergency treatment of accidental infusion leakage in the newborn: report of 14 cases. *Br J Plast Surg* 2001;**54**:396–9.

Davies J, Gault D, Buchdahl R. Preventing the scars of neonatal intensive care. *Arch Dis Child Fetal Neonatal Ed* 1994;**70**:F50–1.

Lehr VT, Lulic-Botica M, Lindblad WJ, *et al.* Management of infiltration injury in neonates using DuoDerm Hydroactive gel. *Am J Perinatol* 2004;**21**:409–14.

Ramasethu J. Pharmacology review: prevention and management of extravasation injuries in neonates. *Neoreviews* 2004;**5**:e491–7.

Raszka WV, Kueser TK, Smith FR, *et al.* The use of hyaluronidase in the treatment of intravenous extravasation injuries. *J Perinatol* 1990;**10**:146–9.

Subhani M, Sridhar S, DeCristofaro JD. Phentolamine use in a neonate for the prevention of dermal necrosis caused by dopamine: a case report. *J Perinatol* 2001;**21**:324–6.

Wilkins CE, Emmerson AJB. Extravasation injuries on regional neonatal units. *Arch Dis Child Fetal Neonatal Ed* 2004;**89**:F274–5.

Use

Hydrocortisone has been in use to manage congenital adrenal abnormality and adrenal insufficiency due to hypopituitarism since 1949. Hypotension in the preterm baby often responds to low-dose intravenous (IV) hydrocortisone. Trials of use to prevent bronchopulmonary dysplasia (BPD) have not delivered much consistent benefit.

Pathophysiology

The adrenal cortex normally secretes hydrocortisone (cortisol) which has glucocorticoid activity and weak mineralocorticoid activity. It also secretes the mineralocorticoid aldosterone. Physiological replacement in adrenal insufficiency is best achieved by a combination of hydrocortisone and the artificial mineralocorticoid fludrocortisone, but where the problem is secondary to pituitary failure, mineralocorticoid replacement is not required because aldosterone production is primarily controlled by the renin–angiotensin system.

Various recessively inherited enzyme deficiencies can cause congenital adrenal hyperplasia, but nearly 95% are due to 21-hydroxylase deficiency, and most of the others to 11-hydroxylase deficiency. Diagnosis is relatively easy in girls because of virilisation and sexual ambiguity, but less easy in boys until the child presents with vomiting, failure to thrive and (ultimately) circulatory collapse: some boys are initially misdiagnosed as having pyloric stenosis. Pelvic imaging, urgent karyotyping, 17-hydroxyprogesterone (17-OHP) measurement and a urinary steroid profile confirm the diagnosis. Congenital adrenal *hypo*plasia can also present in a similar manner, or with hypoglycaemia. It is diagnosed by the presence of salt wasting in the presence of normal urinary tract, the lack of a significant cortisol response to tetracosactide (q.v.) and a normal 17-OHP level.

| Drug | Equivalent activity (mg) | | Biological Half-life (hours) |
	Glucocorticoid	Mineralocorticoid	
Fludrocortisone	0	20	–
Cortisone acetate	25	0·8	8–12
Hydrocortisone	20	1	8–12
Prednisolone	5	<1	12–36
Betamethasone	0.75	0	36–54
Dexamethasone	0.75	0	36–54

Treatment

Early neonatal hypotension: Hydrocortisone often increases blood pressure as effectively as dopamine (q.v.) and may work when a catecholamine does not. 2.5 mg/kg IV every 6 hours is usually enough to reduce the need to use other vasopressor drugs. Try and withdraw treatment within 2–4 days, because steroid use increases the risk of fungal infection and also seems to increase the risk of focal gut perforation, especially if the baby is also given ibuprofen or indometacin.

Preventing BPD: Low-dose trials (0.5 mg/kg IV twice a day for 12 days and half this for 3 days) delivered *no* benefit except to a subgroup with chorioamnionitis. Later development was not affected by such treatment.

Treating BPD: 2.5 mg/kg twice a day for 7 days, and a reducing dose for a further 2 weeks, was as effective as dexamethasone in one study and did not appear to have the latter's detrimental effect on development.

Congenital adrenal hyperplasia: 3–5 mg/m^2 of hydrocortisone once every 8 hours, plus at least 200 micrograms of fludrocortisone once a day, provides a good starting point for neonatal care. Babies with 21-hydroxylase deficiency usually need an additional 2–4 mmol/kg of sodium a day.

Adrenal hypoplasia: Production of cortisol normally averages 6–9 mg/m^2/day, and making allowance for absorption, 8–10 mg/m^2 of hydrocortisone daily in three divided doses given by mouth will meet normal replacement needs (although need may rise severalfold during any acute illness). Give a higher dose in the morning than at other times.

Continued on p. 261

Addisonian crisis: This requires IV glucose and a 10 mg bolus followed by a continuing 100 mg/ m² a day infusion of hydrocortisone. Rapid fluid replacement may be necessary with 0.9% sodium chloride. The high serum potassium almost always corrects itself, but 2 ml/kg of 10% calcium gluconate and/or an infusion of glucose and insulin (q.v.) may be needed if a cardiac arrhythmia develops. In infants of 1–12 months, give IV glucose and an initial 2–4 mg/kg slow IV bolus injection and then 2–4 mg/kg every 6 hours.

Steroid-induced adrenal suppression: See the monograph on dexamethasone.

Supply

100 mg vials of hydrocortisone (as the sodium succinate powder) cost 92p each. Reconstitute with 2 ml of water. An oral suspension can also be provided. Scored 100 microgram fludrocortisone tablets cost 5p each, and small doses can be given with relative ease because the tablets disperse readily in water.

References　　　　　　　　　　　　　　　　　　(See also the relevant Cochrane reviews)

Ng PC, Lee CH, Bnur FL, *et al*. A double-blind, randomized, controlled study of a "stress dose" of hydrocortisone for rescue treatment of refractory hypotension in preterm infants. *Pediatrics* 2006;**117**:367–75. [RCT] (See also pp. 516–8.)

Noori S, Friedlich P, Wong P, *et al*. Hemodynamic changes after low-dosage hydrocortisone administration in vasopressor-treated preterm and term neonates. *Pediatrics* 2006;**118**:1456–66.

Rademaker KJ, de Vries LS, Uiterwaal CSPM, *et al*. Postnatal hydrocortisone treatment for chronic lung disease in the preterm newborn and long-term neurodevelopmental follow-up. *Arch Dis Child Fetal Neonatal Ed* 2008;**93**:F58–63. [SR]

Use

Ibuprofen is an effective alternative to indometacin (see archived monograph), in the management of patent ductus arteriosus, and now widely used instead of paracetamol (q.v.) to control fever in babies and children.

Pharmacology

Ibuprofen (first patented in 1964) seems, in general, to be the NSAID associated with the fewest reported adverse effects when used in adults with rheumatoid arthritis. Using ibuprofen in a child who is dehydrated can cause acute severe renal failure. Gastrointestinal complications are, however, the most common problem, making NSAID treatment inappropriate in any patient with a history of peptic ulceration.

Ibuprofen is generally well absorbed when taken by mouth and excreted in the urine part metabolised. The half-life is extremely variable at birth (10–80 hours) but is similar to that seen in adults (~90 minutes) within 3 months. Oral ibuprofen has a useful role in the management of post-operative pain in childhood. Its interference with bilirubin binding to albumin and variable half-life precludes its use as a neonatal analgesic. Ibuprofen is the most widely used NSAID in children with rheumatoid arthritis.

All NSAIDs inhibit prostaglandin synthesis to some degree. There is, therefore, at least a theoretical risk that high-dose use in the third trimester of pregnancy could cause premature closure of the ductus arteriosus before birth, could prolong or delay labour or could affect post-delivery pulmonary vascular tone (see website commentary). Use around the time of conception doubles the risk of miscarriage, and there may be a marginal increase in the risk of malformation. Manufacturers remain reluctant to recommend the use of any NSAID in pregnancy, and information on recently introduced products is limited. The amount present in breast milk is undetectably small, and there is no contraindication to maternal use during lactation.

Indometacin has for a long time been used to induce ductal closure in preterm babies, because of its ability to inhibit prostaglandin synthesis. However, indometacin also causes a more marked fall in cerebral, renal and gut blood flow than other NSAIDs. While there is no evidence that these changes are of any clinical significance, ibuprofen rather than indometacin is now widely used to effect duct closure in Europe. Indometacin is no longer manufactured in an intravenous (IV) preparation, and supplies were for a time imported at high expense from North America, ironically from the company that made ibuprofen. Like indometacin, early prophylactic ibuprofen reduces the number of very preterm babies eventually undergoing duct ligation. However, there is no evidence that early prophylactic use of either drug improves the long-term prognosis for survivors.

Drug interactions

Babies given steroids while on ibuprofen are at increased risk of focal ischaemic gut perforation.

Treatment

Patent ductus: 10 mg/kg IV, traditionally infused over 15 minutes, should be followed by 5 mg/kg 24 and 48 hours later. Some studies suggest that oral treatment is just as effective. A second course of treatment may be effective when the first course is not.

Fever: An oral dose of 5-8 mg/kg, repeatable after 6 hours, is widely used to control fever in children over 3 months old (and slightly more effective than paracetamol). Avoid use in any child who is dehydrated.

Supply

IV preparations vary greatly in price. The 10 mg/ml preparation used in all the early trials was obtained by asking a local pharmacy to reconstitute one of the 300 mg vials of the lysine salt marketed by Merckle in Germany for intramuscular use with 23.4 ml of water for injection. Such vials cost £1.75 each. Formulations containing lidocaine cannot be substituted for this product. Recordati Rare Diseases (RRD) Inc. markets an IV product (ibuprofen lysine) in America. Orphan Europe markets an IV product, which has a UK licence, dissolved in trometamol, although a trial of prophylactic use raised safety issues. The 10 mg (2 ml) ampoules cost £72. A sugar-free 20 mg/ml oral suspension is available from community pharmacists without prescription (100 ml costs £1.60).

Continued on p. 263

References   (See also the relevant Cochrane reviews and UK guideline **DHUK**)

Cherif A, Khrouf N, Jabnoun S, *et al*. Randomized pilot study comparing oral ibuprofen with intravenous ibuprofen in very low birth weight infants with patent ductus arteriosus. *Pediatrics* 2008;**122**:e1256–61. [RCT]

Dani C, Bertini G, Pezzati M, *et al*. Prophylactic ibuprofen for the prevention of intraventricular hemorrhage among preterm infants: a multicenter, randomised study. *Pediatrics* 2005;**115**:1529–35. [RCT]

Li D-K, Liu L, Odouli R. Exposure to non-steroidal anti-inflammatory drugs during pregnancy and risks of miscarriage: population based cohort study. *Br Med J* 2003;**327**:367–71.

Richards J, Johnson A, Fox G, *et al*. A second course of ibuprofen is effective in the closure of a clinically significant PDA in ELBW infants. *Pediatrics* 2009;**124**:e287–93.

Su B-H, Chiu H-Y, Hsieh H-Y, *et al*. Comparison of ibuprofen and indometacin for early targeted treatment of patent ductus arteriosus in extremely premature infants: a randomised trial. *Arch Dis Child Fetal Neonatal Ed* 2008;**93**:F94–9. [RCT]

Thomas RL, Parker GC, Van Overmeire B, *et al*. A meta-analysis of ibuprofen versus indomethacin for closure of patent ductus. *Eur J Pediatr* 2005;**164**:135–40. [SR]

Van Overmeire B, Touw D, Schepens PJC, *et al*. Ibuprofen pharmacokinetics in preterm infants with patent ductus arteriosus. *Clin Pharmacol Ther* 2001;**70**:336–43.

Use

Imipenem is a useful reserve antibiotic that is active against a very wide range of bacteria. Cilastatin is always administered as well. Meropenem (q.v.) is more appropriate where meningitis is suspected, has fewer adverse effects and is easier to give, but little information on neonatal use is yet available.

Pharmacology

This β-lactam antibiotic, developed in 1983, is active against a very wide range of Gram-positive and Gram-negative aerobic and anaerobic bacteria. Some methicillin-resistant staphylococci, group D streptococci and *Pseudomonas* species are resistant to imipenem. The drug acts synergistically with the aminoglycosides *in vitro* and is sometimes prescribed with an aminoglycoside in the treatment of *Pseudomonas* infection in order to prevent emergence of drug resistance. Like all carbapenems, imipenem is a valuable reserve antibiotic that should only be used on the advice of a consultant microbiologist.

Because imipenem can cause renal toxicity and because it is partially inactivated within the kidney, it is always given in combination with cilastatin, a specific dehydropeptidase enzyme inhibitor that blocks imipenem's renal breakdown. Imipenem is widely distributed in many body tissues and crosses the placenta, but CSF levels are low, and the drug is not recommended for CNS infection. Both imipenem and cilastatin are rapidly eliminated by a combination of glomerular filtration and tubular secretion into the urine in adults, the plasma half-life being under 1 hour. Less is known about drug handling in the neonatal period; the half-life of imipenem is increased threefold, but that of cilastatin increases 11-fold in the first week of life. As a result, any dose regimen that is appropriate for the bactericidal ingredient imipenem will result in the progressive accumulation of cilastatin when the standard product containing equal amounts of both products is used. Whether this matters is not known. A 4:1 imipenem/cilastatin formulation might be better. In its absence prolonged, or high dose, treatment should be employed with caution. Both drugs are rapidly cleared from the body during haemodialysis.

Adverse effects include localised erythema and thrombophlebitis. Neurotoxic reactions including a progressive encephalopathy with seizures have been seen, sometimes preceded by myoclonic twitching, especially in patients with an existing CNS abnormality. For this reason, it is best avoided in meningitis. Meropenem (q.v.) has not been shown to cause seizures in infants with meningitis and so a better alternative in cases with multi-resistant organisms. Rapid infusion may cause nausea and vomiting. Diarrhoea can occur, and this may, on occasion, be the first sign of pseudomembranous colitis.

The manufacturers have advised against the use of imipenem with cilastatin in pregnancy because of increased embryonic loss in animal studies and have not, as yet, been ready to recommend their use in children <3 months old. Substantial placental transfer occurs, but there is no evidence of teratogenicity. Treatment during lactation also seems safe since the baby receives <1% of the weight-related maternal dose and the drug is largely inactivated in the gut.

Drug prescribing

The drug should technically be referred to as 'imipenem with cilastatin', but omitting the words 'with cilastatin' is unlikely to cause misunderstanding, since all commercial preparations contain both drugs. Thus, the dose should be expressed in terms of the amount of imipenem.

Treatment

Give 20 mg/kg of imipenem by intravenous (IV) infusion over 30 minutes once every 12 hours in the first week of life, every 8 hours in babies 1–3 weeks old and every 6 hours in babies 4 or more weeks old. Use with caution in patients with any suspected CNS abnormality. Dosage frequency should be reduced if there is any evidence of renal failure, and treatment stopped altogether if there is anuria unless dialysis is instituted.

Supply and administration

Vials suitable for IV use contain 500 mg of imipenem monohydrate, with an equal quantity of the sodium salt of cilastatin, as a powder ready for reconstitution. Vials cost £12 each. Dilute the content of the 500 mg vial with 100 ml of 10% glucose or glucose saline immediately before use to obtain a solution containing 5 mg/ml. (The drug can be prepared using a less concentrated solution of glucose or glucose saline where necessary.) Shake the vial well until the powder is all

Continued on p. 265

dissolved and then infuse the prescribed dose slowly over 30 minutes. Discard the remaining unused solution promptly. Avoid intramuscular use in young children. A 20 mg/kg dose contains 0.07 mmol/kg of sodium.

References

Lau KK, Kink RJ, Jones DP. Myoclonus associated with intraperitoneal imipenem. *Pediatr Nephrol* 2004;**19**:700–1.

Matsuda S, Suzuki M, Oh K, *et al*. Pharmacokinetic and clinical studies on imipenem/cilastatin sodium in the perinatal period. *Jp J Antibiot* 1988;**41**:1731–41.

Mouton JW, Touzw DJ, Horrevorts AM, *et al*. Comparative pharmacokinetics of the carbapenems: clinical implications. *Clin Pharmacokinet* 2000;**39**:185–201.

Reed MD, Kleigman RM, Yamashita TS, *et al*. Clinical pharmacology of imipenem and cilastatin in premature infants during the first week of life. *Antimicrob Agents Chemother* 1990;**34**:1172–7.

Stuart RL, Turnidge J, Grayson ML. Safety of imipenem in neonates. *Pediatr Infect Dis J* 1995;**14**:804–5.

Zhanel GG, Wiebe R, Dilay L, *et al*. Comparative review of the carbapenems. *Drugs* 2007;**67**:1027–52.

Aim

National policies exist in most countries to provide protection against a range of potentially serious infectious illnesses. Separate monographs are available for BCG vaccination (against TB) and for immunisation against *Haemophilus influenzae*; hepatitis B; measles, mumps and rubella (MMR); meningococcus C; pneumococcus; polio; and diphtheria, tetanus and pertussis (DTP). All the above products (other than the hepatitis B vaccine) are available free of charge in the United Kingdom and in many other countries.

Basic schedule

UK schedules were simplified in 2004 with the introduction of a new five-in-one vaccine, and augmented in 2006 with the addition of the pneumococcal vaccine, and again in 2013 with the introduction of the rotavirus vaccine. Immunisation should never be delayed because of prematurity or low body weight. Whilst most live vaccines should be avoided in a neonatal unit setting because of a theoretical risk to other infants, rotavirus (q.v.) can be given. This and the other routine vaccinations described below should always be started before discharge in babies spending more than 7 weeks in hospital after birth.

Birth	Give selected babies BCG, *and* start hepatitis B vaccination in *at-risk* babies (q.v.)	
8 weeks	DTaP/IPV/Hib (one injection) *and* pneumococcal vaccine (separate injection) *and* rotavirus (orally)	Pediacel® Prevenar 13® Rotarix®
12 weeks	DTaP/IPV/Hib vaccine (second dose) *and* MenC (separate injection) *and* rotavirus (orally)	Pediacel® NeisVac-C® *or* Meningitec® Rotarix®
16 weeks	DTaP/IPV/Hib (third dose) *and* pneumococcal vaccine (separate injection)	Pediacel® Prevenar 13®
Between 12 and 13 months	Hib/MenC (one injection) *and* MMR (separate injection) *and* pneumococcal vaccine (third dose – in a separate injection)	Menitorix® Priorix® *or* MMR II® Prevenar 13®
2–17 years (annually)	Seasonal influenza vaccine (intranasal) – if this is the child's first dose, a second dose is given 4 weeks after the first	Fluenz®
3½–5 years	DTaP/IPV *or* dTaP/IPV *and* MMR vaccine	Repevax® *or* Infanrix-IPV® Priorix® *or* MMR II®
12–13 years (girls only)	Human papillomavirus vaccination (HPV 6,11,16,18) Given in three injections: the second injection is given 1–2 months after the first. The third is given at least 3 to 6 months after second	Gardasil®
13–18 years	Td/IPV vaccine *and* MenC (booster dose) in a separate injection	Revaxis® NeisVac® *or* Meningitec®

DTaP/IPV/Hib, combined diphtheria, tetanus, pertussis, inactivated polio and *Haemophilus* vaccine; MenC, meningococcal C vaccine; Hib/MenC, combined *Haemophilus* and meningococcal C vaccine; MMR, combined measles, mumps and rubella vaccine;
DTaP/IPV, diphtheria, tetanus, pertussis and polio; Td/IPV, tetanus, diphtheria and inactivated polio vaccine.

Foreign travel

Advice for families on immunisation prior to foreign travel is available from pharmacies, general practice surgeries, post offices and travel agents and the Internet (www.nhs.uk/Conditions/Travel-immunisations/Pages/Introduction.aspx and www.fitfortravel.nhs.uk). A sister website, www.travax.nhs.uk (registration required), has information aimed at healthcare professionals. More detailed advice on this and on malaria prophylaxis is also given in the British National

Continued on p. 267

Formulary for Children. Professionals can also get advice from the *National Travel Health Network and Centre* in the United Kingdom by ringing 0845 602 6712 during normal office hours.

Reactions to immunisation

Most reactions to immunisation are not serious. Older children sometimes faint, and a few hyperventilate. Even quite young infants sometimes respond to pain or sudden surprise with a syncopal attack. Blue breath-holding attacks, in which a child cries and then stops breathing, turning limp and unconscious can occur, and can end with a seizure. Attacks of stiffness and pallor, with self-limiting bradycardia or asystole (reflex anoxic seizures), are less common but well documented. Infants prone to these may also have a seizure if they become feverish after immunisation. Sudden brief loss of consciousness and body tone a few hours after vaccination for pertussis is another well-described, but poorly understood, clinical entity (the hypotonic–hyporeflexic episode [HHE] syndrome). Such events should *not* be interpreted as anaphylactic or encephalopathic. Loss of consciousness should only last 5–10 minutes, and recovery is complete without treatment. Such episodes should be managed as though they were a fainting attack.

Anaphylaxis in children under one: True anaphylactic reactions after immunisation are *very* rare and seldom severe. A single 10 micrograms/kg dose of adrenaline (q.v.) given by deep intramuscular (IM), not subcutaneous, injection serves to contain most reactions and is all that can realistically be made available in most community settings. Only a rough estimate of weight is ever needed when giving adrenaline – a standard 150 micrograms dose, repeatable once after 5 minutes, is widely recommended. This is the smallest dose available in the adrenaline auto-injectors (EpiPen® Jr Auto-Injector 0.15 mg, Anapen® 150 and Jext® 150 micrograms). A 1 microgram/kg dose can be given as an intravenous (IV) bolus.

Where urticaria or slowly progressive peripheral oedema is all that develops, it can help to give 250 micrograms/kg of the H_1 histamine antagonist chlorphenamine (q.v.) promptly IM or by slow IV injection (even though the manufacturers have not yet endorsed its use in children).

If there is *serious* stridor, breathing difficulty or progressive angio-oedema, some advocate giving 0.4 ml/kg of a 1 mg/ml (1:1000) solution of L-adrenaline by nebuliser after administering a first IM dose. Then give 250 micrograms/kg of chlorphenamine IM or preferably IV diluted in 5 ml of 0.9% sodium chloride. Give oxygen, and take whatever steps are necessary to ensure that the airway can be secured should this become necessary. The dose of nebulised adrenaline can be repeated after 30 minutes.

Wheeze and bronchospasm (seen particularly in patients with a past history of asthma) respond best to nebulised salbutamol (q.v.); 25 mg of IM or IV hydrocortisone (q.v.) may also be of benefit. Use 0.9% sodium chloride rather than colloid if circulatory collapse makes volume expansion appropriate. Lay the child flat, raise the legs, and send for help, but never leave the patient unattended. While severe anaphylactic shock can cause death, there has not been a single death using any of these products in the United Kingdom since formal monitoring began 25 years ago. Notify all untoward events in the United Kingdom to the Medicines and Health Products Regulatory Agency (http://yellowcard.mhra.gov.uk).

Problems in the preterm baby

Irrespective of weight or gestation at birth, a course of primary immunisation should be started in *every* baby after 8 weeks. While this seems to trigger a marginal increase in self-limiting apnoea for the next 2–3 days, no such increase could be detected in a recent controlled trial involving 190 babies. Although very preterm babies mount a less vigorous antibody response (especially those on dexamethasone for chronic lung disease), immunisation should not be delayed, because such children are likely to become seriously ill if they encounter whooping cough infection in the first year of life. The suggestion that the most vulnerable children should be given a fourth dose of the DTP vaccine at a year has now been discounted, except in countries where diphtheria still occurs with any frequency. The United Kingdom's JCVI advocates immunisation of stable hospitalised infants at the appropriate time, stating that, provided standard infection control precautions are maintained, even administration of the live attenuated rotavirus vaccine to hospitalised infants would be expected to carry a low risk for transmission.

Managing fever

Although giving prophylactic paracetamol (three 15 mg/kg doses over 24 hours) reduces the risk of fever after immunisation, high fever (<39 °C) is very uncommon, and such treatment often reduces the antibody response.

Continued on p. 268

Measles

In communities where measles is still prevalent, a case can be made for offering two doses of the combined measles (MMR) vaccine 4 months apart to all at serious risk once they are 4–5 months old. If an *un*immunised child ≥ 6 months old *does* come into contact with a case of measles (and infectivity lasts from 4 days before to 4 days after the rash appears), a single dose of MMR or measles vaccine will usually prevent overt illness if given within 3 days of exposure. These babies should still be given two further doses of the MMR vaccine at the normal time. Babies less than 6 months old are probably best offered 250 mg of normal human immunoglobulin (q.v.).

HIV infection

Babies with suspected or proven human immunodeficiency virus (HIV) infection need protection from diphtheria, tetanus and whooping cough and from *Haemophilus*, pneumococcal and meningococcal infection like any other child. Consider annual vaccination against the influenza virus. These children should be given the inactivated, rather than the live (oral), polio vaccine and only given the MMR vaccine if the CD4 count is greater than 500 cells/μl. See the monograph on rotavirus vaccine (q.v.) for advice about that vaccine. Babies in the United Kingdom are not routinely given BCG.

Patients with sickle cell disease or no spleen

Babies with *situs ambiguus* and certain cardiac syndromes are often born without a spleen, making them dangerously prone to infection. While haematological features (Howell–Jolly bodies, target cells, etc.) are suggestive, imaging is essential for diagnosis. Give amoxicillin (q.v.) (125 mg twice a day) until the baby is immunised against *H. influenzae* and a similar dose of phenoxymethylpenicillin (penicillin V) once immunised. They benefit from being offered the influenza vaccine and should eventually receive both the available pneumococcal vaccines (q.v.) and all the other usual vaccines. Do the same for children with homozygous (SS or Sb0Thal) sickle cell disease.

Consent

Time must be taken to ensure that parents have had all their questions answered. A record of any issues raised, and of any verbal consent given, should then be placed in the case notes. Prior written consent implies general agreement to the child's inclusion in an immunisation programme, but does not address the issue of current fitness and is no substitute for the presence and involvement of a parent when any vaccine is given.

Documentation

Record the batch number and the site of vaccination in the case notes, and also record what has been done in the family copy of the child's personal health folder. Always tell the family doctor of every vaccination undertaken in a hospital setting as well, in the United Kingdom, as those who maintain the community child health register.

References

(See also the RCPCH 2002 guideline on immunising the immunocompromised child **DHUK**)

AAP. *Red book. 2012 report of the committee on infectious diseases*, 29th edn. Elk Grove Village, IL: American Academy of Pediatrics, 2012.

Collinson A. Safety in numbers: anaphylaxis risk in childhood immunisation. *Arch Dis Child* 2012;**97**:485–6.

Klein NP, Massolo ML, Greene J, *et al.* Risk factors for developing apnea after immunisation in the neonatal intensive care unit. *Pediatrics* 2008;**121**:463–9.

Manillavasagan G, Ramsay M. Protecting infants against measles in England and Wales: a review. *Arch Dis Child* 2009;**94**:681–5.

Pourcyrous M, Korones SB, Arheart KL, *et al.* Primary immunisation of premature infants with gestational age <35 weeks: cardiorespiratory complications and C-reactive protein responses associated with administration of single and multiple separate vaccines simultaneously. *J Pediatr* 2007;**151**:167–72.

Prymula R, Siegrist C-A, Chlibek R, *et al.* Effect of prophylactic paracetamol administration at time of vaccination on febrile reactions and antibody responses in children: two open-label, randomised controlled trials. *Lancet* 2009;**374**:1339–50. [RCT] (See also pp. 1305–6.)

Tse Y, Rylance G. Emergency management of anaphylaxis in children and young people: new guidance from the Resuscitation Council (UK). *Arch Dis Child Educ Pract Ed* 2009;**94**:97–101.

Use

Pooled human immunoglobulin (Ig) can modify the effects of several severe alloimmune ill-nesses and is also used in a number of infectious diseases. Disease-specific Ig are active against only the disease for which use is intended and are used in certain circumstances.

Physiology

Babies produce few antibodies until they are 3–4 months old, although they acquire maternal IgG transplacentally in the last 3 months of pregnancy. Preterm babies have low levels at birth which can decline further, and this may be one reason why they are at risk of nosocomial (hospital-acquired) infection in the first few weeks of life. A systematic review of 19 trials (with >5000 preterm or LBW infants) suggested that *prophylactic use* of intravenous (IV) Ig (often 700 mg/kg IV every 2 weeks) reduced the rate of late-onset infection by 3–4% but had no impact on overall mortality. In contrast, however, another systematic review and one of the largest randomised neonatal trials suggested that when used in the **treatment** of suspected or proven infection, Ig had no benefit.

Pharmacology

Human Ig contains IgG prepared from pooled plasma collected during blood donation. It is screened for hepatitis B surface antigen and for antibodies against hepatitis C virus and HIV types 1 and 2. The final product contains antibodies against a range of common infectious diseases including measles, mumps, varicella, hepatitis A and other common viruses and can be used to provide immediate but short-lasting passive immunity to a range of viral and bacterial illnesses. Donor and PCR screening, heat treatment and alcohol fractionation combine to make HNIG safer than fresh frozen plasma (q.v.) or cryoprecipitate. The process also removes IgM, the main source of anti-T antibody that some have claimed could be a cause of haemolysis in patients with necrotising enterocolitis and *Clostridium difficile* infection. Infusion not infrequently causes a headache and generalised discomfort. Disease-specific Ig for the treatment of hepatitis B (q.v.), rabies, tetanus and varicella zoster (q.v.) as well as anti-D (Rh$_0$) Ig for use in rhesus-negative pregnancies. Use of anti-D (Rh$_0$) Ig can lead to a weakly positive Coombs test in the baby.

Treatment

Fetal thrombocytopenia: Some treat severe alloimmune disease by giving the mother 1 g/kg of IV human Ig weekly. Very severe disease may make fetal platelet transfusions necessary.

Neonatal thrombocytopenia: Babies with immune thrombocytopenia who fulfil the criteria given in the monograph on platelets should be given 400 mg/kg (or even 1 g/kg) of human Ig IV once a day for 1–3 days. Some give oral prednisolone (2 mg/kg every 12 hours for 4–6 days) instead.

Neonatal haemochromatosis: Give women with a previously affected child 1 g/kg IV weekly from 18 weeks to prevent liver damage caused by a materno-fetal alloimmune reaction. Exchange transfusion followed by 1 g/kg of Ig IV may improve the prognosis for babies diagnosed at birth.

Rhesus haemolytic disease: 500 mg/kg IV given over 2 hours reduces the need for photo-therapy and exchange transfusion but increases the likelihood that the baby will need a 'top-up' transfusion.

Supply and administration

A range of IV preparations are available, but all UK use has to be registered because preparations of reliable quality are currently in short supply. A 2.5 or 3 g pack typically costs about £100; other pack sizes are also produced. Storage at 4 °C is recommended for some products. Preparations designed for intramuscular use, though cheaper, must *not* be given IV.

Reconstitute where necessary by adding 20 ml of 0.9% sodium chloride or diluent (as provided) to each gram of lyophilisate immediately before use to obtain a preparation containing 50 mg/ml. Do not shake. Wait until the solution is clear. Start to infuse at a rate of 30 mg/kg/hour (i.e. at 0.6 ml/kg/ hour when using the 50 mg/ml solution), and double the rate twice at half-hourly intervals to a maximum rate of 120 mg/kg/hour, unless there is a systemic reaction (usually vomiting or hypotension). Discard all unused material.

Antibody titres can vary widely between preparations from different manufacturers, and formulations are not interchangeable. Any patient requiring long-term treatment should be maintained on the same formulation throughout.

Continued on p. 270

References (See also relevant national guidelines and the Cochrane reviews)

Elalfy MS, Elbarbary NS, Abaza HW. Early intravenous immunoglobulin (two-dose regimen) in the management of severe Rh hemolytic disease of newborn – a prospective randomized controlled trial. *Eur J Pediatr* 2011;**170**:461–7. [RCT]

INIS Collaborative Group. Treatment of neonatal sepsis with intravenous immune globulin. *N Engl J Med* 2011;**365**:1201–11. [RCT]

Nasseri R, Mamouri GA, Babaei H. Intravenous immunoglobulin in ABO and Rh haemolytic disease of the newborn. *Saudi Med J* 2006;**27**:1827–30. [RCT]

Rand ER, Karpen SJ, Kelly S, *et al.* Treatment of neonatal haemochromatosis with exchange transfusion and intravenous immunoglobulin. *J Pediatr* 2009;**155**:566–71.

Roifman CM, ed. Intravenous immunoglobulin treatment of immunodeficiency. *Immunol Allergy Clin North Am* 2008;**28**(4);691–886.

Salomon O, Rosenberg N. Predicting risk severity and response of fetal neonatal alloimmune thrombocytopenia. *Br J Haematol* 2013;**162**:304–12.

Whitington PF, Kelly S. Outcome of pregnancies at risk for neonatal hemochromatosis is improved by treatment with high-dose intravenous immunoglobulin. *Pediatrics* 2008;**121**:e1615–21.

Use

The influenza virus is an important worldwide cause of serious upper and lower respiratory tract infection which can occur at any time of year but peaks in the winter months. It is a rare cause of CNS infection.

Influenza

Epidemics of influenza, or flu, occur every winter, and the most prevalent subtype varies from year to year, making annual immunisation the only way to provide near-certain protection. Currently available vaccines are trivalent, containing two subtypes of influenza A plus one type B virus. These have provided 70–80% protection, after 10-14 days, from strains that are well matched for those in the vaccine in recent years and provided protection that lasts about a year. Children under 5 (and especially under 2) years old are the most likely to become infected, but it is adults over 65 who are more likely to become seriously ill if they do become infected – the risk being 18-fold higher for those over 85. Women are at slightly more risk during pregnancy and can occasionally become rapidly unwell. A live attenuated intra-nasal vaccine is now incorporated into the UK immunisation schedule for children from the age of 2 years. Vaccination is not contraindicated during lactation.

Indications for giving the inactivated vaccine

Pregnant women: There is good evidence that vaccination is safe during pregnancy and can also provide the baby with significant short-term protection from infection by viral strains against which the vaccine is active.

Children at least 6 months old: These children can be offered the current trivalent inactivated vaccine just before each annual epidemic begins. Ideally, two 0.5 ml doses should be given at least 4 weeks apart the first year that vaccination is offered. A single dose is adequate in subsequent years.

Indications for giving the live attenuated vaccine

Children over the age of 2 years: Children of 2–3 years of age, irrespective of clinical risk, and children of any age in clinical risk groups should be offered the live attenuated intra-nasal vaccine unless it is unsuitable. Young children in the 'at-risk' groups are given two doses in the first year. At other times and in other children, a single dose is sufficient.

Contraindications

Flu vaccine can be given at the same time as other live or inactivated vaccines, but preferably into a different limb, and certainly at least 2.5 cm away from any other injection site. Anaphylactic reactions are rare, but a mammalian cell-based, and *not* a hens' egg-based, product *must* be used if there is a history of egg allergy or of an adverse reaction to any earlier vaccine product.

Documentation

Record the batch number and the site of vaccination in the case notes, and inform the family doctor of any vaccination undertaken in a hospital setting.

Protecting children <6 months old

The manufacturer has not yet sought permission to advocate use in children less than a year old, but there is growing experience of its use in the most vulnerable 6–12-month-old babies. Efficacy is likely to be progressively more limited in babies younger than this. Maternal vaccination during pregnancy does provide some short-term protection. The most effective oral antiviral drug currently available is oseltamivir (q.v.), the usual adult dose being one 75 mg capsule twice a day for 5 days, to be started just as soon as there are clear symptoms. Pregnancy is *not* a contraindication. If the aim is to offer *treatment*, start this within 48 hours of the onset of symptoms regardless of vaccination status, and give a dose twice a day for 5 days, the generally recommended dose being 2 mg/kg (often simplified to 12 mg in children less than 3 months old, 18 mg in babies 3–5 months old and 24 mg at 6–12 months). Reduce the dose in renal failure. There is also some limited support for *prophylactic* use in particularly vulnerable unvaccinated babies who are known to have been exposed to the virus. Give these babies the same dose of oseltamivir once a day for 10 days.

Continued on p. 272

Supply and administration

A range of trivalent and tetravalent inactivated vaccines become available annually (cost £5–£6) in 0.5 ml pre-filled syringes. Tetravalent products are not licensed for use in children <3 years. Shake well before use, and give by deep intramuscular (IM) injection into the anterolateral aspect of the thigh (or deltoid in adults). Store all products in the dark at 2–8 °C.

A trivalent live attenuated vaccine for intra-nasal administration is available in 0.2 ml applicators. 0.1 ml is given via each nostril.

References

(See also the relevant Cochrane reviews and UK guidelines **DHUK**)

Eisenberg KW, Szilagyi PG, Fairbrother G, *et al.* Vaccine effectiveness against laboratory-confirmed influenza in children 6 to 59 months of age during the 2003–2004 influenza seasons. *Pediatrics* 2008;**122**:911–9.

Erlewyn-Lajeurnesse M, Braithwaite N, Lucas JSA, *et al.* Recommendations for the administration of influenza vaccine in children allergic to egg. *Br Med J* 2009;**339**:912–5. [*Br Med J* 2009;**339**:b3680.] (See also correspondence p. 1100.)

Pitman RJ, White LJ, Sculpher M. Estimating the clinical impact of introducing paediatric influenza vaccination in England and Wales. *Vaccine* 2012;**30**:1208–24.

Richards JL, Hansen C, Bredfeldt C, *et al.* Neonatal outcomes after antenatal influenza immunization during the 2009 H1N1 influenza pandemic: impact on preterm birth, birth weight, and small for gestational age birth. *Clin Infect Dis* 2013;**56**:1216–22.

Szilagi PG, Fairbrother G, Griffin MR, *et al.* Influenza vaccine effectiveness among children 6 to 59 months of age during 2 influenza seasons. *Arch Pediatr Adolesc Med* 2008;**162**:943–51.

Zaman K, Roy E, Arifeen SE, *et al.* Effectiveness of maternal influenza immunisation in mothers and infants. *N Engl J Med* 2008;**358**:1555–64. [RCT]

Use

Insulin, first isolated from β cells in the islets of the pancreas in 1922, is used to treat diabetes mellitus. It can also be used to correct unusually high blood glucose levels (hyperglycaemia) in the neonate and to counteract any dangerous rise in the blood potassium level (hyperkalaemia).

Pathophysiology

Inadequate insulin production and abnormal resistance to its secretion cause type 1 and type 2 diabetes respectively. All women with diabetes need to optimise glucose homeostasis during conception and pregnancy, aiming for a glycated haemoglobin (HbA$_{1c}$) level <60 mmol/mol to minimise the risk of congenital malformation and miscarriage. Since insulin does not cross the placenta or appear in human milk, it is the treatment of choice for diabetes during pregnancy and lactation. Some women also become less able to stabilise their blood glucose levels during pregnancy ('gestational' diabetes), and insulin, metformin or a sulphonylurea drug such as glibenclamide will reduce the risk of fetal macrosomia (usually defined as a >4 kg baby) if dietary advice alone does not suffice.

Newborn babies are relatively intolerant of glucose, and the pancreatic response to an intravenous (IV) load is relatively sluggish. Giving 10% glucose at a rate appropriate to normal fluid and calorie needs may sometimes exceed the very preterm child's ability to metabolise glucose or turn glucose into glycogen, and a glucose uptake of more than 14 mg/kg/minute is not called for in the first week of life. While in one trial, use of a continuous IV infusion of insulin in babies receiving parenteral nutrition did result in babies getting 20% more glucose without increasing the incidence of *hyper*glycaemia, there were more episodes of *hypo*glycaemia and more neonatal deaths, so this strategy cannot be endorsed.

Nevertheless, although high levels usually fall quickly if less glucose is given for 6–12 hours, it can be appropriate to give insulin for a time to ***correct*** high blood levels (>12 mmol/l) if they persist once sepsis or some other intercurrent illness has been ruled out. Note that glucose in the *urine* (glycosuria) will not cause excess water loss until the *blood* glucose level exceeds 15 mmol/l.

Arrhythmia due to sudden unexplained neonatal hyperkalaemia (K$^+$>7.5 mmol/l) is occasionally seen in very preterm babies especially in the first 3 days of life. A continuous infusion of glucose and insulin can be used to control this and will usually work quicker than a polystyrene sulphonate resin enema (q.v.). Salbutamol (q.v.) and correction of acidosis with sodium bicarbonate (q.v.) may also help.

Treatment

Hyperglycaemia: Giving an IV infusion of 0.02–0.125 units/kg of insulin per hour, adjusted according to blood glucose levels, can be used to bring down persistently high blood glucose levels (>12 mmol/l).

Hyperkalaemia: Infuse 0.5 units/kg of insulin per hour IV in 10% glucose – watch glucose levels closely.

Neonatal diabetes: This rare condition, which presents with acidosis, dehydration and hyperglycaemia (usually >20 mmol/l), but little ketosis, responds to a very low dose of insulin. Giving 0.5–3.0 units/kg/ day is usually adequate. Try giving this subcutaneously instead of IV if problems persist for more than 2 weeks. Treatment can usually be tailed off within 4–6 weeks, and if evidence of type 1 diabetes does re-emerge, this can usually be controlled by giving 0.1–0.4 mg/kg of glibenclamide by mouth twice a day.

Compatibility

Insulin can be added (terminally) to a line containing TPN (with or without lipid) or containing dobutamine (but not dopamine), glyceryl trinitrate, heparin, midazolam, milrinone, morphine, nitroprusside or propofol.

Supply and administration

10 ml multi-dose vials of human soluble insulin containing 100 units/ml cost approximately £7 each. They are best stored at 4 °C but contain *m*-cresol as a preservative and can be kept for a month at room temperature. Do not freeze. Any short-acting soluble product (such as Humulin S®) can be used for IV or subcutaneous administration. These products should not be used if they appear hazy or coloured. Long-acting slow-release products, containing a cloudy zinc suspension, are only suitable for subcutaneous use.

Continued on p. 274

Take 0.05 ml (5 units) from the vial and dilute to 50 ml with 0.9% sodium chloride to obtain a preparation containing 0.1 unit/ml. An infusion rate of 0.1 ml/kg/hour will give a dose of 0.01 units/kg/hour. The IV solution is stable and does not need to be changed daily, but insulin adheres to plastic, and consistent IV delivery will not be achieved for several hours unless the delivery tubing is first flushed with at least 20 ml of fluid. It is also more consistent if the set is left standing with fluid in it for an hour before it is flushed through. While this is less essential when treatment is first started because the response will determine the initial infusion rate, failure to prime any *replacement* set could well destabilise glucose control.

Pharmacies can provide an oral suspension of glibenclamide on request.

References (See also the relevant Cochrane reviews)

Beardsall K, Vanhaesebrouck S, Ogilvy-Stuart AL, *et al.* Early insulin therapy in very-low-birth-weight infants. *N Engl J Med* 2008;**359**:1873–84. [RCT] (See also pp. 1951–3.)

Cody D. Infant and toddler diabetes. *Arch Dis Child* 2007;**92**:716–9.

Crowther CA, Hiller JE, Moss JR. Effect of treatment of gestational diabetes mellitus on pregnancy outcomes. *N Engl J Med* 2005;**352**:2477–86. [RCT] (See also pp. 2544–6.)

Hey E. Hyperglycaemia and the very preterm baby. *Semin Fetal Neonatal Med* 2005;**10**:377–87.

Pearson ER, Flechter I, Njølstrad PR, *et al.* Switching from insulin to oral sulfonylureas in patients with diabetes due to Kir6·2 mutations. *N Engl J Med* 2006;**355**:467–77. (See also pp. 507–10.)

Use

Ipratropium is an anticholinergic drug used for the treatment of asthma and is frequently prescribed in the wheezy infant including those with bronchiolitis. Ipratropium blocks muscarinic acetylcholine receptors which results in decreased contractility of bronchial smooth muscle.

Pharmacology

Ipratropium is a synthetic quaternary ammonium compound that is structurally similar to atropine but with an isopropyl group at the N atom. Systemic availability is limited to 6.9% when inhaled and 2% when taken orally. This latter aspect is important as ~90% of any inhaled dose tends to be swallowed. The half-life is 3.2–3.8 hours.

There are five muscarinic receptor subtypes (designated M1 through M5), all belonging to the family of transmembrane G-protein-coupled receptors. In the human lung, bronchoconstriction is brought about by stimulation of the M3 receptors on smooth muscle. Ipratropium blocks all muscarinic receptor subtypes with equal affinity which is a potential drawback as blocking M2 receptors significantly potentiates vagally induced bronchoconstriction. This had led to the development of 'selective' muscarinic receptor antagonists like tiotropium which dissociates from the M2 receptor more rapidly than the M3 receptor. Tiotropium has yet to be tested in older children, let alone infants.

The doses of ipratropium used in the treatment of wheeze may be inadequate; although not extensively studied in children, the maximal dilating dose of ipratropium in adult COPD patients is 500 micrograms, yet the dose in each actuation of the metered-dose inhaler is 20 micrograms.

Ipratropium is sometimes used to treat wheeze in infants with established bronchopulmonary dysplasia where they provide some symptomatic relief. The effects of any bronchodilator in acute viral infections (viral-induced wheeze) are highly variable and do not impact on overall hospitalisation rates or length of stay; they may however improve symptoms. Likewise, bronchodilators do not appear to have any major benefits in bronchiolitis. It is not surprising, therefore, that there is considerable variation in practices in treating the wheezy infant (with or without RSV infection).

Maternal use, either during pregnancy or lactation, is usually limited to those women with severe asthma, and because of the poor systemic absorption, it is unlikely to result in either the fetus or breastfed infant being exposed to clinically relevant amounts.

Treatment

Metered-dose inhaler: 20 micrograms three to four times daily via an appropriate spacer.
Nebuliser: 125 micrograms three to four times daily.

Toxicity

Unlike atropine (q.v.), systemic toxic effects are rare; however, use, particularly of the nebulised drug, may result in unilateral (or sometimes bilateral) mydriasis which can alarm parents.

Supply and administration

A 200 dose inhaler providing 20 micrograms of ipratropium bromide per inhalation costs £5.00. A variety of spacers are available, not all of which are compatible with the ipratropium inhaler; one that works is the AeroChamber® plus. This is available in infant (orange) and child (yellow) sizes with a mask and costs £7.40.

Ipratropium bromide nebuliser solution (250 micrograms/ml) is available in 1 ml unit dose vials costing 22p; the solution can be further diluted with 0.9% sodium chloride to make administration easier.

References

(See also the Cochrane review)

Brundage KL, Mohsini KG, Froese AB, *et al*. Bronchodilator response to ipratropium bromide in infants with bronchopulmonary dysplasia. *Am Rev Respir Dis* 1990;**142**:1137–42.
Chavasse RJ, Bastian-Lee Y, Seddon P. How do we treat wheezing infants? Evidence or anecdote. *Arch Dis Child* 2002;**87**:546–7.

Continued on p. 276

De Boeck K, Smith J, Van Lierde S, *et al.* Response to bronchodilators in clinically stable 1-year-old patients with bronchopulmonary dysplasia. *Eur J Pediatr* 1998;**157**:75–9.

Karadag B, Ceran O, Guven G, *et al.* Efficacy of salbutamol and ipratropium bromide in the management of acute bronchiolitis – a clinical trial. *Respiration* 2008;**76**:283–7. [RCT]

Moulton BC, Fryer AD. Muscarinic receptor antagonists, from folklore to pharmacology; finding drugs that actually work in asthma and COPD. *Br J Pharmacol* 2011;**163**:44–52.

Nagakumar P, Doull I. Current therapy for bronchiolitis. *Arch Dis Child* 2012;**97**:827–30.

Yüksel B, Greenough A. Ipratropium bromide for symptomatic preterm infants. *Eur J Pediatr* 1991;**150**:854–7.

Use

Routine supplementation of iron is probably no longer warranted in mothers and infants who receive adequate quantities through their diets, but is essential in countries where maternal nutritional status is poor. In the United Kingdom and most developed countries, the main requirement for oral iron supplements during infancy is in prevention of iron deficiency anaemia during growth in breastfed babies who weighed <2.3 kg at birth. It is also used after birth to correct the iron loss that a few babies suffer as a result of chronic fetal blood loss before birth.

Nutritional factors

Iron is a major constituent of the haemoglobin molecule, and routine supplementation was traditional in pregnancy, although the scientific basis for this is far from convincing and the practice is now actively discouraged except in developing countries where the nutritional status of many women is poor. Here, the baby clearly benefits if the mother takes a regular daily supplement (60 mg of iron and 400 micrograms of folic acid) during pregnancy. Maternal iron deficiency has to be very severe before it causes neonatal anaemia or iron deficiency during infancy. All babies need a further 0.4–0.7 microgram of iron a day to maintain their body stores because the circulating blood volume triples during the 12 months, and this requires a diet containing 1–2 mg/kg of iron a day.

Newborn babies normally have substantial iron stores even when born prematurely (and even in the face of severe maternal iron deficiency). These stores start to become depleted unless dietary intake is adequate by the time the child's blood volume has doubled. Microcytosis (MCV < 96 μm³) at birth is **_never_** a sign of iron deficiency but can be due to a haemoglobinopathy (most commonly some form of thalassaemia).

While there is relatively little iron in breast milk, it is extremely well absorbed (as long as the baby is not also being offered solid food). Absorption from formula milks is only one-fifth as good, and the use of unmodified cow's milk in the first 12 months of life is particularly likely to cause iron deficiency anaemia. It was thought that this might be due to iron loss as a result of occult gastrointestinal bleeding, but recent studies have failed to confirm this. It is possible that the high phosphate content of whole cows' milk may interfere with iron absorption.

Most iron deficiency in the first year of life is iatrogenic; early cord clamping can potentially deprive the baby of 20% of the elemental iron normally present in the body after an intervention-free delivery. The most common cause of anaemia in the neonatal unit is also iatrogenic, from people taking blood for laboratory analysis. These babies, if they become symptomatic, should be offered a top-up transfusion: they do not respond to supplemental iron.

Fortification of artificial feeds with 0.6 mg iron/100 ml is enough to prevent iron deficiency in babies of normal birthweight, and it is now reasonably clear, despite official advice to the contrary, that this is also enough for the preterm baby. Almost all the commonly used formula milks in current use contain at least as much iron as this, making the widespread practice of further supplementation quite unnecessary. Breastfed babies weighing less than 2.3 kg at birth are, however, at risk of developing iron deficiency anaemia 2–3 months after birth due to the rapid expansion of their circulating blood volume with growth. These babies benefit from supplemental iron started within 4–6 weeks of birth. There is no good reason for starting supplemental iron before this because there is some doubt whether the gut absorbs iron in excess of immediate requirement, and there is some reason for believing that the iron-binding protein lactoferrin, present in milk (and particularly in breast milk), only inhibits bacterial growth when not saturated with iron. Some think that early supplementation of breast milk with iron might also unmask latent vitamin E deficiency.

Assessment

A serum ferritin <20 micrograms/l is considered diagnostic of iron deficiency in a 4-month-old infant, especially if the transferrin saturation is <10%. A 10 micrograms/l 'cut-off' can be used after 6 months. Anaemia in young children is very seldom due to iron deficiency, and most babies who are iron deficient are not anaemic.

Prophylaxis and treatment

Healthy term babies: Breastfed babies benefit from supplementation if no other source of iron is introduced into the diet by about 6 months. Term babies fed standard milk formulae do not require further supplementation.

Continued on p. 278

Preterm babies: A daily dose of 5 mg of elemental iron as prophylactic iron supplementation for babies of low birthweight who are solely breastfed is recommended. 1 ml of sodium feredetate (Sytron®), 0.5 ml of ferrous fumarate (Galfer®) or 0.3 ml of ferrous sulphate (Ironorm®) given once daily should provide this recommended amount. Prophylaxis is most logically started 6–8 weeks after birth (or, more simply, at discharge) and sustained until mixed feeding is established. There is no good evidence that *formula*-fed preterm babies benefit from further supplementation after discharge, and excess can have disadvantages.

Babies with anaemia at birth (Hb < 120 g/l): Babies who have suffered *chronic* blood loss from feto-maternal bleeding or twin-to-twin transfusion may benefit once their initial deficit has been corrected by transfusion. Iron supplements are not needed in anaemic babies after *acute* blood loss at birth or in haemolytic anaemia.

Babies on parenteral nutrition: Babies unable to tolerate even partial enteral feeding by 3 months benefit from 100 micrograms/kg of iron a day intravenously (most conveniently given as iron chloride). Babies on erythropoietin (q.v.) also need intravenous (IV) supplementation if they cannot be given oral iron.

Toxicity
Get the stomach emptied and organise prompt lavage if oral ingestion is suspected. Activated charcoal is of no value, but an attempt should be made to identify the amount ingested, and treatment started by giving 15 mg/kg of desferrioxamine mesilate (deferoxamine mesilate [pINNM]) per hour IV for 5 hours if the ingested dose is thought to exceed 30 mg/kg. No universally agreed treatment protocol exists, and advice should be sought from the local poisons centre. Acute toxicity is likely if the serum iron level exceeds 90 μmol/l 4 hours after ingestion. A leucocytosis of over 15×10^9/l, or blood glucose of over 8.3 mmol/l, suggests serious toxicity. Early symptoms include diarrhoea and vomiting followed, after 12–48 hours, by lethargy, coma, convulsions, intestinal bleeding and multi-organ failure. Intestinal strictures may develop 2–5 weeks later.

Supply
It is best to choose a sugar-free preparation requiring no further dilution. Sodium feredetate (previously known as sodium ironedetate) is widely used in the United Kingdom. Each ml of the commercial elixir (Sytron) contains 5.5 mg of elemental iron (38 mg of sodium feredetate). 100 ml bottles cost £1. Ferrous fumarate is one alternative for those concerned that Sytron contains 96% ethanol. Each ml of the commercial syrup (Galfer) contains 9 mg of elemental iron (28 mg of ferrous fumarate). 300 ml of sugar-free syrup costs £5.30. Ferrous sulphate (still widely used in North America) is a second alternative; one widely used commercial formulation (Ironorm) contains 25 mg/ml of iron (15 ml costs £28). Parents can obtain all these similarly priced products from any community pharmacist without a doctor's prescription.

Three IV iron preparations (iron dextran, iron sucrose and ferric carboxymaltose) are available, but none of the manufacturers have endorsed their use in children. Vials containing 500 mg of desferrioxamine mesilate powder (costing £4.30) suitable for reconstitution with 5 ml of water for injection are available.

References (See also the relevant Cochrane reviews)

Andersson O, Hellström-Westas L, Andersson D, *et al*. Effect of delayed versus early umbilical cord clamping on neonatal outcomes and iron status at 4 months: a randomised controlled trial. *Br Med J* 2011;**343**:d7157. [RCT]

Domellöf M. Iron requirements, absorption and metabolism in infancy and childhood. *Curr Opin Clin Nutr Metab Care* 2007;**10**:329–35.

Domellöf M, Dewey KG, Lönnerdal B, *et al*. The diagnostic criteria for iron deficiency in infants should be reevaluated. *J Nutr* 2002;**132**:3680–6.

Friel JK, Andrews WL, Aziz K, *et al*. A randomized trial of two levels of iron supplementation and developmental outcome in low birth weight infants. *J Pediatr* 2001;**139**:254–60. [RCT]

Griffin IJ, Cooke RJ, Reid MM, *et al*. Iron nutritional status in preterm infants fed formulas fortified with iron. *Arch Dis Child Fetal Neonatal Ed* 1999;**81**:F45–9. [RCT]

Hutto EK, Hassan ES. Late vs early clamping of the umbilical cord in full-term neonates: systematic review and meta-analysis of controlled trials. *JAMA* 2007;**297**:1241–52. [SR]

Iannotti LL, Tielsch JM, Black MM, *et al*. Iron supplementation in early childhood: health benefits and risks. *Am J Clin Nutr* 2006;**84**:1261–76. [SR]

Continued on p. 279

Rao R, Georgieff MK. Iron therapy for preterm infants. *Clin Perinatol* 2009;**36**:27–42.

Sankar MJ, Renu S, Kalaivani K, *et al.* Early iron supplementation in very low birth weight infants – a randomized controlled trial. *Acta Paediatr* 2009.**98**:953–8. [RCT]

Sazawal S, lack RE, Ramsan M, *et al.* Effects of routine prophylactic supplemental with iron and folic acid on admission to hospital and mortality in preschool children in a high malaria transmission setting: community-based, randomised, placebo-controlled trial. *Lancet* 2006;**367**:133–43. [RCT]

Taylor TA, Kennedy KA. Randomized trial of iron supplementation versus routine iron intake in VLBW infants. *Pediatrics* 2013;**131**:e433–8. [RCT]

White KC. Anemia is a poor predictor of iron deficiency among toddlers in the United States: for Heme the bell tolls. *Pediatrics* 2005;**115**:315–20.

Zeng L, Dibley MJ, Cheng Y, *et al.* Impact of micronutrient supplementation during pregnancy on the birth weight, duration of gestation, and perinatal mortality in rural west China double blind cluster randomised controlled trial. *Br Med J* 2008;**337**:1211–5. [RCT] (See also pp. 1180–1.)

Ziaei S, Norrosi M, Faghigzadeh S, *et al.* A randomised placebo-controlled trial to determine the effect of iron supplementation on pregnancy outcome in pregnant women with haemoglobin ≥ 13·2 g/dl. *Br J Obstet Gynaecol* 2007;**114**:684–8. [RCT] (See also p. 1308.)

Use
Isoniazid is used, with pyrazinamide (q.v.), in the primary treatment and re-treatment of tuberculosis (TB) which remains a serious notifiable disease. Guidance on dosing in children varies widely (see website commentary). Babies who come into contact with a case of active TB also merit prophylaxis.

Pharmacology
Isoniazid was first isolated in 1912 and found 40 years later to be bacteriostatic and, in high concentrations, bactericidal against *Mycobacterium tuberculosis*. It is active against both intracellular and extracellular bacilli, but because resistance develops when given on its own, when *active* infection is suspected, at least one other drug is always given as well. A 9-month course of isoniazid monotherapy has long been the standard approach for *latent* infection, but studies in adults and children now suggest that a 3- or 4-month course of isoniazid and rifampicin (q.v.) may be better tolerated and better adhered to.

There is no evidence that isoniazid is teratogenic, but treatment increases the excretion of pyridoxine (vitamin B_6), and to counter the risk of peripheral neuropathy, women should take 10 mg of pyridoxine (q.v.) once a day if pregnant or breastfeeding. During lactation, the baby receives up to 20% of the maternal dose, and of the main metabolite, on a weight-for-weight basis, although toxicity has not been seen. In many countries, breastfeeding is discouraged if the mother is still infectious (sputum smear 'positive'). This is unnecessary; any baby so exposed should receive prophylactic isoniazid and pyridoxine for 3 months, once active TB is excluded.

Isoniazid is well absorbed by mouth and excreted in the urine after inactivation in the liver. The half-life is long at birth but is substantially shorter in early childhood than it is in adult life (2–5 hours). However, inactivation is by acetylation, the speed of which is genetically determined (fast acetylators eliminating the drug twice as fast as slow acetylators). Liver toxicity is not common in children but appears related to high-dose treatment and to combined treatment with rifampicin (q.v.). It is probably more common in slow acetylators, but this has yet to be established. Haemolytic anaemia and agranulocytosis are rare complications, while a lupus-like syndrome, liver damage and gynaecomastia have been reported in adults. Treatment should be stopped and reviewed if toxicity is suspected. Use is usually contraindicated in patients with drug-induced liver disease and porphyria.

Malnourished children also benefit from prophylactic pyridoxine, especially in the first year of life.

Maternal tuberculosis
Mothers found to have TB during pregnancy need expert management: they usually get a 10-month course of isoniazid and rifampicin, along with 6 months of pyrazinamide. Some may need 2 months of ethambutol. Fetal infection is only likely if the mother has an extra-pulmonary infection, but the baby is vulnerable to infection after birth from any caregiver with open untreated pulmonary disease and remains at risk of serious generalised ('miliary') infection. Patients are not likely to pass infection to others after they have been on effective treatment for at least 2 weeks, so babies born into such a household only need prophylactic isoniazid as indicated under 'Neonatal prophylaxis'. Where there is a real possibility that the baby has become infected, give both isoniazid and 10 mg/kg of rifampicin (q.v.) once a day for at least 6 months. Pyrazinamide (q.v.) should also be given for the first 2 months under expert supervision (30 mg/kg once a day), especially if there is a possible non-pulmonary focus of infection. Possible meningeal involvement calls for at least a year's expert treatment using four drugs.

Drug interactions
Isoniazid can potentiate the effect of carbamazepine and phenytoin to the point where toxicity develops.

Prophylaxis and treatment
Neonatal prophylaxis: Give babies exposed to infection 5 mg/kg once a day by mouth. Dose adjustment is not necessary for poor renal function. If the baby is tuberculin negative at 3 months, treatment can be stopped and BCG (q.v.) given. Treat for 6 months if the tuberculin test is positive.
Treating latent infection: Give 10 mg/kg of isoniazid *and* 10 mg/kg of rifampicin once a day for 3 months.
Treating overt infection: Give babies over a month old 10 mg/kg once a day by mouth.

Continued on p. 281

Toxicity

Treat any encephalopathy due to an overdose by giving 1 mg of pyridoxine preferably by intravenous (IV) injection, or by mouth, for every milligram of excess isoniazid ingested. Control seizures, acidosis and respiration as necessary.

Supply

An inexpensive sugar-free oral elixir of isoniazid containing 10 mg/ml is available. 2 ml ampoules containing 50 mg (costing £24 each) are suitable for intramuscular or IV injection.

References

Adhikari M. Tuberculosis and tuberculosis/HIV co-infection in pregnancy. *Semin Fetal Neonatal Med* 2009;**14**:234–40.

Bright-Thomas R, Nandwani S, Smith J, *et al.* Effectiveness of 3 months of rifampicin and isoniazid chemoprophylaxis for the treatment of latent tuberculosis infection in children. *Arch Dis Child* 2010;**95**:600–2.

Joint Tuberculosis Committee of the British Thoracic Society. Control and prevention of tuberculosis in the United Kingdom: code of practice 2000. *Thorax* 2000;**55**:887–901.

National Institute for Health and Clinical Excellence. Tuberculosis: clinical diagnosis and management of tuberculosis, and measures for its prevention and control (clinical guideline 117). NICE; 2011. http://guidance.nice.org.uk/CG117

Page KR, Sifakis F, Montes de Oca R, *et al.* Improved adherence and less toxicity with rifampin vs isoniazid for treatment of latent tuberculosis. *Arch Intern Med* 2006;**166**:1863–70.

Roy V, Tekur U, Chopra K. Pharmacokinetics of isoniazid in pulmonary tuberculosis – a comparative study at two dose levels. *Indian Pediatr* 1996;**33**:287–91.

Schaaf HS, Parkin DP, Seifart HI, *et al.* Isoniazid pharmacokinetics in children treated for respiratory tuberculosis. *Arch Dis Child* 2005;**90**:614–8. (See also pp. 551–2.)

Spyridis NP, Spyridis PG, Gelseme A, *et al.* The effectiveness of a 9-month regimen of isoniazid alone versus 3- and 4-month regimens of isoniazid plus rifampin for treatment of latent tuberculosis infection in children: results of an 11-year randomized study. *Clin Infect Dis* 2007;**45**:715–22. [RCT]

Use

Ivermectin has revolutionised the treatment of several chronic parasitic infections. Little is known about use in babies weighing <15 kg because the manufacturer has never supported such use, but there is no good reason to suppose use would be hazardous if called for. Use is currently being explored in treatment of bedbug (*Cimex lectularius*) infestation.

Pharmacology

Ivermectin was isolated in 1980 from a mixture of macrolide antibiotics found in *Streptomyces avermitilis*. It is well absorbed when taken orally and was found to prevent the reproduction of the nematode worm that causes 'river blindness'. The plasma half-life is ~12 hours, and the metabolites are eventually excreted in the stool over the next 2 weeks. It is only teratogenic in animals in near toxic doses. Whole communities have been treated with the drug every 6–12 months for over two decades, and no adverse effect has been detected after unintended exposure during pregnancy. The drug appears in breast milk, but despite a milk/plasma ratio of 0.5, the baby is unlikely to ingest more than 2% of the weight-adjusted maternal dose.

Parasitic infections

The filariform larvae of three relatively common tropical nematode roundworms can cause human infection.

Onchocerciasis: Infection caused by the larvae of *Onchocerca volvulus* transmitted between individuals by the black flies that are common round many fast flowing rivers in Africa and in Central and South America can, if untreated for long enough, eventually cause blindness ('river blindness'). Some 15 million are currently affected and several hundred thousand have been rendered blind. Ivermectin kills the larvae but cannot kill adult worms (which can live for a decade), so repeat dosing is often needed every 6 months.

Filariasis: The larvae of the nematodes *Wuchereria bancrofti*, *Brugia malayi and B. timori* are transmitted between individuals by mosquito bites. Chronic infection is often unnoticed until it causes lymphadenopathy. Ivermectin only kills the larvae, so a cure requires treatment with diethylcarbamazine citrate (1 mg/kg three times a day for 1–2 weeks, starting with a lower dose because larval death can trigger a hypersensitivity reaction).

Strongyloidiasis: Infection by larvae of the nematode *Strongyloides stercoralis* is usually asymptomatic. Larvae in infected soil can enter the skin before migrating elsewhere, even eventually turning into adult worms (sometimes called threadworms in America) in the small intestine – so maintaining the life cycle by auto-reinfection. Treatment with ivermectin may need to be repeated more than once.

Treatment

The generally recommended treatment for all the aforementioned conditions is a single 150–200 micrograms/kg dose of ivermectin, but in babies weighing 15–25 kg, it seems to be acceptable, in practice, to give a single 3 mg dose. The WHO campaign funded by Merck since 1987 has done much to eliminate 'river blindness', but the parasite's extermination still seems a long way off even though man seems to be the parasite's only host.

Management of scabies

The *Sarcoptes scabiei* mite can only survive in contact with man. Covering the whole body overnight with 5% permethrin cream (a potent but poorly absorbed insecticide) will nearly always eradicate infection and seems safe even in the neonate (even though the manufacturer does not recommend use in children less than 2 months old). It can also be used to kill head lice, although wet combing should suffice in a small child. Ivermectin should be used, along with topical treatment, to treat hyperkeratotic 'crusted' scabies – severe infection may need several doses at weekly intervals as the drug is not ovicidal.

Supply and administration

Ivermectin is available in America as a 3 mg tablet. Supplies can be imported into the United Kingdom on request, although the manufacturers have not sought permission to market the product in the United Kingdom. A 30 g tube of 5% permethrin cream is available without prescription for £8.

Continued on p. 283

References

(See also the relevant Cochrane reviews)

Bécourt C, Marguet C, Balguerie X, *et al.* Treatment of scabies with oral ivermectin in 15 infants: a retrospective study on tolerance and efficacy. *Br J Dermatol* 2013;**169**:931–3.

Gann PH, Nreva FA, Gam AA. A randomized trial of single- and two-dose ivermectin versus thiabendazole for treatment of strongyloidiasis. *J Infect Dis* 1994;**169**:1076–9. [RCT]

Goldust M, Rezaee E, Raghifar R, *et al.* Ivermectin vs. lindane in the treatment of scabies. *Ann Parasitol* 2013;**59**:37–41. [RCT]

Goldust M, Rezaee E, Raghifar R, *et al.* Treatment of scabies: the topical ivermectin vs. permethrin 2.5% cream. *Ann Parasitol* 2013;**59**:79–84. [RCT]

Gyopong JO, Chinbuah MA, Gyapong M. Inadvertent exposure of pregnant women to ivermectin and albendazole during mass drug administration for lymphatic filariasis. *Trop Med Int Health* 2003;**8**:1093–101.

Karthikeyan K. Scabies in children. *Arch Dis Child Educ Pract Ed* 2007;**92**:ep65–9.

Katabarwa M, Eyamb A, Hsabomugisha P, *et al.* After a decade of annual dose mass ivermectin treatment in Cameroon and Uganda, onchocerciasis transmission continues. *Trop Med Int Health* 2008;**13**:1196–203.

Ndyomugyenyi R, Kabatereine N, Olsen A, *et al.* Efficacy of ivermectin and albendazole alone and in combination for treatment of soil-transmitted helminths in pregnancy and adverse events: a randomized open label controlled intervention in Masindi district, western Uganda. *Am J Trop Med Hyg* 2008;**79**:856–63. [RCT]

Nwaorgu OC, Okeibunor JC. Onchocerciasis in the pre-primary school children in Nigeria: lessons for onchocerciasis county control programme. *Acta Trop* 1999;**73**:211–5.

Ogbuokiri JE, Ozumba BC, Okonkwo PO. Ivermectin levels in human breast milk. *Eur J Clin Pharmacol* 1994;**46**:89–90.

Pacqué M, Muñoz B, Poetschke G, *et al.* Pregnancy outcome after inadvertent ivermectin treatment during community-based distribution. *Lancet* 1990;**336**:1486–9.

Quarteman MJ, Lesher JL. Neonatal scabies treated with 5% permethrin cream. *Pediatr Dermatol* 1994;**11**:264–6.

Ramaiah KD, Das PK, Vanamail P, *et al.* Impact of 10 years of diethylcarbamazine and ivermectin mass administration on infection and transmission of lymphatic filariasis. *Trans R Soc Trop Med Hyg* 2007;**101**:555–63.

Roberts LJ, Huffam SE, Walton SF, *et al.* Crusted scabies: clinical and immunological findings in seventy-eight patients and a review of the literature. *J Infect* 2005;**50**:375–81.

Sheele JM, Anderson JF, Tran TD, *et al.* Ivermectin causes *Cimex lectularius* (bedbug) morbidity and mortality. *J Emerg Med* 2013;**45**:433–40.

Use
Ketamine given by intravenous (IV) or intramuscular (IM) injection produces a short-lasting trance-like state with profound analgesia and amnesia.

Pharmacology
Ketamine was first developed in 1970, but its mode of action is complex and still unclear. IV administration produces an immediate feeling of dissociation followed, after 30 seconds, by a trance-like state that lasts 8–10 minutes. It produces marked amnesia but is devoid of hypnotic properties. The eyes often remain open, and nystagmus may develop. Functional and electrophysiological dissociation seems to occur between the brain's cortical and limbic systems. Respiration is not depressed, but salivation may increase and laryngeal stridor is occasionally encountered. Muscle tone increases slightly, and random limb movements occasionally require restraint. Serious rigidity is sometimes seen in adults. Tachycardia, systemic hypertension and increases in pulmonary vascular resistance have been reported in adults, but such problems have not been encountered in children. Analgesia persists for a sustained period after the anaesthetic effect has worn off. These characteristics make ketamine a particularly useful drug to give during painful but short-lasting procedures that do not require muscle relaxation. Full recovery can take 2–3 hours, and signs of distress and confusion are sometimes seen in adults during this time. Nightmares and hallucinations have been reported. Midazolam (q.v.) may help if this happens, but these problems are uncommon in children, and there is no evidence that they are common enough to make routine combined use appropriate. Nausea and vomiting are the most common problems. Excessive salivation is only common in children more than a year old. The IV anaesthetic propofol (q.v.) provides an alternative strategy and is also associated with quicker recovery.

Oral administration has been used in older children needing many invasive procedures, but plasma levels only peak after 30 minutes and a 10 mg/kg dose is necessary because bioavailability is low (~16%) because of first-pass liver metabolism. Ketamine is rapidly redistributed round the body ($V_D \sim 2.5$ l/kg) after an IV dose and then cleared from the plasma with a terminal half-life of 3 hours. Clearance is slightly faster in children than adults. Neonatal clearance has not been studied. Ketamine undergoes extensive metabolism in the liver before excretion in the urine, and the metabolic product norketamine has analgesic properties. Overdose may make respiratory support necessary, but has no adverse long-term consequences. Doses lower than those quoted here are adequate when a volatile anaesthetic is also used. Ketamine crosses the placenta, but when given in induction doses prior to caesarean delivery it does not sedate the baby. There are no clear reports of teratogenicity or suggestions that use is incompatible with lactation.

Anaesthesia
'Bolus' IV administration: A 1–2 mg/kg IV dose administered over at least 1 minute will provide about 10 minutes of surgical anaesthesia after about 30 seconds. Have either atropine or glycopyrronium (q.v.) available for prompt IV use because excessive secretions can occasionally become troublesome.

Sustained IV administration: Give a loading dose of 0.5–2 mg/kg IV followed by an infusion of 500 micrograms/kg/hour (2 ml of the dilute preparation described under 'Supply and administration', followed by 1 ml/hour). Four times this dose can be used to produce *deep* anaesthesia when few other options exist.

IM administration: 4 mg/kg given IM will provide dissociative anaesthesia for about 15 minutes after a latent 5–10 minute period. Recovery will usually be complete after 2–3 hours.

Precautions
There are few reports of neonatal use (see web commentary). Complications are uncommon in older children, but stridor and laryngospasm can be encountered especially in response to pharyngeal or laryngeal stimulation. Prolonged apnoea has also been encountered. Because of this, ketamine should *only* be given by an experienced intensivist who is ready and equipped to take immediate control of the airway if necessary (and any such clinician might prefer some other anaesthetic option). Monitoring is essential until recovery is complete. Use is not unwise in patients with head injury as was once thought.

Continued on p. 285

Supply and administration

Ketamine is available in 20 ml vials containing 10 mg/ml costing £5.10 each. To give a continuous infusion of 500 micrograms/kg of ketamine per hour, take 0.5 ml of the 10 mg/ml preparation for each kilogram the baby weighs, dilute to 10 ml with 5% glucose or glucose saline, and infuse at a rate of 1 ml/hour. Multi-dose vials containing 50 and 100 mg/ml are also manufactured.

References   (See SIGN guideline on sedation of children for procedures **DHUK**)

Green SM, Roback MG, Krauss B, *et al.* Predictors of airway and respiratory adverse events with ketamine sedation in the emergency department: an individual-patient meta-analysis of 8,282 children. *Ann Emerg Med* 2009;**54**:158–68. [SR] (See also pp. 169–70 and 171–80.)

Howes MC. Ketamine for paediatric sedation/analgesia in the emergency department. *Emerg Med J* 2004;**21**:275–80. [SR]

Lin C, Durieux ME. Ketamine and kids: an update. *Pediatr Anaesth* 2005;**15**:91–7.

Mistry RB, Nahata MC. Ketamine for conscious sedation in pediatric emergency care. *Pharmacotherapy* 2005;**25**:1104–11. [SR]

Morton NS. Ketamine for procedural sedation and analgesia in pediatric emergency medicine: a UK perspective. *Pediatr Anesth* 2008;**18**:25–9.

Pun MS, Thakur J, Poudyal G, *et al.* Ketamine anaesthesia for paediatric ophthalmology surgery. *Br J Ophthalmol* 2003;**87**:535–7.

Saarenmaa E, Neuvonen PJ, Huttunen P, *et al.* Ketamine for procedural pain relief in newborn infants. *Arch Dis Child Fetal Neonatal Ed* 2001;**85**:F53–6.

Wathen JE, Roback MG, Mackenzie T, *et al.* Does midazolam alter the clinical effects of intravenous ketamine sedation in children? A double-blind, randomised, controlled emergency department trial. *Ann Emerg Med* 2000;**36**:579–88. [RCT]

Use

Labetalol is used to achieve urgent but safe control over high blood pressure in infancy.

Pathophysiology

Judge the need for treatment by measuring the systolic blood pressure in a quiet baby, using a Doppler flow probe or stethoscope, a close fitting cuff that is as wide as possible and an inflatable section that more than surrounds the arm. Resting systolic pressure at 2 weeks varies with gestation at birth; thereafter, 95% of babies have a systolic pressure of between 72 and 112 mmHg throughout the first year of life once they reach a post-menstrual age of 46 weeks.

Serious hypertension in any young child is an emergency. It can be difficult to treat, and overtreatment can cause dangerous hypotension and potentially lethal β-blockade. Treatment should always be discussed with a paediatric nephrologist where possible, because the cause is often renal.

Pharmacology

Labetalol, patented in 1971, is a non-selective α-blocker (causing some decrease in peripheral vascular tone) with additional β-blocking properties like propranolol (q.v.). It is rapidly effective but is soon metabolised by the liver (adult half-life 4–8 hours), so any reactive hypotension quickly corrects itself once the infusion is stopped even though tissue levels exceed plasma levels (V_D ~9 l/kg). The neonatal half-life may be rather longer making reactive hypotension more hazardous. The benefit achieved from controlling hypertension usually outweighs the risk of use in cardiac failure. Glucagon (q.v.) may be of help following an overdose. Hydralazine (q.v.), with or without propranolol, used to be given once the acute situation was under control, but oral nifedipine (q.v.) is now more commonly given.

Oral labetalol is sometimes used to control severe maternal hypertension although it can sometimes make the baby mildly hypotensive, hypoglycaemic and even bradycardic if used shortly before delivery. Use during lactation only exposes the baby to ~1% of the maternal dose on a weight-for-weight basis, although there is one isolated report of this appearing to cause sinus bradycardia. The manufacturers have not yet endorsed the drug's use in children.

Treatment

Initiating treatment: Start by giving 0.5 mg/kg of labetalol per hour (0.5 ml/hour of the dilute solution described under 'Supply and administration'). Measure systolic pressure at least once every 15 minutes, and double the dose given once every 3 hours until an acceptable reduction in pressure has been achieved (aiming for no more than a 25% reduction in a given 24 hour period). The maximum safe dose is 4 mg/kg/hour (4 ml/hour). Once pressure has been reduced as much as seems immediately safe, write down the dose currently being given (X mg/kg) and the pressure limits currently considered acceptable, and initiate a flexible graded maintenance schedule for the next 24 hours using the strategy summarised in the box below.

A FLEXIBLE MAINTENANCE SCHEDULE FOR GIVING INTRAVENOUS (IV) LABETALOL

- Define, once a day, what range of systolic pressure is judged acceptable and write these limits down on the care chart.
- Continue to measure systolic blood pressure twice an hour.
- Continue to give X ml/hour (≡X mg/kg) of labetalol IV while systolic pressure remains within the preset target range.
- Double the dose if systolic pressure goes above, and halve the dose if systolic pressure goes below, this range.
- Stop the infusion if systolic pressure falls below the lower preset limit and the baby is only getting 0.5 ml/hour of labetalol.
- Call for senior review at once if systolic pressure goes more than 10 mm Hg above or below the day's defined target range.

Continued on p. 287

Lowering blood pressure gradually: Modify the defined target range daily, aiming to take 3 days to bring the pressure down to normal unless hypertension is known to be of very recent onset. Start an oral drug and wean from labetalol as soon as practicable.

Supply and administration

20 ml ampoules containing 5 mg/ml of labetalol cost £4.90. Take 10 ml of labetalol for each kilogram the baby weighs from several such ampoules and dilute to 50 ml with 10% glucose or glucose saline to give a solution containing 1 mg/kg/ml of labetalol. Piggyback this into an IV glucose infusion. The drug is stable in solution and does not need to be prepared afresh every 24 hours. Undiluted labetalol is irritant to veins.

References

(See also relevant Cochrane reviews)

Bunchman TE, Lynch RE, Wood EG. Intravenously administered labetalol for treatment of hypertension in children. *J Pediatr* 1992;**120**:140–4.

Crooks BNA, Deshpande SA, Hall C, *et al.* Adverse neonatal effects of maternal labetalol treatment. *Arch Dis Child Fetal Neonatal Ed* 1998;**79**:F150–1.

Deal JE, Barratt TM, Dillon MJ. Management of hypertensive emergencies. *Arch Dis Child* 1992;**67**:1089–92.

Dionne JM, Abitbol CL, Flynn JT. Hypertension in infancy: diagnosis, management and outcome. *Pediatr Nephrol* 2012;**27**:17–32.

Heida KY, Zeeman GG, Van Veen TR, *et al.* Neonatal side effects of maternal labetalol treatment in severe preeclampsia. *Early Hum Dev* 2012;**88**:503–7.

Mirpuri J, Patel H, Rhee H, *et al.* A case of bradycardia in a premature infant on breast milk. *J Invest Med* 2008;**56**:409. [Abstract 203.]

Thomas CA, Moffett BS, Wagner JL, *et al.* Safety and efficacy of intravenous labetalol for hypertensive crisis in infants and small children. *Pediatr Crit Care Med* 2011;**12**:28–32.

Use

Lamivudine is used, in combination with other antiviral drugs, in the control of human immunodeficiency virus (HIV) infection. Short-term use, together with zidovudine and nevirapine (q.v.), in women who are infected but not on any long-term treatment can minimise vertical HIV transmission. Lamivudine is also emerging as one of a number of antivirals showing promise in preventing vertical transmission of hepatitis B in chronically infected women (although vaccination of the newborn baby currently remains the mainstay of prevention – see monograph on hepatitis B vaccine).

Pharmacology

Lamivudine (or 3TC) is an antiviral drug first introduced in 1992 which works, like zidovudine, after intracellular conversion to the triphosphate form, as a nucleoside reverse transcriptase inhibitor (NRTI) to halt retroviral DNA synthesis. Resistance quickly develops if it is used on its own to treat HIV infection, and it is unclear whether sustained low-dose treatment is any better than interferon alfa (q.v.) in the management of chronic hepatitis B infection. Indeed, there is no good information on the use of this drug in young children with hepatitis B infection.

Oral uptake is good and is not reduced (although it is delayed) by ingestion with food. Bioavailability seems, nevertheless, to be rather lower in children than in adults. Most of the drug is rapidly excreted (the half-life is ~2 hours in children) unchanged in the urine, making dosage reduction necessary when there is serious renal failure. It is usually well tolerated though adverse effects include nausea, vomiting and diarrhoea, malaise, muscle pain and a non-specific rash. All the NRTI drugs occasionally cause liver damage with hepatomegaly, hepatic steatosis and potentially life-threatening lactic acidosis. Neuropathy and pancreatitis are only common in children with advanced disease on many other drugs. Lamivudine crosses the placenta. It does not seem to be teratogenic, but there is not enough information to exclude the possibility that it could be embryotoxic if taken at the time of conception. Lamivudine can be detected in breast milk; however, breastfeeding is not recommended in HIV-infected women where formula is available to reduce the risk of neonatal transmission. The low doses used in management of hepatitis B are not expected to cause any serious adverse effects in breastfed infants.

> New information on optimum management becomes available so frequently that communication with a paediatric HIV/infectious diseases specialist is essential. The diagnosis and management must also be discussed with, and supervised by, someone with extensive experience of this condition.

Managing overt HIV infection

Treatment will be influenced by any prior treatment that the mother has received, but will normally include zidovudine and lamivudine together with *either* a protease inhibitor (such as lopinavir or nelfinavir) *or* nevirapine. Other drug strategies can be difficult to use in young babies because no suitable liquid formulation exists.

Emergency intrapartum prophylaxis

An untreated woman presenting in labour at term should be given an immediate dose of nevirapine 200 mg (q.v.). She should be started on one tablet a day of the fixed-dose zidovudine with lamivudine combination tablets and raltegravir (400 mg twice daily). Intravenous zidovudine should be infused for the duration of labour and delivery.

Give the baby 4 mg/kg of zidovudine and 2 mg/kg of lamivudine by mouth once every 12 hours for at least one and preferably 4 weeks. Give the baby 2 mg/kg of nevirapine once a day for 1 week and then 4 mg/kg once a week for 1 week as well.

Treating known HIV infection in infancy

The standard dose is 4 mg/kg by mouth twice a day alone if appropriate or with two or more other antiviral drugs. In the rare situation where treatment is called for in the first month of life, give 2 mg/kg twice a day.

Continued on p. 289

Supply

150 mg lamivudine tablets cost £2.40 each. The fixed-dose zidovudine (300 mg) with lamivudine (150 mg) combination tablets costs £1.20 each.

Stable, oral solutions (banana and strawberry flavoured) containing 10 mg/ml of lamivudine are available costing £16 per 100 ml. The oral syrups contain 0.2 g/ml of sucrose and also contain propylene glycol. Lamivudine cannot be given by intravenous or intramuscular injection.

References

Capparelli E, Rakhamanina N, Mirochnick M. Pharmacotherapy of perinatal HIV. *Semin Fetal Neonat Med* 2005;**10**:161–75.

Han L, Zhang HW, Xie JX, *et al.* A meta-analysis of lamivudine for interruption of mother-to-child transmission of hepatitis B virus. *World J Gastroenterol* 2011;**17**:4321–33.

Johnson MA, Moore KHP, Yuen GJ, *et al.* Clinical pharmacokinetics of lamivudine. *Clin Pharmacokinet* 1999;**36**:41–66.

Moodley D, Moodley J, Coovadia H, *et al.* A multicenter randomised controlled trial of nevirapine versus a combination of zidovudine and lamivudine to reduce intrapartum and early postpartum mother-to-child transmission of human immunodeficiency virus type 1. *J Infect Dis* 2003;**187**:725–35. [RCT]

Moodley JO, Moodley D, Pillay K, *et al.* Pharmacokinetics and antiretroviral activity of lamivudine alone or when coadministered with zidovudine in human immunodeficiency virus type 1-infected pregnant women and their offspring. *J Infect Dis* 1998;**178**:1327–33.

Pan CQ, Lee HM. Antiviral therapy for chronic hepatitis B in pregnancy. *Semin Liver Dis* 2013;**33**:138–46.

Panburana P, Sirinavin S, Phuapradit W, *et al.* Elective cesarean section plus short-course lamivudine and zidovudine for the prevention of mother-to-child transmission of human immunodeficiency virus type 1. *Am J Obstet Gynecol* 2004;**190**:803–8.

Shetty AK, Coovadia HM, Mirochnick M, *et al.* Safety and trough concentrations of nevirapine prophylaxis given daily, twice weekly, or weekly in breast-feeding infants from birth to 6 months. *J Acquir Immune Defic Syndr* 2004;**34**:482–90.

Taylor GP, Anderson J, Clayden P, *et al.* British HIV Association and Children's HIV Association position statement on infant feeding in the UK 2011. *HIV Med* 2011;**12**:389–93.

Taylor GP, Clayden P, Dhar J, *et al.* British HIV Association guidelines for the management of HIV infection in pregnant women 2012. *HIV Med* 2012;**13**(suppl 2):87–157.

UK Group on Transmitted HIV Drug Resistance. Time trends in primary resistance to HIV drugs in the United Kingdom: multicentre observational study. *Br Med J* 2005;**331**:1368–71.

Use

Lamotrigine is used either as sole treatment or as an adjunct to other anti-epileptics, but experience with use in young children is still limited. That treatment has to be introduced gradually is often seen as something of a disadvantage.

Pharmacology

Lamotrigine is a phenyltriazine and structurally unrelated to any other established anti-epileptic drug. It first came into clinical use in 1987 and may work as a sodium channel blocker or by inhibiting excitatory (glutamate) neurotransmitter release. It is well absorbed when taken by mouth and mostly metabolised by the liver. The half-life in adults taking no other drug is 24–36 hours, but it is shorter than this in pregnancy and in children. Tissue levels are high (V_D >1.2 l/kg). A measles-like skin rash is the most common adverse effect. It is usually seen if the dose is too high or is increased too quickly and usually occurs within a few weeks of starting treatment. Combined use with valproate also makes it more likely. More serious toxic skin changes may make it necessary to stop treatment quickly. Fulminant hepatic failure is a further rare hazard.

Lamotrigine has only been formally approved for 'adjunctive' use in young children with refractory partial and general tonic–clonic seizures who are also taking some other anticonvulsant, but it may occasionally be effective in controlling infantile spasms and absence seizures. It is also effective in Lennox–Gastaut syndrome (a severe form of epilepsy in early childhood associated with multiple seizure types in which the waking EEG shows inter-ictal slow spike–wave activity). Lamotrigine is now increasingly thought to be the first anticonvulsant to try when managing partial (focal) epilepsy not only in adults but also in children five or more years old. It may reduce seizure activity in juvenile myoclonic epilepsy, but is of no help in severe myoclonic epilepsy of infancy (Dravet syndrome).

Lamotrigine crosses the placenta (F/M ratio ~1). While anticonvulsants generally double the risk of birth defects, both rodent studies and registry data of lamotrigine monotherapy are reassuring. Combination therapy with other anticonvulsants increases the risk, and use of lamotrigine with valproate is particularly teratogenic. Lamotrigine passes into breast milk, and plasma concentrations in the breastfed infant are ~30% of those in their mother. Few adverse effects are reported, but there is the potential for infant serum levels to reach 'therapeutic ranges' if the maternal dose is high. Apnoea has been reported in one breastfed infant whose mother was receiving high doses.

Drug interactions

All the drugs that increase liver enzyme activity (such as carbamazepine, phenobarbital and phenytoin) greatly speed the elimination of lamotrigine. The dose given often needs to be *increased* as a result. Combined treatment with carbamazepine may increase the risk of toxicity. Combined treatment with valproate, in contrast, (which may confer synergistic benefit) doubles the half-life, probably because both drugs compete for glucuronidation in the liver. A *lower* dose needs to be used in consequence, especially when treatment is first started. The valproate dose will also need to be lowered by 25–35%.

Treatment

Monotherapy: Start by giving 300 micrograms/kg once a day by mouth for 2 weeks and then twice a day for a further 2 weeks. Treatment can then be further 'titrated' upwards as necessary, to maximise seizure control, to a dose that should not, initially, exceed 2 mg/kg twice a day.

Adjunctive (combined) therapy: Children taking other enzyme-inducing drugs (see 'Drug interactions') often require double the usual dose, while those on valproate usually only need a third to a half the usual dose.

Blood levels

Knowledge of the blood level does not help to optimise management, but may reveal failure to take medicine as prescribed. Effective levels are usually 1–4 mg/l (1 mg/l = 3.9 μmol/l) but can be higher.

Supply

Scored dispersible 5 mg tablets of lamotrigine cost 7p each. Although they are only semi-soluble, small doses can be given with reasonable accuracy by adding a tablet to 10 ml of tap water; one ml of liquid will then contain ~500 micrograms of lamotrigine as long as the particulate

Continued on p. 291

matter is kept in suspension. The same dose can also be given into the rectum if oral treatment is not possible. A stable suspension with a 4-week shelf life can be prepared, but it has a very unpleasant taste.

References

(See also the relevant Cochrane reviews)

Cummings C, Stewart M, Stevenson M, *et al.* Neurodevelopment of children exposed in utero to lamotrigine, sodium valproate and carbamazepine. *Arch Dis Child* 2011;**96**:643–7.

Cunnington MC, Weil JG, Messenheimer JA, *et al.* Final results from 18 years of the International Lamotrigine Pregnancy Registry. *Neurology* 2011;**76**:1817–23.

Frank LM, Enlow T, Holmes GL, *et al.* Lamictal (lamotrigine) monotherapy for typical absence seizures in children. *Epilepsia* 1999;**40**:973–9. [RCT]

Marson AG, Al-Kharusi A, Alwaidh M, *et al.* The SANAD study of effectiveness of carbamazepine, gabapentin, lamotrigine, oxcarbazepine, or topiramate for treatment of partial epilepsy: an unblinded randomised controlled trial. *Lancet* 2007;**369**:1000–15. [RCT]

Moore JL, Aggarwal P. Lamotrigine use in pregnancy. *Expert Opin Pharmacother* 2012;**13**:1213–6.

Morrow J, Russell A, Guthrie E, *et al.* Malformation risks of antiepileptic drugs in pregnancy: a prospective study from the UK epilepsy and pregnancy register. *J Neurol Neurosurg Psychiatry.* 2006;**77**:193–8. (See also the editorial p. 145.)

Newport DJ, Pennell PB, Calamaras MR, *et al.* Lamotrigine in breast milk and nursing infants: determination of exposure. *Pediatrics* 2008;**122**:e223–31.

Nordmo E, Aronsen L, Wasland K, *et al.* Severe apnea in an infant exposed to lamotrigine in breast milk. *Ann Pharmacother* 2009;**43**:1893–7.

Pennell PB, Peng L, Newport DL, *et al.* Lamotrigine in pregnancy: clearance, therapeutic drug monitoring and seizure frequency. *Neurology* 2008;**70**:2130–6.

Piña-Garza JE, Levisohn P, Gucuyener K, *et al.* Adjunctive lamotrigine for partial seizures in patients aged 1 to 24 months. *Neurology* 2008;**70**:2099–108.

Use

Levetiracetam is an anticonvulsant commonly used off label in neonates with difficult-to-treat seizures. It is a pyrrolidone derivative and is chemically unrelated to other currently available anticonvulsants. Although the exact mechanism of action is unclear, it has been shown to regulate glutamate release and NMDA receptor-mediated excitatory synaptic transmission. Unlike other anticonvulsants, it does not induce cell death in the developing brain which might offer a theoretical benefit over older established anticonvulsants.

Levetiracetam has a broad antiepileptic activity across different seizure types and syndromes and is licensed in many countries as add-on treatment for partial-onset seizures in children >4 years. In children and adults, the most common side effects are somnolence and behavioural side effects. Case studies and pharmacokinetic studies in newborn babies have suggested that levetiracetam is also safe in this age group, but randomised controlled trials have yet to be published.

Pharmacology

Levetiracetam has linear pharmacokinetics, is mainly excreted unchanged by the kidneys and is metabolised via enzymatic hydrolysis by a plasma esterase. A number of case series suggest that levetiracetam may be safe in the treatment of neonatal seizures. Pharmacokinetic studies in newborns have shown not only longer half-life than in adults and older children but one that changes within the first few days; on day 1, the half-life is ~16–18 hours; however, this decreases during the first week of life to 8–9 hours. There are limited data for dosing in the neonatal population, but levetiracetam may be administered intravenously or orally, and limited data suggest the doses described under 'Treatment'.

There are no studies of levetiracetam in therapeutic hypothermia, although 'cooled' asphyxiated newborns are included in the populations of some of the case studies. The predominantly renal excretion of levetiracetam (two-thirds is eliminated unchanged in the urine and the remaining one-third is hydrolysed in the blood) should mean that hypothermia *per se* should not impact on dosing; however, excretion is affected by renal impairment which is commonly seen in 'cooled' infants as a result of their initial hypoxic insult.

Maternal use

Levetiracetam appears to be a much safer alternative during pregnancy than sodium valproate with a reported low risk of major congenital malformations following first trimester use. Clearance of levetiracetam increases significantly during pregnancy, and serum concentrations may fall as low as 40% of baseline. Serum levels return to normal within the first week after pregnancy. Levetiracetam is excreted into breast milk in considerable amounts, and the mean milk/maternal serum concentration ratio is 1.00; however, serum concentrations in the breastfed infant seem to stay <10–15 μmol/l, and no adverse effects in breastfed infants have been reported.

Treatment

Intravenous (IV): May be given with or without a loading dose depending on the urgency with which seizure control is needed. **Without a loading dose:** start with 10 mg/kg twice daily, increasing by 10 mg/kg/day over 3 days to 30 mg/kg twice daily. **With loading dose:** 40 mg/kg loading dose followed by 10 mg/kg once daily (note: the authors of this study suggested from their pharmacokinetic studies that a maintenance dose of 10 mg/kg eight hourly results in better maintenance of serum levels towards the end of the first week of life).
Oral/enteral: 10 mg/kg/day in one to two divided doses, increase daily by 10 mg/kg over 3 days to 30 mg/kg/day (further increases in doses have been reported up to 60 mg/kg/day).

Interactions

Levetiracetam may increase the effects of methadone and SSRIs. One report in adults suggests phenytoin plasma levels may be increased by up to 52%, but this has not been seen in other studies or in children.

Supply and administration

Levetiracetam is available as an oral sugar-free solution containing 100 mg/ml and in 5 ml vials for IV use containing 100 mg/ml. The IV solution must be mixed prior to administration with 0.9% sodium chloride or dextrose 5%. The manufacturer recommends dilution to 100 ml to give a 5 mg/ml solution for administration; however, a 1:1 dilution of the drug from

Continued on p. 293

the vial with 0.9% sodium chloride or dextrose 5% has been reported without adverse effects in older children and adults. The infusion is given over 15 minutes. Bioavailability is almost 100% after oral administration; there is no need to alter the dose or the dosing frequency when switching between parenteral and enteral routes.

References

Allegaert K, Lewi L, Naulaers G, *et al*. Levetiracetam pharmacokinetics in neonates at birth. *Epilepsia* 2006;**47**:1068–9.

Glauser TA, Mitchell WG, Weinstock A, *et al*. Pharmacokinetics of levetiracetam in infants and young children with epilepsy. *Epilepsia* 2007;**48**:1117–22.

Mawhinney E, Craig J, Morrow J, *et al*. Levetiracetam in pregnancy: results from the UK and Ireland epilepsy and pregnancy registers. *Neurology* 2013;**80**:400–5.

Merhar SL, Schibler KR, Sherwin CM, *et al*. Pharmacokinetics of levetiracetam in neonates with seizures. *J Pediatr* 2011;**159**:152–4.

Ramantani G, Ikonomidou C, Walter B, *et al*. Levetiracetam: safety and efficacy in neonatal seizures. *Eur J Paediatr Neurol* 2011;**15**:1–7.

Sharpe CM, Capparelli EV, Mower A, *et al*. A seven-day study of the pharmacokinetics of intravenous levetiracetam in neonates: marked changes in pharmacokinetics occur during the first week of life. *Pediatr Res* 2012;**72**:43–9.

Shoemaker MT, Rotenberg JS. Levetiracetam for the treatment of neonatal seizures. *J Child Neurol* 2007;**22**:95–8.

Wheless JW, Clarke D, Hovinga CA, *et al*. Rapid infusion of a loading dose of intravenous levetiracetam with minimal dilution: a safety study. *J Child Neurol* 2009;**24**:946–51.

Use

Animal-derived thyroid extracts have been used to treat deficiency since 1890. Synthetic thyroxine was first produced in 1926. Both synthetic- and animal (usually porcine)-derived products are available, although the former are hard to obtain, have variable thyroxine content and are not licensed.

Pathophysiology

Thyroid-stimulating hormone (TSH) produced by the pituitary regulates the release of levothyroxine (T_4) and (to a lesser extent) liothyronine (T_3) from the thyroid gland. T_4 is then converted to T_3 in the tissues. About a third of maternal T_4 (but not TSH and T_3) crosses the placenta, thus explaining why even the fetus that lacks a thyroid gland is asymptomatic at birth.

Subclinical maternal hypothyroidism in early pregnancy may increase the risk of spontaneous abortion and has a deleterious effect on the child's neurodevelopment; the aim of treatment should therefore be to keep maternal TSH ≤2.5 mU/l. Anti-thyroid drugs and maternal thyroid receptor antibodies can cross the placenta causing fetal hypo- and hyperthyroidism. Fetal goitre may be detected by antenatal ultrasound. The mother can be offered an anti-thyroid drug if the fetus is thyrotoxic, while hypothyroidism has, occasionally, been managed by inserting 250–500 micrograms of thyroxine into the amniotic cavity once every 10–14 days (so it can be swallowed by the fetus). Mothers taking thyroxine may breastfeed; small amounts are found in breast milk (but these are too low to treat the hypothyroid baby).

Hypothyroidism at birth

Congenital hypothyroidism occurs in about 1 in 3500 babies and is due to thyroid dysgenesis (~85%) and dyshormonogenesis (~15%). There is considerable clinical and biochemical heterogeneity, but treatment should be started within 2 weeks of birth if outcome is to be optimised. Babies in the United Kingdom are screened for hypothyroidism using the newborn bloodspot screening ('Guthrie') card at 5–7 days of age. Confirmation requires the demonstration of a high TSH and, usually, also a low T_4 in a serum sample. This programme has been very successful, but thyroid function should still be measured if hypothyroidism is suspected because false negatives can occur and because hypothyroidism can evolve.

The normal TSH surge and the rise in the T_3 and T_4 after birth are less marked in the preterm infant. These babies often have low thyroid hormone levels, a trend that may be exacerbated by exposure to the iodine in antiseptics and X-ray contrast media. The risk of developmental delay and cerebral palsy also seems to be increased in preterm babies who had transient low thyroxine levels after birth, but trials have not shown that correction improves long-term outcome.

Newborn bloodspot screening ('Guthrie')

TSH screening for hypothyroidism is generally performed on dried blood samples. Quantitative TSH assays are undertaken by the UK Supra-Regional Assay Service on 200 μl of serum (ca. 600 μl of whole blood). T_4 assays can normally be undertaken on 50 μl of serum (ca.150 μl of whole blood).

Treatment

Neonatal treatment: The usual starting dose is 10–12 micrograms/kg of levothyroxine by mouth once a day. Smaller doses may be needed in babies with significant endogenous thyroid hormone production. Monitor the thyroid hormone and TSH levels after 2 and 4 weeks and then every 1–2 months during the first year of life, aiming for a TSH in the normal range and a free T_4 level in the upper part of the normal range. Because hypothyroidism is occasionally transient, it is usual to reassess the requirement for continued treatment when the child is 2 or 3 years old.

Older children: In older children, a starting dose of 50–100 micrograms/m²/day has been suggested.

Blood levels

Early levels vary, but serum TSH levels >10 mU/l are rare after the first week of life. Free T_4 levels are higher in neonates than in adults (something not always reflected in local laboratory reference ranges).

Continued on p. 295

Age	Free T$_3$	Free T$_4$	TSH
1–30 days	4.5–7.8	12.4–27.4*	1.08–11.8*
31–60 days	5.2–8.0	12.4–21.75	0.68–12.56
61 days–1 year	4.1–7.9	10.8–19.5	0.62–7.3
1–5 years	4.2–7.6	11.7–19.0	0.75–6.57

Values for thyroid hormones from Strich *et al.* (2012).
*T$_4$ and TSH may exceed this in the first 3 days of life.

Interactions

Anticonvulsants, iron preparations and antacids all reduce effect by binding to thyroxine or by delaying or preventing absorption. Soy-based milks and simethicone (Infacol®) which may be started by parents in the absence of medical input may also interfere with thyroxine absorption.

Supply

25, 50 and 100 micrograms tablets of levothyroxine cost between 6 and 9p each. Solutions containing 25, 50 and 100 micrograms/5 ml (costing between £51 and £54 for 100 ml) are available. If treatment has to be given by intravenous or intramuscular injection and no suitable T$_4$ product is available (as in the United Kingdom), treatment with a 2 micrograms/kg dose of liothyronine (T$_3$) twice a day should be considered (although experience with such an approach is very limited).

References

(See also the relevant Cochrane reviews)

American Academy of Pediatrics. Update on newborn screening and therapy for congenital hypothyroidism. *Pediatrics* 2006;**117**:2290–303.

Balapatabendi M, Harris D, Shenoy SD. Drug interaction of levothyroxine with infant colic drops. *Arch Dis Child* 2011;**96**:888–9.

Biswas S, Buffery J, Enoch H, *et al.* A longitudinal assessment of thyroid hormone concentrations in preterm infants younger than 30 weeks' gestation during the first 2 weeks of life and their relationship to outcome. *Pediatrics* 2002;**109**:222–7.

Chung ML, Yoo HW, Kim KS, *et al.* Thyroid dysfunctions of prematurity and their impacts on neurodevelopmental outcome. *J Pediatr Endocrinol Metab* 2013;**26**:449–55.

Dichtel LE, Alexander EK. Preventing and treating maternal hypothyroidism during pregnancy. *Curr Opin Endocrinol Diabetes Obes* 2011;**18**:389–94.

Glinoer D, Abalovich M. Unresolved questions in managing hypothyroidism during pregnancy. *Br Med J* 2007;**335**:300–2.

Hrytsiuk I, Gilbert R, Logan S, *et al.* Starting dose of levothyroxine for the treatment of congenital hypothyroidism. *Arch Pediatr Adolesc Med* 2002;**156**:485–91. [SR]

Kloostra L, Crawford S, van Baar AL, *et al.* Neonatal effects of maternal hypothyroxinemia during early pregnancy. *Pediatrics* 2006;**117**:161–7.

Korada SM, Pearce M, Ward Platt MP, *et al.* Difficulties in selecting an appropriate neonatal thyroid stimulating hormone (TSH) screening threshold. *Arch Dis Child* 2010;**95**:169–73.

Mizuta H, Amino N, Ichihara K, *et al.* Thyroid hormones in human milk and their influence on thyroid function of breast-fed babies. *Pediatr Res* 1983;**17**:468–71.

Neale DM, Cootauco AC, Burrow G. Thyroid disease in pregnancy. *Clin Perinatol* 2007;**34**:54–357.

Polak M. Thyroid disorders during pregnancy: impact on the fetus. *Horm Res Paediatr* 2011;**76**(suppl 1): 97–101.

Srinivasan R, Harigopal S, Turner S, *et al.* Permanent and transient congenital hypothyroidism in preterm infants. *Acta Paediatr* 2012;**101**:e179–82.

Strich D, Edri S, Gillis D. Current normal values for TSH and FT3 in children are too low: evidence from over 11,000 samples. *J Pediatr Endocr Metab* 2012;**25**:245–8.

Valerio PG, van Wassenaer AG, Vijlder JJ, *et al.* A randomized masked study of triiodothyronine plus thyroxine administration in preterm infants less than 28 weeks of gestational age: hormonal and clinical effects. *Pediatr Res* 2004;**55**:248–53. [RCT]

Williams FL, Simpson J, Delahunty C, *et al.* Collaboration from the Scottish Preterm Thyroid Group. Developmental trends in cord and postpartum serum thyroid hormones in preterm infants. *J Clin Endocrinol Metab* 2004;**89**:5314–20.

Use

Lidocaine is a widely used local anaesthetic. A short infusion can sometimes stop neonatal fits resistant to phenobarbital and the benzodiazepines and is occasionally used to control arrhythmia.

Pharmacology

Systemic and subcutaneous use: Lidocaine hydrochloride is a local anaesthetic of the amide group with effects on the central nervous system (where it acts as a sedative in low doses and a stimulant in high doses), on peripheral nerves (where it decreases conduction) and on the heart (where it shortens the duration of the action potential). It was first marketed in Sweden in 1948. Lidocaine is metabolised by the liver cytochromes P450 1A2 and 3A4, but some of the intermediary breakdown products are metabolically active as well as potentially toxic; up to a third is excreted unchanged by the neonatal kidney. Oral administration fails to produce adequate blood levels because of rapid first-pass liver metabolism. The terminal half-life is about 100 minutes in adults and at least twice this in the newborn. Intravenous infusion produces high drug concentrations in those organs with a high blood flow, with later redistribution throughout the body. This volume of distribution is particularly high in the neonatal period ($V_D > 1 \, l/kg$).

Lidocaine has different effects at different serum concentrations: in adults, antiarrhythmic effects are seen at concentrations of 1.5–6 mg/l, and anticonvulsant properties are seen at levels slightly higher than this. Toxic effects are seen at concentrations >9 mg/l, and lidocaine, itself, causes seizures at concentrations >15 mg/l.

That lidocaine is metabolised by the hepatic cytochrome system means that when used during neonatal therapeutic hypothermia, clearance is reduced by almost a quarter; thus, a modified dosing scheme is required to prevent accumulation and adverse effects.

Lidocaine rapidly crosses the placenta. Maternal lidocaine, used to infiltrate the perineum prior to delivery, can be detected in the infant's serum 48 hours later. There are no reports of malformations and rodent teratogenicity studies are reassuring. Lidocaine passes into breast milk, but it is unlikely that breastfed infants ingest clinically relevant amounts.

Analgesic cream: Plain (30%) lidocaine ointment is ineffective when applied to the skin, but a eutectic mixture of local anaesthetics (EMLA®) cream, containing 2.5% lidocaine and 2.5% prilocaine, provides good surface anaesthesia for 1–2 hours in children if applied under an occlusive dressing at least 1 hour in advance of venepuncture but seems less effective in babies (possibly because of rapid skin clearance). Tetracaine gel (q.v.) may provide quicker and marginally better pain relief for venepuncture in infancy. The manufacturers have been reluctant to endorse the use of EMLA cream in children less than a year old, but the prilocaine it contains does not seem to cause significant methaemoglobinaemia (at least in babies of 30 or more weeks' gestation with a reasonably mature epidermis) as had once been feared.

Treatment

Surface anaesthesia: Apply 1 g of EMLA cream to a 2×2 cm area of undamaged skin, and cover with an occlusive dressing for 1 hour. Keep away from the eyes. Tetracaine gel may be a better alternative.
Mucosal anaesthesia: Use no more than 0.1 ml/kg of a 4% lidocaine spray or 0.3 ml/kg of a 2% lidocaine gel on mucosal surfaces. Experience with the spray in small children is limited, and a randomised study showed that use did not reduce the distress displayed by 1–5-year-olds during nasogastric tube insertion.
Infiltrative local anaesthesia: 0.3 ml/kg of 1% plain lidocaine provides excellent anaesthesia for 1–2 hours after 1–2 minutes. Take care not to inject anything into a blood vessel and give no further lidocaine for 4 hours. A 0.6 ml/kg dose of 1% lidocaine in adrenaline will offer pain relief for 3 hours. Bupivacaine (q.v.) can provide pain relief for at least 6 hours but only after a half hour latent period.
Fits and arrhythmia: Dosing depends on prematurity and the presence of therapeutic hypothermia.

A 'traditional' regime for normothermic infants has been:

	Loading phase		Maintenance phase #1	Maintenance phase #2
	10 minutes	6 hours	12 hours	12 hours
Term infants	2 mg/kg	6 mg/kg/hour	4 mg/kg/hour	2 mg/kg/hour

Continued on p. 297

However, modified regimes (aiming to keep plasma concentrations below 9 mg/l) for both normo-thermic and hypothermic patients, and which may be better, were recently described as follows:

Normothermia	Loading phase		Maintenance phase #1	Maintenance phase #2
	10 minutes	4 hours	12 hours	12 hours
Weight 0.8–2.0 kg	2 mg/kg	5 mg/kg/hour	2.5 mg/kg/hour	1.25 mg/kg/hour
Weight 2.0–2.5 kg		6 mg/kg/hour	3 mg/kg/hour	1.5 mg/kg/hour
Weight ≥2.5–4.5 kg		7 mg/kg/hour	3.5 mg/kg/hour	1.75 mg/kg/hour

Hypothermia	Loading phase		Maintenance phase #1	Maintenance phase #2
	10 minutes	3.5 hours	12 hours	12 hours
Weight 2.0–2.5 kg	2 mg/kg	6 mg/kg/hour	3 mg/kg/hour	1.5 mg/kg/hour
Weight ≥2.5–4.5 kg		7 mg/kg/hour	3.5 mg/kg/hour	1.75 mg/kg/hour

Toxicity

Accidental infiltration of the fetal scalp during the injection of lidocaine into the maternal perineum can cause toxic apnoea, bradycardia, hypotension and fits – a cluster of features that can be mistaken for intrapartum asphyxia. Some babies have required ventilatory support, but most have made a complete recovery. Management is as discussed in the monograph on bupivacaine.

Compatibility

Compatibility with other continuously infused drugs is noted, where known, in the monograph for the second product. It can also be added (terminally) to TPN and lipid. It is not compatible with phenytoin.

Supply

A 0.1% (1 mg/ml) solution of lidocaine for infusion in 500 ml of 5% dextrose is available. The initial loading dose can be given using 2 ml/kg of this infusion given at a rate of 12 ml/kg/hour for **10 minutes only**; thereafter, the numerical value for the infusion rate (in ml/hour) is equal to the numerical value of the dose (in mg/kg/hour).

Various size (2–20 ml) ampoules of adrenaline-free 1% (10 mg/ml) lidocaine are available and cost between 28p and 83p each. This can be used to give the loading dose if fluid restriction is necessary; give 0.2 ml/kg of this at a rate of 1.2 ml/kg/hour for **10 minutes only**.

20 ml ampoules of 1% lidocaine with adrenaline (10 mg of lidocaine and 5 micrograms of adrenaline per ml) cost £1.90.

5 g tubes of EMLA cream cost £2.25. Lidocaine as a 5% ointment is available in 15 g tubes costing £6.10 each. A 4% lidocaine jet-spray delivery system for use during laryngoscopy costs £5.

References

(See also the relevant Cochrane reviews)

Babl FE, Goldfinch CM Mandrawa C, *et al.* Does nebulized lidocaine reduce the pain and distress of nasogastric tube insertion in young children? A randomized, double-blind, placebo-controlled trial. *Pediatrics* 2009;**123**:1548–55. [RCT]

Boylan GB, Rennie JM, Chorley G, *et al.* Second-line anticonvulsant treatment of neonatal seizures: a video-EEG monitoring study. *Neurology* 2004;**62**:486–8. [RCT]

Lundqvist M, Ågren J, Hellström-Westas L, *et al.* Efficacy and safety of lidocaine for treatment of neonatal seizures. *Acta Paediatr* 2013;**102**:863–7.

Malingré MM, van Rooij LGM, Rademaker CMA, *et al.* Development of an optimal lidocaine infusion strategy for neonatal seizures. *Eur J Pediatr* 2006;**165**:598–604.

Continued on p. 298

Marcatto Jde O, Vasconcelos PC, Araújo CM, *et al.* EMLA versus glucose for PICC insertion: a randomised triple-masked controlled study. *Arch Dis Child Fetal Neonatal Ed* 2011;**96**:F467–8. [RCT]

Mitani GM, Steinberg I, Lien EJ, *et al.* The pharmacokinetics of antiarrhythmic agents in pregnancy and lactation. *Clin Pharmacokinet* 1987;**12**:253–91.

Ortega D, Viviand X, Lorec AM, *et al.* Excretion of lidocaine and bupivacaine in breast milk following epidural anesthesia for cesarean delivery. *Acta Anaesthesiol Scand* 1999;**43**:394–7.

Shany E, Banzagen O, Watemberg N. Comparison of continuous drip of midazolam or lidocaine in the treatment of intractable neonatal seizures *J Child Neurol* 2007;**22**:255–9.

Tulloch JK, Carr RR, Ensom MH. A systematic review of the pharmacokinetics of antiepileptic drugs in neonates with refractory seizures. *J Pediatr Pharmacol Ther* 2012;**17**:31–44. [SR]

van den Broek MP, Huitema AD, van Hasselt JG, *et al.* Lidocaine (lignocaine) dosing regimen based upon a population pharmacokinetic model for preterm and term neonates with seizures. *Clin Pharmacokinet* 2011;**50**:461–9.

van den Broek MP, Rademaker CM, van Straaten HL, *et al.* Anticonvulsant treatment of asphyxiated newborns under hypothermia with lidocaine: efficacy, safety and dosing. *Arch Dis Child Fetal Neonatal Ed* 2013;**98**:F341–5.

van Donselaar-van der Pant KA, Buwalda M, van Leeuwen HJ. Lidocaine: local anaesthetic with systemic toxicity. *Ned Tijdschr Geneeskd* 2008;**152**:61–5.

van Rooij LG, Hellström-Westas L, de Vries LS. Treatment of neonatal seizures. *Semin Fetal Neonatal Med* 2013;**18**:209–15.

Van Rooij LGM, Toet MC, Rademaker KMA, *et al.* Cardiac arrhythmias in neonates receiving lidocaine as anticonvulsive treatment. *Eur J Pediatr* 2004;**163**:637–41.

Use

This antibiotic should be kept in reserve and only used, on microbiological advice, to treat methicillin-resistant *Staphylococcus aureus* (MRSA) and vancomycin-resistant enterococcal infection. There is little published information on neonatal use and even less on use in the preterm baby.

Pharmacology

Linezolid is an oxazolidinone antibiotic, first marketed in 2000, which inhibits bacterial protein synthesis. It is active against a range of Gram-positive bacteria, including both MRSA and glycopeptide intermediate-resistant *S. aureus* (GISA). Linezolid is also active against vancomycin-resistant enterococci, strains of *Streptococcus pneumoniae* resistant to a range of other antibiotics and some anaerobes, including *Clostridium perfringens*, *C. difficile* and *Bacteroides fragilis*. Linezolid has no clinically significant effect on most Gram-negative bacteria; thus, Enterobacteriaceae and *Pseudomonas aeruginosa* are not susceptible to linezolid, but it has occasionally been used to treat multi-drug-resistant TB.

Linezolid is rapidly and completely absorbed when given orally, and it penetrates the meninges well when these are inflamed. Thirty per cent is excreted unchanged in the urine; the remainder is excreted as inactive metabolites (which could accumulate in severe renal failure). The half-life in children aged 1 week to 10 years old (2–3 hours) is half that seen at birth and again in adults. Reversible myelosuppression (including anaemia, neutropenia and thrombocytopenia) has been reported; thus, a full blood count should be performed weekly if treatment becomes necessary for longer than this. Optic, peripheral and auditory nerve neuropathies and lactic acidosis have also been reported with sustained use. There is also concern that prolonged low-dose use could lead to the development of bacterial resistance (especially with *Enterococcus faecium*).

Linezolid is a weak, reversible, non-selective monoamine oxidase (MAO) inhibitor and can cause hypertension and CNS excitability when used at the same time as (or within 2 weeks of treatment with) a MAO antidepressant. Combined use with a range of other antidepressants could cause a 'serotonin syndrome' with hyperpyrexia and cognitive dysfunction. Very limited information is available on use during pregnancy. Placental transfer is to be expected due to the drug's low molecular weight. It should only be used during pregnancy when the benefit outweighs the potential fetal risks because, although there is no evidence of teratogenicity, increased embryo death, decreased litter size, decreased fetal weight and costal cartilage abnormalities were reported during drug testing in mice. Linezolid enters breast milk. Limited data indicate that the amounts received through breast milk are less than infant doses. If linezolid is required, it is not a reason to discontinue breastfeeding. Manufacturers have not yet recommended use in children under 18.

Drug interactions

Use with care, and monitor blood pressure, during co-administration with any sympathomimetic drug (such as dopamine or dobutamine).

Treatment

Dose: Give 10 mg/kg by slow intravenous (IV) injection. Oral absorption is good in adults and adolescents, but has not yet been studied in young children and infants. Treatment is usually continued for 2 weeks.

Timing: Give once every 12 hours in infants less than a week old (changing to 8 hourly if the clinical response is inadequate) and once every 8 hours after that.

Supply and administration

300 ml bags containing 2 mg/ml of linezolid suitable for IV administration cost £44 each. Do not mix linezolid with, or infuse it into the same line as, any other drug. Do not dilute further before administration. The manufacturers say that adults should receive any IV infusion over at least 30 minutes, but that is because the volume of fluid involved is considerable. Bags should be stored at room temperature, protected from light during storage in the foil overwrap provided and inverted gently two to three times before use. The fluid slowly turns yellow with time, but this does not affect potency. No intramuscular preparation exists. Granules to make up 150 ml of an oral suspension containing 20 mg/ml are available (costing £222). Mix with 123 ml of water to produce 150 ml.

Continued on p. 300

References

Brennan K, Jones BL, Jackson L. Auditory nerve neuropathy in a neonate after linezolid treatment. *Pediatr Infect Dis J* 2009;**28**:169.

Chiappini E, Conti C, Galli L, *et al*. Clinical efficacy and tolerability of linezolid in pediatric patients: a systematic review. *Clin Ther* 2010;**32**:66–88. [SR]

Jungbluth GL, Welshman IR, Hopkins NK. Linezolid pharmacokinetics in pediatric patients: an overview. *Pediatr Infect Dis J* 2003;**22**:S153–7.

Kaplan SL, Deville JG, Yogev R, *et al*. Linezolid *versus* vancomycin for treatment of resistant Gram-positive infections in children. *Pediatr Infect Dis J* 2003;**22**:677–85.

Kearns GL, Andersson T, James LP, *et al*. Impact of ontogeny on linezolid disposition in neonates and infants. *J Clin Pharmacol* 2003;**43**:840–8.

Khairulddin N, Bishop L, Lamagni TL, *et al*. Emergence of methicillin resistant *Staphylococcus aureus* (MRSA) bacteraemia among children in England and Wales, 1990–2001. *Arch Dis Child* 2004;**89**:378–9.

Langgartner M, Mutenthaler A, Haiden N, *et al*. Linezolid for treatment of catheter-related cerebrospinal fluid infections in preterm infants. [Letter] *Arch Dis Child Fetal Neonatal Ed* 2008;**93**:F397.

Mercieri M, Di Rosa R, Pantosti A, *et al*. Critical pneumonia complicating early-stage pregnancy. *Anesth Analg* 2010;**110**:852–4.

Nambiar S, Rellosa N, Wassel RT, *et al*. Linezolid-associated peripheral and optic neuropathy in children. *Pediatrics* 2011;**127**:e1528–32.

Rose PC, Hallbauer UM, Seddon JA, *et al*. Linezolid-containing regimens for the treatment of drug-resistant tuberculosis in South African children. *Int J Tuberc Lung Dis* 2012;**16**:1588–93.

Sagirli O, Onal A, Toker S, *et al* Determination of linezolid in human breast milk by high-performance liquid chromatography with ultraviolet detection. *J AOAC Int* 2009;**92**:1658–62.

Schaaf HS, Willemse M, Donald PR. Long-term linezolid treatment in a young child with extensively drug-resistant tuberculosis. *J Pediatr Infect Dis* 2009;**28**:748–50.

Stalker DJ, Jungbluth GL. Clinical pharmacokinetics of linezolid, a novel oxazolidinone antibacterial. *Clin Pharmacokinet* 2003;**42**:1129–40.

Su E, Crowley K, Carcillo JA, *et al*. Linezolid and lactic acidosis: a role for lactate monitoring with long-term linezolid use in children. *Pediatr Infect Dis J* 2011;**30**:804–6.

Tan TQ. Update on the use of linezolid: a pediatric perspective. *Pediatr Infect Dis J* 2004;**23**:955–6.

Watanabe S, Tanaka A, Ono T, *et al*. Treatment with linezolid in a neonate with meningitis caused by methicillin-resistant *Staphylococcus epidermidis*. *Eur J Pediatr* 2013;**172**:1419–21.

Use

For parenterally fed neonates, lipid emulsions are the only source of the essential fatty acids, linoleic acid and α-linolenic acid. The earliest lipid emulsions, developed in the 1960s, were soybean oil based. Intralipid® is the most widely studied of these lipid products and has been widely used in infants and children requiring parenteral nutrition (q.v.). Subsequent development of lipid emulsions has focused on reducing the amount of soybean oil by replacing it with other oils including coconut oil, olive oil and fish oil.

Pharmacology

Intralipid is an emulsion of soybean oil stabilised with egg phospholipid. It is approximately isotonic and is available as a 10% solution providing 1.1 kcal/ml and as a 20% solution providing 2 kcal/ml. It contains 52% linoleic acid, 22% oleic acid, 13% palmitic acid and 8% α-linolenic acid.
Lipofundin® is a mix of soybean oil and medium-chain triglycerides in equal amounts, and like Intralipid, it is available in 10% (just over 1.0 kcal/ml) and 20% (2 kcal/ml) solutions. It contains 27% linoleic acid, 12% oleic acid, 5% palmitic acid and 4% α-linolenic acid.
ClinOleic® is an 80:20 mixture of olive and soybean oils. It is available as a 20% (2 kcal/ml) solution containing 18.5% linoleic acid, 59.5% oleic acid, 10.8% palmitic acid and 2% α-linolenic acid.
SMOFlipid® is a mixture of soybean oil (30%), olive oil (25%), medium-chain triglycerides (30%) and fish oil (15%). The fish oil contributes omega-3 fatty acids, and early experience has suggested that they may be of benefit in the prevention and treatment of total parenteral nutrition (TPN)-induced cholestasis. SMOFlipid is available as a 20% solution. It contains 18.7% linoleic acid, 27.8% oleic acid, 9.2% palmitic acid and 2.4% α-linolenic acid.

When lipid emulsions were first introduced, they were often only infused for 4–20 hours a day, so that lipaemia could 'clear', but continuous infusion has been shown to improve tolerance and seems more 'physiological'. The 20% products are better tolerated than 10% ones (if available), possibly because the phospholipid content is lower. Infection with *Malassezia furfur* can occur, and this lipid-dependent fungus may escape detection if specific culture techniques are not used, but the fungaemia usually clears if administration is stopped.

Nutritional factors

The use of lipid emulsion enhances protein utilisation and considerably increases calorie provision in babies receiving TPN. The co-infusion of 0.8 ml/kg of a 20% lipid emulsion per hour with an infusion of 6 ml/kg/hour (i.e. 144 ml/kg/day) of an amino acid solution containing 10% glucose increases total calorie intake from 60 to 100 kcal/kg/day. By way of comparison, 160 ml/kg/day of one of the high-calorie preterm milk formulae provides an intake of 130 kcal/kg/day (if no allowance is made for incomplete intestinal absorption). An infusion of 0.1 ml/kg/hour (0.5 g/kg/day) is the minimum needed to meet essential fatty acid needs. Gluconeogenic metabolic pathways also seem to utilise the glycerol generated to make glucose and improve glucose homeostasis.

Intake

Policies still vary widely, but it seems safe to start infusing at least 0.4 ml/kg of 20% lipid emulsion (0.08 g of fat) per hour through a peripheral, central or umbilical line within a day or two of birth once it is clear that the baby is stable. There is no evidence that stepped introduction improves tolerance, but there is good evidence that many babies will develop hyperlipidaemia when intake exceeds 0.8 ml/kg/hour (3.8 g/kg of fat a day). Babies less than a week old, or <28 weeks' gestation at birth, may be marginally less tolerant. Septic, acidotic and post-operative babies should probably not be offered more than 2 g/kg/day.

Administration

1.2 μm lipid filters exist, but lipid emulsions cannot be infused through the 0.2 μm filters normally used for amino acid solutions, so lipid is best only allowed to mix just before it enters the baby. Protection from light may limit hydroperoxide production, but this has not yet been shown to deliver clinical benefit. Some units change the syringe and giving set daily because of concern that lipid emulsion can leach the chemical plasticiser out of syringes.

Blood levels

Serum triglycerides higher than 2 mmol/l (the highest level seen in the breastfed baby) suggest early lipid overload. Plasma turbidity is a much less satisfactory test. Re-emergent lipaemia may suggest early sepsis.

Continued on p. 302

Supply

100 ml bags of 20% emulsions of Intralipid cost £7.30, those of ClinOleic cost £6.30, and those of Lipofundin cost £12.50. SMOFlipid is available in 500 ml bags costing £20.50. Never add anything to lipid emulsions other than compatible vitamin solutions (e.g. Vitlipid®) or co-infuse it with a fluid containing any drug other than heparin, insulin or isoprenaline. Discard all open bags.

References

(See also the relevant Cochrane reviews)

Avila-Figueroa C, Goldmann DA, Richardson DK *et al.* Intravenous lipid emulsions are the major determinant of coagulase-negative staphylococcal bacteremia in very low birth weight newborns. *Pediatr Infect Dis J* 1998;**17**:10–7.

Cairns PA, Wilson DC, Jenkins J, *et al.* Tolerance of mixed lipid emulsion in neonates: effect of concentration. *Arch Dis Child Fetal Neonatal Ed* 1996;**75**:F113–6. [RCT]

Deshpande G, Simmer K. Lipids for parenteral nutrition in neonates. *Curr Opin Clin Nutr Metab Care* 2011;**14**:145–50.

Drenckpohl D, McConnell C, Gaffney S, *et al.* Randomized trial of very low birth weight infants receiving higher rates of infusion of intravenous fat emulsions during the first week of life. *Pediatrics* 2008;**122**: 743–51. [RCT]

Driscoll DF, Bistrian BR, Demmelmair H, *et al.* Pharmaceutical and clinical aspects of parenteral lipid emulsions in neonatology. *Clin Nutr* 2008;**27**:497–503.

Goulet O, Antébi H, Wolf C, *et al.* A new intravenous fat emulsion containing soybean oil, medium-chain triglycerides, olive oil, and fish oil: a single-center, double-blind randomized study on efficacy and safety in pediatric patients receiving home parenteral nutrition. *JPEN J Parenteral Enteral Nutr* 2010;**34**: 485–95. [RCT]

Matlow AG, Kitai I, Kirpalani H, *et al.* A randomised trial of 72- versus 24-hour intravenous tubing changes in newborns receiving lipid therapy. *Infect Control Hosp Epidemiol* 1999;**20**:487–93. [RCT]

Sherlock R, Chessex P. Shielding parenteral nutrition from light: does the available evidence support a randomized, controlled trial? *Pediatrics* 2009;**123**:1529–33.

Tomsits E, Pataki M, Tölgyesi A, *et al.* Safety and efficacy of a lipid emulsion containing a mixture of soybean oil, medium-chain triglycerides, olive oil, and fish oil: a randomised, double-blind clinical trial in premature infants requiring parenteral nutrition. *J Pediatr Gastroenterol Nutr* 2010;**51**:514–21. [RCT]

Use

Protease inhibitors are used with other drugs to control human immunodeficiency virus (HIV) infection. Neonatal use (in both preterm and term infants) of the lopinavir (LPV)/ritonavir (RTV) combination has been associated with reports of adverse cardiac, renal, metabolic and neurological effects thought to primarily be due to the alcohol and propylene glycol. However, a direct effect of the drugs cannot be excluded; as a result, the LPV with RTV combination is best avoided in routine infant post-exposure prophylaxis and should only be prescribed to preterm neonates in exceptional circumstances.

Pharmacology

LPV and RTV are protease inhibitors that bind to HIV protease, causing the formation of immature viral particles that are incapable of infecting other cells. Both came into general clinical use in the late 1990s. Giving a low (and sub-therapeutic) dose of RTV with LPV boosts the effectiveness of LPV. Both drugs are well absorbed orally, especially when given with food. They are metabolised by hepatic cytochrome P450 3A4 (CYP3A4) enzymes and excreted in the faeces. The half-life in adults is 5–6 hours but approximately 3.6 hours in infants.

Both LPV and RTV cross the placenta, and there is some evidence of embryonic and fetal toxicity in animal studies. Registries of use in human pregnancies have yet to find any consistent effects. Diabetes can develop or be exacerbated in patients taking a protease inhibitor; thus, close attention should be paid to women at risk of gestational diabetes. While there is some suggestion of an association with adrenal dysfunction in babies exposed *in utero*, this appears to be confined to those individuals who are also given postnatal treatment. Breastfeeding is not recommended in HIV-infected women where formula is available to reduce the risk of neonatal transmission. In countries where formula is not readily available or safe, ongoing use during breastfeeding is used to reduce transmission. Small amounts of LPV pass into breast milk, and low (sub-therapeutic) levels can be detected in babies, which have the potential nonetheless to cause anaemia in the exposed baby.

Drug interactions

The protease inhibitors are best given with food, but didanosine is best given on an empty stomach. Since LPV and RTV are part metabolised by CYP3A4, their clearance is increased by a wide range of other drugs including carbamazepine, dexamethasone, phenobarbital, phenytoin, rifampicin and theophylline. Protease inhibitors also inhibit the clearance of other drugs; co-treatment with drugs that have a narrow therapeutic range (e.g. antihistamines, benzodiazepines, rifampicin, amiodarone and flecainide) is discouraged because of a variable and unpredictable reduction in clearance of these drugs. Digoxin levels are variably affected. (See www.hiv-druginteractions.org.)

Treatment

> New information on optimum management becomes available so frequently that communication with a paediatric HIV/infectious diseases specialist is essential. The diagnosis and management must also be discussed with, and supervised by, someone with extensive experience of this condition.

LPV with RTV **should not** be used in any baby less than 14 days old (or if they are premature, before they reach 42 weeks post-menstrual age) unless there are good reasons for doing so due to adverse effects thought to primarily be due to the alcohol and propylene glycol the liquid formulation contains.

At ages 14 days to 12 months, a starting dose of 300/75 mg/m² (i.e. 300 mg of the LPV component and 75 mg of the RTV component) twice a day seems to offer adequate serum levels. Older children are usually given 230/57.5 mg/m² of LPV with RTV twice a day, using a higher dose of 300/75 mg/m² when there are issues with resistance.

Supply

These drugs cannot be given intravenously or intramuscularly and are best taken with a little food to minimise gastric irritation.

Continued on p. 304

A solution of LPV with RTV (Kaletra®) is available containing 80 mg/ml of LPV and 20 mg/ml of RTV (100 ml costs £45). It contains 43% alcohol, 15% propylene glycol and fructose corn syrup. The bitter taste can be disguised by giving it with chocolate-flavoured milk. It must *not* be mixed with water and is best kept at 4 °C, but is stable at room temperature for a month.

References

Chadwick EG, Capparelli EV, Yogev R, *et al.* Pharmacokinetics, safety and efficacy of lopinavir/ritonavir in infants less than 6 months of age: 24 week results. *AIDS* 2008;**22**:249–55.

Chadwick EG, Pinto J, Yogev R, *et al.* Early initiation of lopinavir/ritonavir in infants less than 6 weeks of age: pharmacokinetics and 24-week safety and efficacy. *Pediatr Infect Dis J* 2009;**28**:215–9.

Chadwick EG, Rodman JH, Britto P, *et al.* Ritonavir-based highly active antiretroviral therapy in human immunodeficiency virus type 1-infected infants younger than 24 months. *Pediatr Infect Dis J* 2005;**24**: 793–800.

Chadwick EG, Yogev R, Alvero CG, *et al.* Long-term outcomes for HIV-infected infants less than 6 months of age at initiation of lopinavir/ritonavir combination antiretroviral therapy. *AIDS* 2011;**25**:643–9.

Dryden-Peterson S, Shapiro RL, Hughes MD, *et al.* Increased risk of severe infant anemia following exposure to maternal HAART, Botswana. *J Acquir Immune Defic Syndr* 2011;**56**:428–36.

Jullien V, Urien S, Hirt D, *et al.* Population analysis of weight-, age-, and sex-related differences in the pharmacokinetics of lopinavir in children from birth to 18 years. *Antimicrob Agents Chemother* 2006;**50**: 3548–55.

McArthur MA, Kalu SU, Foulks AR, *et al.* Twin preterm neonates with cardiac toxicity related to lopinavir/ritonavir therapy. *Pediatr Infect Dis J* 2009;**28**:1127–9.

Microchnick M, Capparelli E. Pharmacokinetics of antiretrovirals in pregnant women. *Clin Pharmacokinet* 2004;**43**:1071–87.

Nikanjam M, Chadwick EG, Robbins B, *et al.* Assessment of lopinavir pharmacokinetics with respect to developmental changes in infants and the impact on weight band-based dosing. *Clin Pharmacol Ther* 2012;**91**: 243–9.

Oldfield V, Plosker GL. Lopinavir/ritonavir: a review of its use in the management of HIV infection. *Drugs* 2006;**66**:1275–99. [SR]

Pasley MV, Martinez M, Hermes A, *et al.* Safety and efficacy of lopinavir/ritonavir during pregnancy: a systematic review. *AIDS Rev* 2013;**15**:38–48.

Resino S, Bellón JM, Ramos JT, *et al.* Salvage lopinavir-ritonavir therapy in human immunodeficiency virus-infected children. *Pediatr Infect Dis J* 2004;**23**:923–30.

Sáez-Llorens X, Violair A, Deetz CO, *et al.* Forty-eight-week evaluation of lopinavir/ritonavir, a new protease inhibitor, in human immunodeficiency virus-infected children. *Pediatr Infect Dis J* 2003;**22**:216–23.

Simon A, Warszawski J, Kariyawasam D, *et al.* Association of prenatal and postnatal exposure to lopinavir-ritonavir and adrenal dysfunction among uninfected infants of HIV-infected mothers. *JAMA* 2011;**306**:70–8.

Taylor GP, Clayden P, Dhar J, *et al.* British HIV Association guidelines for the management of HIV infection in pregnant women 2012. *HIV Med* 2012;**13**(suppl 2):87–157.

Urien S, Firtion G, Anderson ST, *et al.* Lopinavir/ritonavir population pharmacokinetics in neonates and infants. *Br J Clin Pharmacol* 2011;**71**:956–60.

Use
Several benzodiazepines have been used to arrest seizure activity, and lorazepam is the drug of choice in most guidelines once venous access is established.

Pharmacology
The success of the first benzodiazepine, chlordiazepoxide (Librium®), in 1960 triggered the development of a number of related products including diazepam (licensed in 1963) and lorazepam (licensed a year later). They were widely, and liberally, used to treat anxiety, before it came to be accepted that such use should always be limited to the lowest possible dose for the shortest possible time. Dependence can become a serious problem, even with careful prescribing.

Lorazepam readily crosses the placenta, but there is no clear evidence of teratogenicity. Maternal use, particularly if high doses are used, in the third trimester or during labour may cause hypothermia, lethargy, poor feeding or neonatal withdrawal. Lorazepam is excreted into breast milk in small amounts (~5–10% of the maternal dose). Breastfeeding may further sedate an already affected baby in the immediate postnatal period, but sustained use during lactation does not seem to cause noticeable drowsiness.

The drug is well absorbed when taken by mouth, conjugated to an inactive glucuronide in the liver and then excreted in the urine by glomerular filtration. The half-life in the neonatal period is 30–50 hours (two to three times as long as in adults). Tissue drug levels slightly exceed plasma levels (V_D~1.3 l/kg).

Most benzodiazepines are of limited value in long-term treatment of epilepsy but have an important role in the management of prolonged seizures. Diazepam was the first to be widely used. Clonazepam, lorazepam and midazolam (q.v.) have all been used. There is, however, continuing concern that while the benzodiazepine may well abolish the physical signs of the seizure, electrical seizure activity may still sometimes persist.

Rapid intravenous (IV) administration in the neonate can sometimes precipitate hypotension, respiratory depression and abnormal seizure-like movements, especially in response to the first dose given. Withdrawal symptoms are also very common after sustained use (as they are with midazolam) even if the dose given is lowered slowly.

Treatment
Dose: A single 100 micrograms/kg dose will usually stop all visible seizure activity within 10 minutes. While this can be repeated after 10 minutes, the long half-life in early infancy increases the risks of sedation and respiratory depression.

Route of administration: Lorazepam is normally given IV. Buccal and intra-nasal routes, while not well studied, do seem to be almost equally effective (at least in babies more than a few weeks old). Lorazepam can also be given by mouth, but intramuscular administration is painful and best avoided.

Sustained infusion can cause a progressive accumulation of the potentially toxic excipient propylene glycol.

Antidote
Flumazenil is a specific antidote (as described in the monograph on midazolam).

Supply and administration
1 ml ampoules containing 4 mg of lorazepam cost 35p each. These contain 1 ml of propylene glycol and 0.02 ml of benzyl alcohol, should be protected from light and are best stored at 4 °C. For accurate neonatal administration, it is best to draw the content of the ampoule into a large syringe immediately before use and then dilute this to 40 ml with 0.9% sodium chloride (producing a solution that contains 100 micrograms/ml). For intra-nasal use, dilution to 8 ml is more appropriate (producing a 500 micrograms/ml solution). Absorption after IM administration is not only slow and painful but also rather unpredictable.

A sugar-free oral suspension can be provided.

References
(See also the relevant Cochrane reviews) ◉

Ahmad S, Ellis JC, Kamwendo H, *et al.* Efficacy and safety of intranasal lorazepam versus intramuscular paraldehyde for protracted convulsions in children: an open randomised trial. *Lancet* 2006;**367**:1591–7. [RCT]

Anderson M. Benzodiazepines for prolonged seizures. *Arch Dis Child Educ Pract Ed* 2010;**95**:183–9.

Continued on p. 306

Appleton R, Sweeney A, Choonara I, *et al.* Lorazepam *versus* diazepam in the acute treatment of epileptic seizures and status epilepticus. *Dev Med Child Neurol* 1995;**37**:682–8.

Chess PR, D'Angio CT. Clonic movements following lorazepam administration in full-term infants. *Arch Pediatr Adolesc Med* 1998;**152**:98–9.

Chicella M, Jansen P, Parthiban A, *et al.* Propylene glycol accumulation associated with continuous infusion of lorazepam in pediatric intensive care patients. *Crit Care Med* 2002;**30**:2752–6.

Dominquez KD, Crowley MR, Colemen DM, *et al.* Withdrawal from lorazepam in critically ill children. *Ann Pharmacother* 2006;**40**:1035–9.

Maytal J, Novak GP, King KC. Lorazepam in the treatment of refractory neonatal seizures. *J Child Neurol* 1991;**6**:319–23.

McDermott CA, Kowalczyk AL, Schritzler ET, *et al.* Pharmacokinetics of lorazepam in critically ill neonates with seizures. *J Pediatr* 1992;**120**:479–83.

McElhatton PR. The effects of benzodiazepine use during pregnancy and lactation. *Reprod Toxicol* 1994;**8**:461–75.

Muchohi SN, Obiero K, Newton CRJC, *et al.* Pharmacokinetics and clinical safety of lorazepam in children with severe malaria and convulsions. *Br J Clin Pharmacol* 2008;**65**:12–21.

Sexson WR, Thigpen J, Stajich GV. Stereotypic movements after lorazepam administration in premature neonates: a series and review of the literature. *J Perinatol* 1995;**15**:146–9.

Use

Magnesium sulfate is used for a variety of reasons in the perinatal setting. It is now widely used in acute severe asthma (including during pregnancy). It is encountered more frequently in prevention or control of eclampsia in the mother. While it does not appear to be particularly effective as a tocolytic, maternal administration can reduce the risk of cerebral palsy in babies of less than 30 weeks gestation. In the neonate, it has been used to treat neonatal hypomagnesaemia and late neonatal hypocalcaemia. Other reported uses include treatment of persistent pulmonary hypertension and the prevention of further neurological damage in perinatal asphyxia.

Pharmacology

Magnesium sulfate is the treatment of choice for the mother if she has eclampsia and for *pre-eclampsia* severe enough for urgent delivery to be contemplated. Use reduces the risk of maternal seizures and probably lowers maternal mortality, but it does nothing to lower blood pressure or reduce perinatal mortality. Treatment with magnesium sulfate is still widely used to inhibit preterm labour in North America, although there is no controlled trial evidence of benefit and there is increasing evidence that high-dose treatment may have adverse consequences for the baby. Even short-term use increases fetal magnesium levels, and high serum levels (>4 mmol/l) can cause hypotonia, reduced gastrointestinal motility and respiratory depression after birth. Several trials have, however, now found that brief use reduces the risk of severe cerebral palsy when given for just 12–24 hours to mothers in strong well-established preterm labour. While not well studied during pregnancy, magnesium is an effective bronchodilator in acute severe asthma in the emergency department. It should not be withheld during pregnancy. Breastfeeding should not be discouraged because of maternal treatment.

Symptomatic neonatal hypocalcaemia (serum calcium <1.7 mmol/l) is now rare and usually associated with hypomagnesaemia. Empirical data suggest that treatment with intramuscular (IM) magnesium sulfate improve things more quickly than calcium gluconate (q.v.).

Magnesium is a smooth muscle relaxant and can cause significant pulmonary and systemic vasodilatation. A number of relatively small non-randomised observational studies, most preceding the introduction of inhaled nitric oxide (q.v.), had shown continuous infusions to be effective when other treatments had failed. In the only randomised comparative trial, magnesium was less effective than inhaled nitric oxide, which should be the treatment of choice when it is available. Magnesium is a natural antagonist of N-methyl-D-aspartate (NMDA) glutamate voltage-dependent channels and can reduce the excessive intracellular Ca^{2+} influx following glutamate stimulation following asphyxial injury. Although therapeutic hypothermia has now become a standard of care in developed countries, it is not universally available, and magnesium is a cheap alternative that has shown some benefit in one randomised trial. There is also the suggestion from an animal focal stroke model that there is an additive benefit when magnesium is used with mild hypothermia.

Maternal use

Preventing or treating eclampsia: Give 4 g intravenously over 15 minutes followed by an IV infusion of 1–2 g/hour (according to local guidelines) for up to 24 hours if no seizures. If an eclamptic seizure occurs while on treatment, then give another bolus dose of 2 g and continue the infusion. In countries where sustained intravenous (IV) treatment could be problematic, give 5 g IM once every 4 hours.

Reducing the risk of cerebral palsy: Mothers facing an imminent delivery before 30 weeks gestation should be given a 4 g IV loading dose and then a 1 g/hour infusion until delivery (but for no more than to 24 hours). This has no impact on perinatal mortality, but does significantly reduce the risk of the baby developing serious cerebral palsy. Aim to complete at least 4 hours of infusion prior to delivery, but it should still be given even if delivery is anticipated sooner. Infusion can be repeated at a later date if delivery does not occur.

Acute severe asthma: Consider giving a single 1.2–2 g IV infusion of magnesium sulfate over 20 minutes in patients with acute severe asthma who have not had a good initial response to inhaled bronchodilator therapy or who have life-threatening or near-fatal asthma.

Neonatal use

Hypocalcaemia: Giving 100 mg/kg of magnesium sulfate (0.2 ml/kg of a 50% solution) by deep IM injection on two occasions 12 hours apart will control most cases of symptomatic late neonatal hypocalcaemia.

Continued on p. 308

Hypomagnesaemia: The same dose every 6–12 hours can also be used to treat primary neonatal hypomagnesaemia irrespective of the cause (normal plasma level: 0.75–1.0 mmol/l). This is usually given IV or IM because it is a purgative (like Epsom salts) when given by mouth.
Persistent pulmonary hypertension: If inhaled nitric oxide is not available, consider giving a loading dose of 250 mg/kg of magnesium sulfate IV over 10–15 minutes. If a clinical response is obtained once the serum magnesium level exceeds 3.5 mmol/l, give between 20 and 75 mg/kg an hour for 2–5 days while maintaining a blood level of between 3.5 and 5.5 mmol/l.
Intrapartum asphyxia: If therapeutic hypothermia is not available, consider a 250 mg/kg dose IV once a day for 3 days. Watch for respiratory depression.

Supply and administration

Magnesium sulfate is conventionally prescribed as the heptahydrate. 50% magnesium sulfate contains 0.5 g (4.1 mmol) of magnesium in every millilitre. It is available in 2 and 4 ml ampoules costing £1.05 and £1.50, respectively (pre-filled syringes are available in 4, 5 and 10 ml sizes but cost considerably more). To give a baby a 250 mg/kg IV 'stat' dose, draw 1 gram of magnesium sulfate (2 ml of the 50% solution) for each kilogram the baby weighs into a syringe, dilute to 20 ml with 10% glucose saline to obtain a solution containing 50 mg/kg/ml, and give 5 ml of this solution slowly over 10–15 minutes. To then continue delivering 20 mg/kg/hour, give 0.4 ml/hour of the same solution.

20 ml (4 g) ampoules of a 20% solution costing £17 are available for use in adults.

References   (See also relevant Cochrane reviews and UK guideline on pre-eclampsia)

Barker D, Chin H. Use of magnesium in moderating tachycardia in acute severe asthma in pregnancy. *Br J Anaesth* 2013;**110**:1059.

Bhat MA, Charoo BA, Bhat JI, *et al*. Magnesium sulfate in severe perinatal asphyxia: a randomized, placebo-controlled trial. *Pediatrics* 2009;**123**:e764–9. [RCT]

Dhillon R. The management of neonatal pulmonary hypertension. *Arch Dis Child Fetal Neonatal Ed* 2012;**97**:F223–8.

Greenberg MB, Penn AA, Whitaker KR, *et al*. Effect of magnesium sulfate exposure on term neonates. *J Perinatol* 2013;**33**;188–93.

Grimes DA, Nanda KK. Magnesium sulfate tocolysis. Time to quit. *Obstet Gynecol* 2006;**108**:986–9.

Gurner TL, Cockburn F, Forfar JO. Magnesium therapy in neonatal tetany. *Lancet* 1977;**i**:283–4. [RCT]

Magpie Trial Follow-up Study Collaborative Group. The Magpie trial: a randomised trial comparing magnesium sulphate with placebo for pre-eclampsia. Outcome for children at 18 months. *Br J Obstet Gynaecol* 2007;**114**:300–9. [RCT] (See also pp. 289–9.)

Paradisis M, Osborn DA, Evans N, *et al*. Randomized controlled trial of magnesium sulfate in women at risk of preterm delivery-neonatal cardiovascular effects. *J Perinatol* 2012;**32**:665–70. [RCT]

Rouse DJ, Hirtz DG, Thom E, *et al*. A randomized controlled trial of magnesium sulfate for the prevention of cerebral palsy. *N Engl J Med* 2008;**359**:895–905. [RCT] (See also pp. 962–4.)

Tolsa J-F, Cotting J, Sekarski N, *et al*. Magnesium sulphate as an alternative and safe treatment for severe persistent pulmonary hypertension of the newborn. *Arch Dis Child Fetal Neonatal Ed* 1995;**72**:F184–7.

Use

Mebendazole (methyl 5-benzoyl-1*H*-benzimidazol-2-yl carbamate) is a broad-spectrum benzimidazole used to treat a variety of parasitic infestations including threadworms, roundworms, hookworms and whipworms (described in the monograph on albendazole). It was developed and patented by Janssen in 1971 but later superseded by albendazole (q.v.) which was thought to have fewer side effects. Mebendazole features in the 18th WHO Model List of Essential Medicines published in 2013.

Pharmacology

Mebendazole is poorly soluble in both water and organic solvents. Absorption after oral administration is very limited in man (although it may be improved by co-administration of the drug with a fatty meal). It undergoes extensive first-pass metabolism in both the intestinal wall and the liver, and almost none of the parent drug is excreted unchanged. Clearance is predominantly as metabolites in the bile and urine, but the majority of the drug is excreted unchanged in faeces. The limited amounts absorbed are rapidly metabolised by the liver's cytochrome system to inactive metabolites. Mebendazole shows little toxicity in animals but is rapidly lethal to most nematode worms because of tubulin binding. It is, however, embryotoxic in rats, but there are no reports of teratogenicity in man, and treating serious intestinal helminth infection can improve pregnancy outcome. Very limited data suggest that mebendazole is poorly excreted into breast milk and coupled with the poor absorption orally it is unlikely to adversely affect the breastfed infant. Nonetheless, the manufacturer advises that use is avoided both during pregnancy and lactation. Likewise, they have also yet to endorse use in children under the age of 2 years.

Interactions

Co-administration with cimetidine can lead to increased plasma levels of mebendazole, probably due to inhibition of hepatic first-pass cytochrome P450-mediated metabolism.

Maternal treatment

Community-based studies in an area where severe anaemia from hookworm infection is extremely common have shown that treatment with either albendazole or mebendazole (especially if given with supplemental iron) given in the second and the third trimester can reduce the incidence of severe anaemia, boost birthweight and improve infant survival. The WHO recommends antenatal deworming for pregnant women in areas where the prevalence of hookworm infection exceeds 20–30%.

Treatment in infancy

A single 100mg oral dose of mebendazole will effectively 'deworm' children infected with threadworm (pinworm). The same dose, given twice daily for 3 days, will treat children with roundworms, hookworms and whipworms. Children less than a year old should only be treated if symptomatic because there is, as yet, no evidence on the safety of treatment in children <6months old.

Supply

30 ml of an oral suspension containing 20mg/ml of mebendazole costs £1.60. Chewable 100mg tablets cost 23p each.

References

Bethony J, Brooker S, Albonico M, *et al*. Soil-transmitted helminth infections: ascariasis, trichuriasis and hookworm. *Lancet* 2006;**367**:1521–32.

Brooker S, Hotez PJ, Bundy DA. Hookworm-related anaemia among pregnant women: a systematic review. *PLoS Negl Trop Dis* 2008;**2**:e291. [SR]

Christian P, Khatry SK, West KP. Antenatal anthelmintic treatment, birthweight, and infant survival in rural Nepal. *Lancet* 2004;**364**:981–3.

Dayan AD. Albendazole, mebendazole and praziquantel. Review of non-clinical toxicity and pharmacokinetics. *Acta Trop* 2003;**86**:141–59.

Diav-Citrin O, Shechtman S, Arnon J, *et al*. Pregnancy outcome after gestational exposure to mebendazole: a prospective controlled cohort study. *Am J Obstet Gynecol* 2003;**188**:282–5.

Continued on p. 310

Gyorkos TW, Larocque R, Casapia M, *et al.* Lack of risk of adverse birth outcomes after deworming in pregnant women. *Pediatr Infect Dis J* 2006;**25**:791–4.

Keiser J, Utzinger J. Efficacy of current drugs against soil-transmitted helminth infections: systematic review and meta-analysis. *JAMA* 2008;**299**:193748. [SR]

Kurzel RB, Toot PJ, Lambert LV, *et al.* Mebendazole and postpartum lactation. *N Z Med J* 1994;**107**:439.

Larocque R, Casapia M, Gotuzzo E, *et al.* A double-blind randomized controlled trial of antenatal mebendazole to reduce low birth weight in a hook-worm endemic area of Peru. *Trop Med Int Health* 2006;**11**:1485–95. [RCT]

Montresor A, Awasthi S, Crompton DWT. Use of benzimidazoles in children younger than 24 months for the treatment of soil-transmitted helminthiasis. *Acta Trop* 2003;**86**:223–32. (See also pp. 141–59.)

Montresor A, Stoltzfus RJ, Albonico M, *et al.* Is the exclusion of children under 24 months from anthelmintic treatment justifiable? *Trans R Soc Trop Med Hyg* 2002;**96**:197–9.

Use

Spaced doses of sulphadoxine and pyrimethamine (q.v.) have been shown to reduce the risk of an overt attack of malaria in countries where young children are at high risk, but mefloquine, given the same way, is probably more effective in areas where resistance to this drug combination is now high. Visitors to areas of high resistance to chloroquine (q.v.) are also now, similarly, advised to take a weekly dose of mefloquine.

Pharmacology

Mefloquine hydrochloride is an amino alcohol with a half-life of 2–3 weeks that is concentrated in the red cells. It was developed by the US military as an antimalarial in the 1960s and became generally available in 1986. High-dose treatment can provoke nausea, vomiting, loose stools, headache, abdominal pain and somnolence – symptoms that can be hard to distinguish from malaria itself. At high doses, mefloquine is teratogenic (and sometimes embryotoxic) in rodents. High-dose use should probably be avoided during pregnancy, but prophylactic use (where lower doses are employed) during early pregnancy is not associated with an increased risk of malformations. If indicated, mefloquine should not be withheld as the maternal and fetal risks from untreated malaria are far greater. Little of the drug seems to appear in breast milk, and the baby is unlikely to be exposed to more than 10% of the weight-adjusted maternal dose during lactation, even after allowance is made for the drug's long half-life. However, the amount ingested from breast milk is certainly not enough to reduce the risk of the child becoming infected, and if indicated, the breastfed child should also receive appropriate prophylaxis. It should be noted, however, that the manufacturer has not yet recommended use during pregnancy or in children less than 3 months old.

Drug resistance

UK advice on prophylaxis can be obtained from the Public Health England Malaria Reference Laboratory (www.malaria-reference.co.uk). WHO advice on travel and the prevalence of drug resistance can be found at http://www.who.int/topics/malaria/en/index.html. Go to http://www.cdc.gov/malaria/ for up-to-date advice from the CDC in the America.

Interactions

Mefloquine antagonises the anticonvulsant effect of anti-epileptic drugs and interacts with a number of cardiac drugs, causing in some cases cardiac arrhythmias.

Treatment options in infancy

Intermittent prevention: A single dose every 2–4 months in the first year of life (as, e.g. when seen for vaccination) can substantially reduce the risk of *overt* infection. A 125 mg dose at 2 months, or 250 mg at 9 months, seems safe.

Sustained prevention: Visitors to any area where malaria is endemic should take 5 mg/kg of mefloquine by mouth once a week. Start treatment ideally 3 weeks before entering any endemic area (since most adverse effects will manifest themselves within 3 weeks of starting treatment), and continue treatment for 4 weeks after leaving. There is little experience with sustained use for more than a year, and use is not advised in children with a history of seizures.

Treatment: Mefloquine is now rarely used for the treatment of falciparum malaria because of increased resistance. It is rarely used for the treatment of non-falciparum malaria because better tolerated alternatives are available. Mefloquine should not be used for treatment if it has been used for prophylaxis. If it is used, give 15 mg/kg of mefloquine by mouth followed, after 12 hours, by one further 10 mg/kg dose.

Supply

Scored 250 mg tablets of mefloquine cost £1.80 each. They have a bitter taste, making administration difficult in small children (although the crushed tablet can be mixed with honey jam or other food). No low-dose tablet or liquid formulation exists, making accurate administration to a small baby extremely problematic. Protect from sunlight and humidity once removed from the foil wrapping.

Continued on p. 312

References

Edstein MD, Veenendaal JR, Hyslop R. Excretion of mefloquine in human breast milk. *Chemotherapy* 1988;**34**:165–9.

Gosling PD, Gesase S, Mosha JF, *et al.* Protective efficacy and safety of three antimalarial regimens for intermittent preventive treatment for malaria in infants: a randomised, double blind, placebo controlled trial. *Lancet* 2009;**374**:1521–32.[RCT] (See also pp. 1480–2.)

Nosten F, McGready R, d'Alessandro U, *et al.* Antimalarial drugs in pregnancy: a review. *Curr Drug Saf* 2006;**1**:1–15.

Nosten F, ter Kuile F, Maelankiri L, *et al.* Mefloquine prophylaxis prevents malaria during pregnancy: a double-blind placebo-controlled study. *J Infect Dis* 1994;**169**:595–603. [RCT]

Palmer KJ, Holliday SM, Brogden RN. Mefloquine. A review of its antimalarial activity, pharmacokinetic properties and therapeutic efficacy. *Drugs* 1993;**45**:430–75.

Radloff PD, Phillips J, Nkeyi M, *et al.* Atovaquone and proguanil for Plasmodium falciparum malaria. *Lancet* 1996;**347**:1511–4. [RCT]

Schlagenhauf P, Adamcova M, Regep L, *et al.* Use of mefloquine in children – a review of dosage, pharmacokinetics and tolerability data. *Malar J* 2011;**10**:292.

Schlagenhauf P, Blumentals WA, Suter P, *et al.* Pregnancy and fetal outcomes after exposure to mefloquine in the pre- and periconception period and during pregnancy. *Clin Infect Dis* 2012;**54**:e124–31.

Smoak BL, Writer JV, Keep LW, *et al.* The effects of inadvertent exposure of mefloquine chemoprophylaxis on pregnancy outcomes and infants of US army servicewomen. *J Infect Dis* 1997;**176**:831–3.

Vamhauwere B, Maradit H, Kerr L. Post-marketing surveillance of prophylactic mefloquine (Lariam®) use in pregnancy. *Am J Trop Med Hyg* 1999;**58**:17–21.

Use
Vaccines offer protection from some, but not all, forms of meningococcal meningitis and septicaemia.

Meningococcal disease
Meningococcal infection is a notifiable illness caused by the Gram-negative diplococcus *Neisseria meningitidis*. There are at least 13 serogroups of *N. meningitidis*; groups B, C and Y were historically the most common in the United Kingdom. Other less common serogroups included A, W135, 29E and Z. Before the introduction of the conjugate vaccine, the group C strain accounted for 40% of all meningococcal infection in the United Kingdom but a much higher proportion of all meningococcal deaths. Up to 34% of the population carry meningococci in their nasopharynx.

Group A strains are common in sub-Saharan Africa, where it causes epidemics, and the Indian subcontinent. Serogroup B causes endemic disease in Western Europe, North America and Australasia. Since the introduction of vaccines against serogroup C meningococcus in these areas, it now contributes approximately 80% of total disease burden, at least half of which occurs in children under the age of 2 years. Travel to the Hajj caused the group W135 strain to be seen more widely. Hajj visas will not be issued without proof of vaccination and a valid International Certificate of Vaccination or Prophylaxis; thus, all adults and children (>2 years) must have received a single dose of the quadrivalent A/C/Y/W-135 vaccine between 10 days and 3 years before the date of travel.

Meningococcal infection is spread by droplet and direct contact, the incubation period being 2–7 days. Babies usually present with pyrexia, irritability, vomiting, limpness, pallor and cold extremities: older children with headache, drowsiness and limb pain. The petechial or purpuric rash, which does not blanch on pressure, is seldom an early feature. Infection is most common in children <4 years old, with a second small peak at 15–20 years. Prevention (chemoprophylaxis) is important in close contacts who should normally be given ciprofloxacin (q.v.), or rifampicin (q.v.) when they are known to have ciprofloxacin hypersensitivity. Ceftriaxone (q.v.) can be given to the pregnant woman who is known to be hypersensitive to ciprofloxacin.

Indications
MenC conjugate vaccine: This vaccine, first introduced in 1999, is made from capsular polysaccharide that has been extracted from cultures of *N. meningitidis* serogroup C. The polysaccharide is linked (conjugated) to a carrier protein to increase the immunogenicity. This vaccine is given as part of the child's routine vaccinations at 3 months with a booster during adolescence.

Hib/MenC conjugate vaccine: This vaccine is made from capsular polysaccharides of *H. influenzae* type b (Hib) and *N. meningitidis* group C both conjugated to tetanus toxoid. It boosts the responses to both Hib and MenC when given at 12–13 months of age to children who have received Hib and MenC conjugate vaccines.

Quadrivalent (ACWY) polysaccharide vaccine: This plain vaccine generates little response to the groups C, W135 and Y polysaccharides in infants <18 months old or to the group A polysaccharide in babies <3 months old. In most people, the conjugate MenACWY is now the vaccine of choice.

Quadrivalent (ACWY) conjugate vaccine: The MenACWY vaccine contains capsular polysaccharides from serogroups A, C, W135 and Y. The conjugation improves immunogenicity in young children and older people. Although not yet licensed for children, it is recommended over the plain vaccine in children <5 years because data show a better and longer-lasting antibody response.

4-component meningococcus B (4CMenB) vaccine: The 4-component meningococcus B (4CMenB) vaccine contains four immunogenic components: three recombinant proteins combined with outer membrane vesicles derived from meningococcal NZ98/254 strain. It provides protection against *N. meningitidis* group b, and while licensed for this use in Europe, it has yet to be incorporated into national immunisation schedules due to the cost of the vaccine and absence of cost-effectiveness data, a move that is attracting some criticism.

Contraindications
Immunisation should not be offered to any child who is acutely unwell or has had a severe, proven reaction to a previous injection. Minor infections without fever are not a reason to delay immunisation.

Continued on p. 314

Administration

MenC for children: In the United Kingdom, 0.5 ml of the MenC vaccine is given as part of the second of the primary immunisations (q.v.). A booster is provided in the 12–13-month-old child by giving combined Hib/MenC conjugate vaccine, and a further dose of MenC vaccine during adolescence.

Quadrivalent (ACWY) conjugate vaccine: Children (>2 months old) who have not previously received the ACWY conjugate vaccine should be given a dose if they are travelling to an area that puts them at risk from meningococcal infection. The timing of a booster dose has not been ascertained.

Quadrivalent (ACWY) polysaccharide vaccine: This provides protection against the same serogroups as the quadrivalent (ACWY) conjugate vaccine but offers a less robust and shorter-term protection in children.

4-component meningococcus B (4CMenB) vaccine: The 4CMenB vaccine has yet to be incorporated into any national immunisation schedules. In the United Kingdom, the Joint Committee on Vaccination and Immunisation (JCVI) has advised that the MenB vaccine should be made available free of charge to people with medical conditions that put them at high risk of getting meningococcal disease, including people with asplenia, splenic dysfunction or complement deficiency. Otherwise, it is available privately. In infants under 6 months, it can be given at 2, 3 and 4 months with a booster in the second year of life. In infants of 6–12 months, two doses are given at least 2 months apart. A booster is again given during the second year of life as long as it is at least 2 months after the second dose.

Supply

The MenC conjugate vaccine is available either as a lyophilised powder for reconstitution with a diluent (Menjugate Kit®) or as a suspension in a syringe (NeisVac-C®). After the lyophilised powder is reconstituted, the vaccine must be used within one hour. A third MenC vaccine, Meningitec®, is not recommended in children under 12 months of age because it provides inadequate protection when administered as a single dose in infancy.

Hib/MenC is supplied as a vial of white powder and 0.5 ml of diluent in a pre-filled syringe (Menitorix®). These must be stored at 2–8 °C. Do not freeze.

The meningococcal groups A, C, W135 and Y conjugate vaccine is available in two forms as powder for reconstitution with a vial or syringe of diluent that delivers a 0.5 ml dose (cost £30). The capsular polysaccharide antigens of *N. meningitidis* groups A, C, W135 and Y are conjugated to *Corynebacterium diphtheriae* protein (Menveo®) or to tetanus toxoid protein (Nimenrix®).

0.5 ml vials of the lyophilised ACWY polysaccharide vaccine (ACWY Vax®) with diluent for reconstitution cost approximately £17 each.

The 4CMenB vaccine is available as a pre-filled syringe with 0.5 ml of a suspension for injection (cost £75).

References

(See also the relevant Cochrane reviews and UK guidelines **DHUK**)

American Academy of Pediatrics. Committee on Infectious Diseases. Prevention and control of meningococcal disease: recommendations for use of meningococcal vaccines in pediatric patients. *Pediatrics* 2005;**116**:496–50.

Blanchard-Rohner G, Snape MD, *et al*. Seroprevalence and placental transmission of maternal antibodies specific for Neisseria meningitidis Serogroups A, C, Y and W135 and influence of maternal antibodies on the immune response to a primary course of MenACWY-CRM vaccine in the United Kingdom. *Pediatr Infect Dis J* 2013;**32**:768–76.

Borrow R. Meningococcal disease and prevention at the Hajj. *Travel Med Infect Dis* 2009;**7**:219–25.

Carter NJ. Multicomponent meningococcal serogroup B vaccine (4CMenB; Bexsero®): a review of its use in primary and booster vaccination. *BioDrugs* 2013;**27**:263–74.

Hart CA, Thomson APJ. Meningococcal disease and its management in children. *Br Med J* 2006;**333**:685–90. [SR]

Klein NP, Baine Y, Bianco V, *et al*. One or two doses of quadrivalent meningococcal serogroups A, C, W-135 and Y tetanus toxoid conjugate vaccine is immunogenic in 9- to 12-month-old children. *Pediatr Infect Dis J* 2013;**32**:760–7.

Moxon R, Snape MD. The price of prevention: what now for immunisation against meningococcus B? *Lancet* 2013;**382**:369–70.

Purcell B, Samuelsson, Hahné SJM, *et al*. Effectiveness of antibiotics in preventing meningococcal disease after a case: systematic review. *Br Med J* 2004;**328**:1339–42. [SR]

Continued on p. 315

Stephens DS, Greenwood B, Brandtzaeg P. Epidemic meningitis, meningococcaemia, and *Neisseria meningitidis*. *Lancet* 2007;**369**:2196–210. [SR]

Thompson MJ, Ninis N, Perera R, *et al*. Clinical recognition of meningococcal disease in children and adolescents. *Lancet* 2006;**367**:397–403. (See also pp. 371–2.)

Vesikari T, Esposito S, Prymula R, *et al*. Immunogenicity and safety of an investigational multicomponent, recombinant, meningococcal serogroup B vaccine (4CMenB) administered concomitantly with routine infant and child vaccinations: results of two randomised trials. *Lancet* 2013;**381**:825–35. [RCT]

Use
Mercaptamine is used to reduce the intracellular levels of cystine in cystinosis.

Cystinosis
Cystinosis, first described by Aberhalden in 1903, is a rare autosomal recessive metabolic disorder. The responsible gene, CTNS, encodes cystinosin, an integral membrane protein that transports cystine out of the lysosome. Three clinical types of this disorder are described based on the age at diagnosis and degree of cellular cystine deposition: infantile onset, adolescent onset and adult onset. Patients with infantile cystinosis (the most common and most severe) become symptomatic at 3–18 months of age with polyuria, followed by poor growth, photophobia and, if not diagnosed and treated, renal failure by age 6 years. Although most individuals are not diagnosed until after infancy, occasionally family history hastens postnatal diagnosis or allows prenatal diagnosis based on elevated cystine in amniocytes or chorionic villus samples.

The renal tubular dysfunction leads to classic renal Fanconi syndrome with impaired reabsorption of glucose, phosphate, amino and organic acids and minerals. Renal phosphate losses lead to vitamin D-resistant rickets; chronic losses of sodium bicarbonate and potassium lead to chronic acidosis and hypokalaemia. With ongoing glomerular damage, there is a progressive renal impairment and an end-stage renal disease. There are a variety of ophthalmic abnormalities of which the pathognomonic birefringent refractile corneal deposits are the first to appear.

Pharmacology
Mercaptamine is an amino thiol that depletes lysosomal cystine in a disulphide exchange reaction with cysteine. This results in the formation of a mixed disulphide and cysteine. The mixed disulphide exits lysosomes via a 'system c' transporter, while the remaining cysteine exits via a cysteine carrier. Mercaptamine postpones, and in some cases, even prevents the deterioration of renal function and the development of extra-renal complications. Treatment should be started as soon as the diagnosis of cystinosis is made and continued lifelong, even after renal transplantation, to protect the extra-renal organs.

Sadly, therapy is not straightforward; the free thiol smells (of rotten eggs) and tastes awful, it also needs to be given regularly every 6 hours (although modified-release preparations allow older children and adults to have twice-daily treatment), and gastrointestinal side effects can make tolerance difficult – it causes a threefold increase in gastric acid production and a 50% rise of serum gastrin levels. Excessively high doses can cause skin lesions due to angioendotheliomatosis (these disappear if the dose is reduced). The oral drug has no effect on the corneal cystine crystal accumulation, most likely due to inadequate intraocular levels; thus, an ophthalmic preparation is also required.

The best outcomes are obtained by (1) making an early diagnosis, (2) administering mercaptamine every 6 hours and (3) performing frequent assays of leucocyte cystine.

Treatment

> **Note: Treatment with these products should only be initiated after consultation with a specialist nephrology advisory centre. Regular monitoring is essential.**

Oral treatment: Begin with one-sixth to one-quarter of the expected maintenance dose, increased gradually over 4–6 weeks. The maintenance dose is $1.3\,g/m^2/day$ (~50 mg/kg/day) in four divided doses. Best results are obtained from 6 hourly dosing, but a pragmatic approach is to medicate as soon as the child wakes and before the parents go to bed, with the other two doses given at intermediate times to spread out the medication as close to every 6 hours as possible.
Eye drops: Mercaptamine eye drops are instilled into each eye four to six times a day (at least 2–4 hours apart).

Monitoring treatment
Leucocyte cystine levels are used to determine dosing and compliance once the maintenance dose is achieved and every 3 months thereafter. Blood is obtained 5–6 hours after mercaptamine treatment with the aim to achieve levels <1 nmol/half-cystine/mg protein.

Continued on p. 317

Supply and administration

Mercaptamine capsules are available in 50 mg (cost £70.00 for 100 capsules) and 150 mg strengths (cost £190.00 for 100 capsules). The contents of the capsules can be sprinkled on food (milk, potatoes or starch-based foods) or added to formula milk. Mercaptamine eye drops are available in 0.11 and 0.55% strengths. These are available from 'special-order' manufacturers or specialist importing companies.

References

Besouw MTP, Bowker R, Dutertre J-P, *et al*. Cysteamine toxicity in patients with cystinosis. *J Pediatr* 2011;**159**:1004–11.

Jackson M, Elisabeth Young E. Prenatal diagnosis of cystinosis by quantitative measurement of cystine in chorionic villi and cultured cells. *Prenat Diagn* 2005;**25**:1045–7.

Tsilou ET, Thompson D, Lindblad AS, *et al*. A multicentre randomised double masked clinical trial of a new formulation of topical cysteamine for the treatment of corneal cystine crystals in cystinosis. *Br J Ophthalmol* 2003;**87**:28–31. [RCT]

Wilmer MJ, Schoeber JP, van den Heuvel LP, *et al*. Cystinosis: practical tools for diagnosis and treatment. *Pediatr Nephrol* 2011;**26**:205–15.

Use

Meropenem is a valuable broad-spectrum antibiotic. In many units it is held in reserve, and only used in consultation with a microbiologist or in a research context, when no other satisfactory alternative exists.

Pharmacology

Meropenem is a carbapenem β-lactam antibiotic active against a very wide range of Gram-positive and Gram-negative aerobic and anaerobic bacteria that first came into general clinical use in 1985. Methicillin-resistant staphylococci and *Enterococcus faecium* are resistant to meropenem, as are some strains of *Pseudomonas aeruginosa*. Meropenem is excreted in the urine, mostly unchanged, but partly as an inert metabolite. The elimination half-life in adults is only 1 hour, but a little longer in children 2–6 months old. The initial half-life in the term baby is 2 hours and in the preterm baby 3 hours, but the half-life falls significantly, irrespective of gestation, within 10–14 days of birth.

Meropenem has many of the same properties, and most of the same adverse effects, as imipenem (q.v.), but it seems to cause less nausea. It is also stable to the renal enzyme that inactivates imipenem and does not need, therefore, to be given with cilastatin. It has not been in use as long as imipenem and has not been as extensively studied, but the evidence to date suggests that meropenem is less likely to induce seizures than imipenem with cilastatin (c.v.). Meropenem can also be given as a standard slow intravenous (IV) bolus injection. It penetrates the CSF of patients with bacterial meningitis, and most other body fluids, well.

The limited amounts of meropenem that cross the placenta are insufficient to treat infection in the fetus. Teratogenicity studies and limited reports of use in human pregnancies are largely reassuring. Meropenem passes into breast milk, but there is no reason to withhold breastfeeding.

Treatment

Give 20 mg/kg by slow IV infusion over 15–30 minutes once every 12 hours in the first week of life and once every 8 hours for babies older than this. The dose may be given as an IV injection over 5 minutes if required. Double the dose to 40 mg/kg in children where meningitis, serious infection or *P. aeruginosa* infection is suspected. Intramuscular use is not recommended. Dosage frequency should be halved if there is evidence of renal failure, and treatment stopped altogether if there is anuria unless dialysis is instituted.

Supply

Vials suitable for IV use, containing 500 mg of meropenem as a powder, cost £8. Reconstitute with 9.6 ml of water for injection to give a solution containing 50 mg/ml. The manufacturers recommend prompt use after reconstitution and say that vials are for 'single use only', but they also say that the preparation can be kept for up to 24 hours after reconstitution if kept at 4 °C. A 20 mg/kg dose contains 0.08 mmol/kg of sodium.

References

Baldwin CM, Lyseng-Williamson KA, Keam SJ. Meropenem. A review of its use in the treatment of serious bacterial infections. *Drugs* 2008;**68**:803–38. [SR]

Bradley JS. Meropenem: a new, extremely broad spectrum beta-lactam antibiotic for serious infections in pediatrics. *Pediatr Infect Dis J* 1997;**16**:263–8.

Bradley JS, Sauberan JB, Ambrose PG, *et al*. Meropenem pharmacokinetics, pharmacodynamics, and Monte Carlo simulation in the neonate. *Pediatr Infect Dis J* 2008;**27**:794–9.

Cohen-Wolkowiez M, Poindexter B, Bidegain M, *et al*. Safety and effectiveness of meropenem in infants with suspected or complicated intra-abdominal infections. *Clin Infect Dis* 2012;**55**:1495–502.

Hnat M, Bawdon RE. Transfer of meropenem in the ex vivo human placenta perfusion model. *Infect Dis Obstet Gynecol* 2005;**13**:223–7.

Klugman KP, Dagan R, the Meropenem Meningitis Study Group. Randomised comparison of meropenem with cefotaxime for treatment of bacterial meningitis. *Antimicrob Agents Chemother* 1995;**39**:1140–6. [RCT]

Mouton JW, Touzw DJ, Horrevorts AM, *et al*. Comparative pharmacokinetics of the carbapenems: clinical implications. *Clin Pharmacokinet* 2000;**39**:185–201.

Odio CM, Puig JR, Ferris JM, *et al*. Prospective randomised investigator-blinded study of the efficacy and safety of meropenem vs. cefotaxime in bacterial meningitis in children. *Pediatr Infect Dis J* 1999;**18**:581–90. [RCT]

Padari H, Metsvaht T, Kõrgvee LT, *et al*. Short versus long infusion of meropenem in very-low-birth-weight neonates. *Antimicrob Agents Chemother* 2012;**56**:4760–4.

Continued on p. 319

Sauberan JB, Bradley JS, Blumer J, *et al*. Transmission of meropenem in breast milk. *Pediatr Infect Dis J* 2012;**31**:832–4.

Schuler D, the Meropenem Paediatric Study Group. Safety and efficacy of meropenem in hospitalised children: randomised comparison with cefotaxime, alone and combined with metronidazole or amikacin. *J Antimicrob Chemother* 1995;**36**(suppl A):99–108. [RCT]

van den Anker JN, Pokorna P, Kinzig-Schippers M, *et al*. Meropenem pharmacokinetics in the newborn. *Antimicrob Agents Chemother* 2009;**53**:3871–9.

van Enk JG, Touw DJ, Lafeber HN. Pharmacokinetics of meropenem in preterm neonates. *Ther Drug Monit* 2001;**23**:198–201.

Use

Methadone is widely used in the management of maternal opioid addiction and to control the more severe withdrawal ('abstinence') symptoms seen in some babies born to mothers with such an addiction.

Pharmacology

Methadone hydrochloride is a synthetic opioid analgesic developed in Germany during the 1939–1945 war that is capable of providing sustained pain relief. It is usually taken orally and is less sedating than morphine. Opiate addiction may be associated with reduced fetal growth, but there is no evidence of teratogenicity. Many women who receive methadone continue to abuse other drugs.

Methadone is well absorbed when taken by mouth (90% bioavailability) and largely metabolised by the liver through cytochromes CYP3A4, CYP2B6 and CYP2D6. The elimination half-life of methadone shows substantial inter-individual variability but in most neonates is about 20 hours.

Tissue levels exceed plasma levels (V_D ~6 l/kg). Arrhythmia due to the long QT syndrome is a rare complication and has been seen in the newborn baby of a mother stabilised on methadone. Excessive doses can cause ileus and respiratory depression. However, there appears to be no correlation between the maternal dose at delivery and the baby's risk of neonatal abstinence syndrome, and weaning the maternal dose in the hope that this lessens the fetal and neonatal risks simply increases the likelihood that illicit drugs will also be used.

Use during lactation results in the baby receiving ~3% of the weight-adjusted maternal dose, so in the absence of HIV infection, breastfeeding should be encouraged as there is some evidence that breastfed babies show fewer symptoms of withdrawal and seem less likely to require medication irrespective of the nature of the mother's addiction.

Opiate addiction

Mothers with an opiate addiction are often placed on methadone before delivery in an attempt to reduce illicit opioid usage. Methadone is useful because it can be taken orally, only needs to be taken once or twice a day and has a long-lasting effect. Maternal blood levels are more stable, reducing some of the intoxicating (and potentially damaging) 'swings' to which the fetus of an addicted mother is otherwise exposed. Weaning should not be attempted during pregnancy. In some cases, because of increased clearance, the dose may need to be increased in the last 3 months of pregnancy.

Babies typically start to show some signs of an abstinence syndrome 1–3 days after birth, with restlessness, irritability, rapid breathing, vomiting and intestinal hurry. Feeding problems may exacerbate weight loss. Swaddling and the use of a dummy or pacifier should be enough to control the symptoms in up to half the babies of drug-dependent mothers, but a rapidly reducing dose of methadone or morphine (q.v.) can be given to babies with severe symptoms. Fits are uncommon, seldom seen in the first few days, and more suggestive of a non-opiate drug dependency. Symptoms coming on before 2½ days are more typically seen where the mother is dependent on a hypnotic or sedative (barbiturates, diazepam, etc.). A mixed picture due to the abuse of several drugs is not uncommon and may justify giving phenobarbital (q.v.) as well as methadone (or morphine). Chlorpromazine (q.v.) is an understudied alternative.

Managing neonatal opiate withdrawal

Achieving control: Give one dose every 6 hours by mouth. Start with 100 micrograms/kg, and increase this by 50 micrograms/kg each time a further dose is due until symptoms are controlled.
Maintaining control: Calculate the total dose given in the 24 hours before control was achieved, and give half this amount by mouth once every 12 hours.
Weaning: Once control has been sustained for 48 hours, try and reduce the dose given by 10–20% once each day. Treatment can usually be stopped after 7–10 days although mild symptoms may persist for several weeks.

Antidote

Naloxone (q.v.) is effective but may unmask withdrawal symptoms in an opiate-dependent patient.

Continued on p. 321

Supply and administration

A clear yellow-green non-proprietary oral mixture of this controlled drug, containing 1 mg/ml of methadone hydrochloride, can be provided on request (100 ml costs £2.10). A more dilute solution (100 micrograms/ml) with a month shelf life can sometimes be provided by pharmacies for neonatal use on request.

References

(See also the Cochrane reviews on opiate withdrawal)

Abdel-Latif ME, Pinner J, Clews S, *et al.* Effects of breast milk on the severity and outcome of neonatal abstinence syndrome among infants of drug-dependent mothers. *Pediatrics* 2006;**117**:e1163–9.

Bell J, Harvey-Dodds L. Pregnancy and injecting drug use. [Review] *Br Med J* 2008;**336**:1303–5.

Dryden C, Young D, Hepburn M, *et al.* Maternal methadone use in pregnancy: factors associated with the development of neonatal abstinence syndrome and implications for healthcare resources. *BJOG* 2009;**116**:665–71.

Hussain T, Ewer AK. Maternal methadone may cause arrhythmias in neonates. *Acta Paediatr* 2007;**96**:768–9.

Jansson LM, Choo R, Valez ML, *et al.* Methadone maintenance and breast feeding in the neonatal period. *Pediatrics* 2008;**121**:106–14.

Jarvis M, Schnoll S. Methadone treatment in pregnancy. *J Psychoactive Drugs* 1994;**26**:155–61.

Johnson K, Gerada C, Greenough A. Treatment of neonatal abstinence syndrome. *Arch Dis Child Fetal Neonatal Ed* 2003;**88**:F2–5. [SR]

Jones HE, Kaltenbach K, Heil SH, *et al.* Neonatal abstinence syndrome after methadone or buprenorphine exposure. *N Engl J Med* 2010;**363**:2320–31. [RCT]

Kandall SR, Doberczak TM, Jantunen M, *et al.* The methadone-maintained pregnancy. *Clin Perinatol* 1999;**26**:173–83.

McGlone L, Mactier H, Hassan H, *et al.* In utero drug and alcohol exposure in infants born to mothers prescribed maintenance methadone. *Arch Dis Child Fetal Neonatal Ed* 2013;**98**:F542–4.

Use

Of all the antihypertensive drugs used in pregnancy, methyldopa is the best studied. It was previously used to treat resistant neonatal hypertension but is now rarely used in children.

Pharmacology

Methyldopa interferes with the normal production of noradrenaline (norepinephrine), but also seems to have direct effects on arterioles and on the central vasomotor centre. Methyldopa was first used in the management of hypertension in 1960. It reduces blood pressure and total peripheral vascular resistance without any change in cardiac output or renal blood flow. It has been widely used in the management of maternal hypertension and in patients with pre-eclamptic toxaemia. It readily crosses the placenta, but fetal side effects have not been identified, and the only neonatal effects ever noted have been occasional transient tremor and an equally transient lowering of blood pressure. Neither is there any known contraindication to use during lactation because the baby receives less than 5% of the maternal dose on a weight-for-weight basis.

Oral absorption is variable and incomplete, much of the drug is eliminated by the kidney, and there is some evidence that treatment should be modified in the presence of serious renal failure. The way drug elimination varies with age has not been well studied, but is known to have a biphasic profile: the initial half-life is only about 2 hours, but there is a much more prolonged second phase. The drug's therapeutic action is not, however, related to this half-life: even with intravenous (IV) use, the full effect only becomes apparent after 4 hours, and some effect can still be detected for 10–15 hours, while with oral administration twice a day, the drug's ability to lower blood pressure may not become fully apparent for 2–3 days. Long-term medication induces salt and water retention unless a diuretic is prescribed. Side effects include haemolytic anaemia, thrombocytopenia and gastrointestinal disturbances. Large doses have a sedative effect. If treatment is stopped suddenly, there may be a hypertensive rebound crisis.

Hypertension in pregnancy

The management of a woman already on treatment for hypertension prior to conception does not usually need to be changed, because none of the commonly used drugs are teratogenic. The exception to this is the woman who is on an ACE inhibitor (e.g. captopril) or an angiotensin II receptor antagonist (e.g. losartan and valsartan) as these drugs can cause irreversible fetal renal failure during the third trimester. Diuretic treatment can also be continued if considered appropriate, although continued use does carry disadvantages should pre-eclampsia supervene. If serious hypertension (a blood pressure of 170/110 mmHg or more) is found at booking, it merits immediate treatment, but there is no evidence that early pre-emptive intervention in women with hypertension less serious than this does anything to reduce the eventual incidence of superimposed pre-eclampsia. Hydralazine and, more recently, nifedipine (q.v.) have been the drugs most often used when other symptoms of proteinuric pre-eclampsia become apparent. Short-term atenolol use does not inhibit fetal growth. Labetalol (q.v.), given IV, is probably the drug of choice when it becomes necessary to lower blood pressure in a rapid but controlled way, while magnesium sulfate (q.v.) can be given to minimise the risk of an eclamptic seizure. The only *definitive* treatment for severe pre-eclampsia is delivery, and even after delivery, blood pressure often continues to rise for another 3–5 days before finally returning to normal 2–3 weeks later.

Treatment

Use in pregnancy: Start by giving 250 mg two or three times a day and increase the dose incrementally as necessary not more frequently than once every 3 days. A first 1 g oral loading dose can be given when hypertension needs to be controlled quickly. Doses as high as 1 g four times a day have been used on occasion. Nifedipine is sometimes used as well in patients with pre-eclamptic hypertension.

Supply and administration

5 ml (250 mg) ampoules of methyldopate for IV use are still available in North America and in some other countries but are no longer immediately available from any UK pharmaceutical company (although the product could be imported on request). In order to ensure accuracy, dilute 1 ml (50 mg) from the ampoule with 9 ml of 5% glucose to provide a solution containing 5 mg/ml prior to oral or IV administration. 125, 250 and 500 mg tablets (costing 10–85 p each) remain widely available, and a low-dose oral suspension could be prepared, on request, with a 7-day shelf life.

Continued on p. 323

References

(See also the relevant Cochrane reviews)

Cockburn J, Moar VA, Ounsted M, *et al*. Final report of study of hypertension during pregnancy: the effects of specific treatment on the growth and development of the children. *Lancet* 1982;**i**:647–9. (See also p. 1237.)

Jones HMR, Cummings AJ, Setchell KDR. Pharmacokinetics of methyldopa in neonates. *Br J Clin Pharmacol* 1979;**8**:433–40.

Magee LA, Abalos E, von Dadelszen P, *et al*. How to manage hypertension in pregnancy effectively. *Br J Clin Pharmacol* 2011;**72**:394–401.

Slim R, Ben Salem C, Hmouda H, *et al*. Hepatotoxicity of alpha-methyldopa in pregnancy. *J Clin Pharm Ther* 2010;**35**:361–3.

Solomon CG, Seely EW. Hypertension in pregnancy. *Endocrinol Metab Clin North Am* 2011;**40**:847–63.

White WB, Andreoli JW, Cohn RD. Alpha-methyldopa disposition in mothers with hypertension and their breast-fed infants. *Br J Pharmacol* 1985;**37**:387–90.

Use
Methylthioninium chloride is used to treat methaemoglobinaemia. It has also been used experimentally to treat the refractory hypotension sometimes associated with septic shock.

Methaemoglobinaemia
Methaemoglobin is the oxidised (ferric) form of the haemoglobin molecule, lacking the normal molecule's ability to carry oxygen to the tissues. The condition can be inherited (as a recessive reductase enzyme deficiency or as a dominantly inherited haemoglobinopathy) or occur briefly as a result of drug exposure. Babies are at particular risk because reductase enzyme levels are initially low. Nitric oxide is rapidly inactivated by the haemoglobin molecule forming nitrosylhaemoglobin, which is then converted to methaemoglobin. It is for this reason that excess inhaled nitric oxide (q.v.) can cause methaemoglobinaemia. Aniline dyes (even when absorbed through the skin) can have the same effect, as can the local anaesthetic prilocaine. Excess nitrates in drinking water were once a common cause. If a drop of suspect blood turns chocolate brown rather than red over 30 seconds, when compared to a control sample, as it dries on a filter paper, the suspect specimen almost certainly contains more than 10% of methaemoglobin.

Pharmacology
Methylthioninium chloride is a basic dye first synthesised in 1876. Histologists have used it for more than a century to dye living nerve tissue. It is reduced in the red cell to leuco-methylthioninium (leucomethylene blue) where it then acts to convert methaemoglobin back to haemoglobin. It is therefore used in the treatment of both congenital and acquired methaemoglobinaemia. It has also been used as a dye to monitor reflux, trace fistulas, position tubes, identify premature rupture of membranes and 'mark' the different amniotic sacs in multiple pregnancy, although this last use can cause serious haemolytic anaemia and neonatal jaundice and is claimed to be associated with a high risk of jejunal atresia. Recently, there has been experimental interest in the use of the same drug to control the severe hypotension seen in septic shock when this fails to respond to inotropes and hydrocortisone (q.v.) because this condition seems to be mediated, at least in part, by excess tissue nitric oxide synthesis. Nitric oxide causes vasodilatation by activating soluble guanylate cyclase in smooth muscle cells to produce cyclic guanosine monophosphate, and methylthioninium chloride inhibits this activation.

Methylthioninium chloride is moderately well absorbed when given by mouth and slowly excreted in the urine, after partial conversion to leuco-methylthioninium. Repeated use may be hazardous if renal function is poor. Intravenous (IV) administration can cause a number of adverse reactions including pain, nausea, vomiting, confusion, dizziness, sweating and hypotension. Repeated treatment, or an overdose, can actually *cause* methaemoglobinaemia, haemolysis and hyperbilirubinaemia, and there is no effective treatment for this other than exchange transfusion. Infants with G6PD deficiency are at particular risk in this regard. Long-term treatment has been known to cause haemolytic anaemia. Heinz body formation has also been reported. Methylthioninium chloride turns urine, stools and body secretions blue. The skin also becomes discoloured.

Little is known about the safety of giving IV treatment to a mother during pregnancy or lactation. It crosses the human placenta after intra-amniotic injection and is excreted in the maternal urine. Neonates with G6PD deficiency exposed *in utero* may experience severe haemolysis and hyperbilirubinaemia requiring exchange transfusion. There is some evidence to suggest it can be safely used for lymphatic mapping in breast cancer when this is diagnosed during pregnancy.

Treatment
Give 1 mg/kg IV (1 ml of a solution made up as described under 'Supply and administration') over 1 hour. A repeat dose can be given if necessary after a few hours. Also seek advice from National Poisons Information Service.

Oral treatment has occasionally been used to manage serious congenital methaemoglobinaemia, even though this tends to make the cyanosed patient blue for a different reason! Doses of up to 2 mg/kg once a day by mouth have been used. Oral ascorbic acid (500 mg once a day) may also be effective.

Supply and administration
Methylthioninium chloride is available as a 5 mg/ml solution in 10 ml ampoules costing £39 each; to give 1 mg/kg IV, take 2 ml from the ampoule for each kilogram the baby weighs, dilute to 10 ml with 5% glucose immediately before use, and infuse 1 ml of the resultant solution over

Continued on p. 325

1 hour. More rapid infusions have been given with apparent safety on occasion. Take care to avoid tissue extravasation as this can cause necrotic ulceration.

References

Allergaert K, Miserez M, Naulaers G, *et al*. Enteral administration of methylene blue in a preterm infant. [Abstract] *Pediatr Perinat Drug Ther* 2004;**6**:70.

Crook J. Haemolytic jaundice in a neonate after intra-amniotic injection of methylene blue. *Arch Dis Child* 1982;**57**:872–86.

Driscoll W, Thurin S, Carrion V, *et al*. Effect of methylene blue on refractory neonatal hypotension. *J Pediatr* 1996; **129**:904–8. (See also pp. 790–3.)

Ofoegbu BN, Agrawal RP, Lewis MA. Methylene blue irrigation-treatment of renal fungal balls causing acute renal failure in a preterm infant. *Acta Paediatr* 2005;**96**:939–40.

Pruthi S, Haakenson C, Brost BC, *et al*. Pharmacokinetics of methylene blue dye for lymphatic mapping in breast cancer-implications for use in pregnancy. *Am J Surg* 2011;**201**:70–5.

Use

Metoclopramide provides symptomatic relief from nausea and vomiting in pregnancy when first-line treatment with antihistamines (e.g. diphenhydramine, meclizine, dimenhydrinate) has failed. There are conflicting reports as to its effectiveness as a galactogogue. Although there is some evidence that it reduces symptomatic gastro-oesophageal reflux (GOR) in children a few months old, no neonatal studies have been published, and the risk of neurological effects such as extrapyramidal disorders and tardive dyskinesia has led to it being contraindicated in children <12 months old.

Pharmacology

Metoclopramide hydrochloride is a substituted benzamide related to procainamide. It stimulates motility in the upper gastrointestinal tract without affecting gastric, biliary or pancreatic secretion. It was being evaluated as a possible antiarrhythmic agent when its anti-emetic properties came to light in 1964. It is rapidly absorbed from the intestinal tract, but a variable first-pass metabolism leads to unpredictable plasma levels. Metoclopramide possesses parasympathomimetic activity.

It has been used to control some forms of nausea and vomiting (particularly in patients undergoing cytotoxic treatment or radiotherapy) and in the management of gastric stasis and GOR, but there is good evidence that ondansetron (q.v.) is a better drug to use to control nausea and vomiting in young children.

Metoclopramide is a dopamine receptor antagonist, and idiosyncratic dystonic and dyskinetic extrapyramidal signs are not infrequently seen in children, even at the normally recommended dose. For these reasons, the manufacturers only recommend use in patients under 20 years old to prevent post-operative vomiting, to control the nausea caused by chemotherapy and as an aid to passage of a gastric or similar feeding tube. Domperidone (q.v.) is a related drug which causes fewer dystonic problems. Erythromycin (q.v.) is sometimes used in the neonatal period to stimulate gastrointestinal motility.

Metoclopramide has also been used to treat the severe nausea and vomiting that occasionally occur during pregnancy (hyperemesis gravidarum), and a study of the outcomes of these pregnancies found no evidence of teratogenicity. It has also been given to speed gastric emptying during labour or as a pre-anaesthetic medication to reduce the risk of vomiting. Metoclopramide, like domperidone, stimulates prolactin secretion from the anterior pituitary, but there are conflicting reports as to its ability to enhance lactation (see website commentary). It does not work in all women (possibly because they already have raised prolactin levels), and side effects, such as cramp and diarrhoea, sometimes limit compliance. The drug accumulates in breast milk, but ingestion by the baby would be unlikely to exceed 50 micrograms/kg/day – one-tenth the maximum dose used for medicinal purposes.

Treatment

Mother: Giving 10 (or even 15) mg to the mother by mouth three times a day stimulated milk production in some studies. Taper treatment off over 5–10 days to limit the risk of milk production declining again later.

Baby: Not recommended in children under the age of 12 months due to the risk of neurological effects.

Toxicity

The therapeutic dose is only slightly less than the toxic dose in children. Tachycardia, agitation, hypertonia, feeding problems and diarrhoea have all been reported following a neonatal overdose, together with methaemoglobinaemia which responded to treatment with methylthioninium chloride (q.v.).

Supply and administration

2 ml ampoules containing 10 mg of metoclopramide (costing 27p) are also available for intravenous (IV) or intramuscular use. For IV use, take 1 ml of the liquid formulation in the ampoule, dilute to 50 ml with 0.9% sodium chloride to provide a solution containing 100 micrograms/ml, and give as a slow bolus infusion. Discard discoloured ampoules. Tablets are available in 10 mg strengths costing 3 p each. Metoclopramide is also available as a liquid containing 1 mg/ml (100 ml costs £10) which *must* be protected from light. This can be further diluted with an equal quantity of pure water but should be used within 2 weeks of being dispensed. A sugar-free formulation can be provided on request.

Continued on p. 327

References

(See also the Cochrane review of GOR in infancy)

Bellisant E, Duhamel JF, Guilot M, *et al.* The triangular test to assess the efficacy of metoclopramide in gastro-esophageal reflux. *Clin Pharmacol Ther* 1997;**61**:377–84. [RCT]

Berkovitch M, Elbirt D, Addis A, *et al.* Fetal effects of metoclopramide therapy for nausea and vomiting in pregnancy. *N Engl J Med* 2000;**343**:445–6.

Fife S, Gill P, Hopkins M, *et al.* Metoclopramide to augment lactation, does it work? A randomized trial. *J Matern Fetal Neonatal Med* 2011;**24**:1317–20. [RCT]

Hibbs M, Lorch SA. Metoclopramide for the treatment of gastroesophageal reflux disease in infants: systematic review. *Pediatrics* 2006;**118**:746–52. [SR] (See also pp. 793–4.)

Ingram J, Taylor H, Churchill C, *et al.* Metoclopramide or domperidone for increasing maternal breast milk output: a randomised controlled trial. *Arch Dis Child Fetal Neonatal Ed* 2012;**97**:F241–5. [RCT]

Machida HM, Forbes DA, Gall DG, *et al.* Metoclopramide in gastroesophageal reflux in infancy. *J Pediatr* 1988;**112**:483–7.

Sørensen HT, Nielsen GL, Christensen K, *et al.* Birth outcome following maternal use of metoclopramide. *Br J Clin Pharmacol* 2000;**49**:264–8.

Tolia V, Calhoun J, Kuhns L, *et al.* Randomised, prospective double blind trial of metoclopramide and placebo for gastroesophageal reflux in infants. *J Pediatr* 1989;**115**:141–5. [RCT]

Toppare MF, Laleli Y, Senses DA, *et al.* Metoclopramide for breast milk production. *Nutr Res* 1994;**14**: 1019–23.

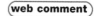

Use

Metronidazole is used in the management of anaerobic bacterial infection (including meningitis) and in the treatment of a range of protozoal infections such as amoebiasis, giardiasis and trichomoniasis. It is also widely used in the United Kingdom after intestinal surgery and in the management of necrotising enterocolitis.

Pharmacology

Metronidazole, a 5-nitroimidazole derivative, is a unique bactericidal antibiotic that first came into clinical use in 1960. It is particularly useful in the treatment of dental, surgical and gynaecological sepsis because of its activity against obligate anaerobes such as *Bacteroides* and *Clostridium* species and facultative anaerobes such as *Gardnerella* and *Helicobacter*. It seems rare for bacterial resistance to develop.

Both partners should be treated when *Trichomonas vaginalis* infection is suspected. Short prophylactic courses, with or without ampicillin, are frequently given during abdominal and pelvic surgery in Europe, but cefoxitin (q.v.) is more often used for this purpose in North America (where metronidazole is still seldom used in children). A reversible sensory neuropathy has been seen in adults after prolonged treatment. Mild gastrointestinal symptoms can occur.

Metronidazole can be given by intravenous (IV) injection but is well absorbed both orally and rectally. The drug has a large volume of distribution (V_D ~0.8 l/kg), penetrates most body fluids (including CSF and ascitic fluid) well and is excreted in the urine after partial breakdown to a product that also has some antimicrobial activity. The plasma half-life is long and inversely related to gestational age at birth. It soon approaches that seen in adults (7–10 hours). The dosage interval may need to be increased where there is hepatic failure, but does not usually require modification in renal failure although some metabolites may accumulate.

Use in pregnancy was long considered controversial because the drug readily crosses the placenta. It is mutagenic in bacteria and carcinogenic in rodents although neither of these effects has been proved in humans. Nor is there any evidence to suggest it is a teratogen, although it can increase the fetotoxic and teratogenic effect of alcohol in mice.

More recently, it has been widely used with apparent safety to treat trichomonal and bacterial vaginitis both during pregnancy and during lactation. While the increased vaginal discharge and the characteristic odour (vaginosis) caused when anaerobic bacteria replace lactobacilli may merit treatment, the PREMET trial suggested treatment with metronidazole might actually *increase* the risk of preterm birth. Oral or vaginal clindamycin (q.v.) seems to be a better alternative. The breastfed baby of any mother on 400 mg twice a day for 7 days will end with a blood level about a quarter of that seen during treatment. While this is said to affect the milk's taste, it seems otherwise harmless. Women can, however, suspend lactation for 24 hours and request an alternative treatment strategy – a single high (2 g) oral dose of metronidazole.

Amoebiasis

Asymptomatic infection is common. It can be difficult to distinguish *Entamoeba histolytica*, which is a worldwide tissue-invasive pathogen, from *E. dispar*, a mere commensal. Intestinal amoebiasis can cause abdominal pain and bloody diarrhoea, while invasive infection can affect the liver, chest or brain. Metronidazole for 5–10 days will treat invasive infection, but diloxanide is necessary to clear the bowel (6.6 mg/kg by mouth three times a day for 10 days) even though the manufacturer has yet to endorse use in young children or during pregnancy.

Drug interactions

Concurrent barbiturate use can decrease the half-life in children, making a higher daily dose necessary. Steroids and rifampicin may have a similar but less marked effect.

Treatment

Give a 15 mg/kg IV loading dose. Then give 7.5 mg/kg, orally or IV, once every 24 hours in babies with a post-menstrual age <26 weeks, once every 12 hours in babies with a post-menstrual age of between 26 and 34 weeks, and every 8 hours in babies with a post-menstrual age ≥34 weeks. Treat infants up to 2 months old using the same regime as neonates with a post-menstrual age ≥34 weeks. Higher doses have been used in meningitis. Slow IV administration is only necessary in older children and adults because of the volume of fluid involved.

Continued on p. 329

Supply

A 20 ml (5 mg/ml) IV ampoule of metronidazole costs £1.60. A 7.5 mg/kg dose contains 0.2 mmol/kg of sodium. Limited solubility precludes intramuscular use as the volume involved would be too large. A 40 mg/ml oral suspension in sucrose is available (100 ml costs £25), and a more dilute suspension can be prepared with a 2-week shelf life. 500 mg tablets of diloxanide cost £3.10, and an oral suspension can be prepared from these.

References

(See also the relevant Cochrane reviews)

Burtin P, Taddio A, Ariburna O, *et al*. Safety of metronidazole in pregnancy: a meta-analysis. *Am J Obstet Gynecol* 1995;**172**:525–9. [SR]

Cohen-Wolkowiez M, Ouellet D, Smith PB, *et al*. Population pharmacokinetics of metronidazole evaluated using scavenged samples from preterm infants. *Antimicrob Agents Chemother* 2012;**56**:1828–37.

Escobedo AA, Almirall P, Alfonso M, *et al*. Treatment of intestinal protozoan infections in children. *Arch Dis Child* 2009;**94**:478–82.

Koss CA, Baras DC, Lane SD, *et al*. Investigation of metronidazole use during pregnancy and adverse birth outcomes. *Antimicrob Agents Chemother* 2012;**56**:4800–5.

Morency A-M, Bujold E. The effect of second trimester antibiotic therapy on the rate of preterm birth. *J Obstet Gynaecol Can* 2007;**29**:35–44. [SR]

Shennan A, Crawshaw S, Briley A, *et al*. A randomised controlled trial of metronidazole for the prevention of preterm birth in women positive for cervicovaginal fibronectin: the PREMET study. *Br J Obstet Gynaecol* 2006;**113**:65–74. [RCT] (See also pp. 976–7.)

Simcox R, Sin WA, Seed PT, *et al*. Prophylactic antibiotics for the prevention of preterm birth in women at risk: a meta-analysis. *Aust NZ J Obstet Gynaecol* 2007;**47**:368–77. [SR]

Suyagh M, Collier PS, Millership JS, *et al*. Metronidazole population pharmacokinetics in preterm neonates using dried blood-spot sampling. *Pediatrics* 2011;**127**:e367–74.

Use

Micafungin, like caspofungin (q.v.), is an echinocandin with established *in vitro* and *in vivo* concentration-dependent fungicidal activity against most *Candida* species. In the European Union and Japan, micafungin is approved for children including neonates for treatment of invasive candidiasis; however, in the United States, approval is for use in children older than 4 months only. Micafungin may be used both prophylactically and to treat established infection.

Pharmacology

Micafungin is a non-competitive inhibitor of β-(1,3)-D-glucan synthase which is necessary for the synthesis of an essential component of the fungal cell wall, β-(1,3)-D-glucan. Fungal cells unable to synthesise this polysaccharide cannot maintain their shape and lack adequate rigidity to resist osmotic pressure, which results in fungal cell lysis. It demonstrates *in vitro* and *in vivo* activity against *Aspergillus* and a range of *Candida* species, including *C. albicans*, *C. parapsilosis*, *C. tropicalis* and *C. glabrata*. Micafungin is not effective in *Zygomycetes* or *Cryptococcus* infection.

Oral absorption is poor and the drug has to be given intravenously. It is highly protein bound and thus is unlikely to penetrate cerebrospinal fluid, intra-vitreal fluid or urine in clinically significant amounts unless used in high doses. Micafungin was found to be embryotoxic and to interfere with visceral organ formation at high doses in pregnant rodents, but nothing, understandably, is yet known about the effect of its use in women during pregnancy or lactation. With a high molecular weight and significant protein binding, it is unlikely that significant amounts will cross the placenta. In the breastfed infant, poor oral bioavailability should further limit exposure.

Micafungin is extensively metabolised in the liver to several metabolites: an M-1 (catechol form), an M-2 (methoxy form of M-1) and an M-5 (hydroxylation at the side chain). These are excreted in an inactive form into bile and to a lesser extent into urine (<1% is in urine in an unchanged form). Although the M-5 part of the metabolism is by cytochrome P450 3A4 (of which micafungin is a weak inhibitor), this is fairly minor, and few drug interactions are described. Clearance in the newborn and premature infants is faster than in older children and adults, and it is believe that age-dependent serum protein binding of micafungin might be responsible for its higher clearance. Side effects include disturbances of liver enzymes, hypokalaemia, hyperbilirubinaemia and hypertension; however, all are rare even at doses up to 15 mg/kg.

Drug interactions

Micafungin increases plasma concentration of amphotericin, itraconazole and nifedipine. Micafungin is not induced by the same drugs that affect caspofungin.

Treatment

Prophylaxis: Give an intravenous (IV) infusion of 1 mg/kg over 60 minutes once daily. Treatment is continued for at least 7 days after the neutrophil count reaches the desirable range.
Treatment: Give an IV infusion of 2 mg/kg over 60 minutes once daily (the dose may be increased to 4 mg/kg daily if the response is inadequate) for at least 14 days.
CNS involvement: *In vivo*-to-clinical bridging studies suggest that dosages greater than those previously mentioned may be required to ensure effective antifungal effect in the CNS. A dose of 10 mg/kg is thought adequate to provide CNS penetration in premature and term neonates. Given that invasive candidiasis usually involves the CNS in premature infants, some argue that this should be the standard dose for all neonates.

Supply and administration

Micafungin comes as a powder ready for reconstitution in 50 mg vials that cost £196 each. The powder is dissolved in 5 ml of 0.9% sodium chloride or 5% glucose. For accurate low-dose administration, further dilute the resultant solution to a concentration of 0.5–2 mg/ml. Infuse over 60 minutes and protect the infusion from light.

References

Ascher S, Smith PB, Benjamin DK Jr. Safety of micafungin in infants: insights into optimal dosing. *Expert Opin Drug Saf* 2011;**10**:281–6.

Benjamin DK Jr, Smith PB, Arrieta A, *et al.* Safety and pharmacokinetics of repeat-dose micafungin in young infants. *Clin Pharmacol Ther* 2010;**87**:93–9.

Continued on p. 331

Hope WW, Mickiene D, Petraitis V, *et al.* The pharmacokinetics and pharmacodynamics of micafungin in experimental hematogenous Candida meningoencephalitis: implications for echinocandin therapy in neonates. *J Infect Dis* 2008;**197**:163–71.

Hope WW, Smith PB, Arrieta A, *et al.* Population pharmacokinetics of micafungin in neonates and young infants. *Antimicrob Agents Chemother* 2010;**54**:2633–7.

Kawada M, Fukuoka N, Kondo M, *et al.* Pharmacokinetics of prophylactic micafungin in very-low-birth-weight infants. *Pediatr Infect Dis J* 2009;**28**:840–2.

Smith PB, Walsh TJ, Hope W, *et al.* Pharmacokinetics of an elevated dosage of micafungin in premature neonates. *Pediatr Infect Dis J* 2009;**28**:412–5.

Yanni SB, Smith PB, Benjamin DK Jr, *et al.* Higher clearance of micafungin in neonates compared with adults: role of age-dependent micafungin serum binding. *Biopharm Drug Dispos* 2011;**32**:222–32.

Use

Miconazole and nystatin (q.v.) are both widely used in the treatment of topical *Candida* infection. There is good controlled trial evidence that miconazole is better than nystatin at eliminating oral thrush.

Pharmacology

Miconazole is an artificial imidazole agent first developed in 1969 which is active against a wide range of pathogenic yeasts and dermatophytes, as well as a range of Gram-positive bacteria (staphylococci and streptococci). These properties make it particularly useful in the treatment of oral and vaginal thrush, candida nappy rash, intertrigo, paronychia, ringworm and athlete's foot. It works by interfering with ergosterol synthesis, damaging fungal cell wall permeability. It is moderately well absorbed when given by mouth (unlike nystatin) and then inactivated by the liver before excretion in the urine, but much of any oral dose is excreted unchanged in the stool. It was, for some years, given by intravenous injection or by mouth in the treatment of a range of systemic fungal infections but is now only used topically to treat infection of the skin, gut or mucous membranes. Miconazole seems to eliminate vaginal candidiasis in pregnancy better than nystatin, and while it is systemically absorbed in very small amounts after vaginal application, there is no evidence that topical use by the mother during pregnancy or lactation poses any hazard to the baby at least when used properly.

Candida dermatitis

Candida can be found in the vagina of a quarter of pregnant women, and a fifth of their babies become colonised at birth, and more over the next month. *Candida* proliferates in moist skin, but overt infection is seldom seen except in babies with excessive intestinal colonisation. It is not surprising, therefore, that overt skin damage (dermatitis) usually starts in the perianal region, especially if the skin is already damaged. Prior prolonged and broad-spectrum antibiotic use makes overt infection more likely.

Use of gentian violet

Gentian violet (also known as 'crystal violet'), a triarylmethane antiseptic dye, is an old-fashioned treatment for *Candida* infection of the skin that is also active against a range of Gram-positive organisms including staphylococci. While it is effective despite its alarming colour, it is no longer used in the United Kingdom (especially on broken skin or mucous membranes) because of theoretical concern about carcinogenicity in mice. The 0.5% aqueous solution is still sometimes used to treat *Candida* infection of the skin elsewhere in the world and is often thought to be the most effective topical product currently available because of its deep penetration. It is probably not wise to apply the solution to mucosal surfaces more than twice a day for 3–4 days. It stains everything it touches, including clothing and skin. It is worth treating the gut with miconazole or nystatin at the same time. Little is known about use during pregnancy or lactation.

Drug interactions

The combination of *oral* miconazole and cisapride (now withdrawn) carried a high risk of arrhythmia. Oral miconazole can affect the anticoagulant effect of warfarin and increase the serum concentrations of carbamazepine and phenytoin.

Treatment

Oral thrush: Smear 1.25 ml of miconazole oral gel round the mouth and gums with a finger after feeds four times a day, and take steps to prevent reinfection as outlined in the monograph on nystatin. Continue treatment for at least 2 days after all the signs of infection have gone (usually 7–10 days in all).

Candida (Monilia) **dermatitis**: Use miconazole nitrate as a cream twice a day for at least 10 days, even if the rash improves quickly. There is a real risk of the problem recurring if treatment is stopped too soon. It may be advisable to treat the gastrointestinal tract as well as the skin if there is evidence of stubborn infection (and nystatin may be better at eradicating *Candida* from the lower bowel).

Supply

One 30 g tube of miconazole skin cream (2% w/w) costs £1.80. A 15 g tube of sugar-free oral gel (24 mg/ml) costs £3 and is also available in the United Kingdom without prescription. The manufacturer does not recommend use in babies less than 4 months old because excessive

Continued on p. 333

administration could cause the baby to choke. The cream and a dusting powder are also available 'over the counter' without prescription.

Inexpensive crystal violet paint (as a 0.5% aqueous preparation) is dispensable on request. Avoid the use of alcoholic solutions and solutions that are more concentrated than this, especially when treating the mouth and tongue.

References

(See also relevant Cochrane reviews)

Ainsworth S, Jones W. It sticks in our throats too. *Br Med J* 2009;**338**:a3178.

Drinkwater P. Gentian violet: is it safe? *Aust NZ J Obstet Gynaecol* 1990;**30**:65–6.

Hoppe JE. Treatment of oropharyngeal candidiasis and candidal diaper dermatitis in neonates and infants: review and reappraisal. *Pediatr Infect Dis J* 1997;**16**:885–94. [SR]

Piatt JP, Bergeson PS. Gentian violet toxicity. *Clin Pediatr* 1992;**31**:756–7.

Rosa FW, Baum C, Shaw M. Pregnancy outcomes after first-trimester vaginitis drug therapy. *Obstet Gynecol* 1987;**69**:751–5.

Wainer S, Cooper PA, Funk E, *et al.* Prophylactic miconazole oral gel for the prevention of neonatal fungal rectal colonization and systemic infection. *Pediatr Infect Dis J* 1992;**11**:713–6.

Use

Midazolam is an effective sedative and a useful first-line anticonvulsant, but it does not relieve pain.

Pharmacology

Midazolam hydrochloride is a short-acting benzodiazepine with hypnotic, anxiolytic, muscle relaxant and anticonvulsant activity. Bioavailability is about 35% when given as a syrup and 50% when absorbed through the nasal or buccal mucosa. Midazolam is metabolised by cytochromes CYP3A4 and CYP2C9 in adults, but these are immature in neonates. Additionally, the main metabolite, 1-hydroxymethyl midazolam, which is also pharmacologically active, is eliminated through the kidney; thus, while the half-life is only 2 hours in adults, it is 12 hours in the neonate. An intravenous (IV) bolus dose in a preterm baby is not recommended as it frequently causes respiratory depression, hypotension and a fall in cerebral blood flow. Myoclonic jerking, not associated with EEG abnormality, and paradoxical agitation have been reported. Sustained use causes drug accumulation, with tissue levels that variably exceed plasma levels (V_D 1–3 l/kg), and withdrawal symptoms have been reported in up to a quarter of all children. Severe encephalopathic features of drowsiness, dystonic posturing and choreoathetosis are sometimes reported 1–2 days after stopping treatment. The manufacturer does not recommend use as a sedative in any child <6 months old, and the Cochrane overview found inadequate evidence to support neonatal use.

Maternal use during the third trimester of pregnancy or during labour may cause neonatal withdrawal or the infant to be hypotonic. However, the drug's rapid clearance means that very little appears in breast milk. Midazolam is now widely used to stop prolonged seizures in children with the rapidity of mucosal absorption from the nose or mouth ('buccal' administration) making IV administration less necessary.

> **Midazolam pharmacokinetics during therapeutic hypothermia have not been established, but as the drug is metabolised extensively by hepatic cytochromes P450 3A4 and 3A5, the half-life is likely to be extended further in cooled infants. Use in hypothermic adults is associated with a fivefold increase in serum levels.**

Treatment

Short-term sedation: A 500 micrograms/kg dose by mouth is often used to premedicate children prior to anaesthesia. A 300 micrograms/kg into the nose can provide sedation during investigational procedures, and 500–700 micrograms/kg into the nose (monitored with an oximeter) relieves stress during suturing.

Continuous sedation: Some units give 60 micrograms/kg/hour to sedate the ventilated baby, but this strategy is now increasingly questioned. The rate of infusion **must** be halved after 24 hours in babies of <32 weeks' postmenstrual age to prevent drug accumulation.

Controlling seizures: A 150–200 micrograms/kg dose given IV over 2 minutes stops most fits in infancy. However, 300 micrograms/kg of the buccal preparation given into the nose or under the tongue will usually achieve this just as quickly (and this can be done outside hospital).

Antidote

All benzodiazepines cause hypotonia, hypotension and coma in excess, but these effects can be reversed by flumazenil, a competitive antagonist with a relatively short (50 minute) half-life. High-dose use may cause respiratory depression. Give one (or two) 10 micrograms/kg IV dose over 15 seconds and assess the effect. If there is a definite but unsustained response, start a continuous IV infusion at 2–10 micrograms/kg/hour for 6–12 hours. Adjust the dose according to response. Use may unmask fits suppressed by benzodiazepines.

Compatibility

Compatibility with other continuously infused drugs is noted, where known, in the monograph for the second product. Midazolam can also be added (terminally) to an IV line containing standard TPN (but not lipid).

Continued on p. 335

Supply and administration

Midazolam: 5 ml ampoules containing either 5 or 10 mg of midazolam cost about 60p. To give 30 micrograms/kg of midazolam per hour as a continuous IV infusion, place 15 mg/kg of midazolam in a syringe, dilute to 50 ml with 10% glucose or glucose saline, and infuse at a rate of 0.1 ml/hour. (A less concentrated solution of dextrose or dextrose saline can be used where necessary.) The drug is stable in solution so it is not necessary to change the infusate daily. Many North American products contain 1% benzyl alcohol.

An oromucosal solution (Buccolam®) containing 5 mg/ml is available in 0.5, 1, 1.5 and 2 ml pre-filled syringes (cost £20–22). The syringes do not need to be refrigerated.

Flumazenil: 5 ml ampoules of flumazenil containing 500 micrograms cost £13.50. Dilute with 5% glucose.

References   (See also the relevant Cochrane reviews)

Anand KJS, McIntosh N, Lagercranz H, *et al.* Analgesia and sedation in neonates who require ventilatory support – results from the NOPAIN trial. *Arch Pediatr Adolesc Med* 1999;**153**:331–8. [RCT]

Aviram EE, Ben-Abraham R, Weinbrioum AA. Flumazenil use in children. *Paed Perinatal Drug Ther* 2004;**5**:202–9.

Ista E, van Diik M, Gamei C, *et al.* Withdrawal symptoms in critically ill children after long term administration of sedatives and or analgesics: a first evaluation. *Crit Care Med* 2008;**36**:2427–32.

McIntyre J, Robertson S, Norris E, *et al.* Safety and efficacy of buccal midazolam versus rectal diazepam for emergency treatment of seizures in children: a randomised controlled trial. *Lancet* 2005;**366**:205–10. [RCT] (See also pp. 182–3.)

Shany E, Benzaqen O, Watemberg N. Comparison of continuous drip of midazolam or lidocaine in the treatment of intractable neonatal seizures. *J Child Neurol* 2007;**22**:255–9.

de Wildt SN, Kearns GL, Hop WC, *et al.* Pharmacokinetics and metabolism of oral midazolam in preterm infants. *Br J Clin Pharmacol* 2002;**53**:390–2.

de Wildt SN, Kearns GL, Hop WCJ, *et al.* Pharmacokinetics and metabolism of intravenous midazolam in preterm infants. *Clin Pharmacol Ther* 2001;**70**:525–31.

Use

Gastro-oesophageal reflux is one of the most common gastrointestinal complaints in infancy, with a reported incidence of 20–40%. Therapeutic options include dietary interventions (smaller, more frequent feeds), positioning (elevating the head of the cot), drugs and, in extreme cases, surgery. Thickened formulae are increasingly being used to treat infants with reflux, driven in large part by the baby food industry. There is no good evidence, as yet, that this approach is of any value in reducing the apnoeic episodes attributed to reflux in the preterm baby. In some babies, it is important to exclude and treat cow's milk protein allergy as the cause of the reflux (see web commentary).

Milk thickeners

A number of thickeners, designed to be added to the milk at the point of use, are available; rice cereal (more popular in North America), carob bean gum, carob seed flour, starches and sodium carboxymethylcellulose are often used. Infant Gaviscon® (q.v.) probably also works in the same way, rather than forming the alginate 'raft' as seen with 'adult' preparations. Care must also be taken to ensure that any products used are designed for use in babies and not older children.

Carob seed flour is a galactomannan refined from the seeds of the carob (or locust) bean tree, *Ceratonia siliqua*. The gum is widely used as a thickening agent and stabiliser in the food industry. Cow & Gate (C&G) Instant Carobel® (a similar product is marketed in some countries as Karicare Aptamil® Feed Thickener) is made from carob seed flour. The powder also contains calcium carbonate, iron sulphate, zinc sulphate and maltodextrin. It is probably wise to monitor the red cell galactose-1-phosphate level in babies with known galactosaemia if using these products. Nestlé Nestargel® is a similar product (available in some countries) but which has less metabolisable carbohydrate and slightly more calcium carbonate. Although these products contain some carbohydrate, they do not add significantly (<1%) to the overall calories of the milk and thus do not replace a high-energy supplement if this is required.

Treatment

Thin formula feeds: Thicken 90 ml (~3 fl.oz) of formula milk with half scoop (1% concentration).
Thicker formula feeds: Thicken 60 ml (~2 fl.oz) with 1 scoop = 1.7 g (3% concentration).
The product requires heat to thicken, so make up the infant formula and immediately add the Instant Carobel. Add gradually and shake vigorously to prevent lumps from forming. Leave to

Composition (per 100 ml) of human milk and anti-reflux formula milks.

	Protein (g)	Fat (g)	CHO (g)	Energy (kcal)	Na (mg)	Ca (mg)	P (mg)	Zn (mg)	Vit D (µg)	Vit K (µg)
Typical mature human breast milk	1.4	4.0	6.6	67	25.3	25	13	0.34	<0.1	0.2
Potato starch thickened										
Nestlé NAN AR®	1.5	3.1	8.2	67	31	77	48	0.5	1.1	5.0
Novalac AR®*	1.7	3.1	7.4	64	22.1	65	50.1	0.5	1	3.9
Rice starch thickened										
Mead Johnson Enfamil AR®	1.7	3.4	7.6	67	27	53	43	0.7	1.0	6.0
Gelatinised maize starch thickened										
SMA Staydown®	1.6	3.6	7	67	22.2	56	44	0.6	1.2	6.7
Carob bean gum thickened										
C&G Anti-reflux®	1.6	3.5	6.8	66	23	77	44	0.59	1.2	4.5
Aptamil Anti-reflux®	1.8	3.6	6.8	66	17.6	56	44	0.6	1.1	6.7
Infacare Anti-reflux®	1.6	3.5	6.8	66	23	77	44	0.59	1.2	4.5

Note: Novalac Digest AR ® is similar but contains hydrolysed proteins.

Continued on p. 337

thicken for 3–4 minutes. Shake again and feed straight away. A teat with a larger hole, for example, 'fast flow', will be required due to the increased thickness of the formula.

Breastfeeding: Mix one scoop of Instant Carobel and 20 ml warm, previously boiled water. Leave to thicken for 3–4 minutes and feed immediately, using a baby spoon.

Anti-reflux milks

Anti-reflux formula milks are marketed by a number of different companies. As with the 'thickeners', the agent used to thicken these milks varies from company to company (see table). These milks are designed to meet the nutritional needs of otherwise healthy term babies and are not suitable for preterm infants. They should not be used with Gaviscon Infant.

There is no evidence to suggest that any one of these formula milks is superior to any other.

Supply

Manufacturers are banned from subsidising the cost of infant formula milks supplied to hospitals or from providing free samples in an attempt to increase their share of the market with newly delivered mothers. The practice has been shown in nine controlled trials to reduce the number of mothers achieving a sustained lactation.

Infant formula milks and modular feeds are a food source and therefore an excellent medium for bacterial and microbial proliferation. Powdered infant formula is a non-sterile product, and there is an inherent risk of infection with pathogenic bacteria such as *Salmonella* and *Enterobacter sakazakii* in preterm, low birthweight and immunocompromised infants who are most at risk. For this reason, most standard term and all preterm infant formula milks are available as ready-made bottles (for use in hospitals) and as either powder or ready-made in cartons for home use. Pre-thickened formula milks are currently not available in a ready-to-feed form.

References

Corvaglia L, Ferlini M, Rotatori R, *et al*. Starch thickening of human milk is ineffective in reducing the gastroesophageal reflux in preterm infants: a crossover study using intraluminal impedance. *J Pediatr* 2006;**148**:265–8. [RCT]

du Toit G, Meyer R, Shah N, *et al*. Identifying and managing cow's milk protein allergy. *Arch Dis Child Educ Pract Ed* 2010;**95**:134–44.

Horvath A, Dziechciarz P, Szajewska H. The effect of thickened-feed intervention on gastroesophageal reflux in infants: systematic review and meta-analysis of randomized, controlled trials. *Pediatrics* 2008;**122**:e1268–77. [SR]

Khoshoo V, Edell D, Thompson A, *et al*. Are we overprescribing antireflux medications for infants with regurgitation? *Pediatrics* 2007;**120**:947–9.

Ludman S, Shah N, Fox AT. Managing cows' milk allergy in children. *Br Med J* 2013;**347**:f5424.

Peter CS, Wiechers C, Bohnhorst B, *et al*. Influence of nasogastric tubes on gastroesophageal reflux in preterm infants: a multiple intraluminal impedance study. *J Pediatr* 2002;**141**:277–9.

Renfrew MJ, Ansell P, Macleod KL. Formula feed preparation: helping reduce the risks; a systematic review. *Arch Dis Child* 2003;**88**:855–8.

The Special Feed Working Group of the Paediatric Group of the British Dietetic Association. *Guidelines for making up special feeds for infants and children in hospital*. London: Food Standards Agency, 2007.

Vandenplas Y, Leluyer B, Cazaubiel M, *et al*. Double-blind comparative trial with 2 antiregurgitation formulae. *J Pediatr Gastroenterol Nutr* 2013;**57**:389–93.

Vandenplas Y, Salvatore S, Hauser B. The diagnosis and management of gastro-oesophageal reflux in infants. *Early Hum Dev* 2005;**81**:1011–24.

Wenzl TG, Schneider S, Scheels F, *et al*. Effects of thickened feeding on gastroesophageal reflux in infants: a placebo-controlled crossover study using intraluminal impedance. *Pediatrics* 2003;**111**:e355–9. [RCT]

Xinias L, Mouane N, Le Luyer B, *et al*. Cornstarch thickened formula reduces oesophageal acid exposure time in infants. *Dig Liver Dis* 2005;**37**:23–7. [RCT]

Use

Milrinone lactate has been most commonly used in the post-operative care of patients with congenital heart disease to treat low cardiac output state and in near-term and term neonates with persistent pulmonary hypertension of the newborn (PPHN) as an adjunct to nitric oxide (q.v.).

Pharmacology

First developed in 1981, milrinone is a selective inhibitor of type 3 cAMP phosphodiesterase (PDE3) isoenzyme in cardiac and vascular muscle. By increasing cAMP concentrations, it enhances myocardial contractility, promotes myocardial relaxation and reduces vascular tone in both systemic and pulmonary vascular beds. There is some evidence that combined short-term use with adrenaline or dobutamine (q.v.) can reduce systemic vascular resistance and increase cardiac output in babies suffering septic shock. A trial of long-term oral use in adults with heart failure in 1991 found an unexpected, and unexplained, increased mortality in those taking milrinone. Sustained use has been avoided ever since, although recent studies have reported safe intravenous (IV) use for up to 8 weeks both in children and in adults with end-stage heart failure awaiting a heart transplant. Neonatal use, other than during recovery from cardiac surgery, has shown no convincing benefits, but there is some suggestion that it may have a role along with inhaled nitric oxide in difficult cases of PPHN. It is thought that milrinone restores the cAMP levels, countering any cAMP-lowering effects of exogenous inhaled nitric oxide as it upregulates PDE3 in the pulmonary vasculature.

Milrinone is actively excreted (largely unmetabolised) by the kidney, the half-life being rather variable (usually 1–2 hours) but five times as long as this immediately after birth. The volume of distribution in young children (V_D >1 l/kg) is substantially more than in adults, making it important to administer an initial loading dose if an early response to treatment is required. An optimal response seems to be achieved when the blood level is ~200 nanograms/ml. Mild thrombocytopenia is common when milrinone is infused for more than 24 hours. Other complications, such as arrhythmia, are rare in children. In animal studies, milrinone crosses the placenta, but there is no evidence of teratogenicity. There are no published reports relating to use during human pregnancy or lactation, and the manufacturers have not yet endorsed the use of milrinone in children.

Treatment

Population pharmacokinetic modelling in preterm infants suggests using a loading infusion of 0.75 micrograms/kg/minute for 3 hours and then a maintenance infusion of 0.2 micrograms/kg/minute for 18 hours to sustain stable blood levels.

In term neonates (and older children), give a loading dose of 50–75 micrograms/kg over 30–60 minutes and then a continuous IV infusion of 30–45 micrograms/kg/hour for 2–3 days (usually for 12 hours after cardiac surgery). Hypotension may occur while the loading dose is being given because the drug causes some vasodilation. Volume expansion and/or low dose dopamine will usually counteract this.

Compatibility

Milrinone can be added (terminally) to a line containing adrenaline, atracurium, dobutamine, dopamine, fentanyl, glyceryl trinitrate, heparin, insulin, isoprenaline, midazolam, morphine, nitroprusside, noradrenaline, propofol, ranitidine or standard TPN (but not furosemide). Compatibility with IV lipid has not been assessed.

Supply and administration

10 ml ampoules containing 10 mg of milrinone (as lactate) cost £19.90. Take 0.6 ml (0.6 mg) of milrinone for each kilogram the baby weighs, and dilute this to 20 ml with 10% glucose or glucose saline. To give 0.5 micrograms/kg/minute, infuse this dilute solution at a rate of 1 ml/hour. Less concentrated solutions of dextrose or dextrose saline can be used. The drug is stable in solution, so a fresh infusion does not need to be prepared every 24 hours.

References

Bailey JM, Hoffman TM, Wessel DL, *et al*. A population pharmacodynamic analysis of milrinone in pediatric patients after cardiac surgery. *J Pharmacokinet Pharmacodyn* 2004;**31**:43–59.

Barton P, Garcia J, Kouatli A, *et al*. Hemodynamic effects of IV milrinone lactate in pediatric patients with septic shock. A prospective, double-blinded, randomized, placebo-controlled, interventional study. *Chest* 1996;**109**:1302–12. [RCT]

Continued on p. 339

Bassler D, Choong K, McNamara P, *et al*. Neonatal persistent pulmonary hypertension treated with milrinone: four case reports. *Biol Neonate* 2006;**89**:1–5.

Cai J, Su Z, Shi Z, *et al*. Nitric oxide and milrinone: combined effect on pulmonary circulation after Fontan-type procedure: a prospective randomized study. *Ann Thorac Surg* 2008;**86**:882–8. [RCT]

Chen B, Lakshminrusimha S, Czech L, *et al*. Regulation of phosphodiesterase 3 in the pulmonary arteries during the perinatal period in sheep. *Pediatr Res* 2009;**66**:682–7.

Hoffman TM, Wernovsky G, Atz AM, *et al*. Efficacy and safety of milrinone in preventing low cardiac output syndrome in infants and children after corrective surgery for congenital heart disease. *Circulation* 2003;**107**:995–1002. [RCT]

McNamara PJ, Laique F, Muang-In S, *et al*. Milrinone improves oxygenation in neonates with severe persistent pulmonary hypertension of the newborn. *J Crit Care* 2006;**21**:217–22.

McNamara PJ, Shivananda SP, Sahni M, *et al*. Pharmacology of milrinone in neonates with persistent pulmonary hypertension of the newborn and suboptimal response to inhaled nitric oxide. *Pediatr Crit Care Med* 2013;**14**:74–84.

Paradisis M, Evans NJ, Kluckow MR, *et al*. Randomised trial of milrinone versus placebo for prevention of low systemic blood flow in very preterm infants. *J Pediatr* 2009;**154**:189–95. [RCT]

Paradisis M, Jiang X, McLachlan AJ, *et al*. Population pharmacokinetics and dosing regimen design of milrinone in preterm infants. *Arch Dis Child Fetal Neonatal Ed* 2007;**92**:F204–9.

Zuppa AF, Nicolson SC, Adamson PC, *et al*. Population pharmacokinetics of milrinone in neonates with hypoplastic left heart syndrome undergoing stage I reconstruction. *Anesth Analg* 2006;**102**:1062–9.

Use

Although gastric ulcer prevention is currently the only marketed indication for misoprostol in most countries, it is also widely used to terminate pregnancy and is a valuable alternative to oxytocin (q.v.) in the control of serious post-partum bleeding. It also has a role (if the dose is kept low) in the induction of labour.

Pharmacology

The only officially recognised use of misoprostol, an orally active prostaglandin E_1 analogue first synthesised in 1973, is to prevent and treat the gastric ulcers that are sometimes caused by non-steroidal anti-inflammatory drug (NSAID) use. The drug's manufacturer has never recommended use for any other purpose or supported the studies needed to evaluate any other use and only makes the drug available in 100 and 200 micrograms tablets (a higher dose than this is usually appropriate when attempting to induce labour in late pregnancy). A 400 micrograms vaginally administered dose of misoprostol is an effective way of preparing the cervix for suction termination, and an 800 micrograms dose given 48 hours after a 200 mg dose of oral mifepristone will effect non-surgical termination of pregnancy during the first trimester. Nausea, abdominal pain, diarrhoea, shivering and fever are the most common transient, dose-dependent side effects. Much lower doses (50 micrograms) usually suffice to induce labour at term, and dangerous uterine hyperstimulation was a common problem with the higher doses before this was recognised. Uterine rupture was frequently reported after use of higher doses in women with a previous caesarean section scar.

The active metabolite, misoprostol acid, is rapidly cleared by the liver, and the half-life with oral administration is less than an hour. Placing a tablet in the posterior fornix of the vagina increases the drug's bioavailability and its half-life. Most women prefer oral treatment, and while the optimum oral dose still requires further study, a recent systematic review found the two approaches to be of comparable efficacy. Because misoprostol is inexpensive, stable at room temperature and available in more than 80 countries, the WHO has incorporated recommendations for misoprostol into its four reproductive health guidelines focused on induction of labour, prevention and treatment of post-partum haemorrhage and management of spontaneous and induced abortion.

Misoprostol should never be used for other reasons during pregnancy, not just because it stimulates uterine activity, but because high-dose first trimester use can cause fetal deformity. Orally administered misoprostol can be detected in colostrum within 1 hour, becoming undetectable by 5 hours. Misoprostol use during established lactation has not been reported. Due to the potential risk of severe drug-induced diarrhoea, the manufacturer advises against use during lactation, although this has not been seen in the breastfed baby.

Treatment

Inducing labour: One approach is to give up to three 25 micrograms oral (or sublingual) doses once every 2 hours, doubling the dose to 50 micrograms every 2 hours if necessary after 6 hours. Treatment is stopped once the uterus is contracting regularly (three 30 second contractions every 10 minutes). An alternative strategy has been to give up to five 100 micrograms doses at four hourly intervals. The existence of a uterine scar is a contraindication to *either* of these strategies, as is the simultaneous use of intravenous (IV) oxytocin.

Post-partum haemorrhage: While IV oxytocin is the drug of choice to control early post-partum bleeding, 600 micrograms of oral (or sublingual) misoprostol is (once absorbed) extremely effective at controlling serious, sustained and life-threatening post-partum bleeding because of its longer half-life.

Supply and administration

The only product currently available in the United Kingdom is a 200 micrograms tablet which costs 17p. Smaller doses can however be given by crushing the tablet and dissolving it in tap water. Any such solution must then be used within 12 hours. Misoprostol has not yet been licensed for obstetric use, but unlike oxytocin, it does not have to be stored in the dark, or kept at 4 °C, to maintain its potency. It is also much cheaper than dinoprostone vaginal gel.

Continued on p. 341

References

(See also the relevant Cochrane reviews and UK guideline on induction of labour **DHUK**)

Crane JMG, Butler B, Young DC, *et al*. Misoprostol compared with prostaglandin E$_2$ for labour induction in women at term with intact membranes and unfavourable cervix: a systematic review. *Br J Obstet Gynaecol* 2006;**113**:1366–76. [SR] (See also pp. 1431–7.)

Hofmeyr GJ, Walraven G, Gülmezoglu AM, *et al*. Misoprostol to treat postpartum haemorrhage: a systematic review. *Br J Obstet Gynaecol* 2005;**112**:547–53. [SR]

Langenbach C. Misoprostol in preventing postpartum hemorrhage: a meta-analysis. *Int J Gynaecol Obstet* 2006;**92**:10–18. [SR]

Pagel C, Lewycka S, Colbourn T, *et al*. Estimation of potential effects of improved community-based drug provision, to augment health-facility strengthening, on maternal mortality due to post-partum haemorrhage and sepsis in sub-Saharan Africa: an equity effectiveness model. *Lancet* 2009;**374**:1441–8. (See also pp. 1400–2.)

Prager M, Eneroth-Grimfors E, Edlund M, *et al*. A randomised controlled trial of intravaginal dinoprostone, intravaginal misoprostol and transcervical balloon catheter for labour induction. *Br J Obstet Gynaecol* 2008;**115**:1443–50. [RCT]

Rahman H, Pradhan A, Kharka L, *et al*. Comparative evaluation of 50 microgram oral misoprostol and 25 microgram intravaginal misoprostol for induction of labour at term: a randomized trial. *J Obstet Gynaecol Can* 2013;**35**:408–16.

Souza ASR, Amorim MMR, Feitosa FEL. Comparison of sublingual versus vaginal misoprostol for the induction of labour: a systematic review. *Br J Obstet Gynaecol* 2008;**115**:1340–9. [SR]

Tang J, Kapp N, Dragoman M, *et al*. WHO recommendations for misoprostol use for obstetric and gynecologic indications. *Int J Gynaecol Obstet* 2013;**121**:186–9.

Vargas FR, Schuler-Faccini L, Brunoni D, *et al*. Prenatal exposure to misoprostol and vascular disruption defects: a case-control study. *Am J Med Genet* 2000;**95**:302–6. (See also pp. 297–301.)

Use

Mivacurium is a useful, quick-acting alternative to atracurium (q.v.) when short-term muscular paralysis is required. It does not blunt the perception of pain.

Pharmacology

Mivacurium is a non-depolarising muscle relaxant that works by competing with acetylcholine at the neuromuscular junction's receptor. Thus, reversal, if required, can be achieved with anticholinesterases such as neostigmine (q.v.). Mivacurium was developed as an analogue of atracurium and introduced into clinical use in 1988. The drug is a mixture of three stereoisomers; only two seem to cause much neuromuscular blockade, but all three are inactivated by plasma cholinesterase. Paralysis is dose related but, after a single bolus dose, seldom lasts >20 minutes (30 minutes in older children). Activity is, however, prolonged by volatile anaesthetics such as isoflurane. Recovery can be prolonged to 2–4 hours in those patients who have pseudocholinesterase deficiency (~0.04% of the population) – a problem not encountered with atracurium. The manufacturers have not yet endorsed the use of mivacurium in children <2 months old, partly because of concern about possible increased sensitivity. Extensive clinical experience suggests that such caution may be unnecessary. There is no contraindication to use during pregnancy or labour, and use during lactation is also almost certainly safe given the drug's short half-life and poor oral absorption.

Atracurium and mivacurium are benzylisoquinolinium non-depolarising muscle relaxants. All drugs in this class (other than cisatracurium) can cause histamine release with flushing, tachycardia, hypotension and (very rarely) an anaphylactoid reaction. Such problems seem less common in children. The risk can also be minimised by avoiding unnecessarily rapid administration.

Treatment

Single-dose administration: A 200 micrograms/kg intravenous (IV) injection provides almost complete muscle relaxation after 1–2 minutes that lasts for about 10–15 minutes. Flush this bolus dose through into the vein slowly over a period of ~30 seconds to minimise the risk of histamine release. A smaller dose is often enough to achieve relaxation prior to tracheal intubation. Paralysis can be sustained longer if necessary by giving further IV doses once every 5–10 minutes.

Continuous infusion: Sustained paralysis generally requires a continuing infusion of about 10 micrograms/kg/minute in early infancy (only slightly more than the amount generally needed in adult life), but some older children require almost twice as much as this. The amount needed is not always predictable and may require individual titration. Recovery is usually rapid once the infusion is stopped.

Antidote

Most of the effects of mivacurium can be reversed by giving 10 micrograms/kg of glycopyrronium (or 20 micrograms/kg of atropine) and 50 micrograms/kg of neostigmine as outlined in the glycopyrronium monograph, but reversal should seldom be called for given mivacurium's short half-life.

Supply and administration

5 ml ampoules containing 10 mg of mivacurium chloride (2 mg/ml) cost £2.80. Multi-dose vials are available in North America, but these should be avoided when treating infants because they contain benzyl alcohol. Store all products below 25 °C, but do not freeze. Protect from light.

Bolus administration: Take 1 ml of mivacurium from the 2 mg/ml ampoule and dilute to 10 ml with 5% glucose or glucose saline to obtain a preparation containing 200 micrograms/ml.

Continuous infusion: To give 10 micrograms/kg/minute, draw 6 mg (3 ml) of mivacurium for each kilogram the baby weighs from the ampoule into a syringe, dilute to 10 ml with 5% dextrose in 0.18% sodium chloride, and infuse at 1 ml/hour. A less concentrated solution of dextrose or dextrose saline can be used if appropriate.

References

Atherton DPL, Hunter JM. Clinical pharmacokinetics of the newer neuromuscular blocking drugs. *Clin Pharmacokinet* 1999;**36**:169–89.

Cerf C, Mesuish M, Gabriel I, *et al.* Screening patients for prolonged neuromuscular blockade after succinylcholine and mivacurium. *Anesth Analg* 2002;**94**:461–6.

Continued on p. 343

Dempsey EM, Al Hazzani F, Faucher D, *et al.* Facilitation of neonatal endotracheal intubation with mivacurium and fentanyl in the neonatal intensive care unit. *Arch Dis Child Fetal Neonatal Ed* 2006;**91**:F279–82.

Guay J, Grenier Y, Varin F. Clinical pharmacokinetics of neuromuscular relaxants in pregnancy. *Clin Pharmacokinet* 1998;**34**:483–96.

Meakin GH. Recent advances in myorelaxant therapy. *Paediatr Anaesth* 2001;**11**:5623–31.

Nauheimer D, Fink H, Fuchs-Buder Th, *et al.* Muscle relaxant use for tracheal intubation in pediatric anaesthesia: a survey of clinical practice in Germany. *Pediatr Anesth* 2009;**19**:225–31.

Plaud B, Goujard E, Orliaguet G, *et al.* Pharmacodynamie et tolérance du mivacurium chez le nourrisson et l'enfant sous anesthésie par halothane-protoxyde d'azote. *Ann Fr Anesth Reanim* 1999;**18**:1047–53.

Rashid A, Watkinson M. Suxamethonium is safe in safe hands: mivacurium should also be considered. *Arch Dis Child Fetal Neonatal Ed* 2000;**83**:F160–1.

Roberts KD, Leone TA, Edwards WH, *et al.* Premedication for nonemergent neonatal intubations: a randomized, controlled trial comparing atropine and fentanyl to atropine, fentanyl, and mivacurium. *Pediatrics* 2006;**118**:1583–91. [RCT]

Use
Morphine is the best studied neonatal analgesic.

Pharmacology
Morphine, the principal alkaloid of opium, has been used for over 2000 years, and a pure extract was obtained from poppy heads in 1805. It is well absorbed when taken by mouth but undergoes rapid first-pass metabolism in the liver (bioavailability ~30%). The half-life in the preterm baby is 6–12 hours but is **very** variable and inversely related to gestational age at birth. Some tissue accumulation occurs with sustained use (V_D ~2 l/kg). Elimination is more rapid in babies older than 2 months, and the half-life in 1–6-year-old children (about 1 hour) is less than in adults. Ordinary doses cause constipation, urinary retention and respiratory depression, and an overdose can cause hypotension, bradycardia and even (rarely) fits. One study suggests that neonatal pain relief may require a blood level of ~120 nanograms/ml, while adverse effects start to appear at levels exceeding 300 nanograms/ml. Lower levels (20–40 nanograms/ml) seem adequate in older children. The high levels required in the newborn may reflect drug receptor differences, and low morphine-6-glucuronide (M6G) metabolite levels. Tolerance may develop with prolonged treatment, and withdrawal symptoms can also occur. Addiction has not been seen with neonatal use for pain relief, but there are concerns that long-term opiate exposure may impact on visual function.

Morphine readily crosses the placenta although maternal clearance shortens the fetal exposure. While there is no evidence morphine is a human teratogen, uncontrolled retrospective studies of neonates chronically exposed to opioids report reduced brain volume at birth. Infants born to opioid-abusing mothers are more often small for gestation and have increased risk of sudden unexpected death in infancy. Neonatal abstinence due to opiate withdrawal produces sleep/wake abnormalities, feeding difficulties, weight loss and seizures. Rodent studies suggest *in utero* exposure causes long-term alterations in the brain and behaviour. Morphine passes into breast milk (M/P ratio ~2.5:1). Although it has poor oral bioavailability, the decreased clearance of morphine during the first few weeks of life means that there is the potential for high maternal doses given over prolonged periods to cause sedation and respiratory depression in breastfed infants.

> Morphine is frequently used in babies undergoing therapeutic hypothermia. Morphine's affinity for the µ-opioid receptors is reduced in hypothermia, rendering it less effective; at least in the early stages, however, as the clearance of morphine is reduced, accumulation may occur if higher doses are given to overcome this. Consider reducing the dose if the baby is adequately sedated after 24–48 hours to lessen the risk of accumulation and toxicity.

Treatment
Neonatal opioid withdrawal: Local guidelines may vary; one approach is to monitor using appropriate withdrawal tool (e.g. modified Finnegan's score every 4 hours). If morphine is required, begin by giving 40 micrograms/kg by mouth every 4 hours. Increase the dose by 20% if scores exceed 24 in total on three consecutive measures or a single score is 12 or greater. After 48 hours of stability (i.e. the sum of the previous three scores is <18 and no single score is >8), wean the dose by 10%. Continue weaning if symptoms are controlled by reducing the dose by 10% every 24–48 hours.

Severe or sustained pain: Provide ventilatory support; give a loading dose of 200 micrograms/kg and then a maintenance infusion of 20 micrograms/kg/hour (10 ml/hour of a solution prepared as described under 'Supply and administration' *for 1 hour*, followed by a maintenance infusion of 1 ml/hour). While this will usually control even severe pain in the first 2 months of life, providing a plasma morphine level of 120–160 nanograms/ml, treatment *has* to be individualised. Staff need discretion to give a further 20 micrograms/kg bolus up to once every 4 hours to control any 'breakthrough' pain.

Sedation while ventilated: Babies given both a loading dose of 100 micrograms/kg and a maintenance infusion of 10 micrograms/kg/hour (i.e. half the doses used for severe pain) seldom breathe out of phase with the ventilator.

Continued on p. 345

Short-term pain relief: Give 100 micrograms/kg by intramuscular (IM) or intravenous (IV) injection (or twice this by mouth). Rapid IV administration does *not* cause hypotension but may cause respiratory depression. A further 50 micrograms/kg dose can usually be given after 6 hours without making ventilator support necessary.

Older children: Drug clearance is more rapid in babies >2 months old, but the plasma morphine level needed to provide pain relief seems to fall. The interplay between these factors has not yet been studied. Use the aforementioned guidance as a starting point and then individualise treatment.

Compatibility

Compatibility with other continuously infused drugs is noted, where known, in the monograph for the second product. Morphine can also be added (terminally) to an IV line containing standard TPN and lipid.

Supply and administration

Ampoules of morphine sulphate containing 10 mg in 1 ml are available at a cost of 72p each. The use of a preservative-free ampoule will reduce the risk of phlebitis. *Always* start by diluting the contents tenfold for accurate neonatal administration. For single bolus doses, 0.1 ml of morphine can be made up to 1 ml with 0.9% sodium chloride, giving a solution of 1 mg/ml. To set up a continuous infusion, dilute the 1 ml of fluid from the ampoule to 10 ml with 0.9% sodium chloride (as previously mentioned), place 1 ml of this diluted preparation for each kilogram the baby weighs in a syringe, dilute to 50 ml with 10% glucose or glucose saline, and infuse at 1 ml/hour to provide an infusion of 20 micrograms/kg/hour. The drug is chemically stable in solution so the infusate does not need to be changed daily.

Oral morphine solutions can be supplied as either morphine hydrochloride or morphine sulphate (Oramorph®) with the strength being adjusted in the pharmacy to suit the neonate. The storage and administration of morphine (other than as an oral solution containing <2.6 mg/ml) are controlled under schedule 2 of the UK Misuse of Drugs Regulations 1985 (Misuse of Drugs Act, 1971).

Reference

(See also the relevant Cochrane reviews)

Anand KJS. Pharmacological approaches to the management of pain in the neonatal intensive care unit. *J Perinatol* 2007;**27**:S4–11.

Anand KJ, Anderson BJ, Holford NH, *et al*. Morphine pharmacokinetics and pharmacodynamics in preterm and term neonates: secondary results from the NEOPAIN trial. *Br J Anaesth* 2008;**101**:680–9.

Anand KJS, Whit Hall R, Desai N, *et al*. Effects of morphine analgesia in ventilated preterm neonates: primary outcomes from the NEOPAIN randomised trial. *Lancet* 2004;**363**:2673–82. [RCT] (See also 2004;**364**:498.)

Carbajal R, Lenclen R, Jugie M, *et al*. Morphine does not provide adequate analgesia for acute procedural pain among preterm neonates. *Pediatrics* 2005;**115**:1494–500.

de Graaf J, van Lingen RA, Simons SH, *et al*. Long-term effects of routine morphine infusion in mechanically ventilated neonates on children's functioning: five-year follow-up of a randomized controlled trial. *Pain* 2011;**152**:1391–7.

McGlone L, Hamilton R, McCulloch DL, *et al*. Neonatal visual evoked potentials in infants born to mothers prescribed methadone. *Pediatrics* 2013;**131**:e857–63.

Menon G, McIntosh N. How should we manage pain in ventilates neonates? *Neonatology* 2008;**93**:316–23.

Olkkola KT, Hamunen K, Maunuksela E-L. Clinical pharmacokinetics and pharmacodynamics of opioid analgesics in infants and children. *Clin Pharmacokinet* 1995;**28**:385–403.

Use

Mupirocin is a topical antibiotic used to treat superficial skin infections and to control spread of methicillin-resistant *Staphylococcus aureus* (MRSA).

Pharmacology

This unusual antibiotic, a fermentation product of the bacterium *Pseudomonas fluorescens*, was formerly called pseudomonic acid. Mupirocin is structurally unlike any other antibiotic and is a mixture of four pseudomonic acids in which a unique hydroxy-nonanoic acid is linked to monic acid.

Mupirocin is bacteriostatic in low concentrations and slowly bactericidal at high concentrations against *Mycoplasma* and most Gram-positive aerobes in an acid environment such as that provided by the skin (pH 5.5). It is non-toxic but rapidly de-esterified and rendered inert by the tissues after parenteral injection, making it only suitable for topical use. The drug first came into clinical use in 1988. Microbiological advice should be taken before using mupirocin, and the product should only be used for a limited period to minimise the risk of drug resistance developing.

There has been one report suggesting that mupirocin may be more effective in treating candidal skin infection than *in vitro* assessments of its sensitivity would suggest, and further controlled studies are probably warranted.

Mupirocin has sometimes, but not always, proved of value in eliminating the chronic nasal carriage of pathogenic staphylococci by healthcare staff. Transient stinging and localised skin reaction can occur. There is no evidence of teratogenicity, and there is nothing to suggest that mupirocin needs to be avoided during pregnancy in situations where its use seems otherwise justified on clinical grounds. Breastfeeding is not contraindicated, because absorption is minimal after topical administration and any of the drug that is ingested is very rapidly metabolised to monic acid.

Treatment

Use mupirocin on the skin (avoiding the eyes) three times a day for not more than 10 days.

Supply

Mupirocin ointment (2% w/w) is available in 15 g tubes costing £4.30 each. This formulation uses a macrogol (polyethylene glycol) base, and it is possible that renal toxicity could result from macrogol absorption through mucous membranes or through extensive application to thin or damaged neonatal skin. In this situation, the equivalent paraffin-based formulation of calcium mupirocin might be preferable; this is currently marketed as an ointment officially designed for nasal use (Bactroban® nasal) in 3 g tubes costing £3.50.

A cream (Bactroban cream) is also available (15 g tubes costing £4.40 each), but this is probably best avoided in the preterm baby because it contains benzyl alcohol.

References

(See also the relevant Cochrane reviews)

Davies EA, Emmerson AM, Hogg GM, *et al*. An outbreak of infection with a methicillin resistant *Staphylococcus aureus* in a special care baby unit: value of topical mupirocin and traditional methods of infection control. *J Hosp Infect* 1978;**10**:120–8.

Fortunov RM, Hulten KG, Hammerman WA, *et al*. Community-acquired *Staphylococcal aureus* infections in term and near-term previously healthy neonates. *Pediatrics* 2006;**118**:874–81.

Gemmell CG, Edwards DI, Fraise AP, *et al*. Guidelines for the prophylaxis and treatment of methicillin-resistant *Staphylococcus aureus* (MRSA) infections in the UK. *J Antimicrob Chemother* 2006;**57**:589–608. [SR]

Graham PL, Morel A-S, Zhou J, *et al*. Epidemiology of methicillin-susceptible *Staphylococcus aureus* in the neonatal intensive care unit. *Infect Control Hosp Epidemiol* 2002;**23**:677–82.

Helai N, Carbonne A, Naas T, *et al*. Nosocomial outbreak of staphylococcal scalded skin syndrome in neonates: epidemiological investigation and control. *J Hosp Infect* 2005;**61**:130–8.

Milstone AM, Budd A, Shepard JW, *et al*. Role of decolonization in a comprehensive strategy to reduce methicillin-resistant *Staphylococcus aureus* infections in the neonatal intensive care unit: an observational cohort study. *Infect Control Hosp Epidemiol* 2010;**31**:558–60.

Muto CA, Jernigan JA, Ostrowsky BE, *et al*. Guideline for preventing nosocomial transmission of multidrug-resistant strains of *Staphylococcus aureus* and *Enterococcus*. *Infect Control Hosp Epidemiol* 2003;**24**:362–86. [SR]

Rode H, de Wet PM, Millar AJW, *et al*. Efficacy of mupirocin in cutaneous candidiasis. *Lancet* 1991;**338**:578.

Saiman L, Cronquist A, Wu F, *et al*. An outbreak of methicillin-resistant *Staphylococcus aureus* in a neonatal intensive care unit. *Infect Control Hospt Epidemiol* 2003;**24**:317–21. (See also pp. 314–6.)

Zakrzewska-Bode A, Mujtjens HL, Liem KD, *et al*. Mupirocin resistance in coagulase-negative staphylococci, after topical prophylaxis for the reduction of colonisation of central venous lines. *J Hosp Infect* 1995;**31**:189–93.

Use
Naloxone reverses the respiratory depression that can be caused by the use of opioids such as codeine, dextropropoxyphene, diamorphine (heroin), fentanyl, meptazinol, methadone, morphine, nalbuphine and pethidine. Use, however, inevitably interferes with their ability to reduce pain. Naloxone can only partly reverse the effects of buprenorphine and pentazocine (which have both agonist and antagonist properties).

Pharmacology
Naloxone is a potent pure opioid antagonist first discovered in 1961. It crosses the placenta rapidly but is not known to be teratogenic. Large doses can be given without apparent toxicity (except in patients dependent on opioids), and repeated use does not cause dependence or tolerance. The drug is largely metabolised by glucuronide conjugation. The plasma half-life is 1–3 hours immediately after birth but approaches that seen in adults (65 minutes) within a few days of birth ($V_D \sim 2.5$ l/kg).

The drug used to be widely used (some might say 'abused') in the 'resuscitation' of babies at birth, although with newborn resuscitation education programmes, this is becoming less of an issue. Naloxone has no role whatsoever during the initial resuscitation of a baby. If the mother has received opiates during labour, then naloxone may be used to check that opioid depression is not causing continued respiratory depression in the apnoeic baby *after* the baby is suitably oxygenated and a reliable cardiac output has been established.

While the potential for maternal opiate use (including that in epidurals) during labour to depress the baby's respiration may have been exaggerated in the past, there is also some evidence that the sedative effect may also have more of an effect on the baby's ability to successfully establish breastfeeding than has generally been appreciated to date. Neonatal opioid depression can last quite a long time. A large maternal dose of pethidine (q.v.) during labour can sometimes make a baby drowsy and reluctant to feed for 2 days. While a single intravenous (IV) dose of naloxone will immediately reverse this depression, any benefit will only be transient because pethidine has such a long half-life and naloxone such a short half-life. On the other hand, a single 100 micrograms/kg intramuscular (IM) dose of naloxone seems to produce a drug 'depot' at the site of the injection that generates effective plasma levels of naloxone for at least 24 hours. Only occasionally is a second IM dose necessary.

A continuous infusion of naloxone is the best way to counteract accidental opiate poisoning in infancy. Such babies present with drowsiness, respiratory depression and pinpoint pupils. Hypotension is not uncommon and fits may occur. Similar infusions have also been used, anecdotally, to counteract the effect of the body's own endogenous opioids (beta-endorphins) when their excessive release in severe septic shock lowers blood pressure and reduces cardiac output. Try the effect of a 50 micrograms/kg IV bolus dose first. Methylthioninium chloride (q.v.) has also been used experimentally for the same purpose.

A 3 micrograms/kg oral dose of naloxone four times a day may help to reduce some of the constipation caused by morphine analgesia in preterm babies.

Treatment
Opioid sedation at birth: 100 micrograms/kg (0.25 ml/kg of 'adult' naloxone) IM has a gradual effect as an opioid antagonist but an effect that is sustained for 24 hours. Treatment may be repeated if necessary. It is not necessary to calculate a precise weight-related dose – an initial 200 micrograms dose (0.5 ml of 'adult' naloxone), irrespective of weight, provides a pragmatic delivery room approach suitable for most babies.

Intravenous use: A 100 micrograms/kg dose is of diagnostic help in opioid poisoning, and a continuous infusion of 50–100 micrograms/kg/hour in glucose or glucose saline will control stupor if it re-emerges.

Contraindications
Administration of naloxone to the baby of an opiate-dependent mother could precipitate withdrawal symptoms. Nevertheless, there is, at the moment, still only one published report of this precipitating seizures during resuscitation (see web commentary). The mother had taken a very high dose of methadone (60 mg) 8 hours earlier, and documented fetal distress complicates the interpretation of this isolated case report.

Continued on p. 348

Supply

1 ml (400 micrograms) ampoules of naloxone marketed for 'adult' use are available costing £4.10 each. 2 ml (40 micrograms) 'neonatal' ampoules are also available but not as useful (cost £5.50). Disposable syringes containing 400 micrograms/ml are available in 1, 2 and 5 ml sizes (cost £13–£20).

References (See also relevant Cochrane reviews)

Akkawi R, Eksborg S, Andersson Å, *et al*. Effect of oral naloxone hydrochloride on gastrointestinal transit in premature infants treated with morphine. *Acta Paediatr* 2009;**98**:442–7.

Furman WL, Menke JA, Barson WJ, *et al*. Continuous naloxone infusion in two neonates with septic shock. *J Pediatr* 1984;**105**:649–51.

Guinsburg R, Wykoff MH. Naloxone during neonatal resuscitation: acknowledging the unknown. *Clin Perinatol* 2006;**33**:121–32. [SR]

Jordan S, Emery S, Bradshaw C, *et al*. The impact of intrapartum analgesia on infant feeding. *Br J Obstet Gynaecol* 2005;**112**:927–34.

Kapadia VS, Wyckoff MH. Drugs during delivery room resuscitation – What, when and why? *Semin Fetal Neonatal Med* 2013;**18**:357–61.

Morland TA, Brice JEH, Walker CHM, *et al*. Naloxone pharmacokinetics in the newborn. *Br J Clin Pharmacol* 1979;**9**:609–12.

Tenenbein M. Continuous naloxone infusion for opiate poisoning in infancy. *J Pediatr* 1984;**105**:645–8.

van Vonderen JJ, Siew ML, Hooper SB, *et al*. Effects of naloxone on the breathing pattern of a newborn exposed to maternal opiates. *Acta Paediatr* 2012;**101**:e309–12.

Werner PC, Hogg MI, Rosen M. Effects of naloxone on pethidine-induced neonatal depression. Part II – intramuscular naloxone. *Br Med J* 1977;**2**:229–31.

Use
Neostigmine metilsulfate (neostigmine methylsulfate [former BAN]) and edrophonium are used to diagnose and treat myasthenia.

Myasthenia
Myasthenia gravis is an acquired autoimmune disorder causing progressive muscle fatigue and weakness. About 10–15% of the babies born to myasthenic mothers are affected by transient neonatal myasthenia due to transplacental transfer of antibodies directed against the acetylcholine receptors of the muscle–nerve junction. Symptoms present within 1–3 days and usually persist for 3–6 weeks. There is no way of knowing before birth whether a baby is going to be affected or not, but most affected babies have mothers with high antibody titres and a history of affected siblings. The presence of polyhydramnios predicts severe involvement. In contrast, maternal disease is sometimes only recognised when the baby presents with symptoms at birth. Symptoms persist for months in the other congenital, recessively inherited forms of myasthenia, although they usually become less severe with time. Respiratory and feeding difficulty may cause prolonged apnoea, aspiration and even death. Hypotonia is common, and stridor can be a problem. Some babies have multiple joint contractures (arthrogryposis) at birth. Ptosis is usually only seen in babies with maternally acquired autoimmune disease. Aminoglycoside antibiotics are hazardous in patients with any of the myasthenic disorders, because they interfere with neuromuscular transmission causing respiratory depression. Some congenital myasthenic syndromes do not respond to neostigmine and pyridostigmine.

Pharmacology
Neostigmine (first developed in 1931) inhibits cholinesterase activity, and therapy prolongs and intensifies the muscarinic and nicotinic effects of acetylcholine, causing vasodilatation, increased smooth muscle activity, lacrimation, salivation and improved voluntary muscle tone. It is therefore the drug of choice in the management of both maternal and neonatal myasthenia gravis. Intravenous (IV) edrophonium has a similar and much more rapid effect, but the response frequently only lasts 5–10 minutes. For this reason, most clinicians now prefer to use intramuscular neostigmine metilsulfate (with or without atropine to control any side effects) both for diagnostic and for maintenance purposes since this produces a response lasting 2–4 hours after a latent period of 20–30 minutes. Other rarer disorders require more complex diagnostic techniques.

Diagnostic use
Always have 15 micrograms/kg of IV atropine on hand to control any undue salivation and equipment to control any unexpected respiratory arrest.
Edrophonium: Give 20 micrograms/kg IV followed, after 30 seconds, by a further 80 micrograms/kg IV if there is no adverse effect. Watch for bradycardia or arrhythmia. Double this dose has been used.
Neostigmine metilsulfate: Use a 150 micrograms/kg intramuscular (IM) test dose.

Treatment
Short-term management: 150 micrograms/kg of neostigmine metilsulfate subcutaneously, or IM, once every 6–8 hours is usually used for maintenance, but twice this dose may be necessary once every 4 hours. Oral treatment with neostigmine bromide can be used once control is achieved. An oral dose that is 10–20 times the IM maintenance dose will need to be given every 3 hours.
Long-term management: Oral pyridostigmine (another anticholinesterase) is preferable in the long-term management of myasthenia because it has a slightly longer duration of action. The usual starting dose is 1 mg/kg by mouth every 4 hours (unless the child is asleep). Adjust later as necessary.
Reversing drug-induced muscle paralysis: The effects of non-depolarising muscle relaxants such as pancuronium can be largely reversed by giving a combined IV injection of 10 micrograms/kg of glycopyrronium and 50 micrograms/kg of neostigmine (as outlined in the monograph on glycopyrronium).

Supply and administration
1 ml (2.5 mg) ampoules of neostigmine metilsulfate for IM use cost 50p each. For accurate administration, take the contents of the ampoule and dilute to 16.5 ml with glucose or glucose saline immediately before use to give a solution containing approximately 150 micrograms/ml. 1 ml ampoules containing 10 mg of edrophonium (costing £19.50) are also available on request.

Continued on p. 350

An oral suspension of neostigmine bromide or pyridostigmine (12 mg/ml) syrup (also contains 5% alcohol) can be made available on request.

References

Kinali M, Beeson D, Pitt MC, *et al.* Congenital myasthenic syndromes in childhood: diagnostic and management challenges. *J Neuroimmunol* 2008;**201-202**:6–12.

Matthes JWA, Kenna AP, Fawcett PRW. Familial infantile myasthenia: a diagnostic problem. *Dev Med Child Neurol* 1991;**33**:924–9.

Morel E, Eymard B, Vernet de Gatabedian B, *et al.* Neonatal myasthenia gravis: a new clinical and immunological appraisal of 30 cases. *Neurology* 1988;**38**:138–42.

Newsom-Davis J. Autoimmune and genetic disorders at the neuromuscular junction. *Dev Med Child Neurol* 1998;**40**:199–206.

Varner M. Myasthenia gravis and pregnancy. *Clin Obstet Gynecol* 2013;**56**:372–81.

Use

Nevirapine sometimes is used to prevent perinatal transmission of human immunodeficiency virus (HIV). Use should always follow current guidelines. Combined treatment with zidovudine (q.v.) costs more but further reduces viral transmission and may make later drug resistance less likely. In resource-poor countries, continued daily prophylaxis (2 mg/kg for 2 weeks and then 4 mg/kg a day) greatly decreases the risk of infection during lactation.

Pharmacology

Nevirapine is a *non*-nucleoside reverse transcriptase inhibitor (NNRTI) that binds to reverse transcriptase, thus inhibiting viral replication. For prophylaxis, use with at least one nucleoside reverse transcriptase inhibitor (NRTI) drug – the most widely studied is zidovudine (q.v.). Nevirapine is well absorbed by mouth, is widely distributed (V_D ~1.2 l/kg), penetrates the CSF well and, because it is lipophilic, is rapidly transferred across the placenta. There is no evidence of teratogenicity. It is extensively metabolised by the cytochrome P450 isoenzyme system in the liver with a half-life of 40–60 hours when treatment is first started. The half-life is almost halved by enzyme autoinduction after 1–2 weeks. It is also reduced in patients on rifampicin but extended in patients taking a range of other drugs including cimetidine, erythromycin and fluconazole. The most important adverse effects with sustained use are skin rash (sometimes severe) and a potentially life-threatening hepatotoxicity (that may make it necessary to suspend or stop treatment); these are most common in the first months of treatment. Hypersensitivity reactions can also be a problem.

Nevirapine can be detected in breast milk; however, breastfeeding is not recommended in HIV-infected women where formula is available to reduce the risk of neonatal transmission. Where formula milk is not available or safe, results from observational studies suggest that nevirapine may reduce, but not totally negate, the risk of HIV transmission through breast milk.

New information on optimum management becomes available so frequently that communication with a paediatric HIV/infectious diseases specialist is essential. The diagnosis and management must also be discussed with, and supervised by, someone with extensive experience of this condition.

Simple intrapartum prophylaxis in a resource-poor setting

The following strategies are *only* appropriate in a previously untreated mother in a resource-poor setting.

If started before delivery: Give a 200 mg oral dose of nevirapine at the start of labour to *all* mothers not on any retroviral drug treatment and one 2 mg/kg dose of nevirapine to the baby 2 days after birth.

If started after delivery: Give the baby one 2 mg/kg dose of nevirapine by mouth as soon as possible after birth and 4 mg/kg of zidovudine by mouth twice a day for 7 days.

Full intrapartum prophylaxis using several drugs

See the recommendations in the monograph on lamivudine.

Post-delivery multi-drug treatment of suspected infection

Neonate: 2 mg/kg once a day for 2 weeks and then 5 mg/kg once a day in babies under 2 months old.

Older babies: Start with 4 mg/kg *once* a day for 2 weeks and then 7 mg/kg *twice* a day unless a rash or other serious side effect develops. Such treatment should only be started where there is at least some provisional evidence that the baby has become infected, as discussed in the monograph on lamivudine.

Supply

200 mg nevirapine tablets cost £2.80 each; 100 ml of a 10 mg/ml suspension in sucrose costs £21.

Continued on p. 352

References

(See also the relevant Cochrane reviews)

Fillekes Q, Mulenga V, Kabamba D, *et al*. Pharmacokinetics of nevirapine in HIV-infected infants weighing 3 kg to less than 6 kg taking paediatric fixed dose combination tablets. *AIDS* 2012;**26**:1795–800.

Ford N, Calmy A, Andrieux-Meyer I, *et al*. Adverse events associated with nevirapine use in pregnancy: a systematic review and meta-analysis. *AIDS* 2013;**27**:1135–43. [SR]

Jackson JB, Musoke P, Fleming T, *et al*. Intrapartum and neonatal single-dose nevirapine compared to zidovudine for prevention of mother-to-child transmission of HIV-1 in Kampala, Uganda: 18 month follow-up of the HIVNET012 randomised trial. *Lancet* 2003;**362**:859–68. [RCT] (See also editorial pp. 842–3.)

Jourdain G, Ngo-Giang-Huong N, La Coeur S, *et al*. Intrapartum exposure to nevirapine and subsequent maternal responses to nevirapine-based antiretroviral therapy. *N Engl J Med* 2004;**351**:229–40. [RCT]. (See also pp. 289–92.)

Kumwenda NI, Hoover DR, Mofenson LM, *et al*. Extended antiretroviral prophylaxis to reduce breast-milk HIV-1 transmission. *N Engl J Med* 2008;**359**:119–29. [RCT] (See also pp. 189–91.)

Mirochnick M, Nielsen-Saines K, Pilotto JH, *et al*. Nevirapine concentrations in newborns receiving an extended prophylactic regimen. *J Acquir Immune Defic Syndr* 2008;**47**:334–7.

Nielsen-Saines K, Watts DH, Veloso VG, *et al*. Three postpartum antiretroviral regimens to prevent intrapartum HIV infection. *N Engl J Med* 2012;**366**:2368–79. [RCT]

Shapiro RL, Holland RT, Capparelli E, *et al*. Antiretroviral concentrations in breast-feeding infants of women in Botswana receiving antiretroviral treatment. *J Infect Dis* 2005;**192**:720–7. (See also pp. 709–12.)

Taha TE, Kumwenda NI, Gibbins A, *et al*. Short postexposure prophylaxis in newborn babies to reduce mother-to-child transmission of HIV-1: NVAZ randomised trial. *Lancet* 2003;**362**:1171–7. [RCT]

Taylor GP, Anderson J, Clayden P, *et al*. British HIV Association and Children's HIV Association position statement on infant feeding in the UK 2011. *HIV Med* 2011;**12**:389–93.

Taylor GP, Clayden P, Dhar J, *et al*. British HIV Association guidelines for the management of HIV infection in pregnant women 2012. *HIV Med* 2012;**13**(suppl 2):87–157.

Use

Nifedipine is a smooth muscle relaxant used to manage hypertension, cardiomyopathy, angina and Raynaud's phenomenon. It seems more effective than betamimetics and as good as atosiban at delaying preterm birth and may well be the best drug to use to delay delivery long enough for betamethasone (q.v.) to speed the maturation of the fetal lung even if the baby is born early.

Pharmacology

Nifedipine, introduced in 1968, causes a reduction in vascular tone (including coronary arteries) by reducing slow-channel cell membrane calcium uptake. All calcium channel blocking drugs also reduce cardiac contractility, but the vasodilator effect of nifedipine is more influential than the myocardial effect. Nifedipine also reduces uterine muscle tone. It is quite well absorbed through the buccal mucosa (having some effect within 5 minutes) and then metabolised by the liver (adult half-life 2–3 hours) before being excreted in the urine. Although there is no evidence of teratogenicity in man, the manufacturers continue to advise against use before 20 weeks' gestation. Nifedipine passes into breast milk, but the nursing infant does not ingest clinically relevant amounts. Nifedipine can also be used to treat Raynaud's phenomenon of the nipple.

Controlling preterm labour

Unexplained spontaneous preterm labour accounts for more than half of all births before 32 weeks' gestation, and obstetric intervention has yet to make any impact on this cause of preterm birth. Indometacin, ethanol (alcohol), nifedipine and the betamimetics, terbutaline and salbutamol (q.v.), are all capable of delaying delivery for 2–3 days, but nifedipine is the only tocolytic that has yet been shown to inhibit labour for long enough to reduce the number of babies requiring intensive care, and use did halve the number delivering within 7 days in one small trial. Atosiban (q.v.), an oxytocin receptor antagonist introduced in 1998, is probably slightly more effective and does not run the risk of causing hypotension, but it is much more expensive and has to be given by intravenous (IV) infusion. Antibiotic treatment does nothing to delay delivery in uncomplicated preterm labour, but treatment with erythromycin (q.v.) *did* delay delivery and improve neonatal outcome in women with preterm pre-labour rupture of membranes. Progesterone (q.v.) prophylaxis may benefit those women with a past history of unexplained very preterm labour with a very short cervix.

Treatment

Controlling preterm labour: Crush one 10 mg capsule between the teeth to achieve sublingual absorption. Up to three further doses may be given at 15 minute intervals while watching for hypotension if contractions persist. If this stops labour, give between 20 and 50 mg of modified-release nifedipine three times a day for 3 days. Some then recommend giving 20 mg three times a day until pregnancy reaches 34 weeks.

Hyperinsulinaemic hypoglycaemia: 100–200 micrograms/kg by mouth once every 6 hours seems to improve glucose control in some patients also taking diazoxide (q.v.). Where there is no response, doubling or tripling the dose may occasionally be helpful. Watch for hypotension.

Hypertension in children: 200–500 micrograms/kg by mouth every 6–8 hours is now increasingly used to control hypertension and to treat angina in Kawasaki disease. Start with the lowest dose and increase as necessary. Consider managing the initial reduction in pressure in a controlled way using IV labetalol (q.v.), especially where hypertension has existed for a sustained, or unknown, time.

Drug interactions

The simultaneous use of magnesium sulfate sometimes causes sudden profound muscle weakness.

Supply

10 mg nifedipine capsules cost 12p each. A range of modified-release tablets and capsules are available. A 20 mg/ml (1 mg per drop) dropper bottle formulation is importable on a 'named-patient' basis for babies. A suspension containing 1 mg/ml can be prepared on request which is stable for a month if protected from light. No IV or intramuscular formulation is available.

Continued on p. 354

References

(See also the relevant Cochrane reviews and UK guideline on tocolysis **DHUK**)

Barrett ME, Heller MM, Stone HF, *et al.* Raynaud phenomenon of the nipple in breast feeding mothers: an underdiagnosed cause of nipple pain. *JAMA Dermatol* 2013;**149**:300–6.

Blaszak RT, Savage JA, Ellis EN. The use of short-acting nifedipine in pediatric patients with hypertension. *J Pediatr* 2001;**139**:34–7.

Giannubilo SR, Bezzeccheri V, Cecchi S, *et al.* Nifedipine versus labetalol in the treatment of hypertensive disorders of pregnancy. *Arch Gynecol Obstet* 2012;**286**:637–42.

Lamont RF, Khan KS, Beattie B, *et al.* The quality of nifedipine studies used to assess tocolytic efficacy: a systematic review. *J Perinat Med* 2005;**33**:287–95. [SR]

Müller D, Zimmering M, Roehr CC. Should nifedipine be used to counter low blood sugar levels in children with persistent hyperinsulinaemic hypoglycaemia? *Arch Dis Child* 2004;**89**:83–5. [SR]

Papatsonis DNM, Kok JH, van Geijn HP, *et al.* Neonatal effects of nifedipine and ritodrine for preterm labour. *Obstet Gynecol* 2000;**95**:477–81. [RCT]

Roos C, Spaanderman ME, Schuit E, *et al.* Effect of maintenance tocolysis with nifedipine in threatened pre-term labor on perinatal outcomes: a randomized controlled trial. *JAMA* 2013;**309**:41–7. [RCT]

Salim R, Garmi G, Nachum Z, *et al.* Nifedipine compared with atosiban for treating preterm labor: a randomized controlled trial. *Obstet Gynecol* 2012;**120**:1323–31. [RCT]

Tsatsaris V, Papatsonis F, Goffinet D, *et al.* Tocolysis with nifedipine or beta-adrenergic agents: a meta-analysis. *Obstet Gynecol* 2001;**97**:840–7. [SR]

Use

Nitazoxanide can be used to treat a range of parasitic infections including, uniquely, the illness caused by the protozoal parasites *Cryptosporidium parvum* and *C. hominis*. Nitazoxanide is under investigation as a treatment (both as monotherapy and in combination) for hepatitis C infection after its antiviral properties were discovered accidentally in HIV- and HCV-co-infected patients who were being treated for cryptosporidiosis.

Pharmacology

Nitazoxanide is a nitrothiazole benzamide (thiazolide) that is recognised as an effective treatment for a wide range of intestinal protozoal and helminthic infections. Originally developed in 1975 as a veterinary drug, it has been used since 1996 to treat children with debilitating diarrhoea due to a range of protozoal infections, including cryptosporidiosis and giardiasis. It seems more effective than albendazole (q.v.) in the treatment of children with whipworm (*Trichuris trichiura*) and as effective (if more expensive) than albendazole in the treatment of ascariasis (*Ascariasis lumbricoides*). It is also effective in fascioliasis (*Fasciola hepatica*), amoebiasis (*Entamoeba histolytica* and *E. dispar*), isosporiasis (*Isospora belli*) and beef tapeworm (*Taenia saginata*) infection. More importantly, it is the first drug to be recognised as effective in the management of cryptosporidiosis, and the manufacturers were permitted to recommend its use in North and South America in 2002 for children with this condition who are at least 12 months old. Use to treat giardiasis was also approved, but this is usually as effectively (and more cheaply) treated with metronidazole (q.v.).

Nitazoxanide and other thiazolides have emerged as a new class of broad-spectrum antiviral drugs and have been shown to inhibit replication of rotavirus and hepatitis B and C in a selective and dose-dependent manner. They have also been reported to be active against a number of other viruses.

Nitazoxanide is a prodrug that is well absorbed orally (especially when taken with food). It is rapidly metabolised by glucuronidation in the liver to the active drug tizoxanide and then cleared from the blood with a terminal half-life of 7 hours. Two-thirds appears in the bile and faeces, and one-third in the urine. Children metabolise the drug in much the same way as adults, but drug handling has not yet been studied in children less than a year old. Adverse effects (abdominal pain and vomiting) seem no more common than with placebo treatment. Animal studies suggest that use during pregnancy is unlikely to be hazardous, and extensive plasma protein binding means that very little active drug will cross the placenta or appear in breast milk.

Treatment

100 mg by mouth twice a day for 3 days was shown to be effective in combating diarrhoea and in reducing mortality in seriously malnourished 1–3-year-old children with severe cryptosporidiosis in one recent small trial. It also eliminated all parasites from the stool. One study used a dose of 7.5 mg/kg twice a day for 3 days in children less than a year old. Albendazole seems more effective in children with HIV infection.

Supply

Although the drug has been in use in North and South America for over 10 years (and has FDA approval), it has not yet been reviewed by UK licensing authorities for any indication. Nitazoxanide is made by Romark Laboratories, Tampa, Florida, and 1.2 g of powder currently costs $60. It can be made available in the United Kingdom on a named-patient basis. Reconstitute with 48 ml of tap water to obtain 60 ml of a sucrose-containing, strawberry-flavoured, 20 mg/ml suspension. Shake before use, and discard after 7 days.

References

Abaza H, El-Zayadi A, Kabil SM, *et al*. Nitazoxanide in the treatment of patients with intestinal protozoan and helminthic infections: a report on 546 patients in Egypt. *Curr Ther Res* 1998;**59**:116–21.

Amadi B, Mwiya M, Musuku J, *et al*. Effect of nitazoxanide on morbidity and mortality in Zambian children with cryptosporidiosis: a randomised controlled trial. *Lancet* 2002;**360**:1375–80. [RCT]

Bailey JM, Errsmouspe J. Nitazoxanide treatment for giardiasis and cryptosporidiosis in children. *Ann Pharmacother* 2004;**38**:634–40. [SR]

Davies AP, Chalmers RM. Cryptosporidiosis. *Br Med J* 2009;**339**:963–7.

Korba BE, Mueller AB, Farrar K, *et al*. Nitazoxanide, tizoxanide and other thiazolides are potent inhibitors of hepatitis B virus and hepatitis C virus replication. *Antivir Res* 2008;**77**:56–63.

Continued on p. 356

Romero-Cabello R, Guerrero LR, Muñóz-Garcia, *et al.* Nitazoxanide for the treatment of intestinal protozoan and helminthic infections in Mexico. *Trans R Soc Trop Med Hyg* 1997;**91**:701–3.

Rossignol JF. Thiazolides: a new class of antiviral drugs. *Expert Opin Drug Metab Toxicol* 2009;**5**:667–74.

Rossignol J-F, Abu-Zekry M, Hussein A, *et al.* Effect of nitazoxanide for treatment of severe rotavirus diarrhoea: randomised double-blind placebo-controlled trial. *Lancet* 2006;**368**:124–9. [RCT] (See also pp. 100–1.)

Rossignol JF, Ayoub A, Ayers MS. Treatment of diarrhea caused by *Cryptosporidium parvum*: a prospective randomized, double-blind, placebo-controlled study of nitazoxanide. *J Infect Dis* 2001;**184**:103–6. [RCT]

Use

Nitisinone is used to prevent the accumulation of toxic metabolites in patients with type 1 tyrosinaemia. Along with a diet low in tyrosine and phenylalanine, the drug is the mainstay of treatment of this condition.

Biochemistry

Type 1 tyrosinaemia is a recessively inherited disorder caused by a deficiency of fumarylacetoacetate hydrolase, the enzyme involved in the fifth step of tyrosine breakdown. It is seen in about 1:100,000 births but is known to be more common in some populations where newborn screening programmes have been implemented to enable early treatment. Symptoms result from the accumulation of fumarylacetoacetate and succinylacetone, which are toxic. The condition is of variable severity but can present within weeks of birth with signs of liver failure, including jaundice (which is often misleadingly mild), diarrhoea, vomiting, oedema, ascites, hypoglycaemia and a severe bleeding tendency. Cirrhosis usually develops over time, and there is a significant long-term risk of hepatocellular carcinoma. Milder cases present later in childhood or early adult life with isolated hepatomegaly, liver failure or hypophosphataemic rickets due to renal tubular dysfunction. Plasma tyrosine levels are usually elevated, but diagnosis depends on demonstrating raised urinary levels of succinylacetone. In a few patients, succinylacetone levels are only slightly raised, and enzyme assay may be needed to confirm the diagnosis. Acute neurological crises can occur, with abdominal pain, muscle weakness and hypertension, when toxic metabolites trigger other problems similar to those seen in acute intermittent porphyria.

Management was transformed in 1992 by the development of nitisinone (2-[2-nitro-4-(trifluoromethyl)benzoyl] cyclohexane-1,3-dione) or NTBC. This inhibits the second enzyme in the pathway of tyrosine metabolism (4-hydroxyphenylpyruvate dioxygenase). However, while this prevents the formation of fumarylacetoacetate and succinylacetone, it causes a marked rise in the plasma tyrosine concentration. Very high tyrosine levels can lead to the deposition of crystals in the cornea, causing photophobia and corneal erosions; it is also possible that high tyrosine levels may cause learning difficulties. Because of this, treatment with nitisinone still needs to be combined with a diet low in tyrosine and phenylalanine. Other adverse effects include transient thrombocytopenia and neutropenia. Treatment should be started as soon as the diagnosis is made, and continued indefinitely. Whether management with nitisinone can completely eliminate the need for liver transplantation will only be known once it is shown that such treatment removes the latent risk of liver cancer. Nitisinone freely crosses the placenta exposing the fetus to similar levels as the mother. At high doses, it has been shown to cause malformations in rodents. Very limited reports of use during human pregnancy have been associated not only with normal neonatal outcomes, but it appears that maternal treatment may also protect an affected fetus from the disease. Experience of use in breastfeeding is equally limited.

Treatment

Initial care: Infants presenting with liver failure when first diagnosed require intensive support and should, if possible, be transferred to a liver unit because a few do not respond to nitisinone and require urgent transplantation.

Continuing care: Start regular maintenance with 500 micrograms/kg of nitisinone twice a day by mouth. Slightly more may sometimes be necessary. The intake of natural protein may need to be restricted and the diet supplemented using an amino acid mixture free of tyrosine and phenylalanine.

Monitoring

Patients should be managed in collaboration with a specialist in metabolic disease. Diet needs to allow normal growth while aiming to keep the plasma tyrosine level below 500 μmol/l. The dose of nitisinone is adjusted by assessing the biochemical response. Some centres also monitor the plasma concentration (the therapeutic nitisinone level usually being between 25 and 50 μmol/l). Serum α-fetoprotein levels should be measured serially, and regular liver scans undertaken to watch for early signs of liver cancer.

Continued on p. 358

Supply and administration

2, 5 and 10 mg capsules of nitisinone (costing £9.40, £18.80 and £34.40 each) are available from Orphan Europe. Divide the daily dose, where possible, into two (not necessarily equal) parts, given morning and evening. The capsules can be opened and the content suspended, immediately before use, in a little water or milk.

References

Chakrapani A, Gissen P, McKiernan P. Disorders of tyrosine metabolism. In: Saudubray J-M, van den Berghe G, Walter JH, eds. *Inborn metabolic diseases. Diagnosis and treatment*, 5th ed. Berlin: Springer-Verlag, 2012: pp. 265–76.

de Laet C, Dionisi-Vici C, Leonard JV, *et al.* Recommendations for the management of tyrosinaemia type 1. *Orphanet J Rare Dis* 2013;**8**:8.

Garcia Segarra N, Roche S, Imbard A, *et al.* Maternal and fetal tyrosinemia type 1. *J Inherit Metab Dis* 2010;**33** suppl 3:S507–10.

Holme E, Lindstedt S. Tyrosinaemia type 1 and NTBC (2-(2-nitro-4-trifluomethylbenzoyl)-1,3,-cyclohexane-dione). *J Inherit Metab Dis* 1998;**21**:507–17.

McKiernan PJ. Nitisinone in the treatment of hereditary tyrosinaemia type 1. *Drugs* 2006;**66**:743–50.

Morrissey MA, Sunny S, Fahim A, *et al.* Newborn screening for Tyr-I: two years' experience of the New York State program. *Mol Genet Metab* 2011;**103**:191–2.

Vanclooster A, Devlieger R, Meersseman W, *et al.* Pregnancy during nitisinone treatment for tyrosinemia type I: first human experience. *JIMD Rep* 2012;**5**:27–33.

Use

Nitric oxide can reduce the need for extracorporeal membrane oxygenation (ECMO) in babies of ≥34 weeks' gestation with persistent pulmonary hypertension (PPHN), but survival is not increased. Echocardiography must be done to confirm pulmonary hypertension and exclude structural heart disease. No trial has yet shown treatment to be of convincing and sustained benefit in babies less mature than this.

Pharmacology

Nitric oxide, recognised in 1987 as a 'relaxing factor' produced in the vessel's endothelial lining cells, is produced endogenously by the conversion of arginine to citrulline by the enzyme nitric oxide synthetase. Nitric oxide stimulates soluble guanylate cyclase activity and increases guanosine 3',5'-cyclic monophosphate (cGMP), leading to vasodilatation. It also inhibits labour by reducing uterine muscle tone, influences macrophage function and acts as a neurotransmitter.

In many ways, nitric oxide is the ideal pulmonary vasodilator, this highly diffusible colourless gas can rapidly reduce the pulmonary vascular tone, and because it only has a very short half-life in the body (2–4 seconds), it lowers pulmonary vascular resistance without lowering systemic blood pressure. Thus, unlike many intravenous or oral pulmonary vasodilators, nitric oxide is more likely to improve rather than exacerbate the effects of ventilation–perfusion mismatch due to its lack of significant systemic effects.

Not all babies (up to 40% in clinical trials) with PPHN respond to treatment with inhaled nitric oxide, and there are few data to support its use in preterm infants. Excess nitric oxide enters the bloodstream where it is quickly inactivated, combining with haemoglobin to produce methaemoglobin. While this molecule is inert, its existence reduces the oxygen-carrying capacity of the blood. The level should therefore be checked an hour after treatment is started and then every 12 hours, aiming to keep the level below 2.5%. Try to reduce the dose of nitric oxide if the level exceeds 4%, and give methylthioninium chloride (q.v.) if it exceeds 7%.

Nitric oxide (NO) reacts with oxygen to form nitrogen dioxide (NO_2), and the level of this needs to be monitored, since some by-products are toxic. Leakage could put staff at risk unless an alarm system exists, and poorly ventilated areas need a gas scavenging system, but most delivery systems address these issues.

Use in babies with persistent pulmonary hypertension

Starting treatment: Start by adding 20 parts per million (ppm) of nitric oxide to the ventilator gas circuit. If this produces a response (a rise of at least 3 kPa in post-ductal arterial pO_2 within 15 minutes while ventilator settings are held constant), the amount given should be reduced, after one hour, to the lowest dose compatible with a sustained response. Wean off treatment promptly if there is no response. Higher doses rarely lead to any further improvement.

Weaning: Failure to use the lowest effective dose causes dependency. So does prolonged use. Try to reduce the dose needed in 'responders' once every 12 hours. Lower the concentration by 10% once every 3 minutes, but reverse any reduction that causes arterial saturation to drop more than 2–3%. Babies sometimes require a low dose (<0.5 ppm) for several days during weaning, even if no response was seen initially. Increasing the inspired oxygen concentration by 20% may facilitate final 'weaning'.

Use in other children

Use can occasionally help to control post-operative pulmonary hypertension in older children after cardiac surgery, but there are *no* other clear-cut indications for use. One trial did find that low-dose use started in preterm babies still ventilated at 7–14 days might marginally increase the number alive and not in oxygen (28 vs. 49%) at 36 weeks. Several other large trials have, however, now shown that, except in the rare baby with overt echocardiographic evidence of pulmonary hypertension, use does **not** improve survival or reduce the incidence of disability at 2 years in babies born more than about 8 weeks early, even when it does initially make the baby slightly less oxygen dependent.

Supply and administration

Nitric oxide was, until recently, an ill-defined therapeutic product, but use in term infants with pulmonary hypertension has now been approved by the regulatory authorities in Europe and in North America. Now that the gas has received formal recognition as a medicinal product, a single

Continued on p. 360

company (INO Therapeutics Inc.) has acquired sole marketing rights, and this company makes uniform delivery and monitoring systems available to hospitals for an hourly fee. Since this arrangement seems to have increased the cost of treatment more than 10-fold, it is going to be important to mount further studies into the cost-effectiveness of this and other strategies for modifying pulmonary vascular tone.

References

(See also the relevant Cochrane reviews)

Askie LM, Ballard RA, Cutter GR, *et al*. Inhaled nitric oxide in preterm infants: an individual-patient data meta-analysis of randomized trials. *Pediatrics* 2011;**128**:729–39. [SR]

Cole FS, Alleyne C, Barks JD, *et al*. NIH Consensus Development Conference statement: inhaled nitric-oxide therapy for premature infants. *Pediatrics* 2011;**127**:363–9.

Dhillon R. The management of neonatal pulmonary hypertension. *Arch Dis Child Fetal Neonatal Ed* 2012;**97**:F223–8.

Hibbs AM, Walsh MC, Martin RJ, *et al*. One-year respiratory outcomes of preterm infants enrolled in the Nitric Oxide (to Prevent) Chronic Lung Disease Trial. *J Pediatr* 2008;**153**:525–9. [RCT]

Kumar P, Committee on Fetus and Newborn. Use of inhaled nitric oxide in preterm infants. *Pediatrics* 2014;**133**:164–70. [SR]

Tanaka Y, Hayashi T, Kitajima H, *et al*. Inhaled nitric oxide therapy decreases the risk of cerebral palsy in preterm infants with persistent pulmonary hypertension of the newborn. *Pediatrics* 2007;**119**:1159–64.

Use

A mixture of 50% nitrous oxide (N_2O) and oxygen provides very safe conscious analgesia in children (although there are few reports of use in infants). Higher concentrations bring little, if any, additional benefit.

History

Humphry Davy, who first described this gas in 1800, was shrewd enough to see that it might be used 'with great advantage in surgical operations where no great effusion of blood takes place'. Despite this, it was the intoxicating and amnesic effect of 'laughing gas' that was exploited for 44 years before Horace Wells first used the drug during dentistry. Although Queen Victoria used chloroform, it was many years before inhalation analgesia became common in childbirth, partly because the early Minnitt machine could leave a woman breathing as little as 10% oxygen. The 'Lucy Baldwin' machine (named after the UK prime minister's wife who did much to champion use by midwives) made safe pain relief available during home birth, but single cylinders containing a 50:50 nitrous oxide/oxygen mixture then came into use in the 1960s.

Pharmacology

Use of a 50% mixture causes conscious analgesia after 3 minutes, and this persists for about 3 minutes after inhalation ceases. Swallowing is depressed but laryngeal reflexes are retained. Use in any patient with an air-containing closed space (such as a pneumothorax or loculated air within a damaged lung) is potentially dangerous because nitrous oxide diffuses into the space, causing a significant increase in pressure. Diffusion hypoxia, due to nitrous oxide returning to the alveoli from the bloodstream more rapidly than it is replaced by nitrogen at the end of the procedure, can be minimised by giving oxygen.

Nurse-supervised use in children to provide short-term analgesia for a range of investigative and treatment procedures can be extremely safe. The only significant problems encountered during procedures lasting up to 30 minutes were mild hypoxaemia, brief apnoea, bradycardia and over-sedation (loss of verbal contact lasting more than 5 minutes), and such problems were only encountered in 0.3% of all procedures. These were, however, slightly more common in children who had also been given both an opioid and a benzodiazepine sedative and in children <1 year old (where 2% experienced some mild adverse effect). Transient dizziness and nausea can be a problem, but only 1% of procedures had to be cancelled because of inadequate sedation or a side effect.

Safe use in young children

Use must be supervised by someone who has undergone appropriate training and should be supervised by a qualified anaesthetist in any child who is drowsy or who has also had another sedative (especially any benzodiazepine or opioid). Do nothing for 4 hours after the child last had milk or solid food (2 hours after clear liquids). Do nothing painful for 3 minutes after starting to give the gas, and stop the procedure if pain relief is inadequate, as may inexplicably happen in 5% of all procedures. Always use a pulse oximeter and have oxygen to hand in case brief diffusion hypoxia occurs during recovery. Use always requires the presence of at least two people, because the person undertaking the procedure for which analgesia is being offered must *never* be the person supervising the administration of nitrous oxide. See the website for a review of use in very young children. Very frequent use in a child could lower body cobalamin (B_{12}) stores.

Pain relief

Maternal pain relief in labour: 50% mixture in oxygen appears uniformly safe and helpful.
Pain relief in infancy: Use in infants and children must be supervised by appropriately trained staff (see 'Safe use in young children').

Supply and administration

Premixed supplies of 50% nitrous oxide in oxygen (Entonox® and Equanox®) come in blue cylinders with a blue and white shoulder. Refills cost about £10. Storage at temperatures below −6 °C can cause the gases to separate; should this happen the cylinder *must* be laid horizontal in a warm room for 24 hours and briefly inverted before use. School-age children should be encouraged to use a mouthpiece or face mask and demand valve, because self-control ensures that use ceases if the patient becomes drowsy. A constant flow system with a blender like the Quantiflex® which shuts down if the oxygen supply fails makes safe administration of a variable

Continued on p. 362

dose possible. Good room ventilation, or a waste gas scavenging system, must be provided where frequent use occurs, to stop the ambient level exceeding 100 ppm, since chronic exposure could interfere with the action of vitamin B_{12} and cause megaloblastic anaemia. There is one report that chronic exposure (once common during dental surgery) might lower female fertility.

References
(See SIGN guidelines on sedation of children for procedures **DHUK**)

Babl FE, Oakley E, Seaman C, *et al*. High-concentration nitrous oxide for procedural sedation in children: adverse events and depth of sedation. *Pediatrics* 2008;**121**:e528–32.

Gall O, Annequin D, Benoit G, *et al*. Adverse events of premixed nitrous oxide and oxygen for procedural sedation in children. *Lancet* 2001;**358**:1514–5.

Mandel R, Ali N, Chen J, *et al*. Nitrous oxide analgesia during retinopathy screening: a randomised controlled trial. *Arch Dis Child Fetal Neonatal Ed* 2012;**97**:F83–7. [RCT]

Medical Research Council. Committee on Nitrous Oxide and Oxygen Analgesia in Midwifery. Clinical trials of different concentrations of oxygen and nitrous oxide for obstetric analgesia. *Br Med J* 1970;**i**:709–13.

Milesi C, Pidoux O, Sabatier E, *et al*. Nitrous oxide analgesia for intubating preterm neonates: a pilot study. *Acta Paediatr* 2006;**95**:1104–8.

Rosen MA. Nitrous oxide for relief of labour pain; systemic review. *Am J Obstet Gynecol* 2003;**186**:S110–26. [SR]

Use

Noradrenaline is a potent vasoconstrictor that is sometimes used to treat severe refractory hypotension (as in patients with septic shock) once any hypovolaemia caused by fluid leaking from damaged capillaries into the extravascular tissue space has been corrected. Milrinone (q.v.) may prove more effective if the hypotension is, at least in part, due to a fall in cardiac output.

Pharmacology

Sympathomimetic agents mimic the actions produced by stimulation of the post-ganglionic sympathetic nerves, preparing the body for 'fight or flight'. Three natural catecholamine agents have been identified: dopamine (primarily a central neurotransmitter), noradrenaline (a sympathetic neurotransmitter) and adrenaline (which has metabolic and hormonal functions). Metabolism is rapid, if variable, so stable concentrations are reached within 10–15 minutes of starting an infusion and clearance is not influenced by renal function. The agents, and their synthetic counterparts, differ in their actions according to the receptors on which they mainly act (though many stimulate most to a varying degree): α_1 smooth muscle receptors, which cause vasoconstriction; α_2 presynaptic nerve receptors, which are thought to inhibit gastrointestinal activity; β_1 receptors, which stimulate cardiac activity; β_2 smooth muscle receptors, which cause vascular and bronchial dilatation; and two CNS dopamine receptors (D_1 and D_2).

Noradrenaline is the main post-ganglionic neurotransmitter in the sympathetic nervous system. Some is also produced along with adrenaline (q.v.) by the adrenal glands in response to stress. It is inactivated when given by mouth and cannot be given by subcutaneous or intramuscular injection because it is such a powerful vasoconstrictor. The main effects are to increase cardiac contractility, heart rate and myocardial oxygen consumption (via β_1 stimulation), but high-dose infusions also cause intense peripheral vasoconstriction (an α_1 agonist effect) unless vasopressin insufficiency (q.v.) has developed. Such peripheral vasoconstriction can sometimes, by increasing the afterload on the heart, counteract the drug's inotropic effect and cause a decrease in cardiac output. Similarly, the increase in myocardial oxygen consumption can exacerbate any existing cardiac failure and compromise ventricular function. For these reasons, the drug should only be used when the need to increase arterial pressure outweighs the risk of lowering cardiac output. Infants with sepsis who are hypotensive but have good cardiac function and adequate vascular volume are the most likely to benefit, though even here the optimum dose calls for careful judgement. Use in babies with persistent pulmonary hypertension may marginally improve oxygenation by changing the balance between pulmonary and systemic artery pressure. Noradrenaline can cause the pregnant uterus to contract.

Drug equivalence

1 mg of noradrenaline acid tartrate contains 500 micrograms of noradrenaline base. The drug is always best prescribed in terms of the amount of **base** to be given to prevent ambiguity.

Treatment

Start with an infusion of 100 nanograms/kg/minute of noradrenaline base (0.1 ml/hour of a solution made up as described under 'Supply and administration') and infuse into a *central* vein. Severe complications can be associated with peripheral infusion as outlined in the monograph on dopamine. The rate of infusion can be increased slowly to a maximum of 1.5 micrograms/kg/minute (1.5 ml/hour), as long as limb perfusion and urine output are watched carefully. Monitor central vascular pressures where possible.

Compatibility

Noradrenaline can be added (terminally) into a line containing dobutamine, heparin, milrinone or standard TPN (with or without lipid). The safety of physical mixture with dopamine remains unassessed.

Supply and administration

Noradrenaline is available in 2 and 4 ml ampoules containing 2 mg/ml of noradrenaline acid tartrate (the equivalent of 1 mg/ml of noradrenaline base) costing £2.20 and £4.40 each. To give an infusion of 100 nanograms/kg/minute of noradrenaline base take 1.5 mg (1.5 ml) of noradrenaline base for each kilogram the baby weighs, dilute to 25 ml with 10% glucose or glucose saline, and infuse at a rate of 0.1 ml/hour. The drug is stable in solutions with a low pH, such as glucose,

Continued on p. 364

but is best prepared afresh every 24 hours unless protected from light. Protect ampoules from light during storage, and discard if discoloured. Tissue extravasation can be dangerous and should be treated as outlined in the monograph on hyaluronidase.

References

Carcillo JA, Fields AI. Clinical practice parameters for hemodynamic support of pediatric and neonatal patients in septic shock. *Crit Care Med* 2002;**30**:1365–78. [SR]

Ceneviva G, Paschall JA, Maffei F, *et al*. Hemodynamic support in fluid refractory septic shock. *Pediatrics* 1998;**102**:e19.

Seri I. Circulatory support of the sick preterm infant. *Semin Neonatol* 2001;**6**:85–95.

Tourneux P, Rakza T, Abazine A, *et al*. Noradrenaline for management of septic shock refractory to fluid loading and dopamine or dobutamine in full-term newborn infants. *Acta Paediatr* 2008;**97**:177–80.

Tourneux P, Rakza T, Bouissou A, *et al*. Pulmonary circulatory effects of norepinephrine in newborn infants with persistent pulmonary hypertension. *J Pediatr* 2008;**153**:345–9.

von Rosensteil N, von Rosensteil I, Adam D. Management of sepsis and septic shock in infants and children. *Paediatr Drugs* 2001;**3**:9–27.

Use

Nystatin is used to treat gastrointestinal and topical *Candida albicans* infection. Low-dose prophylaxis may stop overt infection in 'at-risk' patients. Miconazole gel (q.v.) seems better at eliminating oral infection.

Pharmacology

Nystatin was the first naturally occurring antifungal polyene antibiotic developed in 1951 and is still the most widely used. It is very insoluble and is usually prescribed as a suspension. Nystatin is particularly active against yeast-like fungi and has long been used in the treatment of topical *C. albicans* infection. Full purification is impracticable, and the drug dosage is therefore usually quoted in 'units'. The drug works by combining with the sterol elements of fungal cell membranes causing cell death by producing increased cell wall permeability. Oral absorption is poor. While there is no evidence to suggest that it is unsafe to use nystatin during pregnancy or lactation, treatment with miconazole seems to be a more effective way of eliminating vaginal candidiasis.

The dose usually recommended for oral infection ('thrush') in a baby is 1 ml of the suspension four times a day, but this is not as effective as treatment with oral miconazole gel. A 4 ml dose of nystatin may be more effective, but this still needs controlled trial confirmation. Oral drops can be used to clear *Candida* from the gastrointestinal tract, and ointment used to treat skin infection. Fluconazole (q.v.) costs more and is of similar efficacy, but it should certainly be used if there is tracheal colonisation or systemic infection. Such colonisation can turn into serious overt systemic infection in babies on broad-spectrum antibiotic treatment (because of the resultant change in the normal bacterial flora).

Maternal breast and nipple pain

A tender, lumpy, inflamed breast is best treated for incipient bacterial mastitis with flucloxacillin (q.v.). Local *nipple* pain is usually due to poor positioning (an art that has to be learnt), and this can be rapidly relieved by improved technique. Topical treatments can do more harm than good; some mothers are even sensitive to lanolin cream. Keep the skin dry (while allowing any expressed milk to dry on the nipple).

Candida infection ('thrush') can occasionally be part of the problem and should be suspected if trouble comes on after lactation has been established, especially if the baby has signs of this infection or the mother has vaginitis. Recent antibiotic treatment makes this problem more likely.

Miconazole cream and oral gel (q.v.) may help, but a maternal course of fluconazole is the treatment of choice when there is severe, sustained, stinging or radiating pain, presumably due to duct infection. Give nystatin drops as well to minimise the risk of reinfection if the baby seems to be heavily colonised or more widely infected. Sudden severe pain with marked blanching may be a vasomotor reaction. Anxiety can be one trigger. Local warmth may help; keeping warm may forestall trouble. Some cases seem to be a form of Raynaud's phenomenon, and this occasionally merits pharmacological intervention; giving the mother a 30 mg slow-release tablet of nifedipine once a day often brings rapid relief.

Neonatal treatment

Prophylaxis: 1 ml (100,000 units) of the oral suspension every 8 hours can lower the risk of systemic infection in the very low birthweight baby. Fluconazole once a day is also very affective but more expensive.

Oral candidiasis (thrush): It is standard practice to give 1 ml (100,000 units) by mouth four times a day after feeds, but a larger dose may be more effective.

Candida (*Monilia*) **dermatitis:** Dry the skin thoroughly and apply nystatin ointment at least twice a day for a week. Leave the skin exposed if possible. A cream is better if the skin is broken and wet.

General considerations: Continue to treat for 3 days after a response is achieved to minimise the risk of a recurrence. Consider the possibility of undiagnosed genital infection, especially in the mother of an infected but otherwise healthy full-term baby. Check that the child is not reinfected by a contaminated bottle or teat. Treat the gastrointestinal tract as well as the skin if there is a stubborn monilial nappy (diaper) rash.

Continued on p. 366

Supply

The 30 g tubes of nystatin cream (costing £2.60) contain benzyl alcohol, and some formulations also contain propylene glycol. One 30 ml bottle of the oral suspension (Nystan®) containing 100,000 units/ml costs £1.90 and includes ethanol among its excipients.

References

(See also the relevant Cochrane reviews)

Aydemir C, Oguz SS, Dizdar EA, *et al*. Randomised controlled trial of prophylactic fluconazole versus nystatin for the prevention of fungal colonisation and invasive fungal infection in very low birth weight infants. *Arch Dis Child Fetal Neonatal Ed* 2011;**96**:F164–8. [RCT]

Barrett ME, Heller MM, Stone HF, *et al*. Raynaud phenomenon of the nipple in breast feeding mothers: an underdiagnosed cause of nipple pain. *JAMA Dermatol* 2013;**149**:300–6.

Blyth CC, Barzi F, Hale K, *et al*. Chemoprophylaxis of neonatal fungal infections in very low birthweight infants: efficacy and safety of fluconazole and nystatin. *J Paediatr Child Health* 2012;**48**:846–51. [SR]

Goins RA, Ascher D, Waecker N, *et al*. Comparison of fluconazole and nystatin oral suspensions for treatment of oral candidiasis in infants. *Pediatr Infect Dis J* 2002;**21**:1165–7. [RCT]

Moorhead AM, Amir LH, O'Brien PW, *et al*. A prospective study of fluconazole treatment for breast and nipple thrush. *Breast Feed Rev* 2011;**19**:25–9.

Ozturk MA, Gunes T, Koklu E, *et al*. Oral nystatin prophylaxis to prevent invasive candidiasis in neonatal intensive care unit. *Mycoses* 2006;**49**:484–92. [RCT]

Use

Octreotide is used to treat intractable hypoglycaemia due to persisting neonatal hyperinsulinism when diazoxide (q.v.) fails to abolish all dangerous episodes of hypoglycaemia. It has also found to be useful in the management of persistent pleural effusions caused by lymphatic chyle (chylothorax).

Pharmacology

Octreotide is an analogue of hypothalamic hormone somatostatin, a naturally occurring 14-amino-acid peptide that inhibits the release of several pituitary hormones as well as glucagon and insulin from the pancreas. It also seems to have some influence over the secretion of pepsin, gastrin and hydrochloric acid in the stomach and duodenum and to play some poorly understood role in the perception of pain by the brain. Somatostatin was first isolated in the Salk Institute in 1973, and the potent octapeptide octreotide was synthesised there in 1982. It is rapidly absorbed following subcutaneous injection and then partly metabolised by the liver and partly excreted unchanged in the urine. While its pharmacokinetic behaviour may be non-linear, the normal half-life is about 90 minutes. The drug's main initial use was in the control of acromegaly, in the control of upper intestinal bleeding and in the management of secretory neoplasms. It can help prevent complications during and after pancreatic surgery and has also been found to be of use in the control of both malignant and non-malignant chylous effusions of the chest and abdomen, although the mechanism by which this is achieved is less clear.

Babies who cannot be weaned from intravenous (IV) glucose with diazoxide are likely to require surgical intervention such as subtotal pancreatectomy but may be stabilised while this step is being contemplated by use of octreotide. A dose of 5 micrograms/kg given subcutaneously every 6–8 hours is usually sufficient. Rarely, doses of as much as 7 micrograms/kg every 4 hours may be required to maintain a safe blood glucose level of at least 4 mmol/l. It can also be given as an IV or subcutaneous infusion in a dose of 5–25 micrograms/kg/day. Such treatment should only be contemplated under the direct supervision of a consultant paediatric endocrinologist. There is no animal evidence to suggest that octreotide is fetotoxic or teratogenic and, since the drug is ineffective when given by mouth, no likelihood that use during lactation will prove hazardous.

Babies with persistent chylothorax unresponsive to a medium-chain triglyceride diet or parenteral nutrition may respond to octreotide subcutaneously or by continuous IV infusion. Dosage is titrated against the volume of pleural drainage, and following satisfactory resolution, octreotide is weaned over 2–4 days.

Necrotising enterocolitis has been reported in a neonate following treatment with octreotide for chylothorax following repair of coarctation of the aorta.

Treatment

Hyperinsulinaemic hypoglycaemia: Start with 5 micrograms/kg by subcutaneous injection 6–8 hourly, increasing, incrementally based on response, to 7 micrograms/kg 4 hourly if necessary. Alternatively, consider a dose of 5–25 micrograms/kg/day by subcutaneous or IV infusion.

Chylothorax: Start with 5 micrograms/kg subcutaneously 8 hourly increasing slowly to 20 micrograms/kg if needed. Alternatively give a continuous infusion of octreotide starting at 1 micrograms/kg/hour and increasing incrementally as high as 10 micrograms/kg/hour if required.

Supply

Several strengths of octreotide are available: 1 ml single-dose ampoules containing 50 micrograms (cost £3), 100 micrograms (cost £5.60) or 500 micrograms (cost £27) of octreotide. 5 ml vials containing 200 micrograms/ml cost £56. Ampoules and vials are best stored at 4–8 °C but stable at 25 °C for 2 weeks. Multi-dose vials can be kept for 2 weeks once open.

References

Arnoux JB, de Lonlay P, Ribeiro MJ, *et al*. Congenital hyperinsulinism. *Early Hum Dev* 2010;**86**:287–94.

Chan S, Lau W, Wong WHS, *et al*. Chylothorax in children after congenital heart surgery. *Ann Thorac Surg* 2006;**82**:1650–7.

Helin RD, Angeles STV, Bhat R. Octreotide therapy for chylothorax in infants and children: a brief review. *Pediatr Crit Care Med* 2006;**7**:576–9. [SR]

Continued on p. 368

Hoe FM, Thornton PS, Wanner LA, *et al*. Clinical features and insulin regulation in infants with a syndrome of prolonged neonatal hyperinsulinism. *J Pediatr* 2006;**148**:207–12.

Kapoor RR, Flanagan SE, James C, *et al*. Hyperinsulinaemic hypoglycaemia. [Review] *Arch Dis Child* 2009;**94**:450–7.

Le Quan Sang KH, Arnoux JB, Mamoune A, *et al*. Successful treatment of congenital hyperinsulinism with long-acting release octreotide. *Eur J Endocrinol* 2012;**166**:333–9.

Lindley KJ, Dunne MJ. Contemporary strategies in the diagnosis and management of neonatal; hyperinsulinaemic hypoglycaemia. [Review] *Early Hum Dev* 2005;**81**:61–72.

Roehr CC, Jung A, Proquitté H, *et al*. Somatostatin or octreotide as treatment options for chylothorax in young children: a systematic review. *Intens Care Med* 2006;**32**:650–7. [SR]

Shah D, Sinn JK. Octreotide as therapeutic option for congenital idiopathic chylothorax: a case series. *Acta Paediatr* 2012;**101**:e151–5.

Young S, Dalgleish S, Eccleston A, *et al*. Severe congenital chylothorax treated with octreotide. *J Perinatol* 2004;**24**:2002.

Use

Omeprazole is used to suppress gastric acid secretion when endoscopically proven oesophagitis or peptic ulceration persists despite treatment with ranitidine. Use is not of benefit in most young children with simple gastro-oesophageal reflux.

Pharmacology

Omeprazole, a substituted benzimidazole, was the first proton pump inhibitor (PPI) to come into clinical use in 1983. A number of related drugs are now available, all of which work by inhibiting the last step in the chain of reactions that leads to the secretion of hydrochloric acid by the parietal cells of the stomach. The resultant reduction in gastric acidity, even in the fed state, allows even severe oesophageal erosions to heal. Treatment is only necessary once a day even though the plasma half-life in adults is only about 1½ hours, since a single dose more than halves the secretion of gastric acid for over a day. Side effects are uncommon. Pharmacokinetic studies suggest that children handle the PPIs in much the same way as adults, but the few studies that have been done in children less than a year old suggest that drug accumulation might well occur if a child less than 9 months old is given more than twice the normal starting dose. The plasma half-life is particularly short in later childhood, but this does not, on its own, seem to explain the higher treatment dose sometimes found necessary. Manufacturers have not yet endorsed the intravenous (IV) use of omeprazole in children and only recommend oral use in children over the age of 1 year.

Formal trials (and systematic reviews of those trials) have shown that PPIs do not reduce symptoms of gastro-oesophageal reflux in children. Omeprazole is widely used, with antibiotics (commonly amoxicillin and either clarithromycin or metronidazole) to treat *Helicobacter pylori* gastritis in older children. Omeprazole does not seem to be teratogenic, but less is known about other PPIs during pregnancy. There is only one report of use during lactation, but since the drug is rapidly destroyed by acid (the reason why the drug is formulated in enteric-coated granules), use during lactation is unlikely to affect the baby. Oral bioavailability, even with coating, is only about 65%. Prophylactic IV use has been used to minimise the risk of aspiration pneumonitis (Mendelson's syndrome) before an urgent caesarean delivery under general anaesthesia, but ranitidine (q.v.) seems an equally effective, and better studied, alternative.

Drug interactions

Omeprazole significantly prolongs the half-life of several benzodiazepines.

Treatment

By mouth: Start by giving 0.7 mg/kg by mouth once a day half an hour before breakfast, and double this dose after 7–14 days if this does not inhibit gastric acid production. A few patients may need as much as 2.8 mg/kg a day, but progressive drug accumulation might occur if a baby <3 months old is given more than 1.4 mg/kg. Sustained treatment is hard to justify unless there is continuing evidence of active oesophagitis.

IV use: Give 0.5 mg/kg once a day over 5 minutes (a dose that can be tripled if acid production persists).

Supply and administration

10 and 20 mg dispersible, enteric-coated tablets cost 20p each. Capsules containing enteric-coated granules (Losec MUPS®) are also available at the same cost. Small doses can be given by giving half a tablet dissolved in water or by sprinkling some of the content of a capsule in a small quantity of yoghurt or fruit juice. Powders that can be reconstituted and administered IV are available in 40 mg vials costing £4.20. The granules can block any enteral feeding tube through which they are being administered. Options include diluting the granules in 10 ml of sodium bicarbonate 8.4% (however, this can halve the bioavailability) or diluting in a large volume of warm water and giving immediately, followed by a generous flush of more water.

Omeprazole suspensions may be obtained from 'specials manufacturers' on a named-patient basis; however, those made from omeprazole powder (rather than enteric-coated granules) have reduced bioavailability. Both prescribers and pharmacists take responsibility for the safety and efficacy of the products that patients use and should be aware of the possible risks. These 'specials' of omeprazole suspension are very expensive with the price varying considerably; one report suggested they range from £130 for 60 ml to £1110 for 150 ml. The only absolute indication for the use of omeprazole suspension preparation instead of MUPS is if it is being

Continued on p. 370

administered via a jejunal tube. Other situations where the suspension could be considered are when there is intolerance of the MUPS preparation or the MUPS cause recurrent blockage of an enteral feeding tube.

References

Bishop J, Furman M, Thomson M. Omeprazole for gastroesophageal reflux disease in the first two years of life: a dose finding study with dual-channel monitoring. *J Pediatr Gastroenterol* 2007;**45**:50–5.

Hoyo VC, Venturelli CR, Gonázlez H, *et al.* Metabolism of omeprazole after two oral doses in children 1 and 9 months old. *Proc West Pharmacol Soc* 2005;**48**:108–9.

Majithia R, Johnson DA. Are proton pump inhibitors safe during pregnancy and lactation? Evidence to date. *Drugs* 2012;**72**:171–9.

Matok I, Levy A, Wiznitzer A, *et al.* The safety of fetal exposure to proton-pump inhibitors during pregnancy. *Dig Dis Sci* 2012;**57**:699–705.

Moore DJ, Tao B S-K, Lines DR, *et al.* Double-blind placebo-controlled trial of omeprazole in irritable infants with gastroesophageal reflux. *J Pediatr* 2003;**143**:219–23. [RCT]

Nikfar S, Abdollahi M, Moretti ME, *et al.* Use of proton pump inhibitors during pregnancy and rates of major malformations: a meta-analysis. *Dig Dis Sci* 2002;**47**:1526–9.

Omari TI, Haslam RR, Lundborrg P, *et al.* Effect of omeprazole on acid gastroesophageal reflux and gastric acidity in preterm infants with pathological acid reflux. *J Pediatr Gastroenterol Nutr* 2007;**44**:41–4.

Omari T, Lundborg P, Sandström M, *et al.* Pharmacodynamics and systemic exposure to esomeprazole in preterm infants and term neonates with gastroesophageal reflux disease. *J Pediatr* 2009;**155**:222–8.

Orenstein SR, Hassall E, Furmaga-Jablonska W, *et al.* Multicenter, double-blind, randomized, placebo controlled trial assessing the efficacy and safety of proton pump inhibitor lansoprazole in infants with symptoms of gastroesophageal reflux. *J Pediatr* 2009;**154**:514–20. [RCT]. (See also editorial pp. 475–6 and correspondence pp. 601–2.)

Song JC, Quercia RA, Fan C, *et al.* Pharmacokinetic comparison of omeprazole capsules and a simplified omeprazole suspension. *Am J Health-Syst Pharm* 2001;**58**:689–94.

Use

Ondansetron is now widely used to control post-operative nausea and vomiting. More recently, it has also been shown to be of value in children with gastroenteritis severe enough to merit hospital referral.

Pharmacology

Ondansetron became available in 1990, having been found to be a potent blocker of the neuro-hormone 5-hydroxytryptamine ($5HT_3$) receptors in the gut and central nervous system. Initially, it was only used (together with dexamethasone) to control the nausea and vomiting caused by vagal stimulation when $5HT_3$ is released from intestinal enterochromaffin cells during chemotherapy and radiotherapy. Studies found it to be more effective than metoclopramide (q.v.), and it is now also widely used to pre-empt post-operative vomiting.

More recently, ondansetron has been shown to be of value in the management of the severe vomiting that occasionally accompanies acute gastroenteritis in young children (and the only drug for which there is objective evidence of efficacy). Only about 60% of the drug reaches the circulation when the drug is given by mouth because of first-pass uptake by the liver. The drug is then widely distributed in the body (V_D ~2 kg/l) before being metabolised in a range of different ways in the liver, and because of this, some have argued that a loading dose should probably be considered before starting chemotherapy. Repeat treatment should also be curtailed in patients with severe liver failure. The terminal half-life is about 3 hours. Studies suggest that the clearance is reduced in younger infants (~75% in neonates and ~50% at 3 months). For this reason, it is recommended that patients younger than 4 months receiving ondansetron be closely monitored. A serious overdose can cause seizures and make respiratory support necessary, but recovery occurred within 24 hours in the only case reported to date.

Use in pregnancy

Ondansetron (10 mg every 6 hours) has occasionally been given during pregnancy to control severe nausea and vomiting (hyperemesis gravidarum). One study indicates there is limited evidence to suggest that the risk of cleft palate is increased. Lesser degrees of nausea are most commonly controlled by meclozine which is available without prescription. Nothing is known about the use of ondansetron during lactation, and the drug's small molecular size makes some transfer likely.

Use in infancy

Pre-anaesthetic prophylaxis: Give a single preoperative 100 micrograms/kg oral or slow intravenous (IV) dose.

Severe gastroenteritis: A single 200–300 micrograms/kg oral or slow IV dose is usually used.

During emetogenic chemotherapy: Give 150 micrograms/kg shortly before treatment and two further doses 4 and 8 hours later. Consider giving dexamethasone as well.

Drug interactions

Prolongation of the QT interval has been reported in patients receiving ondansetron; caution should be exercised if there is a history of prolonged QT syndrome or concomitant use of antiarrhythmic drugs known to affect the QT interval. Phenytoin, carbamazepine and rifampicin increase the hepatic metabolism (and thus the clearance) of ondansetron.

Supply and administration

2 ml ampoules containing 4 mg of ondansetron cost £1. Take 2 ml and dilute to 20 ml with glucose or glucose saline to obtain a solution containing 200 micrograms/ml. Rapidly dissolving 4 mg tablets (Zofran Melts®) cost £3.60 each. A pack which, when reconstituted, provides 50 ml of a sugar-free, strawberry-flavoured syrup containing 0.8 mg/ml of ondansetron costs £36. The Zofran® syrup contains sodium benzoate.

References

(See also the relevant Cochrane reviews)

Anderka M, Mitchell AA, Louik C, *et al*. Medications used to treat nausea and vomiting of pregnancy and the risk of selected birth defects. *Birth Defects Res A Clin Mol Teratol* 2012;**94**:22–30.

Bolton CM, Myles PS, Carlin JB, *et al*. Randomized double-blind study comparing the efficacy of moderate-dose metoclopramide and ondansetron for the prophylactic control of postoperative vomiting in children after tonsillectomy. *Br J Anaesth* 2007;**99**:699–703. [RCT]

Continued on p. 372

Culy CR, Bhana N, Plosker GL. Ondansetron: a review of its use as an antiemetic in children *Paediatr Drugs* 2001;**3**:471–9. [SR]

DeCamp LR, Byerley JS, Doshi N, *et al*. Use of antiemetic agents in acute gastroenteritis. A systematic review and meta-analysis. *Arch Pediatr Adolesc Med* 2008;**162**:858–65. [SR] (See also pp. 866–9.)

Einarson A, Maltepe C, Navioz Y, *et al*. The safety of ondansetron for nausea and vomiting of pregnancy: a prospective comparative study. *BJOG* 2004;**111**:940–3.

Freedman SB, Powell EC, Nava-Ocampo AA, *et al*. Ondansetron dosing in pediatric gastroenteritis: a prospective cohort, dose-response study. *Paediatr Drugs* 2010;**12**:405–10.

Mondick JT, Johnson BM, Haberer LJ, *et al*. Population pharmacokinetics of intravenous ondansetron in oncology and surgical patients aged 1–48 months. *Eur J Clin Pharmacol* 2010;**66**:77–86.

Pasternak B, Svanström H, Hviid A. Ondansetron in pregnancy and risk of adverse fetal outcomes. *N Engl J Med* 2013;**368**:814–23.

Sullivan CA, Johnson CA, Roach H, *et al*. A pilot study of intravenous ondansetron for hyperemesis gravidarum. *Am J Obster Gynecol* 1996;**174**:156–58. [RCT]

Szajewska H, Gieruszczak-Bialek D, Dyag M. Meta-analysis: ondansetron for vomiting in acute gastroenteritis in children. *Aliment Pharmacol Ther* 2007;**25**:393–400. [SR]

Use

Giving a solution of salts in glucose by mouth, or down a nasogastric tube, is both the simplest and the best way to rehydrate a child suffering from diarrhoea. Limited initial intravenous (IV) correction is only needed in the few children who present with particularly severe dehydration (>9% acute loss of weight). In all other situations, it is inappropriately invasive, complex and expensive. Ondansetron (q.v.) can help with vomiting.

Recognising dehydration

Dehydration due to diarrhoea currently kills several thousand young children in the world every day and may account for a third of all death in the first year of life. Dehydration has to be recognised clinically – laboratory tests are of no real help. Minor dehydration (<3% loss of body weight) is self-correcting, but loss greater than this calls for corrective action. These children seem irritable, restless and thirsty; their eyes and the anterior fontanelle are slightly sunken; the skin and mucous membranes seem dry; and the extremities are cool. However, the three most reliable signs of significant dehydration (≥5% weight loss) are a raised respiratory rate, delayed (≥2 seconds) capillary refill time and increased skin turgor (delayed recoil when a fold of skin is picked up between thumb and finger). Children who have become lethargic, are reluctant or unable to drink and have weak pulses or an abnormal heart rate have probably suffered a >10% loss.

Pathophysiology

The management of gastroenteritis has four elements: the correction of any dehydration that has already occurred; the replacement of ongoing fluid and electrolyte loss; the continued provision of basic nutrition; and, more selectively, the provision of oral zinc and, where indicated, antimicrobial therapy. Parents can easily come to believe that treatment 'is not working' if the diarrhoea does not stop promptly – they need to be reassured that almost all infectious gastrointestinal illness is self-limiting and that the two key aims of care are first to replace lost water and salts and then to keep the child fed until the illness resolves. Diarrhoea is usually viral, but bloody stools (dysentery) may point to bacterial infection meriting antibiotic treatment once the organism is identified.

Research into the management of cholera in the 1960s showed how oral rehydration could be achieved by harnessing the coupled transport of sodium and glucose molecules across the intestinal brush border. The World Health Organization (WHO) have been extolling the merits of a simple oral rehydration solution (ORS) containing equimolar amounts of sodium and glucose for more than 30 years, and the superiority of this approach is now admitted even in countries addicted to 'high-tech' medicine, although this has not prevented a decline in ORS use in favour of more expensive drugs that caregivers believed to be more effective.

Treatment

Severe dehydration: Babies who have suffered more than a 9% loss of weight need urgent revival with 20–30 ml/kg of 0.9% sodium chloride or, where this is available, compound sodium lactate (Hartmann's) solution given over an hour IV, followed by a further 70 ml/kg of the same solution over the next 5 hours. Hartmann's solution is to be preferred because it provides potassium and also lactate which, metabolised to bicarbonate, corrects acidosis. Nasogastric administration may work if IV access cannot be achieved, but ileus can sometimes make intraosseous (or even intraperitoneal) administration the only remaining option.

Less severe dehydration: Rehydrate with 75 ml/kg of ORS over 4 hours. Then resume breastfeeding or the child's normal diet. Give a further 50–100 ml of ORS for each further episode of diarrhoea or vomiting. Lactose usually remains well tolerated. Avoid carbonated (fizzy) drinks and carbohydrate-enriched juices.

Oral zinc: Adding 40 mg/l of elemental zinc (as gluconate) to ORS speeds recovery in some communities.

Supply

WHO formulation: The WHO has, since 2004, recommended a powder containing 2.6 g of sodium chloride, 1.5 g of potassium chloride, 2.9 g of sodium citrate and 13.5 g of anhydrous glucose which, when added to enough water to give 1 l of fluid, provides a solution containing 75 mmol of sodium, 20 mmol of potassium, 65 mmol of chloride, 10 mmol of citrate and 75 mmol of glucose per litre.

Continued on p. 374

UK formulations: Most commercial UK products differ slightly from the WHO solution, in that they deliver marginally less sodium (usually 50–60 mmol/l rather than 75 mmol/l). Fruit-flavoured powders suitable for children less than a year old include Dioralyte® Relief and Electrolade®. All come in sachets designed for reconstitution just before use with 200 ml of cool, freshly boiled water. Such sachets typically cost 20–30p each. Any of the solution not used promptly can be kept for 24 hours, if it is stored in a fridge.

References
(See also the relevant Cochrane reviews)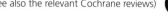

Bahl R, Bhandari N, Saksena M, *et al.* Efficacy of zinc-fortified oral rehydration solution in 6- to 35-month-old children with acute diarrhea. *J Pediatr* 2002;**141**:677–82. [RCT]

Blum LS, Oria PA, Olson CK, *et al.* Examining the use of oral rehydration salts and other oral rehydration therapy for childhood diarrhea in Kenya. *Am J Trop Med Hyg* 2011;**85**:1126–33.

Centres for Disease Control and Prevention. Managing acute gastroenteritis among children: oral rehydration, maintenance, and nutritional therapy. *MMWR* 2003;**52**(no.RR-16):1–16.

Fonseca BK, Holdgate A, Craig JC. Enteral vs intravenous rehydration therapy for children with gastroenteritis: a meta-analysis of randomized controlled trials. *Arch Pediatr Adolesc Med* 2004;**158**:483–90. [SR]

Spanorfer PR, Alessandrini EA, Joffe MD, *et al.* Oral versus intravenous rehydration of moderately dehydrated children: a randomised, controlled trial. *Pediatrics* 2005;**115**: 295–301. [RCT]

Use

Oseltamivir is an oral antiviral prodrug approved for the treatment of acute, uncomplicated influenza in patients 2 weeks of age and older whose flu symptoms have lasted < 2 days. Vaccination with influenza immunisation (q.v.) remains the most effective way of preventing illness from influenza.

Pharmacology

Influenza causes considerable morbidity and mortality each year among children during the seasonal outbreak. Influenza-associated hospitalisations are substantially higher among younger children, especially those aged <2 years, and highest in infants <6 months of age. Oseltamivir is a prodrug for the neuraminidase inhibitor oseltamivir carboxylate, which acts by inhibiting the release of newly formed virions from infected cells and by blocking viral entry into uninfected host cells. Oseltamivir may be used during pandemics to prevent infection in those patients who are not effectively protected by influenza vaccine or to treat those patients who are 'at risk' from the infection if treatment is started within 48 hours of the onset of symptoms.

Oseltamivir is metabolised to the active drug by human carboxylesterase 1 (HCE1), which is expressed predominantly in the liver. The expression of HCE1 increases rapidly during infancy and, as such, neonates may produce smaller amounts of the active metabolite. Oseltamivir is extensively distributed throughout the body, with good penetration into the saliva, nasal mucosa, lung and middle ear. Both oseltamivir and its active metabolite are excreted in the urine. As both the metabolism of oseltamivir and the excretion of the prodrug and active metabolite vary with age, there are considerable differences in the half-life of the active drug oseltamivir carboxylate; this is ~8 hours in older children and adults but is ~15 hours in children <2 years. This is due to the phenomenon known as 'flip-flop kinetics', whereby the metabolite formation rate is slower than its elimination rate, meaning the rate of disappearance from the body is governed by the rate of formation.

Although safety data are limited, oseltamivir can be used during pregnancy and lactation when the potential benefit outweighs the risk (e.g. during a pandemic). Oseltamivir does not appear to cross the placenta. Rodent teratogenicity studies are reassuring. Experience during the 2009/2010 H1N1 epidemic suggests that there is no increased risk of adverse events or outcomes in exposed fetuses. Oseltamivir and its active metabolite, oseltamivir carboxylate, pass into breast milk in clinically insignificant amounts.

Side effects

Gastrointestinal side effects (nausea, vomiting, diarrhoea, stomach pain and cramps) affected ~40% of children in one study of prophylactic use.

Treatment

Age group	Preterm (<37 weeks PMA)	Term neonate	Infant 1–3 months	Infant 3–12 months
Prevention of influenza: Give the drug orally once daily for 10 days post-exposure	1 mg/kg	2 mg/kg	2.5 mg/kg	3 mg/kg
Prevention of influenza: Treatment should be started within 48 hours of the onset of symptoms. Give the drug orally twice a day for 5 days	1 mg/kg	2 mg/kg	2.5 mg/kg	3 mg/kg

Supply

Oseltamivir comes in 30, 45 and 75 mg capsules (costing 77p to £1.50) and 65 ml bottles suitable for reconstitution with water to give a 12 mg/ml sugar-free, 'tutti-frutti'-flavoured suspension (costing £10).

Continued on p. 376

References

(See also the relevant Cochrane reviews)

Acosta EP, Jester P, Gal P, *et al.* Oseltamivir dosing for influenza infection in premature neonates. *J Infect Dis* 2010;**202**:563–6.

American Academy of Pediatrics Committee on Infectious Diseases. Recommendations for Prevention and Control of Influenza in Children, 2013–2014. *Pediatrics* 2013;**132**:e1089–104.

Donner B, Niranjan V, Hoffmann G. Safety of oseltamivir in pregnancy: a review of preclinical and clinical data. *Drug Saf* 2010;**33**:631–42.

Kimberlin DW, Acosta EP, Prichard MN, *et al.* Oseltamivir pharmacokinetics, dosing, and resistance among children aged <2 years with influenza. *J Infect Dis* 2013;**207**:709–20.

Maltezou HC, Drakoulis N, Siahanidou T, *et al.* Safety and pharmacokinetics of oseltamivir for prophylaxis of neonates exposed to influenza H1N1. *Pediatr Infect Dis J* 2012;**31**:527–9.

McPherson C, Warner B, Hunstad DA, *et al.* Oseltamivir dosing in premature infants. *J Infect Dis* 2012;**206**:847–50.

Shinjoh M, Takano Y, Takahashi T, *et al.* Postexposure prophylaxis for influenza in pediatric wards oseltamivir or zanamivir after rapid antigen detection. *Pediatr Infect Dis J* 2012;**31**:1119–23.

Standing JF, Nika A, Tsagris V, *et al.* Oseltamivir pharmacokinetics and clinical experience in neonates and infants during an outbreak of H1N1 influenza A virus infection in a neonatal intensive care unit. *Antimicrob Agents Chemother* 2012;**56**:3833–40.

Xie HY, Yasseen AS 3rd, Xie RH, *et al.* Infant outcomes among pregnant women who used oseltamivir for treatment of influenza during the H1N1 epidemic. *Am J Obstet Gynecol* 2013;**208**:293.e1–7.

Use

Several low molecular weight heparins (LMWHs) are now available. These are derivatives of heparin (q.v.) but have a longer duration of action and are given subcutaneously rather than intravenously. Heparinoids are glycosaminoglycans derived from heparin, but which differ from LMWHs as they contain no heparin fragments and can be used in patients that are allergic to heparin or who develop heparin-induced thrombocytopenia (HIT). Direct thrombin inhibitors (DTIs) are a new class of anticoagulants that may be used in HIT and a small number of other licensed indications in adults. Fondaparinux is a synthetic, antithrombin-dependent inhibitor of factor Xa with several potential advantages over LMWH including a longer half-life, a lower risk for HIT and no effect on bone.

Pharmacology

Low molecular weight heparins: A range of LMWHs are now available, including certoparin, dalteparin sodium (q.v.), enoxaparin (q.v.), reviparin sodium and tinzaparin sodium. All have very similar properties, although the recommended dose of the various products is not always identical. LMWHs have a longer half-life, have a more predictable pharmacodynamic (anticoagulant) effect and cause less osteoporosis and thrombocytopenia than heparin. They have a more profound effect on factor Xa than on thrombin.

The effective dose varies widely and needs to be individually titrated. They are currently the anticoagulant of choice during pregnancy and are used both prophylactically and as treatment for thromboembolism. There is no evidence of teratogenicity, and placenta transfer does not occur. Lactation during treatment is also safe, although if there is need for long-term anticoagulation warfarin may now be used. The molecular weight of the LMWHs makes significant transfer into breast milk very unlikely, and any drug entering the milk would be inactivated in the gut before absorption.

The best studied LMWH in children is enoxaparin; however, there are data for reviparin, dalteparin and tinzaparin use. Neonates generally need a higher dose (as with heparin). Administration by subcutaneous (SC) rather than intravenous injection makes treatment much easier but also makes an overdose less easily treatable.

Heparinoids: Danaparoid sodium is currently the only widely available heparinoid. It is a mixture of porcine-derived glycosaminoglycans (heparan sulphate, dermatan sulphate and chondroitin sulphate). Danaparoid acts primarily by catalysing the inhibition of factor Xa in an antithrombin-dependent fashion. Use is reserved for patients who are allergic to heparin or who have developed thrombocytopenia while taking LMWH. It has a long half-life (~25 hours) which is potentially disadvantageous if patients require urgent surgery or invasive procedures. It also is problematic during serious bleeding because there is no antidote. Elimination via the kidneys means the dose should be reduced in patients with renal function impairment. Although the manufacturers have not endorsed use during pregnancy or lactation, limited experience with danaparoid during pregnancy has, however, largely been safe. It does not appear to cross the placenta and enters breast milk in only small amounts that are likely to be inactivated in the baby's intestine.

Use in childhood has not been endorsed by the manufacturer; however, danaparoid is the most often reported anticoagulant used in paediatric patients (including neonates) with HIT. Treatment is titrated against anti-factor Xa levels (aiming for 0.4–0.8 IU/ml). Occasional cross-reactivity between the drug and a patient's HIT antibodies can occur and should be suspected if there is a new thrombosis and persistent thrombocytopenia during treatment.

Direct thrombin inhibitors: DTIs bind directly to thrombin and block its interaction with its substrates. Hirudins are bivalent DTIs (blocking both the active site of thrombin and exosite 1) and are derived from the 65-amino-acid polypeptide originally isolated from the salivary glands of the medicinal leech *Hirudo medicinalis*. The recombinant hirudins, lepirudin and desirudin, differ very slightly in the amino-terminal composition, but all are antigenic and antibodies are reported in 40–74% of patients. Bivalirudin is a 20-amino-acid synthetic polypeptide analogue of hirudin. Argatroban, dabigatran and melagatran (and its oral precursor, ximelagatran) are univalent DTIs binding only to the active site of thrombin.

There are few reports of use of DTIs during pregnancy or lactation. Three case reports of argatroban (only one where treatment was started during the first trimester) reported successful outcomes. Reports of use of hirudins during pregnancy are equally rare. There are several case reports and series describing children treated with these agents (including prospective studies

Continued on p. 378

evaluating bivalirudin and argatroban) in infants and children, but overall experience with this group of drugs is extremely limited.

Fondaparinux: Experience with this drug in pregnancy and in infants is very limited. A number of case reports and cohort studies suggest use in pregnancy is generally safe and not associated with teratogenicity or adverse fetal outcomes even though small amounts probably do cross the placenta.

Maternal thromboembolism

Prophylaxis: High-risk obstetric patients with thrombophilia, immobility, obesity, pre-eclampsia or a past history of deep vein thrombosis should be assessed for their risk factors and considered for prophylactic LMWH. Doses for dalteparin and enoxaparin are given in their respective monographs. Tinzaparin is given at a dose of 75 units/kg/day, but a simplified dosing scheme for tinzaparin use in pregnant women is given in the table. Doses of 7000 units or higher may be given as two smaller doses, but otherwise, once-daily dosing is appropriate. As with other LMWHs, experience indicates that monitoring of anti-Xa levels is not required during thromboprophylaxis. Stop 24 hours prior to any planned operative (or epidural) delivery until 4 hours after the procedure is over. Women receiving antenatal LMWH should be advised that if they have any vaginal bleeding or once labour begins, they should not inject any further LMWH. There is no need to monitor platelets routinely unless there has been exposure to unfractionated heparin.

Weight (kg) at booking	Total daily dose of tinzaparin
<50	3500 units
50–90	4500 units
91–130	7000 units
131–170	9000 units
>170	75 units/kg

Danaparoid has been used in pregnancy at the standard dose of 750 units given subcutaneously twice daily. Fondaparinux has been used at a dose of 2.5 mg given subcutaneously once a day. There are insufficient data and experience with the various DTIs; if these are used, then use should be in conjunction with a consultant haematologist with appropriate expertise.

Treatment: Doses for dalteparin and enoxaparin are given in their respective monographs. Tinzaparin is given at a dose of 175 units/kg once daily. Routine measurement of peak anti-Xa activity is not usually indicated unless the woman weighs less than 50 kg or more than 90 kg. As with prophylaxis, LMWH should be stopped at the onset of labour or 24 hours before any planned operative delivery or an epidural. Pregnant women who develop HIT or have heparin allergy and require continuing anticoagulant therapy should be managed with danaparoid or fondaparinux under the care of a consultant haematologist with appropriate expertise.

Neonatal treatment

Prophylaxis: Doses for dalteparin and enoxaparin are given in their respective monographs. Tinzaparin is best avoided in neonates due to the presence of benzyl alcohol in the vials. Older infants should receive 50 units/kg of tinzaparin by once-daily SC injection. The other anticoagulants in this monograph have not been used for prophylaxis in children.

Treatment: Doses for dalteparin and enoxaparin are given in their respective monographs. Tinzaparin is best avoided in neonates. Infants of 1–2 months should receive 275 units/kg of tinzaparin once daily (decreasing to 250 units/kg after the age of 2 months) by once-daily SC injection. Bivalirudin has been given either as boluses or as a continuous infusion of 0.125 mg/kg/hour adjusted according to the PTT (aiming for 1.5–2.5 times the baseline). The suggested starting dose for argatroban is 0.1 mg/kg/minute by SC infusion adjusting the dose according to the PTT. Fondaparinux dosing has not been evaluated in children aged <1 year, but a suggested starting dose has been 0.1 mg/kg once daily by SC injection aiming for an anti-Xa level of 0.5–1 mg/l. Treatment of patients requiring bivalirudin, danaparoid, argatroban or fondaparinux should be supervised by a consultant haematologist with appropriate expertise.

Continued on p. 379

Supply and administration

Tinzaparin: Available in 0.5, 0.7 and 0.9 ml pre-filled syringes containing 20,000 units/ml (these between £8.50 and £15.30). A 2 ml (40,000 unit) vial, containing benzyl alcohol, costs £34.20.

Danaparoid: 0.6 ml ampoules containing 750 units (1250 units/ml) cost £26.67.

Bivalirudin: A vial containing 250 mg powder for reconstitution costs £310.00. This should be reconstituted by adding 5 ml water for injection until completely dissolved and the solution is clear. The reconstituted solution should be further diluted to a total volume of 50 ml using 5% glucose or 0.9% sodium chloride to give a final concentration of 5 mg/ml.

Argatroban: 2.5 ml (250 mg) vials of argatroban concentrate for IV infusion cost £249. The concentrate is diluted to a solution of 1 mg/ml by further diluting to a volume of 250 ml using 0.9% sodium chloride or 5% glucose.

Fondaparinux: A range sizes of pre-filled syringes containing either 5 or 12.5 mg/ml fondaparinux sodium are available (cost £6.30 to £11.30).

References   (See also the UK guideline on thromboprophylaxis in pregnancy **DHUK**)

Deitcher SR, Topoulos AP, Bartholomew JR, *et al*. Lepirudin anticoagulation for heparin-induced thrombocytopenia. *J Pediatr* 2002;**140**:264–6.

Lindhoff-Last E, Bauersachs R. Heparin-induced thrombocytopenia-alternative anticoagulation in pregnancy and lactation. *Semin Thromb Hemost* 2002;**28**:439–46.

Magnani HN. An analysis of clinical outcomes of 91 pregnancies in 83 women treated with danaparoid (Orgaran). *Thromb Res* 2010;**125**:297–302.

Nagler M, Haslauer M, Wuillemin WA. Fondaparinux – data on efficacy and safety in special situations. *Thromb Res* 2012;**129**:407–17.

Paidas MJ, Ku D-H W, Arkel YS. Screening and management of inherited thrombophilias in the setting of adverse pregnancy outcome. *Clin Perinatol* 2004;**31**:783–805.

Woo YL, Allard S, Cohen H, *et al*. Danaparoid thromboprophylaxis in pregnant women with heparin-induced thrombocytopenia. *BJOG* 2002;**109**:466–8.

Young G, Tarantino MD, Wohrley J, *et al*. Pilot dose-finding and safety study of bivalirudin in infants <6 months of age with thrombosis. *J Thromb Haemost* 2007;**5**:1654–9.

Young SK, Al-Mondhiry HA, Vaida SJ, *et al*. Successful use of argatroban during the third trimester of pregnancy: case report and review of the literature. *Pharmacotherapy* 2008;**28**:1531–6.

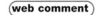

Use

Supplemental oxygen is used to correct hypoxia in babies with pulmonary problems, especially where these are causing a mismatch between the ventilation and the perfusion of the lung.

Pathophysiology

Oxygen deserves its place in any pharmacopoeia because, like any other drug, oxygen can do a lot of harm as well as a lot of good. It needs to be used with care; all use should be documented, and the 'dose' recorded. While lack of oxygen can be damaging, the body can manage with blood that is only about 50–60% saturated as long as the *quantity* of oxygen delivered to the tissues is adequate. Were this not true, the fetus would be in substantial trouble before birth, as would the brain of the baby with cyanotic heart disease. Cardiac output and tissue perfusion matter more than blood pressure, and anaemia can undermine oxygen delivery as much as overt cyanosis. While tissue hypoxia can be damaging, it is the combined effect of CO_2 accumulation and oxygen lack (asphyxia) that is most damaging, causing a respiratory (carbonic acid) as well as a metabolic (lactic acid) acidosis.

Too much oxygen can also be damaging. Prolonged exposure to more than ~60% oxygen can damage the pulmonary epithelium, and hyperbaric oxygen can cause convulsions. Excess oxygen has long been known to be a risk factor for retinopathy of prematurity (ROP). The new understanding of the significance of oxidative stress that emerged towards the ends of the twentieth century contributed to an increased focus on oxygenation in newborn babies both in and beyond the delivery room. The International Liaison Committee on Resuscitation (ILCOR) 2010 guidelines for newborn resuscitation recommended starting a term or near-term newborn needing ventilation on air rather than 100% oxygen. Despite this, we still do not know precisely what constitutes 'excess' oxygen.

Administration

Oxygen may be given into an incubator, especially in small babies, but cot nursing using a nasal cannula is a valuable (and economic) alternative that simplifies parental involvement. Some form of humidification is, however, called for if the baby is getting much oxygen this way. Devices delivering a high flow of warm humidified gas for cannula use are becoming increasingly popular, but there is concern that, at flows of more than 2 l/min, the main benefit derived from their use is caused by the fact that they deliver an unmeasured, uncontrolled and potentially dangerously high form of continuous positive airway pressure (CPAP). A humidified head box is the only satisfactory way of providing more than 50% oxygen to a baby requiring incubator care.

Measurement in air

The amount of oxygen each baby is breathing (as a percentage) should be recorded regularly, and those given oxygen via a nasal catheter should have the ambient concentration needed to provide an equivalent arterial saturation documented periodically, because the relationship between catheter flow and the inspired concentration varies. Equipment should be calibrated regularly against room air (20.9% oxygen) and/or 100% oxygen.

Measuring blood levels

What constitutes a safe range for arterial oxygen pressure is not known. It is said that there must be 50 g/l of desaturated haemoglobin for cyanosis to be visible. Cyanosis is certainly difficult to detect by eye until 25% of the blood is desaturated, and in the neonate, this often only occurs when the arterial partial pressure (PaO_2) is <35 mmHg (or 4.7 kPa). Arterial catheters can reduce the pain and trauma caused by repeated capillary sampling, but there is no evidence that use improves long-term outcome. Transcutaneous pressure and saturation monitors are valuable but not free from error.

A cohort study in 1992 showed an association between the prevalence of acute retinopathy and exposure to transcutaneous oxygen ($TcPO_2$) levels of more than 80 mmHg (~10.7 kPa), and as a result, many units started to aim for $TcPO_2$ levels of 6–10 kPa and to withdraw supplemental oxygen from preterm babies with a $TcPO_2$ level higher than this. Pulse oximetry is widely used to replace monitoring of $TcPO_2$ even though the relationship between PaO_2 and arterial saturation is quite variable in babies (Figure 1a) because of the differing effects of varying shunt and changes in ventilation/perfusion ratio on the curve relating FiO_2 to SaO_2. A more detailed discussion with a link to an interactive algorithm for determining shunt and V_A/Q can be found

Continued on p. 381

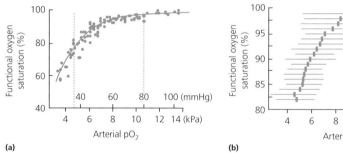
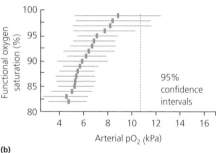

(a)   (b)

Figure 1 The relationship between partial pressure of arterial oxygen and functional oxygen saturation (a) and how this translates to readings on the saturation monitor (b).

in the website commentary. To be certain of keeping TcPO$_2$ (and *PaO$_2$*) below 80 mmHg, the *functional* saturation in babies has to be kept from exceeding 95% (Figure 1b) – equivalent to a *fractional* saturation of 93%. Even this may leave preterm babies at a small risk of 'hyperoxia' as oximeter manufacturers only claim an accuracy of ±3%. Five trials are currently trying to identify what range of saturation optimises long-term outcome.

The Neonatal Oxygen Prospective Meta-analysis (NeOProM) Collaboration is a group of five large masked RCTs of different oxygen saturation targets in extremely preterm infants, and results of outcomes at 18–24 months are expected from meta-analysis of longer-term outcome data from all trials in 2014. Analysis of results to the time of discharge in individual trials (and pooled data from some of the trials) suggests that targeting saturations of 91–95% was associated with a lower mortality rate but at the cost of more infants with severe ROP.

Supply

Piped hospital supplies result in our taking the provision of oxygen for granted: the same is not true in many developing countries. Arrangements for providing oxygen for home use in the United Kingdom have recently undergone a major, and initially unsettling, change. The supply of an oxygen concentrator and of lightweight cylinders by one of four commercial companies must now be authorised by a designated official in each hospital.

Humidification

Piped supplies and cylinders are devoid of water vapour, and humidification is essential to avoid excessive drying of the respiratory tract when giving >40% oxygen. A range of commercial equipment (such as the Vapotherm®) has now become available for delivering a flow of warm well-humidified gas with variable oxygen content. Bubbling gas through water at room temperature however adds 20 g of water to each cubic metre of gas (equivalent to 50% saturation at body temperature), and this is generally adequate unless flow is high or the nose's humidification system has been partially bypassed. For babies breathing high concentrations of head-box oxygen in an incubator, reasonable humidification can be achieved without a heated humidifier by bubbling oxygen through a small bottle situated *inside* the incubator.

References   (See also the relevant Cochrane reviews and the UK guideline on managing ROP **DHUK**)

Balfour-Lynn IM, Primahak RA, Shaw BNJ. Home oxygen for children: who, how and when? *Thorax* 2005;**60**:76–81. (See also the related British Thoracic Society guideline on home oxygen use [and its paediatric supplement]: www.brit-thoracic.org.uk)

Early Treatment for Retinopathy of Prematurity [ET-ROP] Cooperative Group. Revised indications for the treatment of retinopathy of prematurity. *Arch Ophthalmol* 2003;**121**:1684–96. [RCT] (See also pp. 1697–1701 and pp. 1769–71.)

Finer NN. Nasal cannula use in the preterm infant: oxygen or pressure? *Pediatrics* 2005;**116**:1216–7.

Gerstmann D, Berg R, Haskell R, *et al*. Operational evaluation of pulse oximetry in NICU patients with arterial access. *J Perinatol* 2003;**23**:378–83.

Harrison GT, Shaw B. Prescribing home oxygen. *Arch Dis Child Fetal Neonatal Ed* 2007;**92**:F241–3.

Manley BJ, Owen LS, Doyle LW, *et al*. High-flow nasal cannulae in very preterm infants after extubation. *N Engl J Med* 2013;**369**:1425–33.

Continued on p. 382

Quine D, Stenson BJ. Arterial oxygen tension (PaO^2) values in infants <29 weeks of gestation at currently targeted saturations. *Arch Dis Child Fetal Neonatal Ed* 2009;**94**:F51–3.

Rowe L, Jones JG, Quine D, *et al.* A simplified method for deriving shunt and reduced V$_A$/Q in infants. *Arch Dis Child Fetal Neonatal Ed* 2010;**95**:F47–52.

Saugstad OD, Ramji S, Soll RE, *et al.* Resuscitation of newborn infants with 21% or 100% oxygen: an updated systematic review and meta-analysis. *Neonatology* 2008;**94**:176–82. [SR]

Schmidt B, Whyte RK, Asztalos EV, *et al.* Effects of targeting higher vs lower arterial oxygen saturations on death or disability in extremely preterm infants: a randomized clinical trial. *JAMA* 2013;**309**:2111–20. [RCT]

Stenson B, Brocklehurst P, Tarnow-Mordi W. Increased 36-week survival with high oxygen saturation target in extremely preterm infants. UK BOOST II trial; Australian BOOST II trial; New Zealand BOOST II trial. *N Engl J Med* 2011;**364**:1680–2. [RCT]

SUPPORT Study Group of the Eunice Kennedy Shriver NICHD Neonatal Research Network, *et al.* Target ranges of oxygen saturation in extremely preterm infants. *N Engl J Med* 2010;**362**:1959–69. [RCT]

Use

Oxytocin is used (and occasionally misused) in induction or augmentation of labour and to reduce post-partum haemorrhage.

Pharmacology

Oxytocin is a synthetic nonapeptide identical to the naturally occurring hypothalamic hormone. Crude pituitary extracts were first used clinically in 1909 and became commercially available in 1928. The hormone's structure was confirmed in 1953. Oxytocin has for a long time been used to initiate and augment labour (given by continuous intravenous (IV) infusion because uptake is erratic from mucous membranes and the half-life is only 3–4 minutes), but prostaglandin induction (q.v.) is now the preferred option unless the membranes have already ruptured.

A sudden bolus can cause vasodilatation and tachycardia, and secondary hypotension can be dangerous in patients with underlying heart disease. Uterine hyperstimulation can also cause fetal hypoxia, but this can be reversed by stopping the infusion and/or giving a β-mimetic drug. There is some risk of uterine rupture, especially in patients with a uterine scar, even in the absence of cephalopelvic disproportion. Doses greater than 15 mU/minute have an antidiuretic effect, and the risk of symptomatic fetal and maternal hyponatraemia is compounded if the mother ingests excessive fluid in labour. It helps if IV oxytocin is always given through a separate line using a motor-driven syringe pump, but oral intake is also sometimes excessive. Recent studies have not supported earlier claims that oxytocin nasal spray can augment lactation.

While use in mothers delivering under epidural anaesthesia can speed up the second stage of labour, there is no controlled trial evidence that use (with or without early amniotomy) to 'augment' spontaneous labour is of any significant clinical benefit. On the other hand, such augmentation can certainly cause increased pain, and there is a significant risk of uterine hyperstimulation.

A 10 unit dose given when the anterior shoulder is delivered reduces the risk of post-partum haemorrhage and is commonly given IM (although it is only licensed for IV use), while a continuous infusion can be used if bleeding continues after the placenta is delivered. A combined IM injection of oxytocin and ergometrine maleate (Syntometrine®) is marginally more effective in reducing blood loss but causes a transient rise in blood pressure and can cause nausea and vomiting. A 100 micrograms IV dose of carbetocin (a longer-acting synthetic analogue of oxytocin) seems to be equally effective and cause less nausea. Misoprostol (q.v.) is an extremely effective way of containing excessive post-delivery blood when it does occur, especially in a setting where it is difficult to keep supplies of oxytocin refrigerated. Inadvertent administration of Syntometrine to a baby (in mistake for an injection of vitamin K) is known to cause respiratory depression, seizures and severe hyponatraemia, but survivors, luckily, seem to make a complete recovery.

Units used when prescribing oxytocin

Oxytocin is such a potent drug that only a few nanograms are needed. Many staff feel insecure trying to use nanogram units, and for this reason, oxytocin remains (like insulin) one of the few drugs still widely prescribed using the old pharmaceutical unit of potency – the 'unit' – and, because of its small dose, is prescribed in milliunits per minute (often written as mU/minute) to avoid writing *start by giving 0.001 units/minute*.

Treatment

Inducing and augmenting labour: Start with 1 or 2 mU/minute and increase by 1 mU/minute every 30 minutes as necessary using a motor-driven syringe. If more than 4 mU/minute proves necessary, increase the dose by 2 mU/minute increments once every 30 minutes to a maximum of 20 mU/minute.

Post-partum use: Give 10 units of oxytocin (or 1 ml of Syntometrine) IM once the anterior shoulder of the baby is safely delivered. Continuous IV oxytocin will usually limit residual post-partum bleeding.

Supply and administration

Oxytocin comes in 5 or 10 unit (1 ml) ampoules (costing 80p and 90p, respectively). For accurate, continuous dose-adjusted IV administration, dilute 3 units of oxytocin to 50 ml with 0.9% sodium chloride (or Hartmann's solution). This gives a solution containing 60 mU/ml which, when infused at a rate of 1 ml/hour, gives the patient 1 mU/minute of oxytocin (1 unit = 2.2 micrograms

Continued on p. 384

of oxytocin). 1 ml ampoules of Syntometrine contain 5 units of oxytocin and 500 micrograms of ergometrine (cost £1.40). 100 micrograms ampoules of carbetocin (an eight-amino-acid-long oxytocin analogue) cost £17.60. Keep all these products in the dark at 4°C.

References   (See also the relevant Cochrane reviews and UK guideline on induction of labour 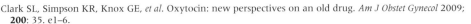)

Clark SL, Simpson KR, Knox GE, *et al*. Oxytocin: new perspectives on an old drug. *Am J Obstet Gynecol* 2009; **200**: 35. e1–6.

Dargaville PA, Campbell NT. Overdose of ergometrine in the newborn infant: acute symptomatology and long-term outcome. *J Paediatr Child Health* 1998; **34**: 83–9.

Fewtrell MS, Loh KL, Blake A, *et al*. Randomised, double blind trial of oxytocin nasal spray in mothers expressing breast milk for preterm infants. *Arch Dis Child Fetal Neonatal Ed* 2006; **91**: F169–74. [RCT]

Hinshaw K, Simpson S, Cummings S, *et al*. A randomised controlled trial of early versus delayed oxytocin augmentation to treat dysfunctional labour in nulliparous women. *Br J Obstet Gynaecol* 2008; **115**: 1289–96. [RCT]

Leung SW, Ng PS, Wong WY, *et al*. A randomised trial of carbetocin versus syntometrine in the management of the third stage of labour. *Br J Obstet Gynaecol* 2006; **113**: 1459–64. [RCT]

Moen V, Brudin L. Rundgren M, *et al*. Hyponatraemia complicating labour – rare or unrecognised? A prospective observational study. *BJOG* 2009; **116**: 552–61.

Su LL, Rauff M, Chan YH, *et al*. Carbetocin versus syntometrine for the third stage of labour following vaginal delivery – a double-blind randomised controlled trial. *BJOG* 2009; **116**: 1461–6. [RCT]

Use

Prophylactic use of palivizumab can reduce the risk of a baby requiring hospital admission with bronchiolitis as a result of respiratory syncytial virus (RSV) infection. Treatment is of no use in babies with established infection.

Respiratory syncytial virus infection

RSV is a negative-sense, single-stranded RNA virus of the family *Paramyxoviridae*, which causes infection in epidemic form every winter. Adults usually only get a mild cold, but babies can develop a respiratory infection severe enough to need hospital admission. A minority need ventilation. Coryza and/or apnoea may be the only symptoms in a preterm baby, but babies can become seriously ill, particularly if they have congenital heart disease or chronic lung disease.

Much can be done to reduce these risks by raising awareness of the extent to which hand washing and limiting 'social' family exposure can lessen cross infection. Barrier nursing and cohorting reduces the risk of infection spreading to other vulnerable inpatients. Most babies merely need brief help with fluid intake and a little oxygen, support that may not always require hospital admission. Nebulised adrenaline (q.v.) lowered the number needing hospital admission in one recent trial, and nebulised hypertonic saline given every 2–4 hours reduced length of stay in four small trials. Corticosteroids, ribavirin, salbutamol and montelukast are of no proven value.

Pharmacology

Palivizumab is a combined human and murine monoclonal antibody produced by recombinant DNA technology that inhibits RSV replication. It has a 20-day half-life. A monthly injection during the seasonal winter epidemic reduces the need for hospitalisation due to RSV infection in 'at-risk' babies. However, use does *not* reduce total health service costs, even when treatment is limited to babies who are still oxygen dependent because of chronic lung disease, unless readmission rates are atypically high. While there is agreement that palivizumab is clinically effective, whether it is cost-effective continues to be debated (see web commentary); the estimated cost is ~£6,000 for the recommended 5 monthly injections in the United Kingdom. Side effects, other than pain and swelling at the injection site, are rare. Use does not interfere with the administration of other vaccines.

Prophylaxis

Some ex-preterm babies who are, or were until recently, oxygen dependent due to chronic lung disease probably merit treatment. So may a few babies with haemodynamically significant congenital heart disease (see web commentary). It should also be considered in children under 2 years old with severe combined immunodeficiency syndrome. Give 15 mg/kg intramuscularly once a month from the start of the winter RSV epidemic. Use the outer thigh (employing two sites where the injection volume exceeds 1 ml).

Supply and administration

The 50 and 100 mg vials of palivizumab (costing £306 and £565) should be stored at 4 °C. Do not freeze. The small 50 mg vial actually contains more than 50 mg of palivizumab, but it is not possible to draw all the drug back out of the vial after reconstitution. This is why the manufacturers recommend that the powder should be dissolved by running 0.6 ml (50 mg vials) or 1 ml (100 mg vials) of water for injection slowly down the side of the vial. Rotate gently for 30 seconds without shaking and then leave it at room temperature for at least 20 minutes until the solution clarifies (it will remain opalescent). The resultant 100 mg/ml solution must be used within 6 hours. Cost can be reduced by using the larger vial and scheduling several babies for treatment on the same day.

References   (See also the Cochrane reviews of the management of bronchiolitis)

American Academy of Pediatrics, Committee on Infectious Diseases. Modified Recommendations for Use of Palivizumab for Prevention of Respiratory Syncytial Virus Infections. *Pediatrics* 2009;**124**:1694–1701.
American Academy of Pediatrics, Subcommittee on Diagnosis and Management of Bronchiolitis. Diagnosis and management of bronchiolitis. *Pediatrics* 2006;**118**:1774–93. (See also 2007;**120**:890–2 and pp. 893–4.)

Continued on p. 386

Gooding J, Millage A, Rye A-K, *et al.* The cost and safety of multidose use of palivizumab vials. *Clin Pediatr* 2008;**47**:160–3.

Isaacs D. Should respiratory care in preterm infants include prophylaxis against respiratory syncytial virus? The case against. *Paediatr Respir Rev* 2013;**14**:128–9.

Jefferson T, Foxlee R, Del Mar C, *et al.* Physical interventions to interrupt or reduce the spread of respiratory viruses: systematic review. *Br Med J* 2008;**336**:77–80. [SR] (See also pp. 55–6.)

King VJ, Viswanathan M, Bordley WC, *et al.* Pharmacologic treatment of bronchiolitis in infants and children. A systematic review. *Arch Pediatr Adolesc Med* 2004;**158**:127–37. [SR] (See also pp. 119–26.)

Kumal-Bahl S, Doshi J, Campbell J. Economic analysis of respiratory syncytial virus immunoprophylaxis in high-risk infants. *Arch Pediatr Adolesc Med* 2002;**156**:1034–41. [SR] (See also pp. 1180–1.)

Kuzik BA, Al Qadhi SA, Kent S, *et al.* Nebulized hypertonic saline in the treatment of viral bronchiolitis in infants. *J Pediatr* 2007;**151**:266–70. [RCT] (See also pp. 235–7.)

Resch B, Resch E, Müller W. Should respiratory care in preterm infants include prophylaxis against respiratory syncytial virus infection? The case in favour. *Paediatr Respir Rev* 2013;**14**:130–6.

Wang D, Bayliss S, Meads C. Palivizumab for immunoprophylaxis of respiratory syncytial virus (RSV) bronchiolitis in high-risk infants and young children: a systematic review and additional economic modelling of subgroup analyses. *Health Technol Assess* 2011;**15**(5).

Use

Pancreatin (pancreatic enzyme supplement) is given to aid digestion in patients with cystic fibrosis (CF).

Cystic fibrosis

CF is a relatively common (affecting ~1:2500 of children born in Europe and North America), recessively inherited genetic disorder associated with abnormal mucus production. It is caused by a primary defect of chloride ion secretion. Pancreatic damage causes malabsorption, while the production of viscid sputum renders patients vulnerable to recurrent bacterial infection. Thick meconium may cause intestinal obstruction (meconium ileus) at birth. Other complications include liver disease (due to biliary tract obstruction) and male infertility. The high chloride content of sweat is diagnostic, and a sample of sweat for laboratory analysis can be obtained by pilocarpine iontophoresis in most term babies more than a few weeks old. Most defective mutant genes are identifiable in the laboratory, and prenatal diagnosis is now possible.

Lung damage, including bronchiectasis, used to limit the number of patients reaching adult life, but survival has now improved significantly. Treatment should start as soon after birth as possible to minimise lung scarring, and management should be supervised from a specialist clinic. Since 2007, all babies born in the United Kingdom have been routinely offered screening for CF as part of the newborn bloodspot screening test.

Nutritional support plays an important part in improving survival. Lung transplantation has been offered to a few patients, but progressive liver disease remains an unsolved problem. Gene therapy offers hope for the future. Lower respiratory tract infection needs prompt and vigorous treatment. Only a few babies need pancreatic supplements at birth, but almost all need supplementation before they are 6 months old.

Pharmacology

Pancreatin is an extract prepared from porcine pancreatic tissue that is given by mouth to aid digestion in patients with CF and pancreatic insufficiency. It contains protease enzymes that break protein down into peptides and amino acids, lipases that hydrolyse fats to glycerol and fatty acids and amylases that convert starch into dextrins and sugars. It is available as a powder, in capsules containing powder, in capsules containing enteric-coated granules, as free granules and as a tablet. Pancreatin should be taken with food, or immediately before food, in order to speed transit into the small intestine, because the constituent enzymes are progressively inactivated by stomach acid. The extent to which the enteric-coated formulations actually improve intact passage into the duodenum is open to some doubt. Buccal soreness can occur if the powdered product is not swallowed promptly. Perianal soreness can be helped by a zinc oxide barrier ointment, but it may be a sign of excessive supplementation. High-dose enteric-coated formulations are best avoided, having occasionally caused colonic strictures in older children.

Treatment

Different formulations are available. The choice should be guided by the local specialist clinic. Creon® Micro granules and Pancrex V® 125 capsules are suitable for neonates. Check the baby's faecal elastase; if less than 500 micrograms elastase per gram of stool, then it is generally assumed there is pancreatic insufficiency. Enzymes (and fat-soluble vitamin supplements) should be prescribed once pancreatic insufficiency is confirmed or even while waiting for test results if pancreatic insufficiency is likely from the clinical history or genotype.

One scoop (100 mg) of Creon Micro granules are given, mixed with a small amount of breast milk or formula feed, before each feed. The powder from one Pancrex V '125' capsule is sprinkled into each feed. The dose is cautiously increased as necessary judging by the amount of undigested fat in the stool.

Supply

Each 100 mg of Creon Micro contains 200 protease units, 5000 lipase units and 3600 amylase units and costs 16p. Pancrex V '125' capsules contain a minimum of 160 protease units, 2950 lipase units and 3300 amylase units per capsule and cost 14p each. Store all products in a cool place.

Continued on p. 388

References

(See the relevant Cochrane reviews of CF care)

Balfour-Lynn IM. Newborn screening for cystic fibrosis: evidence for benefit. *Arch Dis Child* 2008;**93**:7–10.

Borowitz D, Robinson KA, Rosenfeld M, *et al.* Cystic Fibrosis Foundation evidence-based guidelines for management of infants with cystic fibrosis. *J Pediatr* 2009;**155**(suppl):S73–93.

Conway SP, Wolfe SP, Brownlee KG, *et al.* Vitamin K status among children with cystic fibrosis and its relationship to bone mineral density and bone turnover. *Pediatrics* 2005;**115**:1325–31.

Feranchak AP, Sontag MK, Wagener JS, *et al.* Prospective, long-term study of fat-soluble vitamin status in children with cystic fibrosis identified by newborn screen. *J Pediatr* 1999;**135**:601–10.

Littlewood JM, Wolfe SDP. Control of malabsorption in cystic fibrosis. *Paediatr Drugs* 2000;**2**:205–22.

Lu KD, Engmann C, Moya F, *et al.* Cystic fibrosis in premature infants. *J Perinatol* 2011;**31**:504–6.

Minasian C, McCullagh A, Bush A. Cystic fibrosis in neonates and infants. *Early Hum Devel* 2005;**81**:997–1004.

O'Sullivan BP, Baker D, Leung KG, *et al.* Evolution of pancreatic function during the first year in infants with cystic fibrosis. *J Pediatr* 2013;**162**:808–12.e1.

O'Sullivan BP, Freedman SD. Cystic fibrosis. *Lancet* 2009;**373**:1891–904.

Sims EJ, Mugford M, Clark A, *et al.* Economic implications of newborn screening for cystic fibrosis: a cost of illness retrospective cohort study. *Lancet* 2007;**369**:1187–95.

Use

Pancuronium causes sustained muscle paralysis. Ventilated babies should not be paralysed unless they are sedated, and most sedated babies do not need paralysis. Sustained paralysis is usually only offered to babies needing major respiratory support who continue to 'fight' the ventilator despite sedation.

Pharmacology

Pancuronium is a competitive non-depolarising muscle relaxant developed in 1966 as an analogue of curare (tubocurarine), the arrow-tip poison used by South American Indians. Pancuronium competes with acetylcholine for the neuromuscular receptor sites of the motor end plates of voluntary muscles. It is part metabolised by the liver and then excreted in the urine with a half-life that is variably prolonged in the neonatal period. Simultaneous treatment with magnesium sulfate or an aminoglycoside will further prolong the period of blockade. Pharmacokinetic information does not seem to have influenced the empirical dose regimens generally used in neonatal practice. Very little crosses the placenta, but doses of 100 micrograms/kg have been given into the fetal circulation to induce fetal paralysis prior to intrauterine fetal transfusion. Larger doses cause paralysis for 2–4 hours.

Drug	Onset of action (minutes)	Duration of action after initial dose
Atracurium	2–3	20–35 minutes
Cisatracurium	1.5–2	20–35 minutes
Pancuronium	2–3	60–100 minutes
Rocuronium	1–2	22–67 minutes (dose dependent)
Suxamethonium	0.5–1	4–6 minutes
Vecuronium	2.5–3	20–40 minutes

Sedation or paralysis can reduce lung barotrauma in small babies requiring artificial ventilation, reducing the risk of pneumothorax and chronic lung disease, but there are no grounds for routinely paralysing ventilated babies. Paralysis makes it much more difficult to judge whether a baby is in pain, and sedation and paralysis both make it harder to watch for seizures or assess a baby's neurological status. Rocuronium (q.v.) is a related drug largely cleared from the body through the biliary tract rather than the renal tract; it may be a better drug to use where there is renal failure. Atracurium (q.v.) may be the best drug to use in this situation; it is usually given as a continuous infusion because it has a much shorter duration of action. Suxamethonium (q.v.) is the drug to use when paralysis is only required for a few minutes, whereas vecuronium (q.v.) may be a useful alternative if more sustained paralysis is needed.

Never paralyse a non-ventilated baby without first checking that you can achieve face-mask ventilation, and never paralyse a ventilated baby without first checking whether pain, correctable hypoxia, respiratory acidosis, inadequate respiratory support or an inappropriate respiratory rate is the cause of the baby's continued non-compliance. Pancuronium sometimes produces a modest but sustained increase in heart rate and blood pressure, but does not usually have any noticeable effect on gastrointestinal activity or bladder function, and its use does not preclude continued gavage feeding.

Joint contractures have been reported in a few chronically paralysed babies, but these usually resolve spontaneously once the infant is no longer paralysed. More importantly, it has been suggested that the sustained high-dose use of any neuromuscular blocking drug in the neonate may make serious, progressive, late-onset deafness more likely if they are also treated with a loop diuretic such as furosemide (q.v.).

Treatment

First dose: Give 100 micrograms/kg to obtain paralysis within 2–3 minutes.

Further doses: Most babies continue to comply with the imposed ventilatory rate as they 'wake' from the first paralysing dose, but a few require prolonged paralysis. The standard repeat

Continued on p. 390

dose is half the initial dose given by intravenous (or intramuscular) injection as need arises, but some larger and older babies seem to require a higher maintenance dose.

Supply and administration
2 ml ampoules containing 4 mg of pancuronium cost £4 each. Dilute 0.5 ml from the ampoule with 0.5 ml of 0.9% sodium chloride in a 1 ml syringe before use to obtain a preparation containing 100 micrograms in 0.1 ml. Pancuronium is stable for up to 6 weeks at 25 °C, but is best stored, wherever possible, at 4 °C. Open ampoules should not be kept. The US product contains 1% benzyl alcohol.

References   (See also relevant Cochrane reviews)

Besunder JB, Reed MD, Blumer JL. Principles of drug biodisposition in the neonate. A critical evaluation of the pharmacokinetic-pharmacodynamic interface (part ll). *Clin Pharmacokinet* 1988;**14**:261–86.

Church HL, Kong KL, North J. Is the decreasing availability of vecuronium and pancuronium putting patients at risk? *Eur J Anaesthesiol* 2009;**26**:347–8.

Costarino AT, Polin RA. Neuromuscular relaxants in the neonate. *Clin Perinatol* 1987;**14**:965–99.

Fanconi S, Ensner S, Knecht B. Effects of paralysis with pancuronium bromide on joint mobility in premature infants. *J Pediatr* 1995;**127**:134–6.

Robertson CMT, Tyebkhan JM, Peliowski A, *et al.* Ototoxic drugs and sensorineural hearing loss following severe neonatal respiratory failure. *Acta Paediatr* 2006;**95**:214–23.

Use

Paracetamol is a valuable analgesic also sometimes used to control fever. That it can be given orally, rectally and intravenously adds to its usefulness.

Pharmacology

Paracetamol, which has analgesic and antipyretic but no anti-inflammatory properties, was first marketed as an alternative to phenacetin in 1953. Paracetamol has become the most widely used analgesic for children (although dosage is often suboptimal). Intermittent (PRN) administration in response to perceived pain seldom provides optimal relief; however, visceral pain often needs opiate analgesia. Clearance is slightly slower in babies with visible jaundice. Tolerance does not develop with repeated use (as it does with opioid drugs), and respiratory depression is not a problem, but there is an analgesic ceiling that cannot be overcome by using a higher dose. Paracetamol is rapidly absorbed by mouth, widely distributed in the body ($V_D \sim 1\,l/kg$) and mostly conjugated in the liver before excretion in the urine. Optimum pain relief only occurs an hour after the blood level peaks. Paracetamol is metabolised primarily in the liver into toxic and non-toxic products. Three metabolic pathways are notable:

- Glucuronidation accounts for 40–65% of the metabolism of paracetamol in adults.
- Sulphation (sulphate conjugation) may account for 20–40%.
- N-hydroxylation and rearrangement, then glutathione conjugation, account for less than 15%. The hepatic cytochrome P450 enzyme system (CYP2E1, CYP1A2 and CYP3A4) metabolises paracetamol, forming a minor yet significant alkylating metabolite known as N-acetyl-p-benzoquinone imine (NAPQI), which is then irreversibly conjugated with the sulphydryl groups of glutathione.

Due to metabolic immaturity, neonatal clearance of paracetamol is different from adults. Sulphate conjugation is well developed in a neonate and is the major metabolic pathway for paracetamol clearance. Glucuronidation clearance is not well developed and plays a minor role in paracetamol clearance in neonates. With maturation, these clearance pathways for paracetamol change. The usual adult ratio of 2:1 glucuronide to sulphate conjugates of paracetamol is achieved by 12 years of age. The half-life of paracetamol is increased in term neonates (3.5 hours) and especially so in preterm neonates (5.7 hours). Hepatotoxicity in children from paracetamol ingestion has been demonstrated, and there is the potential for this to occur in neonates. Despite the low activity of CYP2E1 (it is still only 80% of the activity of adults at 1 year), NAPQI can still be formed in neonates and occurs somewhat later than might be expected. Toxicity is treated using N-acetylcysteine (q.v.).

Rectal absorption is rapid but incomplete and influenced by the volume given. Paracetamol seems the analgesic of choice in pregnancy (although ductal closure has been reported). Previous suggestions that exposure was associated with talipes and digital abnormalities have not been sustained in large series; however, there does appear to be a link with gastroschisis and small bowel atresia. Low concentrations (0.04–0.23% of the maternal amount) pass into breast milk. If the mother takes the maximum recommended daily dose (4 g), the infant will receive no more than 2.8 mg/kg (or ~5% of infant daily dosage of 60 mg/kg/day). Thus, it is generally considered compatible with breastfeeding.

Management of fever

While paracetamol can give symptomatic relief to a child who is feverish (just as an adult will sometimes take two aspirins and retire to bed!), its use to control fever *per se* is usually uncalled for. One oral 30 mg/kg dose often suffices. Prophylactic use for febrile convulsions is of no proven value. Most children just need to be unwrapped. Forced cooling does not work. Ibuprofen (q.v.) may be preferable for babies over 3 months old because asthma seems more common later on in children who experienced early paracetamol exposure. Although giving prophylactic paracetamol reduces the risk of fever after immunisation, high fever (<39 °C) is uncommon, and such treatment often reduces the antibody response.

Treatment of patent ductus arteriosus

Several reports, and some early randomised controlled trials, have recently been published suggesting that paracetamol might be an alternative to the non-selective COX inhibitors, ibuprofen (q.v.) and indometacin. Both intravenous (IV) and oral paracetamol administration has been investigated, but many questions remain unanswered regarding the safety and suitability of

Continued on p. 392

paracetamol particularly in a preterm population. Most reports to date have used doses that are significantly higher (15 mg/kg 6 hourly for 2–7 days) and longer than the recommended analgesic dose in the preterm population (who are most likely to have a patent ductus arteriosus (PDA)). One group used a lower IV dose (10 mg/kg 8 hourly for 3 days) to apparently equal effect after finding altered liver transaminases in one treated baby using the previous regime.

Until more evidence, including pharmacokinetic and pharmacodynamic data, from prospective randomised controlled trials (especially ones that include a conservative 'no-treatment' arm) becomes available, clinicians should exercise caution with the use of high-dose paracetamol in preterm neonates that require treatment of their PDA. Any such treatment should, for now, ideally be part of a properly designed prospective, randomised controlled trial looking at not only short-term but also long-term outcomes.

Toxicity

Lethal liver damage can occur in adults if the plasma level exceeds 150 mg/l four or more hours after ingestion (1 mg/l = 6.62 mmol/l). The safe threshold after repeated use is much less certain. Toxicity can occur in infants after sustained use even with therapeutic doses.

Although data is limited, it is suggested that intervention with *N*-acetylcysteine following a single IV dose above 60 mg/kg is appropriate as a precautionary measure.

Pain relief/antipyretic use in the neonate
Oral administration:

Post-menstrual age (weeks)	Loading dose (mg/kg)	Subsequent doses (mg/kg)	Dosing interval (hours)	Maximum cumulative daily dose (mg/kg)
28–32	20	10–15	8–12	30
≥32	20	10–15	6–8	60

IV administration (infusion over 15 minutes)

Post-menstrual age (weeks)	Loading dose (mg/kg)	Subsequent doses (mg/kg)	Dosing interval (hours)	Maximum cumulative daily dose (mg/kg)
28–32	20	7.5	8	22.5
33–36	20	10	8	40
≥37	20	10	6	40

Rectal administration:

Post-menstrual age	Loading dose (mg/kg)	Subsequent doses (mg/kg)	Dosing interval (hours)	Maximum cumulative daily dose (mg/kg)
28–32 weeks		20	12	40
33–37 weeks (and term neonates <10 days old)	30	15	8	60
Term neonate ≥10 days old	30	20	6–8	90

Continued on p. 393

Pain relief/antipyretic use in older children

Oral administration:

- **Child 1–3 months:** 30–60 mg every 8 hours as necessary (to a maximum of 180 mg in 24 hours)
- **Child 3–6 months:** 60 mg every 4–6 hours (to a maximum of 240 mg in 24 hours)
- **Child 6–12 months:** 120 mg every 4–6 hours (to a maximum of 480 mg in 24 hours)

IV administration:

Give 15 mg/kg every 4–6 hours (to a maximum of 60 mg/kg in 24 hours).

Supply

100 ml of the 24 mg/ml sugar-free elixir costs 73p. Parents can get this for a baby over 3 months old without a prescription. Using this elixir rectally (instead of a suppository) speeds absorption. Other strengths (50 and 100 mg/ml) of solution exist, and care should be exercised during prescription and administration.

50 ml (10 mg/ml) IV vials cost £1.13. May be diluted to a concentration of 1 mg/ml in 5% glucose or 0.9% sodium chloride 0.9%. If diluted, it should be used within an hour of dilution.

References

(See also the relevant Cochrane reviews)

Allegaert K, Anderson B, Simons S, *et al*. Paracetamol to induce ductus arteriosus closure: is it valid? *Arch Dis Child* 2013;**98**:462–6.

Anderson BJ, Allegaert K. Intravenous neonatal paracetamol dosing: the magic 10 days. *Paediatr Anaesth* 2009;**19**:289–95.

Beringer RM, Thompson JP, Parry S, *et al*. Intravenous paracetamol overdose: two case reports and a change to national treatment guidelines. *Arch Dis Child* 2011;**96**:307–8.

Dang D, Wang D, Zhang C, *et al*. Comparison of oral paracetamol versus ibuprofen in premature infants with patent ductus arteriosus: a randomized controlled trial. *PLoS One* 2013;**8**:e77888. [RCT]

Dart RC, Rumack BH. Intravenous acetaminophen in the United States: iatrogenic dosing errors. *Pediatrics* 2012;**129**:349–53.

Duggan ST, Scott LJ. Intravenous paracetamol (acetaminophen). *Drugs* 2009;**69**:101–13.

Jacqz-Aigrain E, Anderson BJ. Pain control: non-steroidal anti-inflammatory agents. *Semin Fetal Neonatal Med* 2006;**11**:251–9.

Levy G, Khanna NN, Soda DM, *et al*. Pharmacokinetics of acetaminophen in the human neonate: formation of acetaminophen glucuronide and sulfate in relation to plasma bilirubin concentration and d-glucaric acid excretion. *Pediatrics* 1975;**55**:818–25.

Mazer-Amirshahi M, van den Anker J. Is paracetamol safe and effective for ductus arteriosus closure? *Arch Dis Child* 2013;**98**:831.

Oncel MY, Yurttutan S, Erdeve O, *et al*. Oral paracetamol versus oral ibuprofen in the management of patent ductus arteriosus in preterm infants: a randomized controlled trial. *J Pediatr* 2014;**164**:510–4.e1. [RCT]

Palmer GM, Atkins M, Anderson BJ, *et al*. IV acetaminophen pharmacokinetics in neonates after multiple doses. *Br J Anaesth* 2008;**101**:523–30.

Savino F, Lupica MM, Tarasco V, *et al*. Fulminant hepatitis after 10 days of acetaminophen treatment at recommended dosage in an infant. *Pediatrics* 2011;**127**:e494–7.

Simbi KA, Secchieri S, Rinaldo M, *et al*. In utero ductal closure following near-term maternal self-medication with nimesulide and acetaminophen. *J Obstet Gynaecol* 2002;**22**:440–1.

Tekgunduz KS, Ceviz N, Demirelli Y, *et al*. Intravenous paracetamol for patent ductus arteriosus in premature infants - a lower dose is also effective. *Neonatology* 2013;**104**:6–7.

van Lingen RA, Deinum JT, Quak JME *et al*. Pharmacokinetics and metabolism of rectally administered paracetamol in preterm neonates. *Arch Dis Child Fetal Neonatal Ed* 1999;**80**:59–63.

Use

Amino acid solutions, together with glucose and other trace nutrients, are used with or without a lipid emulsion (q.v.) to supplement or replace enteral feeding when milk feeds are contraindicated or poorly tolerated.

Nutritional factors

Intravenous (IV) solutions are capable of providing every nutrient necessary for growth, although enteral feeding is always to be preferred where possible. Serious progressive cholestatic jaundice can occur in the preterm baby who is not offered at least a little milk by mouth, and sepsis can exacerbate this problem. Preterm babies not given at least 1 g/kg of protein a day develop a progressive negative nitrogen balance, and an intake of at *least* 2.5 g/kg a day seems necessary to support growth. If parenteral nutrition is given, and some argue that it is given too often, there should be enough protein to minimise the interruption of growth.

The standard neonatal preparation that is most widely used contains glucose and a mixture of synthetic L-amino acids (Vaminolact®) with trace minerals (7.5 ml/l of Peditrace®), water-soluble vitamins (0.7 of the contents of a vial of Solivito N®) and an extra 30 mg ascorbic acid per litre and a basic quantity of sodium (27 mmol/l), potassium (20 mmol/l), calcium (12.5 mmol/l), magnesium (1.3 mmol/l) and phosphate (12.3 mmol/l). This provides either 2.7 or 3.5 g/l of nitrogen (17 or 22 g/l of protein) and is available formulated so that the final glucose concentration is 10%, 12.5% or 15% (providing 400, 500 or 600 kcal/l of energy). It contains no iron. Solutions containing more than 10% glucose rapidly cause thrombophlebitis unless infused into a large vessel. Lipid emulsion and fat-soluble vitamins (e.g. Vitlipid N® infant) should be added to augment the calorie intake and provide the baby's other nutritional needs. Amino acid solutions with a profile mimicking that provided by the placenta or breast milk are now generally used. These contain taurine and do not produce the high plasma tyrosine and phenylalanine levels previously seen with egg protein-based products. The acidosis that develops when the intake of non-metabolisable chloride exceeds 6 mmol/kg/day can be reduced by substituting up to 6 mmol/kg of acetate. Aluminium (present as a contaminant in some ingredients – notably calcium gluconate) can affect bone density and cause permanent neurological damage.

Intake

Babies taking nothing by mouth can usually be started on 5 ml/kg/hour of the standard 10% solution with 2.7 g/l of nitrogen as soon as they are stable (6 ml/kg in babies over 2 days old). Energy intake can then be increased further *either* by using a formulation containing 12.5 or 15% glucose (if a central 'long line' is available) *or* by increasing the infusion rate to 7 or 8 ml/kg/hour. While this policy provides 2.4 g/kg of protein a day from the outset, the product containing 3.5 g/l of nitrogen will come closer to optimising the protein intake needed for sustained growth. More phosphate (q.v.) may also be needed. Some babies of <30 weeks' gestation need another 2–3 mmol/kg of sodium a day to replace loss due to renal immaturity.

Administration

Individually 'customised' infusions are rarely necessary. Their routine use causes much unnecessary blood sampling, the results are no better, and any such policy doubles the total cost. How beneficial it is to add heparin (q.v.) remains inadequately studied. A few other drugs (as noted in the relevant monographs in this compendium) can be co-infused with the formulation specified here if lack of vascular access so demands, but this may increase the risk of sepsis. These should be infused using a Y connector sited as close to the patient as possible. Add *nothing* to any amino acid solution after it leaves the pharmacy.

Monitoring

Clinically stable children require only marginally more biochemical monitoring than bottle-fed babies when on the standard formulation described here: it is the problem that made parenteral nutrition necessary that usually makes monitoring necessary. Ignore urinary glucose loss unless it exceeds 1%. Liver function should be monitored. Sepsis is the main hazard associated with any reliance on IV nutrition.

Tissue extravasation

'Tissue burns' are much more serious than those caused by a comparable solution of glucose. A strategy for the early treatment is described in the monograph on hyaluronidase (q.v.).

Continued on p. 395

Supply

Pre-prepared standard nominal half-litre bags cost about £28 to produce and remain safe to use for a month. Bags should be changed aseptically after 48 hours; change the bag, filter *and* giving set every 96 hours.

References
(See also the relevant Cochrane reviews)

Beecroft C, Martin H, Puntis JWL. How often do parenteral nutrition prescriptions for the newborn need to be individualized? *Clin Nutr* 1999;**18**:83–5.

Clark RH, Chase DH, Spitzer AR. Effects of two different doses of amino acid supplements on growth and blood amino acid levels in premature neonates admitted to a neonatal intensive care unit: a randomized controlled trial. *Pediatrics* 2007;**120**:1286–96. [RCT] (See also **121**:865–6.)

Embleton ND. Optimal protein and energy intakes in preterm infants. *Early Hum Dev* 2007;**83**:831–7.

Lenclen R, Crauste-Manciet S, Narcy P, *et al.* Assessment and implementation of a standardized parenteral formulation for early nutritional support of very preterm infants. *Eur J Pediatr* 2006;**165**:512–8.

Poindexter BB, Langer JC, Dusik AM, *et al.* Early provision of parenteral amino acids in extremely low birth weight infants: relation to growth and neurodevelopmental outcome. *J Pediatr* 2006;**148**:300–5. (See also pp. 291–4.)

Yeung MY, Smyth JP, Maheshwari R, *et al.* Evaluation of standardized versus individualised total parenteral nutrition regime for neonates less than 33 weeks gestation. *J Paediatr Child Health* 2003;**39**:613–7.

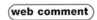

Use

Benzylpenicillin is the treatment of choice for pneumococcal, meningococcal, syphilitic, gonococcal and aerobic and anaerobic streptococcal infection. It is also very adequate for *Listeria* infection, although ampicillin and amoxicillin (q.v.) are better. Flucloxacillin (q.v.) is more appropriate for staphylococcal infection because most strains produce penicillinase. Procaine penicillin is sometimes used to treat syphilis.

Pharmacology

Benzylpenicillin is a naturally occurring bactericidal substance, first used clinically in 1941. It acts by interfering with bacterial cell wall synthesis. Most penicillins cross the placenta to some extent. Rodent teratogenicity studies and epidemiological studies in humans are reassuring. Only trace amounts of benzylpenicillin (penicillin G) and phenoxymethylpenicillin (penicillin V) enter breast milk, and both are generally considered compatible with breastfeeding.

Phenoxymethylpenicillin is acid stable and can be used when giving penicillin by mouth, giving 25 mg/kg doses at similar time intervals as for the intravenous (IV) or intramuscular (IM) drug. One other such situation where this is useful is in sickle cell disease where newborn screening allows for prophylaxis to be instituted before 2 months of age at a dose of 125 mg twice daily.

Active excretion by the renal tubules is the most important factor affecting the serum half-life, which falls from 4 to 5 hours at birth to 1½ hours by 1 month (gestation at birth having only a modest influence on this). Exposure may further stimulate tubular secretion. Very high levels are neurotoxic, making it important to reduce the dose or choose a different drug when there is renal failure. Transient thrombocytopenia can also occur. Allergic reactions are the main hazard in those with a history of prior exposure. The dose regime recommended here allows for the fact that CSF penetration is poor even when the meninges are inflamed. Intrathecal treatment is not advisable.

Group B streptococcal (GBS) infection

A number of similar policies exist for the prevention of early-onset neonatal group B streptococcal (GBS) disease. These may or may not include universal screening of pregnant women at 35–37 weeks' gestation for carriage of GBS. Currently, prevalence in the United Kingdom does not seem to justify the universal screening policy advocated in North America and some other areas. However, half the babies born to carriers also become carriers for a time, and 1–2% go on to develop life-threatening infection within hours of birth. Carriage cannot be eliminated by antenatal treatment, and early neonatal infection often develops too rapidly for post-delivery treatment to be effective, but prophylaxis started at least 4 hours before delivery can reduce the risk of neonatal illness. Most guidelines recommend that known carriers, mothers with a previous baby with early-onset GBS infection, with intrapartum pyrexia (≥38 °C) or whose membranes have been ruptured ≥18 hours, should be given benzylpenicillin every 6 hours as a slow IV injection during labour. Depending on the history of allergy, women allergic to penicillin should receive IV cefazolin or clindamycin (q.v.). Babies only require further investigation or treatment after delivery if they are symptomatic, there was inadequate intrapartum antibiotic prophylaxis or they were born before 37 weeks' gestation.

Treatment

Dose: Give 60 mg/kg per dose IM or (slowly) IV when there could be evidence of meningitis (especially GBS meningitis); 30 mg/kg is more than adequate in all other circumstances. Consider giving gentamicin synergistically as well for 48 hours for infection with group B streptococci or *Listeria*.

Timing: Give one dose every 12 hours in the first week of life, one dose every 8 hours in babies 1–3 weeks old and one dose every 6 hours in babies four or more weeks old. The dose should be halved and the dosage interval doubled when there is renal failure. Give treatment for at least 7–10 days in proven pneumonia and septicaemia and in the management of congenital syphilis. Treat meningitis for 3 weeks and osteitis for 4 weeks. Oral medication is sometimes used to complete a course of treatment.

Supply and administration

A 600 mg (one million units or one 'megaunit') vial costs 92p. Add 5.6 ml of sterile water for injection to get a solution containing 10 mg in 0.1 ml. Slow IV administration has been advocated, but there is no published evidence to support this advice (see web commentary). A 60 mg/

Continued on p. 397

kg dose of the UK product contains 0.17 mmol/kg of sodium (most US products contain the potassium salt). Staff handling penicillin regularly should avoid hand contact as this can cause skin sensitisation. Penicillin V (25 mg/ml) is available as a sugar-free suspension (£14.70 per 100 ml) which is stable for 2 weeks after reconstitution if stored at 4 °C.

References (See the relevant Cochrane reviews of GBS prophylaxis)

Centers for Disease Control and Prevention. Prevention of Perinatal Group B Streptococcal Disease: Revised Guidelines from CDC, 2010. *MMWR Recomm Rep* 2010;**59**(RR-10):1–32.

Colbourn TE, Asseburg C, Bojke L, *et al.* Preventive strategies for group B streptococcal and other bacterial infections in early infancy: cost effectiveness and value of information analysis. *Br Med J* 2007;**335**:655–8. [SR] (See also pp. 622–3.)

Committee on Infectious Diseases; Committee on Fetus and Newborn, Baker CJ, Byington CL, Polin RA. Policy statement—Recommendations for prevention of perinatal group B streptococcal (GBS) disease. *Pediatrics* 2011;**128**:611–6.

Depani SJ, Ladhani S, Heath PT, *et al.* The contribution of infections to neonatal deaths in England and Wales. *Pediatr Infect Dis J* 2011;**30**:345–7.

Matsuda S. Transfer of antibiotics into maternal milk. *Biol Res Pregnancy Perinatol* 1984;**5**:57–60.

Meier ER, Miller JL. Sickle cell disease in children. *Drugs* 2012;**72**:895–906.

Mercer BM, Carr TL, Beazley DD, *et al.* Antibiotic use and drug-resistant infant sepsis. *Am J Obstet Gynecol* 1999;**181**:816–21.

Muller-Pebody B, Johnson AP, Heath PT, *et al.* Empirical treatment of neonatal sepsis: are the current guidelines adequate? *Arch Dis Child Fetal Neonatal Ed* 2011;**96**:F4–8.

Oddie S, Embleton ND. Risk factors for early onset neonatal group B streptococcal sepsis: case control study. *Br Med J* 2002;**325**:308–11.

Pacifici GM. Placental transfer of antibiotics administered to the mother: a review. *Int J Clin Pharmacol Ther* 2006;**44**:57–63.

Schrag SJ, Zywicki S, Farkey MM, *et al.* Group B streptococcal disease in the era of intrapartum antibiotic prophylaxis. *N Eng J Med* 2000;**342**:15–20.

Use

Pethidine remains widely used to relieve pain during labour, although evidence of efficacy is limited. Use in infancy has received little study, and toxic quantities of the active metabolite norpethidine can accumulate with repeated usage. Morphine (q.v.) remains by far the best studied neonatal analgesic.

Pharmacology

Pethidine is a synthetic opioid developed in Germany during a review of the many analogues of atropine in 1939. The dose required to provide analgesia is variable. It is only a tenth as potent as morphine, and its analgesic effect is not as well sustained. It was originally hoped that because it bears no chemical similarity to morphine, it would not be addictive, but this is not so. Oral bioavailability is limited (about 50%) because of rapid first-pass clearance by the liver, where the drug undergoes hydrolysis or demethylation and conjugation before excretion. Tissue levels markedly exceed plasma levels (V_D about 7 l/kg), and clearance in the first 3 months is much slower than later in infancy. The average half-life in young babies is about 11 hours but is also *very* variable (range 3–60 hours). In contrast, in babies 3–18 months old, the half-life may be even lower than it is in adults (half-life ~3½ hours). Similar half-life changes have been documented for morphine. This variation between patients and over time, and the lack of any clear evidence as to what constitutes an effective analgesic dose, makes it difficult to recommend the use of pethidine in young children. The active metabolite, norpethidine, is renally excreted. It has an extended half-life, and neurotoxic quantities can accumulate with repeated usage, particularly if there is renal failure.

Increased scepticism is being voiced about the drug's central place in the management of pain relief in labour, but for a long time, it remained the only parenteral analgesic that midwives in many countries could give on their own authority. It often causes more drowsiness, disorientation and nausea than genuine relief from pain. Pethidine crosses the placenta rapidly; it can be detected in cord blood 2 minutes after maternal intravenous (IV) injection and remains in the infant's body for at least 24–48 hours. Use during labour attracts some criticism; it is only about one-tenth as potent as morphine and use can lead to poor feto-maternal gas exchange and fetal acidosis. It frequently causes respiratory depression in infants who are born more than 60 minutes after administration (greatest risk is to those born 2–3 hours after administration). Repeated maternal doses adversely affect the newborn due to accumulation and variable half-life of 3–60 hours at that age.

Feeding in exposed babies may be slow, and some babies show impaired behavioural responses and EEG abnormalities for 2–3 days after birth. Maternal use during lactation only exposes the baby to about 2% of the weight-related maternal dose. There is no evidence of teratogenicity.

Pain relief

Maternal pain relief in labour: 50–100 mg, repeated 1–3 hours later if necessary. Subject to a maximum of 400 mg in 24 hours.

Pain relief in infancy: A dose of 1 mg/kg given as an intramuscular (IM) or IV injection has been used but usually only in babies receiving ventilatory support. No repeat dose should be given for 10–12 hours in babies <2 months old (or for 4–6 hours in infants more than 3 months old) if drug accumulation is to be avoided.

Antidote

Neonatal respiratory depression is readily reversed by naloxone (q.v.). Opiate use during labour can also cause sustained neonatal drowsiness and interfere with the early initiation of lactation, and there are many who argue that IM naloxone should be used more widely to counter this problem.

Supply and administration

1 and 2 ml ampoules containing 50 mg/ml are available. They cost approximately 45p each. Take 0.2 ml (10 mg) from the ampoule and dilute to 1 ml with glucose, glucose saline or saline to obtain a preparation containing 10 mg/ml for accurate IM or IV administration. The storage and administration of pethidine are controlled under schedule 2 of the UK Misuse of Drugs Regulations 1988 (Misuse of Drugs Act 1971).

Continued on p. 399

References

(See also the relevant Cochrane reviews)

Armstong PJ, Bersten A. Normeperidine toxicity. *Anaesth Analg* 1986;**65**:536–8.

Bricker L, Laender T. Parenteral opioids for labour pain relief: a systematic review. *Am J Obstet Gynecol* 2002;**186**:S94–109. [SR]

Hogg MI, Wiener PC, Rosen M, *et al.* Urinary excretion and metabolism of pethidine and norpethidine in the newborn. *Br J Anaesth* 1977;**49**:891–9.

Pokela M-L. Pain relief can reduce hypoxia in distressed neonates during routine treatment procedures. *Pediatrics* 1994;**93**;379–83. [RCT]

Pokela M-L, Olkkola KT, Koivisto M, *et al.* Pharmacokinetics and pharmacodynamics of intravenous meperidine in neonates and infants. *Clin Pharmacol Ther* 1992;**52**:342–9.

Reynolds F. The effects of maternal labour analgesia on the fetus. *Best Pract Res Clin Obstet Gynaecol* 2010;**24**:289–302.

Saneto RP, Fitch JA, Cohen BH. Acute neurotoxicity of meperidine in an infant. *Pediatr Neurol* 1996;**14**:339–41.

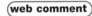
Use
Phenobarbital remains perhaps the most widely used anticonvulsant in neonatology and is still, for many, the first-line treatment for seizures in cooled and non-cooled infants.

Pharmacology
Phenobarbital, first marketed as a hypnotic in 1904, was widely used as an anticonvulsant for many years. Use in children then declined sharply because sustained exposure was thought to have an adverse effect on behaviour, although subsequent trials failed to detect the supposed parallel adverse effect on cognition. Many adults certainly still remain well controlled on long-term medication.

Oral phenobarbital is only slowly absorbed, and IM absorption can take 2–4 hours, so the drug must be given intravenous (IV) if a rapid response is required. An overdose can cause drowsiness, vasodilatation, hypotension and dangerous respiratory depression. Therapeutic hypothermia has been shown to double the half-life.

Phenobarbital is largely metabolised by multiple hepatic cytochromes, but a quarter is excreted unchanged in the urine in the neonatal period. The plasma half-life is so long in the neonatal period (*2–4 days*) that treatment once a day is perfectly adequate. The half-life decreases with age and is halved after 1–2 weeks of medication because the drug also acts to induce liver enzymes. This enzyme-inducing property has been used to speed hepatic conjugation and excretion of bilirubin. Phenobarbital also influences the metabolism and half-life of a number of other drugs. Phenobarbital, phenytoin and carbamazepine all induce hepatic microsomal enzymes, speeding the metabolism of oestrogens and progestogens, making it unwise for women to rely on any low-dose oral contraceptive when taking any of these anticonvulsants.

> **Phenobarbital pharmacokinetics are affected by therapeutic hypothermia as the drug is metabolised extensively by hepatic CYP450. There is reduced clearance during hypothermia – some reports suggest a doubling of the half-life – however this does not appear to have a clinically relevant effect. Give a single loading dose as outlined under 'Treatment'. A second dose should probably be considered before other anticonvulsants, but avoid maintenance if possible.**

Maternal use
Fetal consequences: Barbiturates rapidly cross the placenta, the fetal blood level being two-thirds the maternal level. Although there is some dispute whether barbiturate use is associated with a higher than expected incidence of oral clefts and cardiac malformations, most pregnancies (including otherwise healthy women attempting suicide with high-dose barbiturates) do not experience an increase in adverse outcomes. The hazards associated with uncontrolled epilepsy are, however, likely greater than the hazards associated with continued medication.

Neonatal consequences: Babies of mothers taking phenobarbital are occasionally hypoprothrombinaemic at birth, but this bleeding tendency can be easily corrected by giving the baby 100 micrograms/kg of vitamin K (q.v.) IM at birth. (A standard 1 mg dose is widely used.) Neonatal withdrawal can occur after exposure during the third trimester. Giving phenobarbital during labour can cause the baby to be rather sleepy and feed poorly for 2–3 days. Some authorities feel that breastfeeding may be unwise in mothers taking phenobarbital on a regular basis, and calculations suggest that neonatal blood levels could approach or exceed those seen in the mother. More information is needed, because few problems have been reported in practice. Drowsiness has occasionally been alluded to however, and there is one report of a baby who appeared to develop severe withdrawal symptoms when breastfeeding was stopped abruptly at 7 months.

Use to prevent neonatal jaundice: Maternal treatment (typically 100 mg a day) reduces the chance that neonatal jaundice will need treatment, and neonatal treatment (typically 5–8 mg/kg a day for 2–7 days) may work, but this is not widely used. Phototherapy (q.v.) usually suffices and avoids any issues with side effects.

Continued on p. 401

Neonatal use

Intrapartum asphyxia: Animal evidence suggests that phenobarbital reduces the amount of damage caused by cerebral anoxia (independent of its anticonvulsant effect), and the evidence from one small trial using a prompt 40 mg/kg loading dose suggests it may also be of clinical value, although another small study, and a small trial of the barbiturate thiopental (q.v.), failed to find evidence of clinical benefit.

Cholestatic jaundice: Phenobarbital (5 mg/kg/day) will improve bile flow and can sometimes alleviate pruritus, although ursodeoxycholic acid (q.v.) is usually more effective. Additional vitamin K will be required. Vitamins A, D and E (q.v.) may be needed if jaundice is prolonged.

Maternal drug dependency: Babies of mothers who are dependent on other drugs as well as opiates who are suffering *serious* withdrawal symptoms sometimes benefit from a short 4–6-day course of phenobarbital. Start with the same loading as for seizure control (see following text).

Seizures: There is no evidence that failure to control *all* seizure activity puts the baby at increased risk of long-term cerebral damage. Nonetheless, electroencephalographic (EEG) seizure activity often occurs in the absence of visible motor activity in the newborn baby, and when such activity is semi-continuous, it is potentially damaging. Animal evidence certainly points in that direction.

Although some babies who fail to respond to a standard loading dose of phenobarbital seem to respond clinically to a higher loading dose, it is not yet clear how often this actually stops EEG seizure activity. While high-dose treatment (with a loading dose up to 40 mg/kg) has its advocates, it can make many babies drowsy enough to render neurological assessment more difficult, if not impossible, and cause some preterm babies to become ventilator dependent. Where a high loading dose *has* been used, no daily maintenance dose should be started for at least 3–4 days (especially if there has been intrapartum asphyxia and use of therapeutic hypothermia). Seizures that fail to respond to phenobarbital may respond to phenytoin (q.v.) or lidocaine (q.v.). Clonazepam and midazolam (q.v.) seldom arrest EEG evidence of seizure activity if phenobarbital has not been successful. Pyridoxine dependency (q.v.), biotin deficiency (q.v.) and folinic acid-responsive seizures *must* be considered if unexplained seizures do not respond to phenobarbital.

Isolated seizures, in a baby who appears alert, awake and normal when not actually fitting, are usually well controlled by phenobarbital. These babies usually have a normal inter-ictal EEG, and their long-term prognosis is usually good. If phenobarbital and phenytoin fail, carbamazepine (q.v.), valproate (q.v.) or vigabatrin (q.v.) may work. It is seldom necessary to use more than one drug. Most babies given an anticonvulsant in the early neonatal period can usually be weaned from all treatment within 14 days, and few need medication at discharge from hospital.

Treatment

Give 20 mg/kg as a slow IV loading dose over 20 minutes to control seizures (once any biochemical disturbance, such as hypoglycaemia, has been excluded or treated) followed by 4 mg/kg once a day IV, IM or by mouth. Increase this to 5 mg/kg once a day if treatment is needed for more than 2 weeks. While higher loading doses have been used (see under 'Intrapartum asphyxia'), these can cause respiratory depression in the preterm baby and can cause prolonged sedation in babies undergoing therapeutic hypothermia.

Blood levels

The therapeutic level in the neonatal period is 20–40 mg/l (1 mg/l = 4.42 µmol/l), which is higher than the range generally quoted for use in later childhood. Drowsiness is common, especially if levels exceed 50 mg/l, and respiratory depression becomes progressively more likely. Some clinicians aim for a free (unbound) level of approximately 25 mg/l. Because of the long half-life, timing is not critical.

Supply and administration

IV ampoules contain viscid propylene glycol (80–90% w/v). 1 ml (30 mg) ampoules costing £6.70 are convenient for neonatal use; dilution with an equal quantity of water (giving a 15 mg/ml solution) makes injection through a fine (24 gauge) cannula easier. Greater dilution, though widely recommended, is *not* necessary with slow administration when this strength ampoule is used (and no dilution is necessary when the 15 mg/ml ampoule is used), but slow administration is important to minimise the risk of shock, hypotension or laryngospasm. Extravasation is also

Continued on p. 402

damaging because of the solution's high osmolality and high pH (10–11). A 3 mg/ml non-proprietary oral elixir is available, but its alcohol content (38%) is potentially toxic to the neonate. An aqueous, sugar-free preparation with a 2-week shelf life can usually be made in various strengths on request.

References

(See also the relevant Cochrane reviews)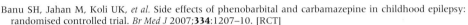

Banu SH, Jahan M, Koli UK, *et al.* Side effects of phenobarbital and carbamazepine in childhood epilepsy: randomised controlled trial. *Br Med J* 2007;**334**:1207–10. [RCT]

Bio LL, Siu A, Poon CY. Update on the pharmacologic management of neonatal abstinence syndrome. *J Perinatol* 2011;**31**:692–701.

Chawla D, Parmar V. Phenobarbitone for prevention and treatment of unconjugated hyperbilirubinemia in preterm neonates: a systematic review and meta-analysis. *Indian Pediatr* 2010;**47**:401–7. [SR]

Filippi L, la Marca G, Cavallaro G, *et al.* Phenobarbital for neonatal seizures in hypoxic ischemic encephalopathy: a pharmacokinetic study during whole body hypothermia. *Epilepsia* 2011;**52**:794–801.

Hall RT, Hall FK, Daily DK. High-dose phenobarbital therapy in term newborn infants with severe perinatal asphyxia: a randomised, prospective study with three-year follow-up. *J Pediatr* 1998;**132**:345–8. [RCT]

Hellstrom-Westas L, Blennow G, Londroth M, *et al.* Low risk of seizure recurrence after withdrawal of antiepileptic treatment in the neonatal period. *Arch Dis Child Fetal Neonatal Ed* 1995;**72**:F97–101.

Murray DM, Boylan GB, Ali I, *et al.* Defining the gap between electrographic seizure burden, clinical expression and staff recognition of neonatal seizures. *Arch Dis Child Fetal Neonatal Ed* 2008;**93**:F187–91.

Painter MJ, Scher MS, Stein AD, *et al.* Phenobarbital compared with phenytoin for the treatment of neonatal seizures. *N Engl J Med* 1999;**341**:485–9.

Shellhaas RA, Ng CM, Dillon CH, *et al.* Population pharmacokinetics of phenobarbital in infants with neonatal encephalopathy treated with therapeutic hypothermia. *Pediatr Crit Care Med* 2013;**14**:194–202.

Thoresen M, Stone J, Hoem NO, *et al.* Hypothermia after perinatal asphyxia more than doubles the plasma half-life of phenobarbitone. [abstract]. In: *Pediatric Academic Societies 2003 annual meeting.* Seattle (WA), May 3–6, 2003. EPAS 2003–137.

van den Broek MP, Groenendaal F, *et al.* Pharmacokinetics and clinical efficacy of phenobarbital in asphyxiated newborns treated with hypothermia: a thermopharmacological approach. *Clin Pharmacokinet* 2012;**51**:671–9.

Use

Phenytoin controls acute neonatal seizures as effectively as phenobarbital (q.v.), but phenytoin is seldom the first anticonvulsant used because of its very unpredictable half-life.

Pharmacology

Phenytoin was first developed and used as an anti-epileptic drug in 1936. Cosmetic changes, such as gum hypertrophy, acne, hirsutism and facial coarsening have now reduced the popularity of phenytoin as a drug of choice in the long-term management of epilepsy. Unwanted psychological changes, such as aggression, sedation, depression and impaired memory, are also common. Phenytoin may control the arrhythmia seen with digoxin toxicity. An overdose can cause restlessness or drowsiness, vomiting, nystagmus and pupillary dilatation, but symptoms resolve without specific intervention when treatment is stopped. **Fosphenytoin** is a related prodrug (1.5 mg of fosphenytoin = 1 mg of phenytoin) and is less irritant, but neonatal experience is limited and prescribing this drug in 'phenytoin-equivalent' units risks causing confusion.

Pharmacology in pregnancy

Phenytoin crosses the placenta freely, and there is an increased risk of congenital malformation (cleft palate and congenital heart defects) which is thought to be related, at least in part, to medication rather than the epilepsy. It may also cause fetal arrhythmias and long-term neurodevelopmental delay in children exposed *in utero*. Exposure can depress fetal vitamin K-dependent clotting factor levels, but the risk of haemorrhage in the neonate can be avoided by giving intramuscular (IM) vitamin K at birth. Mothers who need to remain on phenytoin during pregnancy may need to take more in the third trimester because of pharmacodynamic changes. Phenytoin passes into breast milk in relatively low amounts and is generally considered safe for breastfeeding.

Pharmacology in the first year of life

The pharmacology of phenytoin is already complicated in the neonate due to a variable rate of elimination and a highly variable volume of distribution. It exhibits non-linear (saturable) metabolism via hepatic cytochromes P450 2C9 and 2C19 as well as being affected by other drugs such as phenobarbital. The elimination process is saturated at plasma levels near the upper end of the therapeutic range, and at this point, small changes in the amount prescribed can have a disproportionate effect on the plasma level once clearance exceeds half the maximum rate possible (the Michaelis constant) prolonging the half-life ('zero-order' kinetics). An initial intravenous (IV) loading dose of 18 mg/kg and then a dose of 2.5–5 mg/kg by mouth twice a day are now considered the optimum strategy for children more than 4–6 months old. However, because the volume of distribution is almost twice as high in young babies (V_D ~1.2 l/kg) as it is in later life, a higher loading dose seems appropriate in babies less than 6 months old. Similarly, because the rate of elimination is so variable, treatment should only be sustained for more than a couple of days if plasma levels can be measured.

> **Therapeutic hypothermia prolonged the already variable half-life of phenytoin, and levels in cooled infants are likely to be higher than in normothermic infants. Maintenance treatment is best avoided unless levels can be closely monitored.**

Treatment

A loading dose of 20 mg/kg given IV over 10–20 minutes (to prevent hypotension, arrhythmia and pain at the injection site) will usually control acute status epilepticus at any age. The optimum maintenance dose is variable, but 2 mg/kg IV every 8–12 hours will usually maintain a therapeutic level in the first week of life, and the same maintenance dose usually works when given by mouth (at least in babies over 2 weeks old). Older babies may require two or three times as much as this (i.e., 10–20 mg/kg/day). Crystallisation makes the IM route unsatisfactory.

Continued on p. 404

Blood levels

The optimum plasma concentration is usually 10–20 mg/l (1 mg/l = 3.96 µmol/l) but 20% less than this in the first 3 months of life because of reduced protein binding. Levels must be measured if phenytoin is given for more than 2–3 days in babies only a few months old.

Supply and administration

5 ml (250 mg) ampoules of phenytoin cost £2.40. Give IV through a filter ***always*** preceded and followed by a bolus of 0.9% sodium chloride because crystals form when phenytoin comes into contact with any solution containing glucose. To give IV maintenance treatment accurately, first draw 1 ml of fluid from the ampoule into a syringe and dilute to 10 ml with 0.9% sodium chloride to get a solution containing 5 mg/ml. The fluid is very alkaline (pH 12). Ampoules contain 2 g propylene glycol and 10% alcohol. An oral suspension in sucrose contains 6 mg/ml (100 ml costs £4.30). 750 mg (10 ml) vials of fosphenytoin (which can be given IV or IM) cost £40.

References (See also the relevant Cochrane reviews)

Bourgeois BFD, Dodson WE. Phenytoin elimination in newborns. *Neurology* 1983;**33**:173–8.

Cheng A, Banwell B, Levin S, *et al.* Oral dosing requirements for phenytoin in the first three months of life. *J Popul Ther Clin Pharmacol* 2010;**17**:e256–61.

Frey OR, von Brenndorff AI, Probst W. Comparison of phenytoin serum concentrations in premature neonates following intravenous and oral administration. *Ann Pharmacother* 1998;**32**:300–3.

Harden CL, Pennell PB, Koppel BS, *et al.* Management issues for women with epilepsy—focus on pregnancy (an evidence-based review): III. Vitamin K, folic acid, blood levels, and breast-feeding: Report of the Quality Standards Subcommittee and Therapeutics and Technology Assessment Subcommittee of the American Academy of Neurology and the American Epilepsy Society. *Epilepsia* 2009;**50**:1247–55.

Meador K, Reynolds MW, Crean S, *et al.* Pregnancy outcomes in women with epilepsy: a systematic review and meta-analysis of published pregnancy registries and cohorts. *Epilepsy Res* 2008;**81**:1–13. [SR]

Painter MJ, Scher MS, Stein AD, *et al.* Phenobarbital compared with phenytoin for the treatment of neonatal seizures. *N Engl J Med* 1999;**341**:485–9. [RCT]

Takeoka M, Krishnamoorthy KS, Soman TB, *et al.* Fosphenytoin in infants. *J Child Neurol* 1998;**13**:537–40.

Use

Supplemental phosphate (as oral sodium phosphate) can be used prophylactically to prevent neonatal rickets due to phosphate deficiency in the very low birthweight baby.

Nutritional factors

The transplacental fetal uptake of calcium and phosphate is high especially in the second trimester of pregnancy, and comparable intakes are hard to achieve in the preterm neonate. The mineral content of breast milk is particularly inadequate, but ordinary standard milk formulae are also deficient. Most preterm milk formulae and breast milk fortifiers (q.v.) contain additional calcium and phosphate for this reason.

Deficient mineral intake after birth compromises subsequent bone growth. Poor bone mineralisation leads to osteopenia, and pathological fractures can develop once bone growth starts to accelerate after 6–8 weeks; severe deficiency can also cause rickets with fraying and cupping of the bony metaphyses on X-ray. When breast milk is used, phosphate deficiency is normally the limiting factor. Low plasma phosphate levels are associated with increased hydroxylation of 25-hydroxycholecalciferol to 1,25-dihydroxycholecalciferol (the metabolically active form of vitamin D), increased phosphate absorption from the gut, maximum renal retention of phosphate and hypercalciuria (which is corrected by phosphate supplementation). Parenterally fed babies develop similar problems. Formula-fed babies can, on the other hand, sometimes develop a calcipenic type of rickets with marginal hypocalcaemia and no renal calcium spill, but secondary hyperparathyroidism with hyperphosphaturia. There is evidence of a prenatal deficiency of phosphate in some VLBW babies possibly as a result of pre-eclampsia and/or placental insufficiency. A controlled trial of oral phosphate supplementation in babies with a low plasma phosphate level and a high initial urinary calcium loss shortly after birth found that early supplementation can prevent the development of osteopenia of prematurity. Post-discharge supplementation does not seem necessary.

Treatment

Oral administration: VLBW babies developing a plasma phosphate level of <1.5 mmol/l in the first few weeks of life should be offered ~500 μmol/kg of extra phosphate twice a day by mouth. Some babies benefit from supplementation three times a day.

Intravenous administration: The low solubility of inorganic calcium and phosphorus can compromise bone growth in LBW babies needing prolonged parenteral nutrition (q.v.). Intake can be increased to 1.5 mmol/kg/day by using the soluble organic salt, sodium glycerophosphate.

Monitoring

Treatment can be reduced or stopped when the plasma phosphate level exceeds 1.8 mmol/l and/or the tubular reabsorption of phosphate in the urine falls below 95% (in the absence of acute tubular necrosis). The renal tubular phosphate reabsorption (% TPR) can be calculated from the formula

$$FE_{Na}\left(\%\right) = 1 - \left(\left(\frac{Urinary\,sodium}{Plasma\,sodium}\right) \times \left(\frac{Plasma\,creatinine}{Urinary\,creatinine}\right)\right) \times 100$$

Supply

An oral solution containing 1 mmol/ml of phosphate (with 1.28 mmol/ml Na and 0.2 mmol/ml K) can be obtained by dissolving a 500 mg Phosphate-Sandoz® tablet (costing 16p) in water and then making the resultant solution up to 16 ml.

References

Catache M, Leone CR. Role of plasma and urinary calcium and phosphorus measurements in early detection of phosphorus deficiency in very low birthweight infants. *Acta Paediatr* 2003;**92**:76–80.

Costello I, Powell C, Williams AF. Sodium glycerophosphate in the treatment of neonatal hypophosphataemia. *Arch Dis Child Fetal Neonatal Ed* 1995;**73**:F44–5.

Harrison CM, Johnson K, McKechnie E. Osteopenia of prematurity: a national survey and review of practice. *Acta Paediatr* 2008;**97**:407–13.

Continued on p. 406

Holland PC, Wilkinson AR, Diaz J, *et al*. Prenatal deficiency of phosphate, phosphate supplementation, and rickets in very-low-birthweight babies. *Lancet* 1990;**335**:697–701. [RCT]

Kurl S, Heinonen K, Lansimies E. Randomized trial: effect of short versus long duration of calcium and phosphate supplementation on bone mineral content of very low birth weight (VLBW) infants born <32 weeks gestation. [Abstract] *Pediatr Res* 2004;**55**:448A.

Pohlandt F. Prevention of postnatal bone demineralisation in very low-birth-weight infants by individually monitored supplementation with calcium and phosphorus. *Pediatr Res* 1994;**35**:125–9.

Ryan S. Nutritional aspects of metabolic bone disease in the newborn. *Arch Dis Child Fetal Neonatal Ed* 1996;**74**:F145–8.

Tinnion RJ, Embleton ND. How to use...alkaline phosphatase in neonatology. *Arch Dis Child Educ Pract Ed* 2012;**97**:157–63.

Use

Piperacillin is a ureidopenicillin originally intended as an anti-pseudomonal antibiotic; it is now only available as an 8:1 combination with the β-lactamase inhibitor tazobactam. Tazobactam is a β-lactam sulphone that possesses little intrinsic antibacterial activity itself but which has high affinity for many non-chromosomally mediated β-lactamases. The resulting piperacillin/tazobactam combination has a broad spectrum of activity encompassing most Gram-positive and Gram-negative aerobic and anaerobic bacteria, including many producing β-lactamases. This broad spectrum, and the role of such antibiotics in the emergence of multi-resistant *Enterobacteriaceae* strains, make it unsuitable as first-line antibiotic therapy in early- or late-onset neonatal sepsis.

Pharmacology

Piperacillin has been used in neonates since the 1980s, although degradation by bacterial β-lactamases limited its clinical usefulness as monotherapy for many infections. The half-life of piperacillin is variable and is altered by prematurity and age; in the newborn, the elimination half-life ranges from 3.5 to 14 hours, whereas between 1 and 6 months of age, the half-life is about 47 minutes. In preterm infants, the half-life ranges from 1.7 to 4.3 hours and was inversely proportional to gestational age, postnatal age and birthweight. Both piperacillin and tazobactam are approximately 30% bound to plasma proteins. Both components are eliminated via the kidney by glomerular filtration and tubular secretion. Piperacillin is largely excreted rapidly as unchanged substance, with 68% of the administered dose appearing in the urine. Small amounts are metabolised to a minor microbiologically active desethyl metabolite. Tazobactam and its metabolite are eliminated primarily by renal excretion, with 80% of the administered dose appearing as unchanged substance and the remainder as the single metabolite. Piperacillin, tazobactam and desethyl piperacillin are also secreted into the bile. Piperacillin crosses both the inflamed and non-inflamed blood–brain barrier albeit in unpredictable amounts; however, CSF penetration of the β-lactamase inhibitor tazobactam is modest; for this reason, piptazobactam is not recommended as a treatment for CNS infections. The combination has a high sodium content (5.58 mmol per 2.25 g vial) and may contribute to hypernatraemia.

Treatment

Neonate:	
Gestational age at birth <36 weeks	
Postnatal age 0–7 days	90 mg/kg every 12 hours
Postnatal age 8–28 days	90 mg/kg every 8 hours
Gestational age at birth ≥36 weeks	
Postnatal age 0–7 days	90 mg/kg every 8 hours
Postnatal age 8–28 days	90 mg/kg every 6 hours
Infants 1 month to 1 year:	90 mg/kg every 6–8 hours

> **Note: Doses are expressed as a combination of piperacillin and tazobactam (both as sodium salts) in a ratio of 8:1. Thus, 90 mg/kg of the piperacillin/tazobactam combination is equivalent to 80 mg/kg of piperacillin and 10 mg/kg tazobactam.**

Compatibility

Avoid mixing with aciclovir, aminoglycosides, amphotericin, dobutamine, ganciclovir, vancomycin and sodium lactate compound (Hartmann's or Ringer lactate solution). Whenever piperacillin/tazobactam is used concurrently with another antibiotic (e.g. aminoglycosides), these must be administered separately. The mixing of β-lactam antibiotics with an aminoglycoside *in vitro* can result in substantial inactivation of the aminoglycoside. Flush the line between administration of piperacillin/tazobactam and other drugs.

Continued on p. 408

Supply and administration

Available as 2.25 g powder for injection (a 4.5 g vial is also available but is unnecessary in the neonatal unit). Each 2.25 g vial contains piperacillin 2 g and tazobactam 250 mg both as sodium salts. Reconstitute the contents of the 2.25 g vial with 8.4 ml of 0.9% sodium chloride solution or water for injection to give a solution of 225 mg/ml. Further dilute 1 ml of this 225 mg/ml piptazobactam solution with 9 ml of compatible fluid (to a total volume of 10 ml). The resulting solution contains 22.5 mg/ml piptazobactam. Infuse 4 ml of this solution for every kilogram of body weight over a period of 20–30 minutes. This reconstituted solution remains stable for up to 48 hours when stored in a refrigerator at 2–8 °C.

References

Berger A, Kretzer V, Apfalter P, *et al*. Safety evaluation of piperacillin/tazobactam in very low birth weight infants. *J Chemother* 2004;**16**:166–71.

Flidel-Rimon O, Friedman S, Gradstein S, *et al*. Reduction in multiresistant nosocomial infections in neonates following substitution of ceftazidime with piperacillin/tazobactam in empiric antibiotic therapy. *Acta Paediatr* 2003;**92**:1205–7.

Gin A, Dilay L, Karlowsky JA, *et al*. Piperacillin-tazobactam: a beta-lactam/beta-lactamase inhibitor combination. *Expert Rev Anti Infect Ther* 2007;**5**:365–83.

Kacet N, Roussel-Delvallez M, Gremillet C, *et al*. Pharmacokinetic study of piperacillin in newborns relating to gestational and postnatal age. *Pediatr Infect Dis J* 1992;**11**:365–9.

Li Z, Chen Y, Li Q, *et al*. Population pharmacokinetics of piperacillin/tazobactam in neonates and young infants. *Eur J Clin Pharmacol* 2013;**69**:1223–33.

Reed MD, Goldfarb J, Yamashita TS, *et al*. Single-dose pharmacokinetics of piperacillin and tazobactam in infants and children. *Antimicrob Agents Chemother* 1994;**38**:2817–26.

Sullins AK, Abdel-Rahman SM. Pharmacokinetics of antibacterial agents in the CSF of children and adolescents. *Paediatr Drugs* 2013;**15**:93–117.

Use

There are few established indications for using plasma albumin; 0.9% sodium chloride can be used for emergency volume expansion at lower cost, fresh frozen plasma (FFP) is more appropriate (q.v.) when there is coagulopathy, and hypotension is often better managed with an inotrope.

Blood levels

Plasma albumin increases proportionate to gestation; values of between 10 and 30 g/l are normal at 28 weeks' gestation, whereas 95% of healthy term babies have a plasma albumin of between 20 and 40 g/l. The fetal liver, however, has a higher absolute synthesis rate in premature than in mature fetuses, suggesting that the protein intake of many preterm neonates remains inadequate to meet their needs.

Products

Human albumin solution is predominantly derived from donated human plasma, although time-expired blood and, in some countries, placental material have been used as sources. Albumin was traditionally purified using a cold ethanol fractionation process first described in 1946, but since the 1980s, many manufacturers have used chromatographic purification and filtration steps instead. These carry a number of potential advantages; the processes lend themselves better to automation, there is less damage to the protein, and there are higher yields (80–85% vs. 60–70%) and greater purity (>98% vs. 95%). Pasteurisation at 60 °C for 10 hours inactivates a range of viruses including hepatitis A, B and C, as well as HIV. Octanoate (caprylate) and/or N-acetyl tryptophan stabilisers prevent albumin being denatured during the pasteurisation process. An isotonic solution with a similar colloid osmotic pressure to plasma contains 3–5% albumin. A hyperoncotic, isotonic 20% solution is also available.

Indications

Hypovolaemia: The value of plasma infusions in the neonatal period is highly questionable. Persistent hypotension at birth, once acidosis has been corrected, can, rarely, be due to acute hypovolaemia, and this is best treated by blood transfusion. Most cases are more appropriately treated with an inotrope such as dopamine and/or dobutamine (q.v.). Trials in adults with burns or trauma found that crystalloids (like Ringer lactate) reduce mortality more than an albumin infusion. In neonates, albumin infusions do not confer any advantage over crystalloids in the acute treatment of hypovolaemia.

Hypoproteinaemia: Underproduction due to liver failure, or to excess gut or renal loss, can cause oedema and hypovolaemia, triggering a compensatory retention of salt and water. Where this does not respond to a diuretic, 20% albumin may produce a diuresis, although the effect will be relatively short lived because most of the body's albumin is in the extravascular space, intercompartmental exchange is rapid and plasma protein turnover is high (25%/day). Use of albumin to treat hypoproteinaemia actually *increased* the risk of death in one recent systematic review.

Polycythaemia: A partial (dilutional) exchange transfusion is sometimes done in a symptomatic baby if the venous haematocrit is over 75%. There is no evidence that this improves the long-term outcome, and it can occasionally cause necrotising enterocolitis. 4.5% albumin has occasionally been used, but 0.9% sodium chloride is just as effective. In most babies, the haematocrit will start to fall within 6–12 hours anyway.

Treatment

20 ml/kg of 4.5% albumin or 5 ml/kg of 20% albumin may be piggybacked terminally into an existing glucose infusion: stopping the glucose will merely precipitate reactive hypoglycaemia. Infusion (distal to any filter) into a line containing an amino acid solution (TPN) increases the risk of bacterial proliferation but may have to be accepted. Any 20% albumin **must** be given slowly to prevent vascular overload.

Supply

4.5 and 5% human albumin solution is available in a number of different sized vials (50–500 ml), whereas 20% human albumin solution is available only in 50 and 100 ml vials. Blood grouping is not necessary. Preparations contain 120–150 mmol/l of sodium and small amounts of potassium and are stable for 3 years at room temperature. Do not use if turbid.

Continued on p. 410

References

(See also the relevant Cochrane reviews)

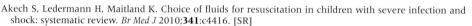

Akech S, Ledermann H, Maitland K. Choice of fluids for resuscitation in children with severe infection and shock: systematic review. *Br Med J* 2010;**341**:c4416. [SR]

Cochrane Injuries Group Albumin Reviewers. Human albumin administration in critically ill patients: systematic review of randomised controlled trials. *Br Med J* 1998;**317**:235–40. [SR]

Dempsey EM, Barrington K. Short and long term outcomes following partial exchange transfusion in the polycythaemic newborn: a systemic review. *Arch Dis Child Fetal Neonatal Ed* 2006;**91**:F2–6. [SR]

de Waal KA, Baerts W, Offringa M. Systematic review of the optimal fluid for dilutional exchange transfusion in neonatal polycythaemia. *Arch Dis Child Fetal Neonatal Ed* 2006;**91**:F7–10. [SR]

Greenough A, Emery E, Hird MF, *et al.* Randomised controlled trial of albumin infusion in ill preterm infants. *Eur J Pediatr* 1993;**152**:157–9.

Haynes GR, Navickis RJ, Wilkes MM. Albumin administration – what is the evidence of clinical benefit? A systematic review of randomised controlled trials. *Eur J Anaesthesiol* 2003;**20**:771–93. [SR]

Matejtschuk P, Dash CH, Gascoigne EW. Production of human albumin solution: a continually developing colloid. *Br J Anaesth* 2000;**85**:887–95.

Morris I, McCallion N, El-Khuffash A, *et al.* Serum albumin and mortality in very low birth weight infants. *Arch Dis Child Fetal Neonatal Ed* 2008;**93**:F210–2. (See also p. F326.)

So KW, Fok TF, Ng PC, *et al.* Randomised controlled trial of colloid or crystalloid in hypotensive preterm infants. *Arch Dis Child Fetal Neonatal Ed* 1997;**76**:F43–6.

van den Akker CH, Schierbeek H, Rietveld T, *et al.* Human fetal albumin synthesis rates during different periods of gestation. *Am J Clin Nutr* 2008;**88**:997–1003.

Use

Plasma substitutes (colloids) can be used to expand intravascular volume in patients with impending or established shock. Although artificial products are generally as effective as 4.5% human albumin (q.v.) and significantly cheaper, there is, however, ongoing debate across all ages about the most suitable fluid. Hydroxyethyl starch solutions are no longer recommended and have been withdrawn in many countries.

Pharmacology

Gelatin is a purified protein obtained by the partial hydrolysis of BSE-free bovine collagen. A sterile saline solution containing 40 g/l of modified gelatin has the same properties and uses as dextran 40 (a polymer of glucose), but gelatin, unlike dextran, does not interfere with subsequent blood grouping and compatibility testing procedures. A range of products, of which Gelofusine® is the best known, are available. The gelatin in Gelofusine (molecular weight 30,000) has only a 4 hour half-life and is rapidly excreted unchanged in the urine. Anaphylactic reactions have been described, but are rare in young children. Immediate and delayed-type hypersensitivity reactions have sometimes occurred after immunisation with vaccines containing gelatin (e.g. the MMR vaccine) in pre-sensitised children.

Etherified starches are artificial colloids with a mean molecular weight (~200,000) three times that of plasma albumin. The starches are glucose polymers containing mainly amylopectin (branched glucose chains) that has been etherified with hydroxyethyl groups. Several starches are available, and they differ in the degree of etherification; **hexastarch** is more etherified than **pentastarch**, which, in turn, is more etherified than **tetrastarch**.

Hetastarch is a mixture of different starches. While the smaller molecules are rapidly excreted in the urine, the larger molecules remain in the bloodstream for some days undergoing slow enzymatic degradation. While use can cause a sustained expansion of the intravascular volume, even in the presence of capillary leak of albumin, this product was associated with an *increased* risk of transient renal failure in adults with septic shock when compared to gelatin in one recent trial. Large volumes interfere with coagulation. The manufacturers of these starches stress that little is known about use of any of these products during pregnancy or childhood.

Indications for use

A major systematic review in 1998 suggested that the indiscriminate use of **any** colloid in the management of hypovolaemia actually does more harm than good. However, this may be because the product is being used inappropriately rather than because it is inherently dangerous. Gelatin can be used to reconstitute packed red cells. It may also be the best colloid to use during routine surgery because it has the least effect on *in vitro* tests of coagulation, but 20 ml/kg is the largest dose known to have been used in any 1 day in the neonatal period. Naturally, where blood has been lost, it will often be more appropriate to replace this as soon as practicable. Early neonatal hypotension without hypovolaemia is more appropriately treated with dobutamine and/or dopamine (q.v.), or hydrocortisone (q.v.), while fresh frozen plasma (q.v.) should be used where there is a significant clotting factor deficiency. See the web commentary for further information.

Treatment

20 ml/kg of gelatin infused over 5–15 minutes should correct all but the most severe hypovolaemia. The effect of giving more than a total of 30 ml/kg in the first week of life has not been studied.

Supply

500 ml bags of 4% gelatin (Gelofusine) in 0.9% sodium chloride cost £4.70. 500 ml bags of 6 or 10% pentastarch in 0.9% sodium chloride cost £12.50 and £16.50, respectively. These products contain 154 mmol/l of sodium. They should not be kept once they have been opened because they contain no preservative. Do not use any material that looks cloudy or turbid.

References   (See also the relevant Cochrane reviews) ◑

Akech S, Ledermann H, Maitland K. Choice of fluids for resuscitation in children with severe infection and shock: systematic review. *Br Med J* 2010;**341**:c4416. [SR]

Continued on p. 412

Boluyt N, Bollen W, Bos AO, *et al.* Fluid resuscitation in neonatal and pediatric hypovolaemic shock: a Dutch Pediatric Society evidence-based clinical practice guideline. *Intensive Care Med* 2006;**32**:995–1003.

Roberts JS, Bratton SL. Colloid volume expanders. Problems, pitfalls and possibilities. *Drugs* 1998;**55**:621–30.

Schortgen F, Lacherade J-C, Bruneel F, *et al.* Effects of hydoxyethylstarch and gelatin on renal function in severe sepsis: a multicentre randomised study. *Lancet* 2001;**357**:911–16. [RCT] (See also **358**:581–3.)

Shierhout G, Roberts I. Fluid resuscitation with colloid or crystalloid solutions in critically ill patients: a systematic review of randomised trials. *Br Med J* 1998;**316**:961–4. [SR]

Veldman A. Complications of hydroxyethyl starch in paediatric patients. *Eur J Anaesthesiol* 2010;**27**:86–7.

Veldman A. Is hydroxyethyl starch safe in neonates? *Pediatr Crit Care Med* 2004;**5**:202–3.

Wilkes MM, Navickis RJ, Sibbald WJ. Albumin versus hydroxyethyl starch in cardiopulmonary surgery: a meta-analysis of postoperative bleeding. *Ann Thorac Surg* 2001;**72**:527–33. [SR]

Wills BA, Dung NM, Loan HT, *et al.* Comparison of three fluid solutions for resuscitation in dengue shock syndrome. *N Engl J Med* 2005;**353**:877–89. [RCT] (See also pp. 941–4.)

Use

Platelet concentrates are used when bleeding occurs in the presence of severe thrombocytopenia.

Pathophysiology

Thrombocytopenia is one of the most common haematological findings among babies in the neonatal unit; up to 30% of all NICU patients (and up to 75% of ELBW babies) will have a low platelet count at some point during their hospital stay. Previously, it was accepted that neonates shared the same 'normal' values as adults (i.e. $150–450 \times 10^9/l$); however, more recently, it has been accepted that the lower limits are as low as $105 \times 10^9/l$ for infants ≤32 weeks' gestation and as low as $125 \times 10^9/l$ for near-term and term infants. Neonatal thrombocytopenia is generally defined as severe when the platelet count is $<50 \times 10^9/l$, and many would prophylactically transfuse, even the seemingly well baby, once the platelet count drops to $20–30 \times 10^9/l$. When faced with a low platelet count, always check first that the 'thrombocytopenia' is not due to clots or platelet clumping in the sample. Causes of neonatal thrombocytopenia can usually be determined by the clinical history and presentation. In particular, the gestation, the timing of onset of thrombocytopenia, maternal and neonatal history and the FBC and blood film can be used to identify the cause in the vast majority of neonates. These can be incorporated into a diagnostic algorithm for both preterm and term neonates.

In **preterm neonates**, the majority of early-onset cases of thrombocytopenia are due to conditions that cause placental 'insufficiency' and/or intrauterine growth restriction. Such cases are usually self-limiting, with the platelet count falling to a nadir of $>50 \times 10^9/l$ approximately 4–7 days after birth before spontaneously improving within 10–14 days. Other haematological features – transient neutropenia, increased nucleated red cells, polycythaemia and Howell–Jolly bodies – are often also present. Sepsis, perinatal hypoxia and congenital viral infections may also cause early-onset thrombocytopenia. In late-onset thrombocytopenia, NEC and sepsis are the most common causes. Heparin (q.v.) occasionally causes a dangerous thrombocytopenia that is made worse if platelets are given.

In **term neonates**, neonatal alloimmune thrombocytopenia (NAIT) is the most important cause of thrombocytopenia. In the otherwise well but thrombocytopenic term neonate where there is no history to suggest maternal systemic lupus erythematosus (SLE) or idiopathic thrombocytopenic purpura is causing an autoimmune thrombocytopenia. NAIT should be excluded by serological and genetic testing, as soon as possible. Maternal antibodies, produced as a result of transplacental sensitisation, attack fetal platelets (in a process analogous to the red cell destruction that occurs in rhesus haemolytic disease), treatment with immunoglobulin (q.v.) may be appropriate, and fully compatible platelets are required (i.e. they must lack the antigen against which the antibodies are directed). The transfusion service can usually provide platelets that are both HPA-1a and HPA-5b negative (the antibodies responsible for 95% of all problems). These will almost always be suitable and can be used if the situation is urgent before platelet grouping and any formal confirmation of the diagnosis are possible. Maternal washed and irradiated platelets can be used on those rare occasions when the blood transfusion service finds itself unable to provide suitable donor platelets.

A few term and preterm neonates (<1%) have persistent thrombocytopenia and should have further specialised investigations performed. Some may well have diagnostic or suggestive dysmorphic features to suggest syndromes, such as trisomy 21, 13 or 18 or thrombocytopenia-absent radii (TAR) syndrome.

Administration

10 ml/kg of platelets from a single ABO- and Rh-compatible CMV-negative donor will usually suffice unless there is alloimmune thrombocytopenia. Here more is given, and a higher minimum count aimed for, because platelet function is poorer. To minimise loss, draw the contents of the pack into a 50 ml syringe through a special platelet or blood transfusion set with a 170–200 μm filter and then infuse over 30 minutes, using a narrow bore extension set linked (near the patient) to an intravenous line primed with 0.9% sodium chloride.

Supply

Leucodepleted 50 ml single-unit packs containing 60×10^9 platelets are available from hospital blood banks. Packs for intrauterine use are irradiated and further concentrated before issue. Platelets need to be stored under special conditions, kept at room temperature and used *promptly* on receipt. They quickly lose their therapeutic power if this is not done, and bacterial contamination also becomes increasingly likely.

Continued on p. 414

References

(See also the UK website guidelines)

Baer Vl, Lambert DK, Henry E, *et al.* Severe thrombocytopenia in the NICU. *Pediatrics* 2009;**124**:e1095–100.

Birchall JE, Murphy MF, Kaplan C, *et al.* European Fetomaternal Alloimmune Thrombocytopenia Study Group. European collaborative study of the antenatal management of feto-maternal alloimmune thrombocytopenia. *Br J Haematol* 2003;**122**:275–88.

British Society for Haematology. Guidelines for the use of platelet transfusions. *Br J Haematol* 2003;**122**:10–23.

Killie MK, Kjeldsen-Kragh J, Husebekk A, *et al.* Cost-effectiveness of antenatal screening for neonatal alloimmune thrombocytopenia. *Br J Obstet Gynaecol* 2007;**114**:588–95. (See also **115**:412–4.)

Porcelijn L, Van den Akker ESA, Oepkes D. Fetal thrombocytopenia. *Semin Fetal Neonatal Med* 2008;**13**:223–30.

Risson DC, Davies MW, Williams BA. Review of neonatal alloimmune thrombocytopenia. *J Paediatr Child Health* 2012;**48**:816–22.

Roberts I, Murray NA. Neonatal thrombocytopenia. *Semin Fetal Neonatal Med* 2008;**13**:256–64.

Sola MC, Del Vecchio A, Rimsza LM. Evaluation and treatment of thrombocytopenia in the neonatal intensive care unit. *Clin Perinatol* 2000;**27**:655–79.

Wiedmeier SE, Henry E, Sola-Visner MC, *et al.* Platelet reference ranges for neonates, defined using data from over 47,000 patients in a multihospital healthcare system. *J Perinatol* 2009;**29**:130–6.

Use

Two types of vaccines are now available offering protection from some, but not all, forms of pneumococcal meningitis, septicaemia, pneumonia and otitis media.

Pneumococcal infection

A range of serious bacterial infections are caused by the encapsulated Gram-positive coccus, *Streptococcus pneumoniae*. 84 capsular forms have been identified, but 8–10 of these are responsible for 85% of the cases currently seen in the United Kingdom. It often causes community-acquired pneumonia and is now the most common cause of lethal or disabling bacterial meningitis. Patients with impaired immunity are at particular risk. Penicillin remains the drug of choice except in areas where the minimum inhibitory concentration for penicillin is now >2 micrograms/ml.

Infants at **high risk** include those with homozygous sickle cell disease, with no spleen (or a poorly functioning spleen) or with congenital or acquired immunodeficiency (including HIV infection). Such patients should be offered prophylactic antibiotics, because the current vaccines only offer protection from *some* of the capsular types of pneumococcal infection. They may also benefit from being given the multivalent plain polysaccharide vaccine when 2 years old, and such immunisation should also be offered to patients 2 weeks ahead of any planned splenectomy or chemotherapy.

Products

Plain polysaccharide vaccine: An unconjugated vaccine, active against 23 of the more commonly encountered capsular types of pneumococcal infection, has been available for some years. Because this vaccine offers relatively little protection when given to children under 2 years old, it has generally only been offered to adults and to older children considered to be at particularly high risk of infection.

Conjugate vaccine: A new 13-valent conjugated protein–polysaccharide vaccine (active against the 1, 3, 4, 5, 6A, 6B, 7F, 9V, 14, 18C, 19A, 19F and 23F strains) was introduced for use in young children in 2010. This has replaced the previous available 7-valent conjugated vaccine which caused a 70% decrease in invasive pneumococcal disease in young children in 3 years. While cases due to vaccine-related serotypes fell by almost 80%, disease was then largely caused by the extra 6 serotypes which are now covered by 13-valent conjugated vaccine.

Contraindications

Avoid immunisation during an acute infection and while pregnant. Patients already immunised with the plain 23-valent vaccine (or the earlier 12- or 14-valent vaccines) do not need to be re-immunised with the present 23-valent vaccine for 3–5 years.

Interactions

The conjugate vaccine can be given (into a different limb) at the same time as any other childhood vaccine, but parents who seem unhappy at the thought of their child facing more than one 'needle' at a single clinic visit can, if necessary, be offered a different staged plan. The plain vaccine should not be given until at least 8 weeks after the new conjugate vaccine has been given. Anaphylaxis is extremely unlikely – its management is discussed in the monograph on immunisation.

Administration

Plain vaccine: High-risk children (i.e. those with conditions listed in the second paragraph of 'Pneumococcal infection') who are 2 or more years old should still be offered a single 0.5 ml deep intramuscular injection of the plain 23-valent vaccine, because it provides broader protection from pneumococcal infection.

Conjugate vaccine: Young children who have not yet started their primary course of immunisation should be offered three 0.5 ml doses of the new conjugate 13-valent vaccine. Children in the United Kingdom are offered this when 2, 4 and 12 months old, and the WHO has now made use a priority in all countries where mortality is high.

Supply

Plain polysaccharide vaccine is available as 0.5 ml vials (Pneumovax II®) cost £8, whereas 0.5 ml vials of the conjugate vaccine (Prevenar13®) cost £49. A 10-valent conjugate vaccine (Synflorix®) is also available (cost £28) but is not as widely used. Always store at 4 °C.

Continued on p. 416

References

(See also the relevant Cochrane reviews and UK guidelines)

Ampofo K, Pavia AT, Chris S, *et al*. The changing epidemiology of invasive pneumococcal disease at a tertiary children's hospital through the 7-valent pneumococcal conjugate vaccine era: a case for continuous surveillance. *Pediatr Infect Dis J* 2012;**31**:228–34.

Cardoso MRA, Nascimento-Carvalho CM, Ferrero F, *et al*. Penicillin-resistant pneumococcus and risk of treatment failure in pneumonia. *Arch Dis Child* 2008;**93**:221–5.

Grijalva CG, Nuorti JP, Arbogast PG, *et al*. Decline in pneumonia admissions after routine childhood immunisation with pneumococcal conjugate vaccine in the USA: a time-series analysis. *Lancet* 2007;**369**:1179–86. (See also pp. 1144–5.)

Kaplan SL, Barson WJ, Lin PL, *et al*. Early trends for invasive pneumococcal infections in children after the introduction of the 13-valent pneumococcal conjugate vaccine. *Pediatr Infect Dis J* 2013;**32**:203–7.

O'Brien KL, Wolfon LJ, Watt JP, *et al*. Burden of disease caused by *Streptococcus pneumoniae* in children younger than 5 years: global estimates. *Lancet* 2009;**374**:893–902. (See also pp. 854–6.)

Sinha A, Levine O, Knoll MD, *et al*. Cost-effectiveness of pneumococcal conjugate vaccination in the prevention of child mortality: an international economic analysis. *Lancet* 2007;**369**:389–96. (See: www.gavialliance.org.)

Van der Poll T, Opal SM. Pathogenesis, treatment and prevention of pneumococcal pneumonia. *Lancet* 2009;**374**:1543–56.

Whitney CG, Pilishvilli T, Farley MM, *et al*. Effectiveness of seven-valent pneumococcal conjugate vaccine against invasive pneumococcal disease: a matched case-control study. *Lancet* 2006;**368**:149–502. (See also pp. 1469–70.)

Use
Polio vaccine gives lasting immunity to the three polio viruses.

Poliomyelitis
Poliomyelitis is a notifiable infectious illness that has now been eradicated from most of the world, but cases were still being recorded in Afghanistan, Chad, Ethiopia, northern India, Indonesia, Pakistan, Nigeria and Yemen in 2005. The World Health Organization launched a global 15-year plan to rid the world of this disease in 1988, and one country – northern Nigeria – now accounts for almost half of all the new cases being reported across the world each year. Infection may be clinically silent but may also produce aseptic meningitis and severe lasting paralysis. An injectable formaldehyde-inactivated triple-strain (Salk) vaccine first became available in 1958; a live, attenuated, triple-strain oral (Sabin) vaccine was introduced in 1962; and a more potent monovalent product was licensed for use in India in 2005. The Salk vaccine is now the only product used in North America and being used with increasing frequency in most parts of Europe (the Sabin vaccine was still used in the United Kingdom until September 2004). Overall, however, there is now a global move towards greater use of the inactivated Salk vaccine. The two products have, between them, certainly made the eventual global eradication of polio a realistic aim. While polio (and measles) could eventually, with sustained commitment and good management, be eradicated from the world, just as smallpox was in 1980, it is not proving easy.

Indications
Inactivated parenteral vaccine (IPV): With the arrival of a combined injectable vaccine that also offers protection from diphtheria, tetanus, whooping cough and *Haemophilus* (Hib) infection, this is now becoming the product of choice worldwide. Give three doses by intramuscular (IM) injection at least 4–8 weeks apart, starting at least 6 weeks (and usually 2 months) after birth. Because the live and inactivated products are interchangeable, there is nothing to stop the inactivated vaccine being used to complete a course of treatment started using the live, oral vaccine.
Live oral vaccine (OPV): Give three doses by mouth at monthly intervals (as with the inactivated vaccine). Remember however that children excrete the live virus in their stools for up to 6 weeks after immunisation, putting other unimmunised and immunocompromised patients and family contacts at risk. This product should never, therefore, be used in a maternity hospital setting. There is also a one in a million chance of the live, attenuated vaccine itself causing paralytic disease.

Contraindications
Early pregnancy, immunodeficiency, immunosuppression, reticuloendothelial malignancy and high-dose corticosteroid treatment (the equivalent of more than 1 mg/kg prednisolone a day or 2 mg/kg for more than 1 week in the last 6 weeks) are contraindications to the use of any live vaccine (but **not** for the inactivated polio vaccine (IPV)). Children should not be immunised while febrile or given the oral vaccine while suffering from diarrhoea or vomiting. For anaphylaxis (rare even with the IM product), see under immunisation.

Interactions
Polio vaccine can be given at the same time as other live and inactivated vaccines. The live vaccine should not, ideally, be given less than 3 weeks before or 3 months after a dose of normal immunoglobulin.

Administration
Inactivated vaccine: Give 0.5 ml by deep IM injection into any limb not simultaneously being used to give some other vaccine using a fresh syringe and a 25 mm, 23 gauge needle.
Oral live vaccine: The normal dose is three drops by mouth. Repeat if regurgitated. Older children have, traditionally, been offered the drops on a sugar cube.

Documentation
Tell the family doctor every time a child is immunised in hospital, and record what was done in the child's own personal health booklet. Community-based registers of vaccine uptake also need to be informed.

Continued on p. 418

Supply

The combined (DTaP/IPV/Hib) vaccine (Pediacel®) made by Aventis Pasteur is the IPV now used in the United Kingdom. Always shake each 0.5 ml vial before use. A monovalent inactivated vaccine is also available on request. The live oral polio vaccine (OPV) remains available in some countries in 10-dose containers (which should be discarded at the end of any session) and in 10× single-dose packs. Store all products in the dark at 2–8 °C.

References   (See also full UK website guidelines **DHUK**)

Advisory Committee on Immunization Practices. Updated ACIP recommendations regarding routine poliovirus vaccination. *Morb Mortal Wkly Rep* 2009;**58**:829–30.

American Academy of Pediatrics. Committee on Infectious Diseases. Poliomyelitis prevention: revised recommendations for use of only inactivated poliovirus vaccine for routine immunisation. *Pediatrics* 1999;**104**:1404–6.

Ehrenfeld E, Chumakov K. Monovalent oral poliovirus vaccines – a good tool but not a total solution. [Editorial] *N Engl J Med* 2008;**359**:1726–7.

Ehrenfeld E, Glass RI, Agol VI, *et al.* Immunisation against poliomyelitis: moving forward. *Lancet* 2008; **371**:1385–7.

Grassly NC, Wenger J, Durrani S, *et al.* Protective efficacy of a monovalent oral type 1 poliovirus vaccine: a case-control study. *Lancet* 2007;**369**:1356–62. (See also pp. 1320–2, and **370**:129–33.)

MacLennan C, MacLennan J. What threat from persistent vaccine-related poliovirus? *Lancet* 2005;**366**:351–3. (See also pp. 359–60 and 394–6.)

Thompson KM, Duintjer Tebbens RJ. Eradication versus control for poliomyelitis: an economic analysis. *Lancet* 2007;**369**:1363–71.

Use

Sodium and calcium polystyrene sulfonate are cation-exchange resins administered orally or rectally in the treatment of severe hyperkalaemia (plasma potassium ≥7.5 mmol/l). Intravenous (IV) salbutamol (q.v.) may provide a more immediate, and an IV glucose infusion with insulin (q.v.) a more reliable, way of achieving a sustained lowering of the plasma potassium level in the neonatal period by causing influx of potassium into cells. However, neither salbutamol nor glucose and insulin will remove potassium from the body.

Pharmacology

Sodium and calcium polystyrene sulfonate are cation-exchange resins used to draw potassium out of the body and into the gut in exchange for sodium or calcium, thus effecting the elimination of potassium from the body in the faeces. Faecal impaction has been reported following rectal administration in children, as have gastrointestinal concretions when the drug is given by mouth in early infancy, especially if there is already some degree of intestinal ileus for any reason.

Because none of the exchange resins are entirely selective for potassium, it is best to choose a calcium resin if the plasma calcium level is already low, since a sodium resin will further deplete the body's calcium. Calcium resin is also preferred if the plasma sodium level is already high, because the sodium resin can exacerbate hypernatraemia, which if it becomes severe (plasma sodium ≥160 mmol/l) may cause serious neurological damage. Each gram of sodium resin is capable, in practice, of extracting about 1 mmol of potassium from the body (as much as 3 mmol in theory). The equivalent weight of the calcium resin is marginally less effective.

Do not attempt *any* treatment for hyperkalaemia without first checking that the high plasma potassium level is not merely due to potassium leaking from damaged red cells ('haemolysis') into the plasma sample sent for laboratory analysis. Neonates seem to tolerate high plasma potassium levels much better than older patients, but treatment should be considered urgently if there are significant electrocardiographic changes. Correct any hypocalcaemia with 10% IV calcium gluconate (q.v.) and give 1 mmol/kg of IV sodium bicarbonate (q.v.) to reduce the risk of sudden, potentially life-threatening cardiac arrhythmia. IV or nebulised salbutamol and IV glucose and insulin are both capable of lowering plasma potassium levels more rapidly than any cation-exchange resin, but they do not rid the body of excess potassium. An exchange transfusion with *fresh* blood (or washed red cells), although it may take a little time to set up, is probably the best way of achieving a *sustained* fall in the plasma potassium level in the neonatal period, while a cation-exchange resin may be the more appropriate strategy in older children where bowel complications are less likely. Peritoneal dialysis, or haemodialysis, is an even better option in centres with the necessary expertise to do this, although such a strategy is usually only necessary when there is renal failure and/or fluid overload. Consider adrenal failure (usually due to congenital adrenal hyperplasia) if there is hyponatraemia, hypoglycaemia and/or hypotension, and treat as outlined in the monograph on hydrocortisone.

Treatment

Give 500 mg/kg as a retention enema. Ensure evacuation by colonic irrigation after 8–12 hours (6 hours in the case of Sorbisterit®) in order to ensure complete recovery of the resin. This is preferably done with the aid of X-ray image intensification. Treatment may be repeated after 12 hours if necessary. Double this dose can be employed in severe hyperkalaemia. Do *not* give polystyrene sulfonate resins orally in the neonatal period; they may, however, be considered in the same dose later on in conditions where dietary restriction of potassium impacts on nutritional intake. Monitor the plasma electrolytes to minimise the risk of overtreatment.

Supply and administration

Sodium polystyrene sulfonate (Resonium A®) is available as a powder costing about 15p per gram, and calcium polystyrene sulfonate (Calcium Resonium®), also as a powder, costs about 23p per gram. A further calcium polystyrene sulfonate preparation, Sorbisterit®, may also be available (cost 10p per gram), but this has a variable sucrose content (50–250 micrograms/g of powder). The sodium resin contains approximately 4.5 mmol of sodium per gram. Some pharmacies can prepare the enema in advance using a mixture of water and 9% methylcellulose (the latter acts as a faecal softener), but the resin can be prepared on the ward immediately prior to use if necessary using 6 ml/kg of water. In the United States, polystyrene sulfonate resins are usually made up in a solution of 25% sorbitol rather than in water and methylcellulose.

Continued on p. 420

References

Cameron JC, Kennedy D, Feber J, *et al.* Pretreatment of infant formula with sodium polystyrene sulfonate: focus on optimal amount and contact time. *Paediatr Drugs* 2013;**15**:43–8.

Filippi L, Cecchi A, Dani C, *et al.* Hypernatraemia induced by sodium polystyrene sulphonate (Kayexalate®) in two extremely low birth weight newborns. *Paediatr Anaesth* 2004;**14**:271–5.

Hu P-S, Su B-H, Peng C-T, *et al.* Glucose and insulin infusion versus kayexalate for the early treatment of non-oliguric hyperkalaemia in very-low-birth-weight infants. *Acta Paediatr Taiwan* 1999;**40**:314–8.

Malone TA. Glucose and insulin versus cation-exchange resin for the treatment of hyperkalaemia in very low birth weight infants. *J Pediatr* 1991;**118**:121–3.

Masilamani K, van der Voort J. The management of acute hyperkalaemia in neonates and children. *Arch Dis Child* 2012;**97**:376–80.

O'Hare FM, Molloy EJ. What is the best treatment for hyperkalaemia in a preterm infant? *Arch Dis Child Fetal Neonatal Ed* 2008;**93**:174–6. [SR]

Yaseen H, Khalaf M, Dana A, *et al.* Salbutamol versus cation-exchange resin (kayexalate) for the treatment of nonoliguric hyperkalemia in preterm infants. *Am J Perinatol* 2008;**25**:193–7.

Use

Potassium is an essential nutrient, and potassium chloride is often used to correct bodily depletion.

Pathophysiology

An intake of 2 mmol/kg of potassium per day is more than enough to meet all the body's normal needs. Breast milk, artificial milk formulae and standard neonatal parenteral nutrition solution (q.v.) all contain more than enough potassium to meet basic needs. Hypokalaemia in the neonatal period is more often the result of potassium redistribution than any true body deficit.

While urinary sodium loss (as summarised in the monograph on sodium chloride) can vary widely in the neonatal period, potassium loss seldom varies very much. Most healthy preterm and term babies remain in positive potassium balance throughout the neonatal period. Stressed, ventilator-dependent preterm babies sometimes show a raised renal potassium loss during the first 2 days of life, although this almost always resolves spontaneously within 3–4 days and seldom causes a serious fall in plasma level.

There are a few conditions associated with excessive renal potassium loss that can produce severe hypokalaemia. Some diuretics, if used for a sustained period, can induce significant urinary potassium loss, while chronic diarrhoea can also induce a significant body potassium deficit.

Potassium is the most important intracellular cation in the body, and a cellular deficit causes ileus, urinary retention, neuromuscular weakness and ECG changes (including ST segment depression, a low-voltage T wave and U wave changes). Alkalosis drives extracellular potassium into the cells, making the plasma level a poor marker of whole body depletion. Insulin (q.v.) can have a similar effect. Compartmental shifts are the most common cause of apparent neonatal hypokalaemia; true depletion requiring replacement is really quite rare. Overtreatment, on the other hand, can easily cause hyperkalaemia.

A dose of 3 mmol/kg has been used to cause immediate cardiac asystole in those rare situations where fetocide is deemed necessary.

Treatment

Oral treatment: This is the preferred route for correcting any potassium deficit. Start with a total of 2 mmol/kg a day given in a series of small divided doses with feeds to minimise gastric irritation. The oral rehydration fluid (q.v.) recommended by the World Health Organization provides both the simplest and the quickest way of correcting the salt and fluid loss caused by diarrhoea.

Intravenous treatment: Correct any true body deficit slowly over 1–2 days, using a solution that does not contain more than 40 mmol of potassium per litre, given at a rate of no more than 0.2 mmol/kg/hour (a higher rate of up to 0.5 mmol/kg/hour may rarely be justified if there is severe potassium depletion). Exceptionally, for example, in the fluid-restricted baby, 80 mmol of potassium per litre may be given via a central line. ECG monitoring is recommended during infusion in some centres. Concentrated solutions can cause thrombophlebitis and pain at the injection site, while extravasation can cause tissue necrosis. *Always check the dose carefully: an overdose can be rapidly fatal.*

Supply and administration

A sugar-free oral 7.5% solution of potassium chloride (Kay-Cee-L®) containing 1 mmol (75 mg) per millilitre is available from the pharmacy on request (100 ml costs £1.40).

10 ml ampoules of strong 15% potassium chloride contain 1.5 g (or ~20 mmol) of potassium for intravenous (IV) use usually stored with the controlled drugs in most units. These cost 48p each. Note that ampoules are also available in a range of *other* strengths. Strong potassium chloride must normally be *diluted at least 50-fold* with 0.9% sodium chloride (or a mixture of 0.9% sodium chloride in glucose) prior to administration.

For peripheral line administration, dilute prior to use to 1 mmol in 25 ml (40 mmol/l); in fluid-restricted babies, a more concentrated solution of 1 mmol in 12.5 ml (80 mmol/l) may be given via **a central line** only. The resultant solution should be mixed with some care in order to make quite sure that the potassium does not separate or 'layer' out prior to administration.

The inadvertent use of potassium chloride instead of sodium chloride during the reconstitution of other IV drugs has caused several deaths. There are strong grounds for insisting that all potassium chloride ampoules should be stored well away from all other routinely used ampoules. Many hospitals keep all such ampoules with the controlled drugs.

Continued on p. 422

References

Brem AS. Electrolyte disorders associated with respiratory distress syndrome and bronchopulmonary dysplasia. *Clin Perinatol* 1992;**19**:223–32.

Engle WD, Arant BS Jr. Urinary potassium excretion in the critically ill neonate. *Pediatrics* 1984;**74**:259–64.

John E, Klavdianou M, Vidyasagar D. Electrolyte problems in neonatal surgical patients. *Clin Perinatol* 1989;**16**:219–32.

Tubman M, Majumdar SR, Lee D, *et al.* Best practices for safe handling of products containing concentrated potassium. *Br Med J* 2005;**331**:274–7.

Use

Praziquantel is an oral anthelminthic that was originally discovered by Merck during the 1970s while screening for tranquilisers. It was later co-developed with Bayer (Germany) and became available in 1979. It has been the mainstay of schistosomiasis control programs for decades. Despite widespread use in older children and adults, it is only recently that attention has turned to the treatment of infants and preschool children. A mistaken assumption that preschool children (under 5 years) are at low risk for infection because they have little direct contact with schistosome cercariae-infested water has led to a 'treatment gap' in this group of children, and initial registrations of this drug with the FDA and other drug safety agencies excluded them from the product license. This was addressed, in part, in 2012 when the WHO formally recognised that infants and preschool children are at significant risk of schistosomiasis and thus qualify for treatment with praziquantel; however, there are few suitable formulations available.

Praziquantel, when taken with albendazole (q.v.), is also highly effective in the treatment of intestinal, liver and lung fluke infections including those due to *Fasciolopsis buski*, *Metagonimus yokogawai*, *Heterophyes heterophyes*, *Clonorchis sinensis*, *Echinostoma* spp., *Opisthorchis viverrini*, *O. felineus* and various species of *Paragonimus*.

Schistosomiasis

Schistosomiasis is a tropical disease also known as bilharzia after Theodor Bilharz. It is caused by blood-dwelling trematodes (flatworms) of the genus *Schistosoma* and is estimated to affect over 200 million people in tropical countries, 20 million of whom have severe illness. *S. haematobium*, *S. mansoni* and *S. intercalatum* are found in sub-Saharan Africa. *S. mansoni* is also endemic in parts of South America and the Caribbean. *S. japonicum* infection occurs in China, the Philippines and parts of Indonesia, while *S. mekongi* is found in Cambodia and Laos. Although the mortality rate is low, schistosomiasis is a chronic illness that can damage internal organs and, in children, impair growth and cognitive development. The urinary form of schistosomiasis is associated with increased risks for bladder cancer in adults. *S. mansoni*, *S. japonicum*, *S. intercalatum* and *S. mekongi* cause intestinal disease, whereas *S. haematobium* causes urinary disease. Schistosome transmission requires contamination of water by faeces or urine containing eggs, a specific freshwater snail as intermediate host and human contact with water inhabited by the intermediate host snail. Acute schistosomiasis (Katayama syndrome) can present as fever, malaise, myalgia, fatigue, non-productive cough, diarrhoea (with or without blood), haematuria (when the infection is due to *S. haematobium*) and right upper quadrant pain. Chronic and advanced disease results from the host's immune response to deposition of schistosome eggs in tissues and the granulomatous reaction to antigens they secrete.

Pharmacology

The commercial preparation of praziquantel is a racemic mixture, of which only the 'laevo' isomer has schistosomicidal activity either *in vivo* or *in vitro*. It is rapidly absorbed when taken orally; it undergoes first-pass metabolism. Over 80% of the dose is excreted as metabolites in the urine within 24 hours. Trematode worms, in contrast, absorb praziquantel through calcium channels but cannot metabolise it. They contract immediately after exposure and gradually disintegrate. While the drug is effective against most stages in the life cycle of the schistosome, juvenile worms are harder to eradicate, and this may be a factor in the poor cure rates and treatment failures observed in some areas.

Maternal disease

In 2002, the WHO reversed its previous decision to exclude pregnant and lactating women from eradication programmes on the basis that the balance of risk supported including pregnant and lactating women in such mass treatment programmes. The Entebbe Mother and Baby Study found praziquantel adversely affected the incidence of eczema among infants of mothers with *S. mansoni*. Only small levels of praziquantel appear in breast milk. Expert opinion holds that lactation should not be a contraindication to maternal treatment. Minimisation of the infant's exposure can be achieved by giving a dose just before the infant's longest sleep period if expressed stored breast milk or formula milk cannot be safely substituted for 48 hours after administration.

Treatment

Maternal treatment: 20 mg/kg followed after 4–6 hours by one further dose of 20 mg/kg (20 mg/kg given three times on 1 day for *S. japonicum* infections).

Continued on p. 424

Infant treatment: 40 mg/kg of either tablet or syrup (see under 'Supply'). The tablet (or portion of tablet) may be swallowed whole or crushed prior to administration.

Supply
Bayer makes praziquantel tablets in Germany. These are available as scored 600 mg tablets that can easily be broken into ½ or ¼ tablets aiming to give the child a dose within the 'acceptable' range of 30–60 mg/kg. A liquid formulation containing 600 mg in 5 ml is made by the Egyptian International Pharmaceutical Industries Company (EIPICO), but the aniseed taste can be off-putting for children and supplies are known to be variable due to its *ad hoc* production. A public–private partnership between Merck, Astellas Pharma, the Swiss Tropical and Public Health Institute and TI Pharma are currently developing an alternative suitable for children aged 3 months to 6 years that will enter clinical development by 2014.

References
(See also the relevant Cochrane reviews)

Castro N, Medina R, Sotelo J, *et al*. Bioavailability of praziquantel increases with concomitant administration of food. *Antimicrob Agents Chemother* 2000;**44**:2903–4.

Coulibaly JT, N'gbesso YK, Knopp S, *et al*. Efficacy and safety of praziquantel in preschool-aged children in an area co-endemic for *Schistosoma mansoni* and *S. haematobium*. *PLoS Negl Trop Dis* 2012a;**6**:e1917.

Coulibaly JT, N'gbesso YK, Knopp S, *et al*. Performance and safety of praziquantel for treatment of intestinal schistosomiasis in infants and preschool children. *PLoS Negl Trop Dis* 2012b;**6**:e1917.

Doenhoff MJ, Cioli D, Utzinger J. Praziquantel: mechanisms of action, resistance and new derivatives for schistosomiasis. *Curr Opin Infect Dis* 2008;**21**:659–67.

Elliott AM, Mpairwe H, Quigley MA, *et al*. Helminth infection during pregnancy and development of infantile eczema. *JAMA* 2005;**294**:2032–4.

Elliott AM, Ndibazza J, Mpairwe H, *et al*. Treatment with anthelminthics during pregnancy: what gains and what risks for the mother and child? *Parasitology* 2011;**138**:1499–507.

Gray DJ, Ross AG, Li YS, *et al*. Diagnosis and management of schistosomiasis. *Br Med J* 2011;**342**:d2651.

Hotez PJ, Savioli L, Fenwick A. Neglected tropical diseases of the Middle East and North Africa: review of their prevalence, distribution, and opportunities for control. *PLoS Negl Trop Dis* 2012;**6**:e1475.

Olds GR. Administration of praziquantel to pregnant and lactating women. *Acta Trop* 2003;**86**:185–95.

Stothard JR, Sousa-Figueiredo JC, Betson M, *et al*. Closing the praziquantel treatment gap: new steps in epidemiological monitoring and control of schistosomiasis in African infants and preschool-aged children. *Parasitology* 2011;**138**:1593–606.

Stothard JR, Sousa-Figueiredo JC, Betson M, *et al*. Schistosomiasis in African infants and preschool children: let them now be treated! *Trends Parasitol* 2013;**29**:197–205.

Wu W, Wang W, Huang YX. New insight into praziquantel against various developmental stages of schistosomes. *Parasitol Res* 2011;**109**:1501–7.

Use

Probiotics can be used to restore a healthy balance of bowel microorganisms in individuals troubled by diarrhoea. Several controlled trials have also shown that use reduces the risk of necrotising enterocolitis (NEC). Maternal use during pregnancy and lactation seems safe and may help to 'normalise' the range of bacteria present in the vagina, but has not yet been shown to reduce the risk of preterm birth.

Microbiological issues

Interest in the use of lactic acid-producing bacteria to retain or restore a healthy balance of microorganisms in the gut has grown steadily in the last 20 years, and commercially available live cultures of these organisms are now often called 'probiotics'. *Lactobacillus delbrueckii* subsp. *bulgaricus* (formerly known as *L. bulgaricus* and which occurs in naturally soured milk) was the first organism to be widely studied, but this does not grow well in the human gut. Various other lactobacilli including *L. acidophilus*, a normal commensal of the gut, and *L. casei* are now more commonly used. Other organisms studied include *Saccharomyces boulardii, Streptococcus thermophilus* and various *Bifidobacterium* species.

Early studies focused on the ability of these microbial supplements to re-establish a more normal bowel flora in children suffering for serious diarrhoea, and other studies looked to see if use could enhance growth in early infancy. More recently, studies have, more importantly, looked to see whether early prophylactic use can minimise the risk of excessive, unbalanced, early colonisation of the gut by potentially pathogenic organisms in the vulnerable preterm baby. The few trials done as yet to see whether use can reduce disease severity in babies with severe atopic dermatitis have had inconsistent outcomes.

Sustained close contact with the mother helps the normal baby acquire a balance of healthy gut bacteria at birth, as can breastfeeding. The gut of the unfed, antibiotic-treated, preterm baby is at high risk of being colonised by potentially pathogenic bacteria, and this may be one of the main factors that render the baby vulnerable to NEC. Reduced gut blood flow in the period immediately before and after birth (which is particularly common after intra-uterine growth restriction) puts the baby at even greater risk. Serious NEC currently occurs in about 7% of babies born at gestations ≤28 weeks and is one of the most common causes of death after the respiratory problems seen in the first week of life. Even in survivors, the need for surgery, and for further respiratory support, can have a serious impact on subsequent growth and development, especially if surgery involved the removal of a significant length of the gut. The use of breast milk seems to reduce the risk of NEC. Hope is rising that probiotic priming, and the more consistent use of breast milk, could greatly reduce the incidence of NEC; however, there are several unanswered questions in relation to dose, timing and species as well as concerns about long-term effects on the developing intestinal ecosystem. These concerns are likely to remain until large, multicentre trials adequately designed to address safety are completed.

Prophylactic neonatal use

While it is increasingly clear that treatment is beneficial in babies ≤30 weeks' gestation, the best product to use is not yet clear. A 125 mg/kg dose of Infloran® (a mixture of *L. acidophilus* and *Bifidobacterium bifidum*) was given twice a day in the two largest trials reported to date. Start prophylaxis as soon as feeds are started, and give for 6 weeks. Other studies have reported the use of five drops (containing 10^8 colony-forming units) of BioGaia ProTectis® which contains *Lactobacillus reuteri*. The PiPS (trial of probiotic administered early to prevent infection and NEC) is using 10^9 colony-forming units of *Bifidobacterium breve* strain BBG.

Supply and administration

Infloran is imported into the United Kingdom from Austria by IDIS World Medicines. Twenty 250 mg capsules (which should be stored at 4 °C) cost £14. Mix half the content of one capsule with milk immediately before it is given. The Infloran capsule is stable for 24 hours after accessing the powder inside; therefore, one capsule can be used for two doses in a 24-hour period. BioGaia ProTectis® is available direct from the manufacturer and a number of pharmacies (cost £15 for 5 ml).

References   (See also the relevant Cochrane reviews) ◑

Braga TD, da Silva GA, de Lira PI, *et al*. Efficacy of *Bifidobacterium breve* and *Lactobacillus casei* oral supplementation on necrotizing enterocolitis in very-low-birth-weight preterm infants: a double-blind, randomized, controlled trial. *Am J Clin Nutr* 2011;**93**:81–6. [RCT]

Continued on p. 426

Deshpande G, Rao S, Keil A, *et al.* Evidence-based guidelines for use of probiotics in preterm neonates. *BMC Med* 2011;**9**:92–105.

Deshpande G, Rao S, Patole S. Probiotics for prevention of necrotising enterocolitis in preterm neonates with very low birth weight: a systematic review of randomised controlled trials. *Lancet* 2007;**369**:1614–20. [SR] (See also pp. 1578–80.)

Deshpande G, Rao S, Patole S, *et al.* Updated meta-analysis of probiotics for preventing necrotizing enterocolitis in preterm neonates. *Pediatrics* 2010;**125**:921–30. [SR]

Embleton ND, Yates R. Probiotics and other preventative strategies for necrotising enterocolitis. *Semin Fetal Neonatal Med* 2008;**13**:35–43.

Fallon EM, Nehra D, Potemkin AK, *et al.* A.S.P.E.N. clinical guidelines: nutrition support of neonatal patients at risk for necrotizing enterocolitis. *JPEN J Parenter Enteral Nutr* 2012;**36**:506–23.

Jenke A, Ruf A-M, Hoppe T, *et al.* Bifidobacterium septicaemia in an extremely low-birthweight infant under probiotic therapy. *Arch Dis Child Fetal Neonatal Ed* 2012;**97**:F217–8.

Kitajima H, Sumida Y, Tanaka R, *et al.* Early administration of *Bifidobacterium breve* to preterm infants: randomised controlled trial. *Arch Dis Child Fetal Neonatal Ed* 1997;**76**:F101–7. [RCT]

Manzoni P, Mostert M, Leonessa ML, *et al.* Oral supplementation with *Lactobacillus casei* subspecies *rhamnosus* prevents enteric colonization by *Candida species* in preterm neonates: a randomized study. *Clin Infect Dis* 2006;**42**:1735–42. [RCT]

Van Neil CW, Feudtner C, Garrison MM, *et al.* Lactobacillus therapy for acute infectious diarrhea in children: a meta-analysis. *Pediatrics* 2002;**109**:678–84. [SR]

Use

Progesterone may be used to augment low endogenous levels during the luteal phase in some women undergoing induction of ovulation or assisted conception. This may be continued into the first trimester. Several trials are currently studying prophylactic use in women with a previous history of preterm labour, or who are found, during mid-pregnancy screening, to have an unusually short cervix. As yet, the RCOG only recommends using progesterone in high-risk women as part of clinical trials.

Pharmacology

The chemical structure of progesterone, a natural hormone produced by the ovary's corpus luteum, was first determined in 1934. It was synthesised artificially soon afterwards and used, intermittently, for many years to treat various menstrual disorders despite very little objective evidence of benefit. It has also been intermittently used, since 1960, to reduce the risk of miscarriage. While there was no evidence that it reduces the general miscarriage rate in a Cochrane review of 14 small trials in 2003, there did seem to be a case for mounting a further trial in women who had already suffered at least three miscarriages. The PROMISE study (first trimester progesterone therapy in women with a history of unexplained recurrent miscarriage) is due to publish its data in October 2014.

A systematic review undertaken in 1990 suggested that progesterone might also have a role in reducing the risk of preterm labour in women with a strong prior history of this problem, and interest in this approach to the prevention of recurrent preterm labour has increased significantly in recent years. Some early small trials suggested that use reduced the risk of preterm birth in women who have already experienced preterm birth, but larger trials failed to replicate these findings. In one trial where mid-pregnancy screening revealed a very short cervix (≤15 mm), use almost halved delivery before 34 weeks, and a retrospective review also suggested beneficial effect in women with a mid-trimester cervical length of <28 mm. Although a reduction in preterm birth seems attractive, there is little evidence as yet for short-term benefit to the baby, even if progesterone does prevent preterm delivery. Furthermore, there is no evidence of long-term benefit for the baby. This may not just be 'absence of evidence' as it is becoming increasingly recognised that a delay in delivery could have negative effects if the fetus remains in an adverse intrauterine environment. Treatment is not effective in twin pregnancy.

Warnings about exposure to any progestogen in early pregnancy were issued in the 1960s after reports appeared saying that this could cause masculinisation of the female fetus, but it seems, in retrospect, that most cases were caused by exposure to norethisterone rather than progesterone. There would seem to be a threefold increase in the risk of second- or third-degree hypospadias in boys after first trimester use, but later use does not seem to be associated with any general excess of congenital abnormality. Use as a contraceptive during breastfeeding found no evidence effect on lactation, and the effects of progesterone on the breastfed infant are believed to be minimal due to the poor oral bioavailability. Gynaecomastia has been reported on rare occasions.

Management of infertility due to inadequate luteal phase

Vaginal gel (containing progesterone 90 mg per application) may be used either after documented ovulation or on day 18–21 of cycle. In some centres, after *in vitro* fertilisation, daily application of the gel is continued for 30 days after laboratory evidence of pregnancy. An intramuscular (IM) preparation or vaginal capsule (containing 200 mg) may also be offered as an alternative after *in vitro* fertilisation or gamete intra-fallopian transfer.

Prophylaxis in a singleton pregnancy

Nightly insertion of a 200 mg progesterone capsule into the vagina from the 24th to the 34th week of pregnancy nearly halved the risk of preterm birth in women found to have a short cervix on mid-pregnancy screening in one recent trial. 250 mg depot injections of hydroxyprogesterone caproate given IM once a week from the 20th to the 36th week of pregnancy reduced the risk of recurrent preterm delivery in one small trial.

Supply and administration

Vaginal gel: Vaginal gel applicators containing 90 mg of progesterone (Crinone®) cost approximately £2 each.

Continued on p. 428

Vaginal capsules: Capsules containing 200 mg of micronised progesterone (Utrogestan®) cost £1 each. These contain arachis (peanut) oil.

IM prophylaxis: 1 and 2 ml ampoules containing 50 mg/ml of progesterone (Gestone®) cost £4.50 each

References

(See also the relevant Cochrane reviews)

Borna S, Sahabi N. Progesterone for maintenance tocolytic therapy after threatened preterm labour: a randomised controlled trial. *Aust N Z J Obstet Gynaecol* 2008;**48**:58–63. [RCT]

Conde-Agudelo A, Romero R, Nicolaides K, *et al.* Vaginal progesterone vs. cervical cerclage for the prevention of preterm birth in women with a sonographic short cervix, previous preterm birth, and singleton gestation: a systematic review and indirect comparison metaanalysis. *Am J Obstet Gynecol* 2013;**208**:42.e1–8. [SR]

Daya S. Efficacy of progesterone support for pregnancy in women with recurrent miscarriage: a meta-analysis of controlled trials. *Br J Obstet Gynecol* 1989;**96**:275–80. [SR]

DeFranco EA, O'Brien JM, Adair CD, *et al.* Vaginal progesterone is associated with a decrease in the risk of early preterm birth and improved neonatal outcome in women with a short cervix: a secondary analysis from a randomized, double blind, placebo-controlled trial. *Ultrasound Obstet Gynecol* 2007;**30**:697–705. [RCT]

Fonseca EB, Celik E, Parra M, *et al.* Progesterone and the risk of preterm birth among women with a short cervix. *N Engl J Med* 2007;**357**:462–9. [RCT] (See also pp. 498–501)

Hassan SS, Romero R, Vidyadhari D, *et al.* Vaginal progesterone reduces the rate of preterm birth in women with a sonographic short cervix: a multicenter, randomized, double-blind, placebo-controlled trial. *Ultrasound Obstet Gynecol* 2011;**38**:18–31. [RCT]

Nath A, Sitruk-Ware R. Progesterone vaginal ring for contraceptive use during lactation. *Contraception* 2010;**82**:428–34.

Norman JE, Mackenzie F, Owen P, *et al.* Progesterone for the prevention of preterm birth in twin pregnancy (STOPPIT): a randomised, double blind, placebo-controlled study and meta-analysis. *Lancet* 2009;**373**:2034–40. [RCT] (See also pp. 2000–2.)

Pabuccu R, Akar ME. Luteal phase support in assisted reproductive technology. *Curr Opin Obstet Gynecol* 2005;**17**:277–81.

Rouse DJ, Caritis SN, O'Brien JM, *et al.* Progesterone vaginal gel for the reduction of recurrent preterm birth: primary results from a randomized, double-blind, placebo-controlled trial. *Ultrasound Obstet Gynecol* 2007;**30**:687–96. [RCT]

Use
A dose of chloroquine (q.v.) once a week was for many years the most widely used strategy for preventing malaria, but a combination of weekly chloroquine and daily proguanil is now the more widely recommended option. Proguanil with atovaquone, or mefloquine (q.v.), is now the strategy that has to be used for prophylaxis in many parts of the world where most parasites have become resistant to chloroquine.

Pharmacology
Proguanil is a biguanide first developed in the United Kingdom during World War II as the result of a collaboration instigated by the MRC's Joint Chemotherapy Committee. It is rapidly absorbed when taken orally and quickly metabolised in the liver to the active metabolite cycloguanil. Both are then excreted largely in the urine (the somewhat variable half-life in adults being about 20 hours).

Atovaquone is an antiprotozoal developed in the early 1990s that is sometimes used to prevent or treat *Pneumocystis* infection in patients unable to tolerate co-trimoxazole (q.v.) and, along with proguanil, in the prevention and treatment of malaria. It has a plasma half-life of 2–3 days (probably because of enterohepatic recycling) before it is excreted largely unchanged in the stool. Almost nothing is yet known about the use of atovaquone during pregnancy or lactation.

Malarone® is a widely used fixed combination tablet of proguanil hydrochloride with atovaquone.

Other prophylactic strategies
Nets impregnated with permethrin offer substantial night-time protection. Diethyltoluamide (DEET) sprays and lotions are effective for 5–10 hours. Use a formulation with <30% DEET to minimise the risk of toxicity. Long sleeves and trousers lessen the risk after dusk.

Prophylaxis
In pregnancy: Malaria can be a devastating disease during pregnancy, and prophylaxis with proguanil is known to be of considerable value in areas where infection is endemic. Side effects are minimal with the standard prophylactic dose (200 mg once a day), and there is no evidence of teratogenicity. Consider giving a daily folate supplement as well. More needs to be learnt about maternal use during lactation, but use certainly exposes the baby to much less drug than would result from standard prophylactic treatment (5 mg/kg once a day). Less is known about combined use with atovaquone, one retrospective study suggests that it is not a major teratogen, and most would argue that the combination should only be employed if no other alternative is available. No authority has yet recommended the use of Malarone during lactation.

In infancy: Start giving Malarone once a day 1–2 days before entering any area where malaria is prevalent and continue treatment for 1 week after leaving. It is probably safe to give children weighing at least 6 kg half of one paediatric tablet (i.e. 12.5 mg of proguanil and ~41 mg of atovaquone) if the risk of infection is high but better to use other strategies to avoid exposure and treat any signs of infection promptly if these do occur. Children weighing over 10 kg can certainly take one crushed tablet once a day.

Treatment
One option is to give any small child with overt signs of infection two crushed tablets of the paediatric strength Malarone once a day for 3 days. There is little experience of treating babies weighing <5 kg as yet.

Supply
Proguanil: Scored 100 mg tablets (which only cost 9p) can be quartered, crushed and administered on a spoon or down a nasogastric tube. A suspension could be prepared, but its 'shelf life' is not yet certain, and there is no evidence that the greater precision this might offer is important.

Proguanil with atovaquone: Malarone® provides an alternative approach to prophylaxis and treatment, but the manufacturers have not yet recommended prophylactic use in early infancy. The standard paediatric tablet (which may be crushed and mixed with food or milky drink) contains 25 mg of proguanil hydrochloride, and 62.5 mg of atovaquone costs 52p. No suspension exists.

Continued on p. 430

References

Gilveray G, Looareesuwan S, White NJ, *et al.* The pharmacokinetics of atovaquone and proguanil in pregnancy in women with acute falciparum malaria. *Eur J Clin Pharmacol* 2003;**59**:545–52.

Lell B, Luckner D, Ndjavé M, *et al.* Randomised placebo-controlled study of atovaquone plus proguanil for malaria prophylaxis in children. *Lancet* 1998;**351**:709–13. [RCT]

Marra F, Salzman JR, Ensom MH, *et al.* Atovaquone-proguanil for prophylaxis and treatment of malaria. *Ann Pharmacother* 2003;**37**:1266–75.

Nakato H, Vivancos R, Hunter PR. A systematic review and meta-analysis of the effectiveness and safety of atovaquone-proguanil (Malarone) for chemoprophylaxis against malaria. *J Antimicrob Chemother* 2007;**60**:929–36. [SR]

Taylor WRJ, White NJ. Antimalarial drug toxicity: a review. *Drug Saf* 2004;**27**:25–61.

Pasternak B, Hviid A. Atovaquone-proguanil use in early pregnancy and the risk of birth defects. *Arch Intern Med* 2011;**171**:259–60.

Use

Propofol is a rapid-acting intravenous anaesthetic. Adults needing intensive care are often sedated with a continuous infusion, but serious (sometimes lethal) metabolic complications were encountered when this strategy was used in children. Pain control requires an opiate, such as remifentanil (q.v.), as well.

Pharmacology

Propofol is a clear colourless insoluble phenolic compound supplied in an isotonic, oil-in-water, lipid emulsion that came into use as a useful short-acting IV anaesthetic in 1984. It is unrelated, chemically, to any other anaesthetic agent but behaves rather like ketamine (q.v.). Recovery from propofol is, however, rather more rapid, and 'hangovers' are less common. The drug is rapidly redistributed into fat and other body tissues and more than half leaves the circulation within 10 minutes even after neonatal IV administration (V_D ~4 l/kg). Propofol is then conjugated and metabolised in the liver. The elimination half-life in older children is 5–10 hours although, with sustained use, elimination from deep stores may take 2–3 days. In neonates, propofol mainly undergoes hydroxylation to quinol metabolites with only limited glucuronidation. Clearance in neonates is ~32% that in 1-year-olds, and while there is some general correlation between clearance and both post-menstrual and postnatal age, there is considerable inter-individual variability.

Propofol crosses the placenta readily but is neither teratogenic nor fetotoxic in animals. The manufacturers do not recommend use during pregnancy or delivery, although it is used during caesarean section. Substantial quantities appear in breast milk, but a baby taking milk from the breast 12 hours after the mother's delivery under propofol anaesthesia would ingest <1% of the weight-related maternal dose. It was thought to be the cause for green discolouration of breast milk in one woman.

There is significant inter-individual variability in the pharmacokinetics of propofol in neonates, and its use has led to transient decreases in heart rate and oxygen saturation and more prolonged (60 minutes) hypotension even in what might be considered standard doses in older children. The drug was used as a sedative in paediatric intensive care for 15 years before any controlled trials were undertaken, and it was several years before reports of unexpected metabolic acidosis, and rhabdomyolysis, with sudden life-threatening cardiac and renal failure started to appear. It is now clear that prolonged infusion can sometimes cause a myopathy due to impaired fatty acid oxidation in patients of *any* age which is only reversible by stopping treatment at once and offering prompt haemoperfusion. Maintaining a generous glucose infusion may make this hazard less likely by limiting the tendency of the body to mobilise energy stores from fat.

Use during neonatal intubation

2.5 mg/kg of propofol given IV over 10 seconds will usually cause relaxation without apnoea and render the baby oblivious to the stress of intubation, but some babies need a second dose. The addition of a 3 micrograms/kg bolus of remifentanil can be used to provide pain-free working conditions within 90 seconds, but this can cause brief apnoea, and intubation on its own should cause relatively little pain.

Use for continuous IV sedation or anaesthesia

Maintenance anaesthesia: Anaesthesia for any procedure lasting >10–15 minutes requires a maintenance infusion of propofol. Evidence suggests that this should **never** be given to any young child at a rate exceeding 4 mg/kg/hour. Where (as is often the case) this fails to provide adequate pain relief, an opiate, such as remifentanil, should be given as well – the dose of propofol should not be increased.

Prolonged sedation: Propofol is now widely used to provide sustained sedation for older patients requiring intensive care, but it should **not** be used in this way, especially in children <3 years old because there is a small, but currently unpredictable, risk of sudden 'propofol infusion syndrome' collapse.

Precautions

Propofol use must be supervised by an experienced anaesthetist/intensivist, and recovery monitored until it is complete.

Continued on p. 432

Supply and administration

20 ml ampoules of a 0.5% IV emulsion (contains 5 mg/ml) cost £3.50. This may be administered undiluted or diluted to a concentration not <1 mg/ml with 5% glucose or 0.9% sodium chloride. Store ampoules at room temperature, shake before use, and do not freeze. The lipid content makes it important to protect any line used for sustained infusion from microbial contamination.

References

Allegaert K, de Hoon J, Verbesselt R, *et al.* Maturational pharmacokinetics of single intravenous bolus of propofol. *Pediatr Anesth* 2007a;**17**:1028–34.

Allegaert K, Peeters MY, Verbesselt R, *et al.* Inter-individual variability in propofol pharmacokinetics in preterm and term neonates. *Br J Anaesth* 2007b;**99**:864–70.

Birkholz T, Eckardt G, Renner S, *et al.* Green breast milk after propofol administration. *Anesthesiology* 2009;**111**:1168–9.

Cornfield DN, Tegtmeyer K, Nelson MD, *et al.* Continuous propofol infusion in 142 critically ill children. *Pediatrics* 2002;**110**:1177–81.

Ghanta S, Abdel-Latif ME, Lui K, *et al.* Propofol compared with the morphine, atropine, and suxamethonium regimen as induction agents for neonatal endotracheal intubation: a randomized, controlled trial. *Pediatrics* 2007;**119**:e1248–55. [RCT]

Kam PCA, Cardone D. Propofol infusion syndrome. *Anaesthesia* 2007;**62**:690–701. [SR]

Meyer S, Grundmann U, Gottschling S, *et al.* Sedation and analgesia for brief diagnostic and therapeutic procedures in children. *Eur J Pediatr* 2007;**166**:291–302.

Tsui BCH, Wagner A, Usher AG, *et al.* Combined propofol and remifentanil anesthesia for pediatric patients undergoing magnetic resonance imaging. *Pediatr Anesth* 2005;**15**:397–401.

Use

Oral propranolol is used to manage hypercyanotic spells in tetralogy of Fallot, in neonatal thyrotoxicosis and (with hydralazine) in the control of dangerous hypertension. It is sometimes used to control arrhythmia, to manage the long QT syndromes, and, recently, has seen an expanding role in the management of severe infantile haemangiomas.

Pharmacology

Propranolol hydrochloride was the first non-selective β-adrenoreceptor blocking agent. It reduces the rate and force of contraction of the heart and slows cardiac conduction. The hypotension and bradycardia seen with an overdose are best treated with glucagon (q.v.). Respiratory depression and fits can also occur. Caution is essential when the drug is used in the presence of heart failure. The half-life in children and adults is 3–6 hours; the neonatal half-life is substantially longer at 14–15½ hours.

Propranolol has been used extensively during pregnancy for the treatment of maternal hypertension, arrhythmia and migraine headache. Use is generally considered safe. Propranolol crosses the placenta. Use during the second and third trimesters has been associated with fetal growth restriction, and the exposed fetus may display signs of β-blockade after delivery. Propranolol passes into breast milk in small amounts that do not cause any clinically significant effects in the breastfed infant.

Propranolol can be given by intravenous (IV) injection the initial management of arrhythmia and cyanotic 'spells'. Patients started on IV propranolol will need significantly more once oral treatment is started because of high first-pass liver metabolism.

Neonatal thyrotoxicosis

This rare but potentially fatal disorder, seen in 1–2% of the offspring of mothers with Graves' disease, results from the transplacental passage of thyrotropin receptor antibody. Neonatal problems are most frequently seen in babies of mothers with a high antibody titre. This can occur even after the mother has been rendered medically or surgically euthyroid. Propylthiouracil (5 mg/kg every 12 hours) should be given to symptomatic babies. Propranolol is a further mainstay of treatment in severe cases. It may need to be continued for 3–12 weeks after delivery. Lugol iodine (which contains 130 mg/ml of iodine) provides the most easily obtained source of iodine for inhibiting thyroid function. Sedation is occasionally called for. Always seek the advice of an experienced paediatric endocrinologist if symptoms are severe.

Infantile haemangiomas

Infantile haemangiomas are the most common vascular tumours of childhood and affect ~5% of all infants. Although most proliferate and then spontaneously involute with minimal consequences, a small minority can be disfiguring, functionally significant or, rarely, life-threatening. Until recently, corticosteroids were the mainstay of treatment, but these are not without side effects. Indeed, it was after one infant developed complications from the steroids used to treat a haemangioma that the beneficial effects of propranolol were fortuitously discovered; the initiation of propranolol to treat that infant's cardiomyopathy resulted in rapid flattening and fading of the haemangioma. More than 170 reports and studies have subsequently appeared. Systematic review of 41 of these studies showed a response rate, defined as an improvement after starting treatment, of 98% (range 82–100%). Given that many would involute anyway, it is easy to be sceptical; however, evidence from one small randomised trial supports the fact that propranolol speeds the natural resolution, at least in infants.

Although propranolol seems efficacious, side effects are cause for concern in some infants; these include symptomatic hypoglycaemia, hypotension, wheeze and bronchial hyperreactivity, seizure, restless sleep and constipation. For this reason, and the benign outcomes of conservative management, propranolol is best reserved for those haemangioma that are likely to cause problems.

Treatment

Neonatal thyrotoxicosis: Give 250–750 micrograms/kg every 8 hours by mouth to control symptoms, with one drop of Lugol iodine every 8 hours to control the transient neonatal thyrotoxicosis.

Arrhythmia: Try 20 micrograms/kg IV over 10 minutes with ECG monitoring and increase this, in steps, to a cumulative total of 100 micrograms/kg if necessary. Give the effective dose IV once every 8 hours for maintenance. The same strategy may also work for the 'spells' sometimes seen

Continued on p. 434

in severe tetralogy of Fallot (with oxygen, morphine and, if necessary sodium bicarbonate, to correct serious acidosis). For sustained oral maintenance, try 250–500 micrograms/kg every 8 hours, adjusted according to response to a maximum of 1 mg/kg every 8 hours.

Neonatal hypertension: Start with 250 micrograms/kg every 8 hours by mouth together with hydralazine (q.v.) and increase as necessary to a maximum of 2 mg/kg/dose.

Infantile haemangiomas: The target dose for treatment is 1–3 mg/kg/day in three divided doses. Begin with the lowest possible dose and titrate upwards according to the response; many haemangiomas will respond to even small doses. This is best done under inpatient supervision especially in younger infants.

Blood levels

The therapeutic blood level in adults is said to be 20–100 mg/l (1 mg/l = 3.9 μmol/l), but it is best to judge the amount of drug to give by reference to the patient's blood pressure and response to treatment.

Supply and administration

1 mg (1 ml) ampoules of propranolol are available from 'specials' manufacturers or from specialist importing companies. For accurate IV use, dilute to 10 ml with 10% glucose to get a 100 micrograms/ml solution.

Propranolol is available as an oral solution in several strengths (1 ml may contain 1, 2, 4 or 10 mg). 150 ml costs between £12.50 and £20 depending on the strength.

References

Chen TS, Eichenfield LF, Friedlander SF. Infantile hemangiomas: an update on pathogenesis and therapy. *Pediatrics* 2013;**131**:99–108.

Datta S, Kitzmiller JL, Ostheimer GW, *et al.* Propranolol and parturition. *Obstet Gynecol* 1978;**51**:577–81.

Drolet BA, Frommelt PC, Chamlin SL, *et al.* Initiation and use of propranolol for infantile hemangioma: report of a consensus conference. *Pediatrics* 2013;**131**:128–40.

Filippi L, Cavallaro G, Fiorini P, *et al.* Propranolol concentrations after oral administration in term and preterm neonates. *J Matern Fetal Neonatal Med* 2013;**26**:833–40.

Gardner LI. Is propranolol alone really effective in neonatal thyrotoxicosis? *Arch Dis Child* 1980;**134**:707–8. (See also pp. 819–20.)

Hogeling M, Adams S, Wargon O. A randomized controlled trial of propranolol for infantile hemangiomas. *Pediatrics* 2011;**128**:e259–66. [RCT]

Hussain T, Greenhalgh K, McLeod KA. Hypoglycaemia syncope in children secondary to beta-blockers. *Arch Dis Child* 2009;**94**:968–9.

Maguiness SM, Frieden IJ. Management of difficult infantile haemangiomas. *Arch Dis Child* 2012;**97**:266–71.

Marqueling AL, Oza V, Frieden IJ, *et al.* Propranolol and infantile hemangiomas four years later: a systematic review. *Pediatr Dermatol* 2013;**30**:182–91.

Mehta AV, Chidambraram B. Efficacy and safety of intravenous and oral nadolol for supraventricular tachycardia. *J Am Coll Cardiol* 1992;**19**:630–5.

Moss AJ, Zareba W, Hall WJ, *et al.* Effectiveness and limitations of beta-blocker therapy in congenital long-QT syndromes. *Circulation* 2000;**101**:616–23.

Ogilvy-Stuart AL. Neonatal thyroid disorders. *Arch Dis Child Fetal Neonatal Ed* 2002;**87**:F165–71.

Sans V, Dumas de la Roque E, Berge J, *et al.* Propranolol for severe infantile hemangiomas: follow-up report. *Pediatrics* 2009;**124**:e423–31.

Shannon ME, Malecha SE, Cha AJ. Beta blockers and lactation: an update. *J Hum Lact* 2000;**16**:240–5.

Villain E, Denjoy I, Lupoglazoff JM. Low incidence of cardiac events with β-blocking therapy in children with long QT syndrome. *Eur Heart J* 2005;**25**:1405–11.

Use

Prostaglandin E_2 (PGE_2) gels and vaginal tablets are widely used to initiate and augment labour. PGE_1 and PGE_2 are both used to maintain patency of the ductus arteriosus pending surgery in babies with a duct-dependent congenital heart defect, but they can take several hours to become fully effective.

Pharmacology

PGE_1 (alprostadil) and PGE_2 (dinoprostone) are potent vasodilators originally isolated from prostate gland secretions that inhibit platelet coagulation and stimulate uterine contractility. PGE_2 was first synthesised in 1970 and is still occasionally used to terminate pregnancy by extra-amniotic administration, while tablets, gels and pessaries are now very widely used to ripen the cervix and/or initiate labour at term. Misoprostol (q.v.), an analogue of PGE_1, is also sometimes used to initiate labour and is more widely used to control post-partum bleeding, although the manufacturers have not yet sought permission to market the drug for use in this way. Caution must be employed before using prostaglandins (PG) and oxytocin simultaneously because each potentiates the effect of the other.

PG were first used experimentally to maintain ductal patency in 1975, and continuous intra-venous (IV) infusions are now frequently employed in the early preoperative management of duct-dependent congenital heart disease. While PGE_1 is the licensed preparation, a similar dose of PGE_2 is equally effective and considerably cheaper. Because of rapid inactivation during passage through the lung, the half-life during IV infusion is less than a minute. No loading dose is necessary. Monitor oxygen saturation. Respiratory depression and apnoea are common with high-dose treatment (some texts still recommend a dose that is much higher than necessary) and may occur, even with the dose recommended here, especially in the cyanosed or preterm baby. High-dose treatment causes vasodilatation and hypotension and has rarely caused diarrhoea, irritability, seizures, tachycardia, pyrexia and metabolic acidosis. Watch for hypoglycaemia. Continued IV use for >5 days can cause gastric outlet obstruction due to reversible antral hyperplasia, and long-term use can cause hyperostosis of cortical bone.

Sustained oral administration is still sometimes used, but it is rarely employed because delay is not thought to render surgery any less technically difficult. Start with 25 micrograms/kg by mouth once an hour and double this if necessary. Some babies manage with treatment every 3–4 hours, but many need a dose every 2 hours to remain stable. Watch for renal electrolyte loss.

Inhaled or aerosolised PGE_1 has, like epoprostenol (PGI_2), has been used to treat persistent pulmonary hypertension (PPHN). Use has largely been supplanted by inhaled nitric oxide (q.v.). IV infusions, largely to maintain ductal patency but where PPHN coexists, have also been described as having some potential benefit in reducing the amount of PPHN that existed. In this case, pulmonary vasodilatation and the patent duct acting as a 'blow-off' valve improve function in the pressure and volume-loaded right ventricle.

Treatment

Maternal: 1 mg of vaginal gel (2 mg if the cervix is unfavourable) inserted high into the posterior fornix, or a 3 mg vaginal tablet similarly positioned is now the most widely used method of inducing labour. A second dose of either can be given, if necessary, after 6–8 hours.

Neonatal: Start with a 5 nanograms/kg/minute IV infusion through a secure line (0.3 ml/kg/hour of a solution made up as described under 'Supply and administration') and leave this dose running for a few hours before using oxygen saturation to adjust this dose up, or down, as necessary. Always aim to use the lowest effective dose – a dose as high as 40 nanograms/kg/minute is very rarely necessary.

Preventing neonatal apnoea

Use the minimum effective dose of PG. If high-dose treatment *is* necessary, the risk of apnoea can be reduced by giving IV aminophylline (see the archived monograph for theophylline). Caffeine (q.v.) would probably be equally effective.

Compatibility

PGE_2 (dinoprostone) is very unstable in solution and should never be infused with any other drug. In contrast, it *may* be acceptable to add PGE_1 (alprostadil) (terminally) when absolutely necessary, into a line containing adrenaline, dopamine, glyceryl trinitrate, heparin, lidocaine, midazolam, morphine or nitroprusside, although the manufacturers remain reluctant to endorse this advice.

Continued on p. 436

Supply and administration

Alprostadil: A 1 ml IV ampoule (containing 0.5 mg/ml) of alprostadil (Prostin VR®) costs £75. To give an infusion of 5 nanograms/kg/minute, dilute 0.3 ml (150 micrograms) for every kilogram the baby weighs with 5% glucose or 0.9% saline to make a 50 ml solution. Start the infusion at a rate of 0.1 ml/hour.

Dinoprostone: A 0.75 ml IV ampoule (containing 1 mg/ml) of dinoprostone (Prostin® E2) costs £8.50. To give an infusion of 5 nanograms/kg/minute, add 0.5 ml of dinoprostone from this ampoule to 500 ml of 10% glucose or glucose saline to produce a solution containing 1 micrograms of dinoprostone per ml, and infuse this at a rate of 0.3 ml/kg/hour.

Note: *10 mg/ml* ampoules are sometimes stocked for use in termination of pregnancy.

Store ampoules at 4 °C, and prepare a fresh IV solution daily. A sugar-free oral solution with a 1-week shelf life can be prepared on request.

Vaginal gels and tablets are widely used to induce labour; the two are *not* strictly bioequivalent. The cost is approximately the same (£13).

References

(See also the Cochrane reviews of obstetric use)

Brodie M, Chaudari M, Hasan A. Prostaglandin therapy for ductal patency: how long is too long? *Acta Paediatr* 2008;**97**:1303–4.

Browning Carmo KA, Barr P, West M, *et al.* Transporting newborn infants with suspected duct dependent congenital heart disease on low-dose prostaglandin E$_1$ without routine mechanical ventilation. *Arch Dis Child Fetal Neonatal Ed* 2007;**92**:F117–19.

Gupta N, Kamlin CO, Cheung M, *et al.* Prostaglandin E$_1$ use during neonatal transfer: potential beneficial role in persistent pulmonary hypertension of the newborn. *Arch Dis Child Fetal Neonatal Ed* 2013;**98**:F186–8.

Kaufman MB, El-Chaar GM. Bone and tissue changes following prostaglandin therapy in neonates. *Ann Pharmacother* 1996;**30**:269–77.

Lálosi G, Katona M, Túri S. Side-effects of long-term prostaglandin E$_1$ treatment in neonates. *Pediatr Int* 2007;**47**:335–40.

Madar RJ, Donaldson T, Hunter S. Prostaglandins in congenital heart disease. *Cardiol Young* 1995;**5**:202–3.

Meckler GD, Lowe C. To intubate or not to intubate? Transporting infants on prostaglandin E$_1$. *Pediatrics* 2009;**123**:e25–30.

Nakwan N, Wannaro J. Persistent pulmonary hypertension of the newborn successfully treated with beraprost sodium: a retrospective chart review. *Neonatology* 2011;**99**:32–7.

Sood BG, Delaney-Black V, Aranda JV, *et al.* Aerosolized PGE1: a selective pulmonary vasodilator in neonatal hypoxemic respiratory failure results of a phase i/ii open label clinical trial. *Pediatr Res* 2004;**56**:579–85.

Use

Deficiency of pulmonary surfactant can cause considerable mortality and morbidity in the preterm population. Antenatal steroids and exogenous pulmonary surfactants (of synthetic and animal origin) have improved the outcomes in preterm babies considerably since they became more widely used.

Physiology

Although rare inherited congenital defects may render a few term babies permanently unable to make surfactant, the main use for surfactant replacement is in the preterm baby with respiratory distress syndrome (RDS). The lung of the very preterm baby may contain as little as 10 mg/kg of surfactant at birth (a 10th of the amount at term). While labour and/or birth triggers a surge of endogenous surfactant, this takes 48 hours to become fully effective. Care needs to be exercised during this time, as both acidosis and hypothermia interfere with this process, while alveolar collapse increases surfactant consumption. The development of artificial and natural products to bridge this time gap, and their rigorous evaluation, has been one of the major achievements of neonatal medicine.

Endogenous surfactant has a half-life of about 12 hours, after which some is recycled and some is degraded. The baby who is deficient at birth, therefore, needs to be given 100 mg/kg as soon as possible to prevent atelectasis (alveolar collapse) from developing, and if destruction initially exceeds production, one (and occasionally two) further dose 12 and 24 hours later. Inactivation seems to occur more rapidly when there is established RDS, infection or meconium aspiration, rendering a larger dose appropriate.

It is now widely accepted that if non-invasive respiratory support can be provided for babies who are surfactant deficient at birth, this will reduce the numbers of babies with chronic oxygen dependency. The first critical step is to aerate the lung as gently as possible at birth using pressure sustained for several seconds to achieve initial lung expansion before even thinking to 'ventilate' the baby. The second critical step is to prevent atelectasis by using nasal CPAP, non-invasive positive pressure ventilation (NIPPV) or high flow oxygen. The more vulnerable babies may also benefit from early surfactant, but everything should be done to minimise the need to provide ongoing respiratory support using a tube through the larynx.

There remains a naïve belief that because all births at 37–41 weeks' gestation are referred to as 'term' births, there is no risk of these babies being surfactant deficient at birth. Unfortunately, this is not true; babies delivered electively at 37 weeks' gestation by caesarean section can also be surfactant deficient.

Indications for use

Trials conducted in the current era of non-invasive ventilation for respiratory support suggest that there is no particular merit in planning intubation for prophylactic surfactant treatment. However, babies <30 weeks' gestation merit a first dose as soon as possible after intubation if this is required or if a diagnosis of RDS is suspected, particularly if this means that they can be extubated quickly back to CPAP. The cost of treating babies more mature than this is harder to justify until it is clear that they need >40% oxygen to sustain an arterial PaO_2 above 7 kPa (or 90% SaO_2). Babies needing ventilation for pneumonia or meconium aspiration merit consideration for treatment with a product containing surfactant proteins (see web commentary).

Treatment

Poractant alfa: Give 200 mg/kg (2.5 ml/kg) into the trachea as soon as the decision has been made that surfactant is likely to be required. Give a second dose (100 mg/kg) after 4–6 hours if the baby continues to need ventilation with a mean airway pressure of >7 cm H_2O and >40% oxygen, or if there are signs of pneumonia. Consider giving a smaller first dose of 100 mg/kg if surfactant is being given prophylactically in delivery suite, for example, in extremely preterm infants for whom there has not been time to receive antenatal steroids.

Beractant: Give 100 mg/kg (4 ml/kg) in the same way as for poractant alfa but in two to three aliquots. The manufacturer says up to three further doses can be given, at least 6 hours apart, within the next 48 hours.

Optimising usage

Surfactant treatment can be very cost-effective but remains expensive, and a lot can be done to limit redundant and unnecessary treatment. If the lung disease is more severe, there is much to recommend giving subsequent doses of surfactant earlier than the manufacturers recommend.

Continued on p. 438

Likewise, there is little to be gained by giving surfactant to a ventilated baby needing ≤ 30% oxygen when the mean airway pressure is <7 cm H_2O.

Administration

It is traditional to instil the prescribed dose down an endotracheal tube using a fine catheter with the baby supine after clearing any mucus and pre-oxygenating the lungs to minimise cyanosis during administration.

For many years, it was assumed that if surfactant was required, then the baby would need both intubation and sustained respiratory support – neither of these assumptions is necessarily correct. Surfactant can be given using the *IN*tubation *SUR*factant *E*xtubation (INSURE) procedure or even via a fine catheter passed 1.5 cm through the larynx of the unintubated, spontaneously breathing infant.

A 1–2 mg/kg intravenous dose of remifentanil (q.v.) given 60 seconds before attempting intubation will blunt any pain and cause muscle relaxation, but the 2 mg/kg dose will often depress respiration enough to make it wise to delay extubation for 10–20 minutes. It is widely thought that giving the appropriate dose of surfactant in a small volume of fluid will cause fewer cardiovascular disturbances, but a larger volume leads to a more even dispersal within the lung. Surfactant can be given in less than a minute (rather than 4 minutes, as manufacturers often recommend) without causing bradycardia or cyanosis. Ignore any that subsequently reappears in the tracheal tube. Hand ventilate, or reintubate, if the tube seems to have become blocked. Natural surfactants increase lung compliance and oxygenation rapidly – be prepared to reduce the ventilator settings and, more especially, the amount of oxygen quite soon after they are given.

Supply

Poractant alfa comes in 1.5 and 3 ml ready-to-use vials containing 120 and 240 mg of phospholipid costing £280 and £550 each. Beractant comes in 8 ml vials containing 200 mg of phospholipid which cost £310; 4 ml (100 mg) vials are also available in some countries. Store vials at 4 °C, but warm to room temperature before use, and invert gently without shaking to resuspend the material. Do not use, or return vials to the refrigerator, more than 8 hours after they reach room temperature.

References
(See also the relevant Cochrane reviews)

Broadbent R, Fok T-F, Dolovich M, *et al.* Chest position and pulmonary disposition of surfactant in surfactant depleted rabbits. *Arch Dis Child Fetal Neonatal Ed* 1995;**72**:F84–9.

Buckmaster AG, Arnolda G, Wright IMR, *et al.* Continuous positive airway pressure therapy for infants with respiratory distress in non-tertiary care centers: a randomized controlled trial. *Pediatrics* 2007;**120**:509–18. [RCT]

Dargaville PA, Aiyappan A, De Paoli AG, *et al.* Minimally-invasive surfactant therapy in preterm infants on continuous positive airway pressure. *Arch Dis Child Fetal Neonatal Ed* 2013;**98**:F122–6.

Göpel W, Kribs A, Ziegler A, *et al.* Avoidance of mechanical ventilation by surfactant treatment of spontaneously breathing preterm infants (AMV): an open-label, randomised, controlled trial. *Lancet* 2011;**378**:1627–34. [RCT]

Kattwinkel J, Bloom BT, Delmore P, *et al.* High- versus low-threshold surfactant retreatment for neonatal respiratory distress syndrome. *Pediatrics* 2000;**106**:282–8. [RCT]

Moya M, Maturana A. Animal-derived surfactants versus past and current synthetic surfactants: current status. *Clin Perinatol* 2007;**34**:145–77.

Polin RA, Carlo WA and Committee on Fetus and Newborn. Clinical report: surfactant replacement therapy for preterm and term neonates with respiratory distress. *Pediatrics* 2014;**133**:156–63. [SR]

Schaschini M, Nogee LM, Sassi I, *et al.* Unexplained neonatal respiratory distress caused by congenital surfactant deficiency. *J Pediatr* 2007;**15**:649–53.

Speer CP, Sweet DG, Halliday HL. Surfactant therapy: past, present and future. *Early Hum Dev* 2013;**89**(suppl 1):S22–4.

Sweet DG, Bevilacqua G, Carnielli V, *et al.* European consensus guidelines on the management of neonatal respiratory distress syndrome. *J Perinat Med* 2007;**35**:175–86. [SR]

Sweet DG, Carnielli V, Greisen G, *et al.* European consensus guidelines on the management of neonatal respiratory distress syndrome in preterm infants–2013 update. *Neonatology* 2013;**103**:353–68.

te Pas AB, Walther FJ. A randomized, controlled trial of delivery-room respiratory management in very preterm infants. *Pediatrics* 2007;**120**:322–9. [RCT]

Victorin LH, Deverajan LV, Curstedt T, *et al.* Surfactant replacement in spontaneously breathing babies with hyaline membrane disease – a pilot study. *Biol Neonate* 1990;**58**:121–6.

Welzing L, Kribs A, Huenseler C., *et al.* Remifentanil for INSURE in preterm infants: a pilot study for evaluation of efficacy and safety aspects. *Acta Paediatr* 2009;**98**:1416–20.

Use

Pyrazinamide is used in the first phase treatment of tuberculosis (TB). To minimise the risk of drug resistance developing, management should always be overseen by a clinician with substantial experience of this condition. Of the infants infected *in utero* or at the time of delivery, half of those who **are not** treated and 22% of those who **are** treated die from congenital TB; therefore, early diagnosis and treatment are critical.

Pharmacology

Pyrazinamide, like isoniazid (q.v.), to which it is chemically related, is bacteriostatic or bactericidal against *Mycobacterium tuberculosis* depending on the dose used. Other mycobacteria, including *M. bovis*, are resistant. Sixty years after its discovery in 1952, its mode of action is still poorly understood, but the metabolite, pyrazinoic acid, is now known to bind to ribosomal protein S1 (RpsA) which prevent the trans-translocation mechanism whereby the organism can cope with damaged DNA and problems in its replication processes. Resistance develops rapidly if other drugs are not taken at the same time. It is well absorbed orally and should always be used when TB meningitis is a possibility because it rapidly penetrates all body tissues. The half-life in adults is 9–10 hours, but it does not seem to have been studied in children.

Excretion is impaired in severe renal failure, but drug accumulation does not occur during peritoneal dialysis. Liver toxicity is the main hazard, so liver function should be checked before treatment is started and repeated at intervals if there is pre-existing liver disease. Review treatment at once if any sign of liver toxicity (such as nausea, vomiting, drowsiness or jaundice) develops during treatment. Manufacturers in the United States have endorsed use in children, but no such move has been made in the United Kingdom.

Pyrazinamide has an excellent safety record during pregnancy. Despite its widespread use, it is not known if pyrazinamide crosses the placenta. In any case, because untreated TB poses a greater health risk to mother and fetus, treatment should not be withheld. Pyrazinamide passes into breast milk in small amounts that are unlikely to be of clinical significance in the breastfed infant.

Infants exposed to a case of infectious TB

Babies born to mothers with TB: See the monograph on isoniazid for maternal treatment. Give the baby 5 mg/kg of isoniazid as chemoprophylaxis once a day for 3 months, and then do a Mantoux test. If this test is negative and the mother is no longer infectious, BCG can be given and treatment stopped: if it is positive, give 10 mg/kg of isoniazid for a further 3 months. Do not discourage breastfeeding. Congenitally acquired infection usually becomes symptomatic in 2–3 weeks. Treat evidence of active disease as summarised in the following text.

Babies not previously given BCG: Give 10 mg/kg of isoniazid for 6 weeks and then do a Mantoux test. Give a further 20 weeks of isoniazid if this is positive or if the interferon gamma test is positive (where facilities exist for performing this test). Offer full active treatment (see following text) if there are X-ray changes.

Babies previously given BCG: Offer isoniazid for 6 months if the Mantoux test is strongly positive or if it becomes so on retesting 6 weeks later. Offer full treatment if there is evidence of active disease.

Treating overt TB in infancy

TB can progress rapidly in young children. Generalised (or miliary) TB is a real possibility if treatment is not started promptly, infecting bone or the meninges around the brain. Treatment is a two-stage process – an initial 2-month phase using three (or even four) drugs designed to reduce bacterial load to a minimum and minimise the risk of drug resistance developing and a 4-month maintenance phase using just two drugs.

Pyrazinamide: Give 35 mg/kg of pyrazinamide by mouth once a day for the first 2 months of treatment. It is critically important to ensure that the dose is correct and that treatment is taken every day as prescribed. There is a very real risk that dangerous drug-resistant bacteria will evolve and put both the patient, and the community, at risk if this is not done.

Other drugs: Give 10 mg/kg of isoniazid and 10 mg/kg of rifampicin (q.v.) as well by mouth once a day for at least 6 months. Any possible meningeal involvement calls for at least a year's expert treatment and the use of a fourth drug for the first 2 months. A 15 mg/kg dose of ethambutol given once a day for 2 months is the most commonly employed option. While this drug can occasionally cause serious visual loss which can become permanent if not recognised promptly,

Continued on p. 440

there are no well-attested reports of this occurring in a young child with the dose recommended here. A 20–30 mg/kg intramuscular dose of streptomycin once a day for 2 months may be the most acceptable alternative (checking periodically that the trough level does not exceed 5 mg/l).

Supply

500 mg tablets of pyrazinamide cost £1, and 100 mg tablets of ethambutol cost 20p each. Sugar-free oral suspensions can be provided with a four-week shelf life. 1 g vials of streptomycin cost £15 each in the United Kingdom.

References

Bothamley G. Drug treatment for tuberculosis during pregnancy: safety considerations. *Drug Saf* 2001;**24**:553–65.

Donald PR, Maritz JS, Diacon AH. Pyrazinamide pharmacokinetics and efficacy in adults and children. *Tuberculosis (Edinb)* 2012;**92**:1–8.

Joint Tuberculosis Committee of the British Thoracic Society. Control and prevention of tuberculosis in the United Kingdom: code of practice 2000. *Thorax* 2000;**55**:887–901.

Marais BJ, Pai M. Recent advances in the diagnosis of childhood tuberculosis. *Arch Dis Child* 2007;**92**:446–52.

National Institute for Health and Clinical Excellence. *Tuberculosis: clinical diagnosis and management of tuberculosis, and measures for its prevention and control* (clinical guideline 117). NICE, 2011. (See http://guidance.nice.org.uk/CG117. Accessed 13 May 2014).

Patel S, DeSantis ER. Treatment of congenital tuberculosis. *Am J Health Syst Pharm* 2008;**65**:2027–31.

Raju B, Schluger NW. Tuberculosis and pregnancy. *Semin Respir Crit Care Med* 1998;**19**:295–306.

Shi W, Zhang X, Jiang X, *et al.* Pyrazinamide inhibits trans-translation in *Mycobacterium tuberculosis*. *Science* 2011;**333**:1630–2.

Skevaki CL, Kafetzis DA. Tuberculosis in neonates and infants: epidemiology, pathogenesis, clinical manifestations, diagnosis, and management issues. *Pediatr Drugs* 2005;**7**:219–34.

Teo SSS, Riordan A, Alfaham M, *et al.* Tuberculosis in the United Kingdom and Republic of Ireland. *Arch Dis Child* 2009;**94**:263–7.

Vallejo JG, Ong LT, Starke JR. Clinical features, diagnosis, and treatment of tuberculosis in infants. *Pediatrics* 1994;**94**:1–7.

Use

Pyridoxine and its active metabolite, pyridoxal phosphate, are used to treat two inborn errors of metabolism that cause convulsions in early infancy. Pyridoxine is also used in the management of homocystinuria.

Biochemistry

Pyridoxine is widely available in most foodstuffs, and nutritional deficiency is extremely rare. Pyridoxine is converted in the body to pyridoxal phosphate, which is a cofactor for a number of enzymes. Pyridoxine dependency is an autosomal recessive condition associated with mutations in the antiquitin (ALDH7A1) gene. This defect leads to the accumulation of piperideine-6-carboxylate, which binds and inactivates pyridoxal phosphate. Pyridoxine dependency should be considered in any baby with severe seizures even if they seem to have a clear cause (e.g. asphyxia). Most cases present soon after birth, and seizures have even been sensed *in utero*. Development may still be delayed even though pyridoxine controls the fits. The diagnosis can be confirmed by measuring CSF plasma or urine alpha-aminoadipic semialdehyde (α-AASA).

Pyridoxine is converted to pyridoxal phosphate by pyridox(am)ine phosphate oxidase, and patients with the rare recessive defect of *this* enzyme present with neonatal seizures that respond to pyridoxal phosphate, but *not* to pyridoxine. It should be noted that pyridoxine and pyridoxal phosphate also display anticonvulsant activity in some patients who do not have either of these conditions for reasons that are not yet understood. In neonates with resistant seizures, the initial intravenous (IV) pyridoxine may induce non-specific EEG responses that neither identify nor exclude pyridoxine-dependent epilepsy, and all such neonates should probably receive pyridoxine until this diagnosis is fully excluded by metabolic and/or DNA analysis.

Homocystinuria most commonly results from cystathionine β-synthase deficiency. Pyridoxal phosphate is the cofactor for this enzyme, and many patients improve biochemically and clinically with pharmacological doses of pyridoxine. Cases of homocystinuria detected by neonatal screening programmes, however, tend not to be pyridoxine responsive. Other patients present with developmental delay or subsequently with dislocated lenses, skeletal abnormalities or thromboembolic disease.

Diagnostic use

Defects of pyridoxine metabolism: One 100 mg IV dose of pyridoxine stops most fits within minutes. Watch for apnoea. The test is best conducted while the EEG is being monitored (although visible seizure activity may cease some hours or even days before the EEG trace returns to normal), but this test should not be delayed if monitoring proves hard to organise. If the response is negative, or equivocal, and pyridoxine dependency is a likely diagnosis, then oral pyridoxine should be given for 2 weeks. Finally, a trial of pyridoxal phosphate (using the doses detailed under 'Fits later in Infancy') should be considered in patients who do not respond to pyridoxine.

Fits later in infancy: Some patients with pyridoxine dependency present when more than 4 weeks old. All infants with infantile spasms or drug-resistant seizures merit a trial of pyridoxine or pyridoxal phosphate (50 mg/kg of either drug by mouth once a day for a minimum of 2 weeks).

Homocystinuria: Pyridoxine responsiveness should be assessed by measuring plasma methionine and homocysteine under basal conditions, and during a 2–3-week trial of pyridoxine, while ensuring a constant protein intake. Start by giving 100 mg a day (although a dose of up to 250 mg a day may deliver added benefit). Give 5 mg folic acid a day to be sure the response is not impaired by folate deficiency.

Treatment

Fits: Infants with fits that respond to pyridoxine should then receive 50–100 mg indefinitely once a day if tests show excess α-AASA in the urine. The prognosis for siblings may be improved if mothers with a pyridoxine-dependent child take 100 mg of pyridoxine daily in any subsequent pregnancy.

Homocystinuria: Pyridoxine-responsive infants are usually given 50 mg twice a day; older patients are usually given 50–250 mg twice a day, depending on their response. Most patients take 5 mg of folic acid once a day. If this does not completely correct the abnormality, treatment can be combined with a low methionine diet, betaine (q.v.) and/or vitamin B$_{12}$ (q.v.). These treatments can also be used in patients unresponsive to pyridoxine.

Continued on p. 442

Adverse effects

The first dose of pyridoxine or pyridoxal phosphate in a neonate can cause hypotonia or apnoea requiring support. High doses in adults have caused a sensory neuropathy (and might be neurotoxic in children), so long-term management should be overseen by a paediatric neurologist or metabolic physician.

Supply

Pyridoxine: All units should have access to a stock of 2 ml (50 mg/ml) IV ampoules. They cost about £1 each. A sugar-free oral suspension is available, as are 10, 20 and 50 mg tablets (costing 2p each).

Pyridoxal phosphate: 50 mg tablets cost 12p each; a sugar-free suspension is also available.

References
(See also the relevant Cochrane reviews)

Bok LA, Halbertsma FJ, Houterman S, *et al*. Long-term outcome in pyridoxine-dependent epilepsy. *Dev Med Child Neurol* 2012;**54**:849–54.

Bok LA, Maurits NM, Willemsen MA, *et al*. The EEG response to pyridoxine-IV neither identifies nor excludes pyridoxine-dependent epilepsy. *Epilepsia* 2010;**51**:2406–11.

Clayton PT, Surtees RAH, DeVile C, *et al*. Neonatal epileptic encephalopathy. *Lancet* 2003;**361**:1614.

Mills PB, Struys E, Jakobs C, *et al*. Mutations in antiquitin in individuals with pyridoxine-dependent seizures. *Nat Med* 2006;**12**:307–9.

Rahman S, Footitt EJ, Varadkar S, *et al*. Inborn errors of metabolism causing epilepsy. *Dev Med Child Neurol* 2013;**55**:23–36.

Rankin PM, Harrison S, Chong WK, *et al*. Pyridoxine-dependent seizures: a family phenotype that leads to severe cognitive deficits, regardless of treatment regime. *Dev Med Child Neurol* 2007;**49**:300–5.

Wang H-S, Kuo M-F, Chou M-L, *et al*. Pyridoxal phosphate is better than pyridoxine for controlling idiopathic intractable epilepsy. *Arch Dis Child* 2005;**90**:512–5. (See also pp. 441–2.)

Use

Pyrimethamine is used, with sulphadiazine (q.v.), to treat toxoplasmosis and, with sulphadoxine, to treat malaria (as an alternative to co-trimoxazole [q.v.]) in areas where resistance has not yet developed.

Pharmacology

Pyrimethamine is a di-aminopyrimidine that blocks nucleic acid synthesis in the malaria parasite. It also interferes with folate metabolism. It was developed in 1951 and is still widely used in the treatment of toxoplasmosis (the natural history of which is briefly summarised in the monograph on spiramycin) although the only proof of efficacy comes from trials in patients where toxoplasmosis was a complication of HIV infection. Prolonged administration can depress haemopoeisis. Other side effects are rare, but skin rashes may occur and high doses can cause atrophic glossitis and megaloblastic anaemia. Folinic acid (the 5-formyl derivative of folic acid) is used to prevent this during pregnancy because folinic acid does not interfere with the impact of pyrimethamine on malaria and *Toxoplasma* parasites. Pyrimethamine is well absorbed by mouth and slowly excreted by the kidney, the average plasma half-life being about 4 days. Tissue levels exceed plasma levels ($V_D \sim 3 \, l/kg$). The efficacy of pyrimethamine in treating toxoplasmosis is increased eightfold by sulphadiazine. Other sulphonamides are not as effective. Efficacy in treating malaria is also improved by giving sulphadoxine. For this reason, a sulphonamide should *always* be prescribed when pyrimethamine is used to treat a baby for malaria or toxoplasmosis unless there is significant neonatal jaundice, even though the manufacturer only endorses such use in children over 5 years old. Long-term administration can sometimes cause problems (as outlined in the monograph on sulphadiazine). Lactation can continue during treatment, even though the baby receives about a third of the maternal dose on a weight-for-weight basis.

Treatment of malaria

During pregnancy: A single three-tablet dose of Fansidar® (a total of 75 mg of pyrimethamine and 1.5 g of sulphadoxine) and a 3-day course of amodiaquine (q.v.) effectively eliminate tissue parasites. Some think this is unwise in the first trimester, but the teratogenicity seen in animals seems absent in man.

In infancy: Uncomplicated malaria was once commonly treated with one dose of a synergistic mixture of 1.25 mg/kg of pyrimethamine and 25 mg/kg of sulphadoxine (i.e. Fansidar), but resistance to these two drugs has now rendered this strategy ineffective in many parts of the world, and an artemether-based approach (q.v.) has now been adopted in many countries. Quinine (q.v.) remains the best studied way of treating children with *severe* malaria, although an artemether-based approach may be equally effective.

Treatment of toxoplasmosis

During pregnancy: Spiramycin (q.v.) is often used to try and prevent transplacental spread. If fetal infection is thought to have occurred, sustained maternal treatment with 50 mg of pyrimethamine once a day and 1 g of sulphadiazine three times a day by mouth may possibly lessen disease severity.

In infancy: Give an oral loading dose of 1 mg/kg of pyrimethamine twice a day for 2 days followed by maintenance treatment with 1 mg/kg once a day for 8 weeks if there is evidence of congenital infection. Treatment with 50 mg/kg of oral sulphadiazine once every 12 hours should be started at the same time. Check weekly for possible thrombocytopenia, leukopenia and megaloblastic anaemia.

Older children: It is not known whether a year's sustained treatment improves the outcome. Dormant cysts, which often give rise to ocular disease in later life, cannot be eradicated by such an approach. Some centres intersperse continued treatment as outlined in the treatment of congenital infection with 4–6 week courses of spiramycin.

Ocular disease: Clindamycin (q.v.) is sometimes given in babies with ocular disease. Consider photocoagulation for choroidal scars. Prednisolone (2 mg/kg once a day) remains of uncertain value.

Prophylaxis with calcium folinate, leucovorin (USAN)

Give 15 mg by mouth twice a week during pregnancy to prevent pyrimethamine causing bone marrow depression. Exactly the same dose is often given to infants on long-term pyrimethamine treatment.

Continued on p. 444

Supply and administration

Pyrimethamine: 25 mg tablets compounded with sulphadoxine as Fansidar® (see preceding text) cost 25p each. Suspensions can be provided on request, but dosage is not critical and it is often good enough to give small babies a quarter or half tablet.

Calcium folinate: 15 mg tablets and 3 mg (1 ml) ampoules cost £4.50 and £4, respectively.

References   (See also the relevant Cochrane reviews)

Aponte JJ, Schellenberg D, Egan A, *et al*. Efficacy and safety of intermittent preventive treatment with sulfadoxine-pyrimethamine for malaria in African infants: a pooled analysis of six randomised, placebo-controlled trials. *Lancet* 2009;**374**:1533–42.

Fegan GW, Noor AM, Akhwale WS, *et al*. Effect of expanded insecticide-treated bednet coverage on child survival in rural Kenya: a longitudinal study. *Lancet* 2007;**370**:1035–9. (See also pp. 1009–10.)

Omari A, Garner P. Severe life threatening malaria in endemic areas. *Br Med J* 2004;**328**:154. [SR] (See also p. 155.)

Plowe CV, Kublin JG, Dzinjalamala FK, *et al*. Sustained clinical efficacy of sulphadoxine-pyrimethamine for uncomplicated falciparum malaria in Malawi after 10 years of first line treatment: five year prospective study. *Br Med J* 2004;**328**:545–8. (See also pp. 534–5.)

Use
Quinine remains the best studied drug for treating severe malaria in the very young child, but in a child well enough to take treatment by mouth, an artemisinin (see the monographs on artemether with lumefantrine or amodiaquine with artesunate) may – where affordable – prove an even more reliable strategy.

Pharmacology
Four hundred years ago, Jesuit priests noted that an extract from the bark of the cinchona tree had long been valued in Peru as a specific cure for marsh or '4-day' (quaternary) fever. It contains the alkaloid quinine, which kills malarial schizonts when they enter the blood stream. G6PD deficiency is not a contraindication; haemolysis may occur in exposed fetuses with G6PD deficiency. Quinine crosses the placenta (F/M ratio ~0.32). Teratogenic effects are seen in some animal models but not others. Congenital malformations (predominantly deafness and auditory nerve hypoplasia) have been reported in humans but were associated with large doses (up to 30 g) that were taken to trigger abortion. The oxytocic effects are not seen with the smaller doses used to treat malaria. Only small amounts of quinine are secreted into breast milk, and with the exception of infants with G6PD deficiency, no adverse effects are seen.

Managing severe malaria
Malaria can be rapidly fatal, especially in children less than a year old, and symptoms may be nonspecific. There may be vomiting, diarrhoea and weakness or drowsiness as well as fever, and speedy intervention can make the difference between life and death. Many severely ill children are hypovolaemic and benefit from an immediate transfusion of 20 ml/kg of plasma albumin (q.v.) or, if this is not available, 0.9% sodium chloride. Then correct severe anaemia (haematocrit <15%) with blood (q.v.) or, if the anaemia is gross or >10% of the red cells are parasitised, by exchange transfusion. Monitor, prevent and treat hypoglycaemia with sublingual or, if necessary, intravenous (IV) glucose (q.v.). Give lorazepam (q.v.) for seizures and, if this fails, paraldehyde (q.v.). IV mannitol is not helpful, but shock may suggest there is both malaria and septicaemia (with or without meningitis) – start treatment for both if the situation is unclear and review later. Transplacentally acquired infection may only manifest itself 2–8 weeks later with fever, jaundice, anaemia, respiratory symptoms and a large spleen.

Initial treatment
By mouth: See that those well enough to take quinine sulphate (or dihydrochloride) by mouth take 10 mg/kg once every 8 hours for a full 7 days (repeating the dose if vomiting occurs within an hour).
As an IV infusion: Give a loading dose of 20 mg/kg of quinine dihydrochloride (2 ml/kg of a solution made up as specified under 'Supply and administration') over 4 hours. This should be followed by further doses of 10 mg/kg infused over 2–4 hours at 12 hourly intervals. Always use a pump or in-line infusion chamber to avoid cardiotoxicity from rapid administration. Follow with a full course of oral treatment with quinine or any artemisinin combination, for example, artemether and lumefantrine (q.v.).
Intramuscular (IM) administration: 10 mg/kg once every 12 hours for 3 days (or until oral treatment is possible).
Rectal administration: Give 20 mg/kg of quinine, as outlined in the following text, once every 12 hours for 3 days (or until the 7-day course can be completed by mouth). IV artesunate is now becoming the treatment of choice, but an early rectal dose of quinine or artemether can be lifesaving when skilled care is hours away.

Secondary treatment
Complete treatment as soon as oral medication is possible by giving doxycycline or clindamycin or, alternatively, in those areas where the parasites are still sensitive, pyrimethamine and sulphadoxine:
Doxycycline: Give 2.5 mg/kg of this tetracycline by mouth once every 12 hours for 7 days.
Clindamycin: A 10 mg/kg dose of clindamycin (q.v.) given by mouth once every 8 hours for 7 days is an alternative that avoids the risk of dental staining caused by tetracycline use.
Pyrimethamine and sulphadoxine: Give a quarter tablet of Fansidar® on the last day of treatment. Babies 3 or more months old can have half a tablet. For more information, see the monograph on pyrimethamine.

Continued on p. 446

Supply and administration

Quinine: Quinine sulphate is available as dividable 200 mg tablets (cost 7p each) and as an IV product (quinine dihydrochloride) from 'special-order' manufacturers or specialist importing companies in 1 and 2 ml ampoules containing 300 mg/ml. Take 1 ml of this preparation, and dilute it to 30 ml with 5 or 10% glucose saline to get an IV solution containing 10 mg/ml. IM injection is painful, but quinine can also be given into the rectum – just draw up the dose required, dilute to 4 ml with water, and give using a syringe. A less painful buffered product containing four cinchona alkaloids (Quinimax®) is widely used in Africa.

Doxycycline: 50 mg capsules cost 6p each. Scored 100 mg dispersible tablets cost 60p. A 5 mg/ml suspension and a 10 mg/ml syrup (Vibramycin®) are available in America.

References (See also the relevant Cochrane reviews)

Achan J, Talisuna AO, Erhart A, *et al.* Quinine, an old anti-malarial drug in a modern world: role in the treatment of malaria. *Malar J* 2011;**10**:144.

Achan J, Tibenderana JK, Kyabayinze D, *et al.* Effectiveness of quinine versus artemether-lumefantrine for treating uncomplicated falciparum malaria in Ugandan children: randomised trial. *Br Med J* 2009;**339**:b2763. [RCT]

Barennes H, Balima-Koussoubé T, Nagot N, *et al.* Safety and efficacy of rectal compared with intramuscular quinine for the early treatment of moderately severe malaria in children: randomised clinical trial. *Br Med J* 2006;**332**:1055–7. (See also p. 1216.) [RCT]

Dondorp A, Nosten F, Stepniewska K, *et al.* (SEAQUAMAT Trial Group). Artesunate versus quinine for treatment of severe falciparum malaria: a randomised trial. *Lancet* 2005;**366**:717–25. [RCT]

Dondorp AM, Fanello CI, Hendriksen IC, *et al.* Artesunate versus quinine in the treatment of severe falciparum malaria in African children (AQUAMAT): an open-label, randomised trial. *Lancet* 2010;**376**:1647–57. [RCT]

Maitland K, Nadel S, Ollard AJ, *et al.* Management of severe malaria in children: proposed guidelines for the United Kingdom. *Br Med J* 2005;**331**:337–41.

Maitland K, Pamba A, English M, *et al.* Randomized trial of volume expansion with albumin or saline in children with severe malaria: preliminary evidence of albumin benefit. *Clin Infect Dis* 2005;**40**:538·45. [RCT]

Phillips RE, Looareesuwan S, White NJ, *et al.* Quinine pharmacokinetics and toxicity in pregnant and lactating women with falciparum malaria. *Br J Clin Pharmacol* 1986;**21**:677–83.

van der Torn M, Thuma PE, Mabeza GF, *et al.* Loading dose of quinine in African children with cerebral malaria. *Trans R Soc Trop Med Hyg* 1998;**92**:325–31.

Use
Ranitidine is used to treat symptomatic oesophagitis, gastritis and peptic ulceration. Omeprazole (q.v.) may sometimes be more effective.

Pharmacology
Ranitidine (first developed in 1979) reduces stomach acidity by blocking the H_2 histamine receptors in the stomach that control the release of gastric acid. A low-dose 75 mg tablet is now available without prescription for the short-term treatment of heartburn and indigestion in adults. A higher dose is used to treat peptic ulceration but does little for stress-related upper gastrointestinal bleeding. No measurable benefit has yet been seen in trials of prophylaxis in children or adults requiring intensive care.

The pharmacology of ranitidine is very similar to that of cimetidine, but ranitidine does not interact with the metabolism of other drugs in the same way, and it has no antiandrogenic properties. Higher doses have to be used when the drug is given by mouth because of rapid first-pass metabolism in the liver (oral bioavailability being about 50% but rather variable in the neonate). Tissue levels exceed plasma levels (neonatal $V_D \sim 1.8 \, l/kg$). Most of the drug is excreted in the urine. The half-life is 3½ hours at birth but closer to 2 hours (as in adults) by 6 months. It is even longer, at first, in the preterm baby. Most neonatal reports of the use of ranitidine relate to intravenous (IV) administration (a route the manufacturers are not yet ready to recommend in children <6 months old). Necrotising enterocolitis may be more common in babies given an H_2-blocker, and one report has suggested that neonatal use is associated with a higher risk of late-onset sepsis. The dosing interval should be doubled in renal failure or during ECMO treatment.

Ranitidine crosses the placenta. Although the manufacturer advises use should be avoided during pregnancy, epidemiological study reveals no increased prevalence of adverse fetal outcomes. Rodent teratogenicity studies are reassuring. Ranitidine is widely used, with or without an antacid, to minimise the risk of potentially life-threatening pneumonitis that can result from the maternal aspiration of gastric fluid during delivery (Mendelson's syndrome). The standard maternal dose for this is 150 mg by mouth, repeatable after 6 hours. A liquid non-particulate antacid, such as 30 ml of 0.3M sodium citrate, is often given as well if a general anaesthetic becomes necessary. Such a strategy has been shown to reduce gastric acidity and seems safe for the baby, but because the complication is so uncommon, it is difficult to prove that this reduces the threat of serious pneumonitis, and aspiration can still occur despite prophylaxis. Ranitidine passes into breast milk, but the breastfed infant receives only sub-therapeutic amounts.

Treatment
By mouth
Neonate: 2 mg/kg every 8 hours. May be increased to a maximum of 3 mg/kg every 8 hours. Variable first-pass metabolism affects uptake in the term baby.
Infant 1–6 months: Start at 1 mg/kg every 8 hours. May be increased to 3 mg/kg every 8 hours.
Infant 7–12 months: 2–4 mg/kg twice daily.

IV administration
Neonate: 500 micrograms/kg given slowly IV twice a day will usually keep the gastric pH >4 in babies <32 weeks' gestation in the first week of life. Term babies may need 1 (or even 1.5) mg/kg every 6–8 hours. Rapid administration can (rarely) cause an arrhythmia.
Infant 1–6 months: 1 mg/kg every 6–8 hours
Continuous IV infusion: This is rarely used (or necessary). Give a 1.5 mg/kg loading dose, followed by a maintenance infusion of 50 micrograms/kg/hour. Half this dose is more than adequate in the very preterm baby soon after birth.

Compatibility
Ranitidine can be added (terminally), when necessary, into a line containing adrenaline, atracurium, dobutamine, dopamine, fentanyl, glyceryl trinitrate, heparin, insulin, isoprenaline, midazolam, milrinone, morphine, nitroprusside, noradrenaline or vancomycin or with standard TPN (with or without lipid).

Supply and administration
2 ml ampoules containing 25 mg/ml of ranitidine hydrochloride for IV or intramuscular use are available costing 54p. For accurate IV administration, take 1 ml (25 mg) from this ampoule and dilute to 50 ml with 5% glucose to get a preparation containing 500 micrograms/ml. To give a

Continued on p. 448

continuous infusion of 50 micrograms/kg/hour, take 1 ml (25 mg) of drug from the ampoule and dilute to 10 ml with 5% glucose. Then take 1 ml of this diluted solution for each kilogram the baby weighs, make this up to 50 ml with 5% glucose, and infuse at a rate of 1 ml/hour. The drug is stable in solution, so a fresh infusion is not needed every day.

A 15 mg/ml sugar-free syrup, which should not be diluted further, is available (100 ml costs £2.70). Some brands contain alcohol, and care should be taken with young and preterm babies.

References

Bianconi S, Gudavalli M, Sutija VG, *et al.* Ranitidine and late onset sepsis in the neonatal intensive care unit. *J Perinat Med* 2007;**35**:147–50.

Fontana M, Massironi E, Rossi A, *et al.* Ranitidine pharmacokinetics in newborn infants. *Arch Dis Child* 1993;**68**:602–3.

Garbis H, Elefant E, Diav CO, *et al.* Pregnancy outcome after exposure to ranitidine and other H_2 blockers. A collaborative study of the European Network of Teratology Information Services. *Reprod Toxicol* 2005;**19**:453–8.

Guillet R, Stoll BJ, Cotten M, *et al.* Association of H_2-blocker therapy and higher incidence of necrotizing enterocolitis in very low birth weight infants. *Pediatrics* 2006;**117**:e137–42. (See also pp. 531–2.)

Kearns GL, McConnell RF Jr, Trang JM, *et al.* Appearance of ranitidine in breast milk following multiple dosing. *Clin Pharm* 1985;**4**:322–4.

Kuusela A-L. Long term gastric pH monitoring for determining optimal dose or ranitidine for critically ill pre-term and term neonates. *Arch Dis Child Fetal Neonatal Ed* 1998;**78**:F151–3.

Matok I, Gorodischer R, Koren G, *et al.* The safety of H_2-blockers use during pregnancy. *J Clin Pharmacol* 2010;**50**:81–7.

Messori A, Trippoli S, Vaiani M, *et al.* Bleeding and pneumonia in intensive care patients given ranitidine and sucralfate for prevention of stress ulcer: meta-analysis of randomised controlled trials. *Br Med J* 2000;**321**:1103–6. [SR]

Salvatore S, Hauser B, Salvatoni A, *et al.* Oral ranitidine and duration of gastric pH >4.0 in infants with per-sisting reflux symptoms. *Acta Paediatr* 2006;**95**:176–81.

Tighe MP, Afzal NA, Bevan A, *et al.* Current pharmacological management of gastro-esophageal reflux in children: an evidence-based systematic review. *Pediatr Drugs* 2009;**11**:185–202. [SR]

Use

Remifentanil is a very short-acting opiate related to fentanyl (q.v.) that can be used to titrate pain relief during surgery without causing troublesome post-operative respiratory depression. It is always given by intravenous (IV) injection. A single dose is now starting to be used to reduce pain and relax the muscles during neonatal intubation.

Pharmacology

Remifentanil hydrochloride is a short-acting μ-receptor opioid agonist that was first developed in 1991. It achieves its peak analgesic effect within a minute of administration (three or four times faster than fentanyl and very much faster than morphine). Unlike the other opioid drugs currently in clinical use, it is rapidly hydrolysed by non-specific blood and tissue esterases within minutes into a carboxylic acid metabolite which has almost no biological activity, 95% of which is then excreted in the urine. Indeed, it was specifically designed with these properties in mind. The half-life, both in infancy and in later life, is just 5 minutes. Clinical recovery is, therefore, rapid, and it is thought that, because of this, many of the problems of drug dependence and progressive drug accumulation often seen with other opioid drugs can be avoided.

Sustained use does however seem to cause tolerance to develop. A single IV dose provides pain relief within 1 minute that normally only lasts for 5–10 minutes irrespective of the magnitude of the dose given. As a result, sustained analgesia for longer operative procedures requires the administration of a continuous infusion. The most common side effects of such use are nausea, vomiting and headache. While these problems are less often seen when midazolam (q.v.) is given as well, dual treatment significantly increases the risk of respiratory depression. High-dose treatment may cause muscle rigidity of the type sometimes seen with fentanyl. Brief bradycardia is also not uncommon. The manufacturers have not yet recommended use in children less than a year old.

Remifentanil crosses the placenta. Rodent teratogenicity studies have been reassuring, but there are limited data about use during the first trimester. Use during delivery may result in neonatal sedation and respiratory depression. It is not known if remifentanil enters breast milk. However, considering the indication for use and very short half-life, one-time remifentanil use is unlikely to pose a clinically significant risk to the breastfed neonate.

As well as the rapid hydrolysis by non-specific blood and tissue esterases, N-dealkylation of remifentanil by cytochrome P450 also occurs, and there are no published data of remifentanil use in neonatal therapeutic hypothermia. Data from adults undergoing hypothermia during coronary artery bypass grafting show that for each degree fall in temperature below 37 °C, there is a proportional decrease of 6.4% in remifentanil clearance. Care should therefore be exercised if remifentanil is used during hypothermia and the dose titrated against the baby's need.

Treatment

Short term pain relief: 1 microgram/kg IV provides 5–10 minutes of pain relief after 60 seconds but may also briefly cause some respiratory depression. Giving 2 micrograms/kg provides as much muscle relaxation as suxamethonium.

Sustained pain relief: Start by giving 1 microgram/kg/minute IV, after taking control of the child's respiratory needs, and double this if necessary for a while to give 'real-time' control over operative pain of variable intensity. Even higher doses have been used. Remember that pain relief will only last a few minutes once the infusion is stopped or interrupted and that most other analgesics take time to become effective.

Sedation during ventilation: A 10th this dose (0.1 microgram/kg/minute) sedates the preterm baby.

Antidote

Naloxone (q.v.) is an effective antidote, but remifentanil's short half-life should render use unnecessary.

Continued on p. 450

Compatibility

Remifentanil can be added (terminally) to a line containing fentanyl, midazolam or morphine.

Supply and administration

Reconstitution: Prescribing conventionally refers to the amount of remifentanil base, and the product is supplied in vials of varying strength. A vial containing 1 mg of remifentanil base (or ~1.1 mg of remifentanil hydrochloride) costs £4.60. Reconstitute the lyophilised powder in this with 1 ml of sterile water.

Dilution for single dose use: Take 0.1 ml of the reconstituted powder and dilute to 10 ml with 0.9% sodium chloride to get a solution containing 10 micrograms/ml.

Preparing to give a sustained infusion: Take 0.2 ml (200 micrograms) of the reconstituted powder for each kg the baby weighs, and dilute to 10 ml with 0.9% sodium chloride to get a solution that delivers 1 microgram/kg/minute when infused at a rate of 3 ml/hour (for sustained pain relief) or 0.1 microgram/kg/minute when infused at a rate of 0.3 ml/hour (for sedation).

References

Choong K, AlFaleh K, Doucette J, *et al.* Remifentanil for endotracheal intubation in neonates: a randomised controlled trial. *Arch Dis Child Fetal Neonatal Ed* 2010;**95**:F80–4. [RCT]

Crawford MW, Hayes J, Tan JM. Dose-response of remifentanil for tracheal intubation in infants. *Anesth Analg* 2005;**100**:1599–604.

e Silva YP, Gomez RS, Marcatto J de O, *et al.* Early awakening and extubation with remifentanil in ventilated premature neonates. *Pediatr Anesth* 2008;**18**:17683. [RCT]

e Silva YP, Gomez RS, Marcatte J de O, *et al.* Morphine versus remifentanil for intubating preterm neonates. *Arch Dis Child Fetal Neonatal Ed* 2007;**92**:F293–4. [RCT]

Giannantonio C, Sammartino M, Valente E, *et al.* Remifentanil analgosedation in preterm newborns during mechanical ventilation. *Acta Paediatr* 2009;**98**:1111–5.

Norman E, Wikström S, Hellström-Westas L, *et al.* Rapid sequence induction is superior to morphine for intubation of preterm infants: a randomized controlled trial. *J Pediatr* 2011;**159**:893–9.e1. [RCT]

Van de Velde M, Keunkens A, Kuypers M, *et al.* General anaesthesia with target controlled infusion of propofol for planned caesarean section: maternal and neonatal effects of a remifentanil-based technique. *Int J Obstet Anesth* 2004;**13**:153–8.

Weale NK, Rogers CA, Cooper R, *et al.* Effect of remifentanil infusion rate on stress response to the by-pass phase of paediatric cardiac surgery. *Br J Anaesth* 2004;**92**:187–94.

Welzing L, Kribs A, Huenseler C, *et al.* Remifentanil for INSURE in preterm infants: a pilot study for evaluation of efficacy and safety. *Acta Paediatr* 2009;**98**:1426–20.

Welzing L, Roth B. Experience with remifentanil in neonates and infants. *Drugs* 2006;**66**:1339–50. [SR]

Use

An immunoglobulin used to prevent rhesus (Rh) (D) isoimmunisation.

Product

A human immune globulin (currently collected by apheresis from the plasma of donors with high levels of anti-D antibody in the United States) has been used since 1970 to prevent Rh (D)-negative mothers from developing antibodies to transplacentally acquired Rh (D)-positive fetal red cells during childbirth. It is also used after miscarriage, threatened miscarriage and abortion after 12 weeks' gestation or any other obstetric manoeuvre such as chorionic villus biopsy, amniocentesis, fetal blood sampling and external cephalic version that could be associated with feto-maternal bleeding. Other events such as ectopic pregnancy, antepartum haemorrhage and blunt abdominal trauma (from, e.g. seat belt injury) should also be covered. The product works by eliminating fetal red cells from the circulation before they can stimulate active maternal antibody production. While it should be given within 72 hours, if possible, with a view to preventing Rh isoimmunisation compromising any future pregnancy, it still offers some protection if given within 12 days. A monoclonal IgG$_3$ antibody is still under development.

Approximately 1% of Rh-negative mothers develop Rh antibodies late in their first pregnancy (but before delivery) in the absence of any recognisable sensitising event. Furthermore, these 'hypersensitive' mothers seem to be at risk of having a baby with disease of atypical severity in any subsequent pregnancy. Antenatal treatment at 28 and 34 weeks more than halves this risk, but there may be better ways to use the money this would cost in communities where such problems are rare.

Up to about 15% of Rh (D)-positive babies born to Rh (D)-negative women who have received Rh (D) immunoglobulin may have a 'positive' direct antibody (Coombs) test. This is usually only 'weakly' positive but some units do not grade the degree of response; a blood film should distinguish between passive and immune anti-D as a cause of a positive test.

Indications

The amount of anti-D (Rh$_o$) immunoglobulin actually required is proportional to the size of the feto-maternal bleed. For events occurring before 20 weeks' gestation, it has been traditional to give 250 units (50 micrograms) of anti-D immunoglobulin. Later in pregnancy and after delivery, the usual dose is 500 units (100 micrograms), but this should be increased if a Kleihauer test on the mother's blood shows more than one fetal cell per 500 adult red cells (equivalent to 4–5 ml of packed fetal red cells). Such bleeds should be quantified by flow cytometry and an additional 150 units of anti-D immunoglobulin given for each millilitre by which the transplacental bleed exceeds 4 ml of packed fetal red cells.

Contraindications

There are no known contraindications. Use of the UK product has never caused the acquisition of any blood-product-transmitted infection such as hepatitis B or HIV, and current supplies come from America where there is minimal risk of the donor having latent variant Creutzfeldt–Jakob disease. Simultaneous rubella (or MMR) vaccination is acceptable as long as separate syringes are used and the products injected into different limbs. Treat any reaction as outlined in the monograph on immunisation.

Administration

During pregnancy: All Rh (D)-negative women should be offered an intramuscular injection at 28 and 34 weeks' gestation (500 unit seems adequate, but a 1250 unit dose is widely used) to stop the baby becoming immunised before birth unless (a) antenatal tests have shown that the fetus is Rh negative, *or* (b) the mother knows this is going to be her last pregnancy, *or* (c) she knows that the child's father is Rh negative. Injections are usually given into the deltoid muscle.
After delivery: Give at least 500 units IM to Rh-negative mothers whose babies are Rh positive (or whose blood group is unknown). It is pointless to treat mothers who have already started to produce antibodies to the D antigen but important to remember that mothers with *other* antibodies (anti-c, anti-Kell, etc.) may still require protection from the D antigen if they are Rh (D) negative.

Continued on p. 452

Supply and administration

A range of commercial and volunteer donor products are now available in vials and prefilled syringes containing from 250 to 1500 units of anti-D immunoglobulin. 500 units of a non-proprietary product costs £34. Most need to be stored at 4 °C, but lyophilised powders (which should be reconstituted with 0.9% sodium chloride) are safe for a month at room temperature. The products need prescribing, but maternity units in the United Kingdom have now developed Patient Group Directions, because these give midwives a more proactive role in ensuring that all Rh-negative mothers have easy access to prophylaxis.

References   (See also the relevant Cochrane reviews and UK guidelines)

Egbor M, Knott P, Bhide A. Red-cell and platelet alloimmunisation in pregnancy. *Best Pract Res Clin Obstet Gynaecol* 2012;**26**:119–32.

Finning K, Martin P, Summers J, *et al.* Effect of high throughput *RHD* typing of fetal DNA in maternal plasma on use of anti-RhD immunoglobulin in RhD negative pregnant women: prospective feasibility study. *Br Med J* 2008;**336**:816–8.

James RM, McGuire W, Smith DP. The investigation of infants with RhD-negative mothers: can we safely omit the umbilical cord blood direct antiglobulin test? *Arch Dis Child Fetal Neonatal Ed* 2011;**96**:F301–4.

Kumar S, Regan F. Management of pregnancies with RhD alloimmunisation. *Br Med J* 2006;**330**:1255–8 and 1485.

Pilgrim H, Lloyd-Jones M, Rees A. Routine antenatal anti-D prophylaxis for RhD-negative women: a systematic review and economic evaluation. *Health Technol Assess* 2009;**13**(10):1–103. [SR]

Roberts IAG. The changing face of haemolytic disease of the newborn. *Early Hum Dev* 2008;**84**:515–24.

Smits-Wintjens VEHJ, Walther FJ, Lopiore E. Rhesus haemolytic disease of the newborn: postnatal management, associated morbidity and long-term outcome. *Semin Fetal Neonat Med* 2008;**13**:265–71.

Use

Ribavirin was once widely used to reduce the severity of bronchiolitis, but lack of significant benefits has led to its use being restricted to high-risk cases. Combined treatment with interferon alfa (see archived monograph) controls viraemia and slows disease progression in children with chronic hepatitis C infection.

Pharmacology

Ribavirin (first synthesised in 1972) is a stable, white, synthetic nucleoside with *in vitro* antiviral properties against the respiratory syncytial virus and some adenoviruses as well as the influenza, parainfluenza and measles viruses. A significant amount of drug is absorbed systemically after aerosol administration, and the concentration in respiratory secretions is particularly high.

While ribavirin is teratogenic and embryolethal, there is limited published experience (case reports) of use during pregnancy (for the treatment of maternal hepatitis C), and while no adverse effects have been reported, data are too limited to draw any conclusions. Animal studies suggest increased prevalence of limb, eye and brain defects. There is some evidence that it can be mutagenic in cell culture and may (with chronic exposure) induce benign glandular tumours.

Clinical use is therefore currently limited to high-risk children (children with congenital heart disease, existing bronchopulmonary dysplasia or immunodeficiency) with proven lower respiratory tract viral infection. There is only one study suggesting that use speeds recovery in ventilator-dependent infants, and there is little evidence that it reduces the time it takes for patients to stop shedding live virus particles. The only common adverse effect in children with standard treatment is conjunctivitis, but little is known about possible long-term morbidity or toxicity.

Perinatal hepatitis C infection

When viral RNA can be detected in the mother's blood on PCR testing during pregnancy, there is about a 5% risk of the baby becoming infected, and this increases if the woman also has HIV. There is, however, no reason to undertake caesarean delivery or advise the woman not to breastfeed unless there is HIV. One study suggests that delaying membrane rupture as long as possible once the woman goes into labour may minimise the risk of transmission.

If the woman is anti-HCV antibody positive and viral RNA is not detectable, it is very rare for the baby to become infected. When perinatal (rather than antenatal) infection occurs, viral RNA may take 2–3 months to become detectable in the baby, but if it does appear, this indicates active infection and merits referral to a supra-regional liver centre. Other babies should be watched until they become anti-HCV negative. The prognosis for those babies who do become actively infected is variable. It looks as though complete viral elimination occurs in a quarter, but a minority develop progressive disease meriting treatment with ribavirin and interferon alfa to stop liver fibrosis eventually progressing to frank cirrhosis.

Treatment

Nebulised administration: Administer 60 mg/ml of ribavirin for 2 hours three times a day using a small particle aerosol generator (SPAG) for 3–7 days, preferably using a modified Easy Vent® CPAP device. Early treatment *may* be appropriate in high-risk children with a proven viral lower respiratory tract infection to try and reduce the chance of their needing ventilator support. There is no good evidence that use shortens the duration of treatment in children already ill enough to be receiving respiratory support, and such use can easily cause the ventilator to become clogged.

Intravenous (IV) administration: This may be considered in life-threatening RSV, parainfluenza virus and adenovirus infection in immunocompromised children. Give 33 mg/kg as a single dose, then 16 mg/kg every 6 hours for 4 days and then 8 mg/kg every 8 hours for 3 days. Each dose is given as an IV infusion over 15 minutes.

Oral administration: Children with progressive chronic hepatitis C infection have been treated with 15 mg/kg of ribavirin by mouth once a day for 6 or even 12 months. While such treatment is of little benefit on its own, combined treatment with subcutaneous interferon alfa-2b frequently abolishes all detectable evidence of viraemia during treatment and for at least 6 months after treatment stops, especially in patients with genotype 2 or 3 infection. The dose of interferon used has usually been 3 million units/m² of the standard preparation three times a week or 15 micrograms/kg of the pegylated (polyethylene glycol-conjugated) product once a week. Such treatment has *not* yet been attempted in children less than a year old.

Continued on p. 454

Supply and administration

Ribavirin comes in vials containing 6 g of lyophilised drug costing £350 per vial. For nebulised administration, dissolve the powder with 300 ml of sterile water for injection free of all preservatives. Any of the reconstituted solution not used within 24 hours of preparation should be discarded. 10 ml (100 mg/ml) vials for IV administration are available on a named-patient basis from Valeant Pharmaceuticals International Inc. A bubble gum-flavoured oral solution containing 40 mg/ml of ribavirin costs £67 for 100 ml.

References   (See also the relevant Cochrane reviews)

Davison SM, Mieli-Vergani G, Sira J, *et al.* Perinatal hepatitis C virus infection: diagnosis and management. *Arch Dis Child* 2006;**91**:781–5.

Fischler B. Hepatitis C virus infection. *Semin Fetal Neonat Med* 2007;**12**:168–73.

Gonzalez-Peralta R, Kelly DA, Haber B, *et al.* Interferon alfa 2b in combination with ribavirin for the treatment of chronic hepatitis C in children: efficacy, safety and pharmacokinetics. *Hepatology* 2005;**42**:1010–18.

Guerguerian A-M, Gauthier M, Lebel M, *et al.* Ribavirin in ventilated respiratory syncytial virus bronchiolitis. *Am J Respir Crit Care Med* 1999;**160**:829–31. [RCT]

Hu J, Doucette K, Hartling L, *et al.* Treatment of hepatitis C in children: a systematic review. *PLoS One* 2010;**5**:e11542. [SR]

Schuh S. Update on management of bronchiolitis. *Curr Opin Pediatr* 2011;**23**:110–4.

Smedsaas-Löfvenberg A, Nilsson K, Moa G, *et al.* Nebulisation of drugs in a CPAP system. *Acta Paediatr* 1999;**88**:89–92.

Wirth S, Pieper-Boustani H, Lang T, *et al.* Peginterferon alfa-2b plus ribavirin treatment in children and adolescents with chronic hepatitis C. *Hepatology* 2005;**41**:1013–8.

Use

Rifampicin is used with isoniazid (q.v.) to treat tuberculosis and with vancomycin or teicoplanin (q.v.) to treat severe staphylococcal infection. Although largely superseded by ciprofloxacin (q.v.) as prophylaxis in contacts of meningococcal disease, it remains the drug of choice in preventing secondary cases of *Haemophilus* infection. It also has a role in the treatment of cholestatic pruritus.

Pharmacology

This bactericidal antibiotic, first developed in 1966, interferes with DNA-dependent RNA polymerase. It has activity against many mycobacteria, *Neisseria meningitidis* and *N. gonorrhoeae* and is the most active anti-staphylococcal agent known. However, since resistant strains of *Mycobacterium* or *Staphylococcus* emerge quickly if rifampicin is used alone, it is recommended that rifampicin should always be used in combination with a second antibiotic except when the drug is used prophylactically to eliminate bacterial carriage and reduce the risk of meningitis. Rifampicin is readily absorbed when given by mouth. It is highly protein bound and undergoes enterohepatic recirculation. Up to 30% may be excreted unchanged, but the metabolites are excreted in the urine and bile. Dose intervals do not need to be modified in the presence of renal failure. Rifampicin colours urine and other secretions red. The half-life is 3–4 hours but twice this in the first month of life. Transient jaundice can be ignored, but treatment must be stopped at once if thrombocytopenia, nausea and vomiting or other signs of more serious liver toxicity develop. Such adverse effects are rare in children unless there is prior liver disease.

Rifampicin crosses the placenta, but its use is not contraindicated in pregnancy, although use in the third trimester is said to be associated with an increased risk of neonatal bleeding meriting routine intramuscular (IM) vitamin K prophylaxis (q.v.). Some authorities prescribe supplemental maternal vitamin K (10 mg/day) for the last 4–8 weeks of pregnancy. Very little of the drug appears in breast milk.

Drug interactions

Rifampicin induces microsomal liver enzymes and therefore affects the metabolism of a wide range of other drugs. Chloramphenicol, corticosteroids, most benzodiazepines, digoxin, fluconazole, nifedipine, phenobarbital, phenytoin, theophylline, warfarin and zidovudine are all metabolised more rapidly, and dosage levels may need adjustment. Rifampicin also induces its own metabolism, and as a result, clearance increases markedly during the first 2 weeks of use. Treatment of HIV infection with the protease inhibitors nelfinavir and ritonavir greatly increases the clearance of rifampicin, making co-treatment more complex.

Treatment

Synergistic use with teicoplanin or vancomycin: Experience remains limited. Give 10 mg/kg by slow intravenous (IV) infusion (1 ml/kg of dilute solution made up as described under 'Supply and administration') slowly once every 12 hours piggybacked onto an existing IV infusion of glucose or glucose saline for 10 days or 20 mg/kg once a day by mouth.

Treatment of tuberculosis: Seek expert advice. Give 10 mg/kg once a day by mouth (20 mg/kg if meningitis is suspected), together with isoniazid (q.v.). Warn parents that the urine may turn red. Give 1 mg of IM vitamin K if the child is <3 months old to minimise the risk of vitamin K deficiency bleeding.

Secondary prophylaxis against *Haemophilus* infection: Household contacts of index cases should be offered chemoprophylaxis. Give a 10 mg/kg dose to any infant <3 months old and 20 mg/kg to any infants older than 3 months. These doses are given once a day for 4 days up to 4 weeks after onset of illness in the index case.

Secondary prophylaxis against meningococcal infection: Ciprofloxacin is the first choice drug here but rifampicin may be used at a dose of 5 mg/kg every 12 hours for 2 days.

Preventing continued group B streptococcal carriage: 20 mg/kg once a day by mouth for 7 days will reduce, but not eliminate, the risk of continued carriage. Give carrier mothers 600 mg twice a day as well.

Pruritus due to cholestasis: Give 5 (or 10) mg/kg twice a day. Monitor liver function for the first month.

Supply and administration

Rifampicin is available as a powder for IV use in 600 mg vials (costing £7.70) normally dispensed with 10 ml of solvent. Reconstitute the 600 mg vial with 9.6 ml of the solvent and shake well. Take 60 mg of rifampicin (1 ml of the fluid from a 600 mg vial), dilute to 10 ml with 5 or 10%

Continued on p. 456

dextrose to obtain a solution containing 6 mg/ml of rifampicin, and use within 6 hours. Slow infusion over 30–60 minutes is recommended in adults because of the volume involved and because there is some slight risk of hypotension and phlebitis. Do not co-infuse with any alkaline solution. Rifampicin should not be given IM. A 20 mg/ml raspberry flavoured syrup is also available with an undiluted shelf life of 3 years (120 ml costs £3.60).

References
(See also the relevant Cochrane reviews)

Acocella G. Clinical pharmacokinetics of rifampicin. *Clin Pharmacokinet* 1978;**3**:108–27.

American Academy of Pediatrics. Committee on Infectious Diseases. Chemotherapy for tuberculosis in infants and children. *Pediatrics* 1992;**69**:161–5.

Fernandez M, Rench MA, Albanyan EA, *et al.* Failure of rifampin to eradicate group B streptococcal colonisation in infants. *Pediatr Infect Dis J* 2001;**20**:371–6.

Gregorio GV, Ball CS, Mowat AP, *et al.* Effect of rifampicin in the treatment of pruritus in hepatic cholestasis. *Arch Dis Child* 1993;**69**:141–3.

Pullen J, Stolk LML, Degaeuwe PLJ, *et al.* Pharmacokinetics of intravenous rifampicin (rifampin) in neonates. *Ther Drug Monit* 2006;**28**:654–61.

Rosenfeld EA, Hageman JR, Yogev R. Tuberculosis in infancy in the 1990s. *Pediatr Clin North Am* 1993;**40**:1087–103.

Shama A, Patole SK, Whitehall JS. Intravenous rifampicin in neonates with persistent staphylococcal bacteraemia. *Acta Paediatr* 2002;**91**:670–3.

Soukka H, Rantakokko-Jalava K, Vähäkuopus S, *et al.* Three distinct episodes of GBS septicemia in a healthy newborn during the first month of life. *Eur J Pediatr* 2010;**169**:1275–7.

Tan TQ, Mason EO, Ou C-N, *et al.* Use of intravenous rifampicin in neonates with persistent staphylococcal bacteremia. *Antimicrob Agents Chemother* 1993;**37**:2401–6.

Use

Rocuronium can be used instead of suxamethonium (q.v.) to provide rapid muscle paralysis during tracheal intubation, but recovery is much slower. Vecuronium (q.v.) is a similarly long-acting paralytic agent but takes longer to work. Atracurium and mivacurium (q.v.) are useful (but slower acting) alternatives when short-term paralysis is all that is required but are more likely to trigger histamine release.

Pharmacology

Rocuronium is a monoquaternary aminosteroidal muscle relaxant of relatively low potency that first came into clinical use in 1994. It works, like the other non-depolarising muscle relaxants, by competitively attaching itself to the cholinergic receptors on the 'end plates' responsible for transmitting nerve signals to the body's voluntary muscles. Conditions for undertaking laryngeal intubation are achieved almost as quickly with intravenous (IV) rocuronium as they are with IV suxamethonium, but recovery takes much longer, rendering use hazardous if unexpected difficulties are encountered in securing the airway. However, if the drug has to be given by intramuscular (IM) injection, effective muscle relaxation takes much longer to achieve with rocuronium than with suxamethonium (5–10 vs. 3–4 minutes). Rocuronium is mostly eliminated by the liver and the biliary system, but up to a quarter is excreted unchanged in the urine. The half-life in infancy (~1.3 hours) is marginally longer than it is in older children and not greatly affected by renal dysfunction. The manufacturer has not yet endorsed the use of rocuronium in babies less than a month old.

Manufacturers have been reluctant to recommend the use of rocuronium during pregnancy or lactation, and nothing is known about use during the first trimester. Rocuronium crosses the placenta, but it and other neuromuscular blocking agents do not, as a group, seem to pose a significant risk to the embryo or fetus. Rodent teratogenicity studies are reassuring. In women undergoing rapid-sequence induction of general anaesthesia, the F/M ratio is ~0.18 at delivery. No clinical sequelae are noted in the neonate. There is no published experience during lactation; however, considering the indication and dosing, limited use of rocuronium is unlikely to pose a clinically significant risk to the breastfed infant.

Treatment

Brief use to effect intubation: 450 micrograms/kg of rocuronium provides the muscle relaxation needed to effect easy laryngeal intubation within a minute in babies less than a year old, but recovery may take an hour. A larger dose does not speed the onset of paralysis and may double recovery time in a young baby.

Use to provide sustained paralysis: Start by giving 600 micrograms/kg of rocuronium IV. Most babies continue to comply with the imposed ventilator rate as they wake from this first paralysing dose (especially if a moderately fast rate and a relatively short inspiratory time are used), but a few require prolonged paralysis. The standard repeat dose is ¼ to ½ the initial dose IV (or IM) every 2–4 hours as necessary, but some older babies seem to require a higher maintenance dose. Paralysed babies should always be sedated. An infusion of 300–600 micrograms/kg/hour (adjusted according to response) is an alternative to intermittent dosing.

Antidote

Give a combination of 10 micrograms/kg of glycopyrronium (or 20 micrograms/kg of atropine) and 50 micrograms/kg of neostigmine IV, as outlined in the monograph on glycopyrronium.

Sugammadex, a modified γ-cyclodextrin with a lipophilic core and a hydrophilic periphery, is a specific antidote sometimes used to reverse the neuromuscular blockade induced by rocuronium in older children and adults. Information about use in infants, let alone in neonates, is sparse. The manufacturers have yet to endorse its use in children under 2 years of age.

Supply and administration

Rocuronium comes in 5 ml vials containing 10 mg/ml of rocuronium bromide. They cost £3 each. Take 0.1 ml and dilute to 1 ml with 0.9% sodium chloride or 5% glucose to obtain a solution containing 100 micrograms in 0.1 ml for accurate neonatal administration.

Sugammadex is available in 2 ml ampoules containing 100 mg/ml (cost £60). The dose in older children is 2 mg/kg; similar doses appear to be effective in infants in the few case reports to date.

Continued on p. 458

References

Atherton DP, Hunter DM. Clinical pharmacokinetics of the newer neuromuscular blocking drugs. *Clin Pharmacokinet* 1999;**36**:169–89.

Buchanan CC, O'Donnell AM. Case report: sugammadex used to successfully reverse vecuronium-induced neuromuscular blockade in a 7-month-old infant. *Paediatr Anaesth* 2011;**21**:1077–8.

Chambers D, Paulden M, Paton F, *et al*. Sugammadex for reversal of neuromuscular block after rapid sequence intubation: a systematic review and economic assessment. *Br J Anaesth* 2010;**105**:568–75.

Feltman DM, Weiss MG, Nicoski P, *et al*. Rocuronium for nonemergent intubation of term and preterm infants. *J Perinatol* 2011;**31**:38–43. [RCT]

Kaplan RF, Uejima T, Lobel G, *et al*. Intramuscular rocuronium in infants and children: a multicenter study to evaluate tracheal intubating conditions, onset, and duration of action. *Anesthesiology* 1999;**91**:633–8.

Plaud B, Meretoja O, Hofmockel R, *et al*. Reversal of rocuronium-induced neuromuscular blockade with sugammadex in pediatric and adult surgical patients. *Anesthesiology* 2009;**110**:284–94.

Playfor S. Neuromuscular blocking agents in critically ill children. *Paediat Perinat Drug Ther* 2002;**5**:35–46.

Rapp H-J, Altenmueller CA, Waschke C. Neuromuscular recovery following rocuronium bromide single dose in infants. *Pediatr Anaesth* 2004;**14**:329–35.

Zelicof-Paul A, Smith-Lockridge A, Schnadower D, *et al*. Controversies in rapid sequence intubation in children. *Curr Opin Pediatr* 2005;**17**:355–62.

Use

Rotaviruses are the leading cause of severe, dehydrating diarrhoea in children under 5 years of age, causing ~450,000 gastroenteritis-associated child deaths worldwide, over 95% in resource-poor developing countries. Two very effective oral vaccines were introduced in 2006; neither seems to cause intussusception like the first licensed vaccine (RotaShield®) was found to do before its eventual withdrawal from the market in 1999.

Rotaviruses were first discovered in 1973, and it soon became clear that almost every child becomes infected with this virus at least once in their first 5 years. The peak age for infection is 3–30 months, and most infection is caused by the oral intake of faecal contaminants, although respiratory (aerosol) spread may occur. Young and malnourished children are always the most seriously affected. An attenuated monovalent live human rotavirus vaccine (Rotarix®), when tested in a trial involving 20,000 children in Latin America and Finland, reduced serious rotavirus gastroenteritis by 85% and 'all-cause' gastroenteritis by 40%. A pentavalent bovine–human vaccine (RotaTeq®) proved at least as effective when tested on 68,000 American and European children. Surveillance of use of both these vaccines in North America since 2006 has shown a clustering of intussusception events during days 3–6 after the first-dose vaccination, with an estimated excess risk of approximately 0.79 intussusception events for every 100,000 vaccinated infants.

Despite the work of the GAVI Alliance, the communities most in need of these vaccines are those least able to afford them. Development of vaccines for resource-poor countries has been a WHO priority, and one attenuated monovalent bovine–human rotavirus vaccine (Rotavac) has recently undergone a phase 3 trial in India and looks likely to offer the same protection for a fraction of the cost. A Vietnamese product (Rotavin-M1) is being investigated in phase 2 trials.

Because infection is particularly dangerous in a very young child, the logical time to start immunisation is 6–8 weeks after birth. Because of lingering concern that intussusception might still be a problem, the vaccines are currently only licensed for use in children <6–8 months old.

Contraindications

Give thought to the balance of risk before giving either vaccine to a child with gastrointestinal symptoms or to a child who is in close contact with an immunodeficient person. Despite its live attenuated nature, studies in HIV-infected children have shown no additional adverse events. Vaccination is advised not only in infants born to HIV-positive mothers in whom the HIV status is 'indeterminate' but also in infants known to be infected.

Preterm infants

There is no evidence that administration should be delayed or avoided because of preterm birth, although because of the live attenuated nature of the vaccine, the North American ACIP advises the vaccine is best given after discharge from the neonatal unit (as long as the first dose is *before* 15 weeks of age). In contrast, the United Kingdom's JCVI and the Australian ATAGI both advocate the immunisation of stable hospitalised infants at the appropriate time stating that, provided standard infection control precautions are maintained, administration of rotavirus vaccine to hospitalised preterm infants would be expected to carry a low risk for transmission.

Interactions

Other intramuscular paediatric vaccines can be given safely and effectively at the same time as an oral rotavirus vaccine. Concurrent administration with oral polio vaccine can reduce the immune responses (i.e. the antibody levels) to rotavirus vaccination but does not appear to affect the protective efficacy of the vaccine.

Administration

Rotarix: Give two doses by mouth at least 4 weeks apart. Rotarix is now part of the routine immunisation schedule in the United Kingdom (see monograph on immunisation).

RotaTeq: Give three doses by mouth (at 2, 4 and 6 months). The first dose should be given 6–12 weeks after birth, and other two doses should then be given 4–10 weeks apart. Do not repeat if spat out.

Rotavac: Give three doses by mouth at 6–7 weeks, with further doses at least 4 weeks apart.

Continued on p. 460

Supply

Rotarix: This product from GSK comes as a lyophilised powder that needs to be stored at 2–8 °C and reconstituted with buffered diluent. Vials (with a syringe containing 1 ml of the necessary diluent) cost £41.

RotaTeq: This product from Merck comes as a buffered pale-yellow liquid in 2 ml ready-to-use, squeezable, plastic dosing tubes that cost $55 each. Store and transport at 2–8 °C and protect from light.

Rotavac: This Indian product from Bharat Biotech International Limited has yet to receive a licence and is not yet available for use outside clinical trials. It is expected to cost ~55 INR per dose.

References

American Academy of Pediatrics Committee on Infectious Diseases. Prevention of rotavirus disease: updated guidelines for use of rotavirus vaccine. *Pediatrics* 2009;**123**:1412–20.

Dang DA, Nguyen VT, Vu DT, *et al*. A dose-escalation safety and immunogenicity study of a new live attenuated human rotavirus vaccine (Rotavin-M1) in Vietnamese children. *Vaccine* 2012;**30**(suppl 1):A114–21.

Dennehy PH, Bretrand HR, Silas PE, *et al*. Coadministration of RIX4414 oral human rotavirus vaccine does not impact on immune response to antigens contained in routine infant vaccine in the United States. *Pediatrics* 2008;**122**:e1062–6.

Giaquinto C, Dominiak-Felden G, Van Damme P, *et al*. Summary of effectiveness and impact of rotavirus vaccination with the oral pentavalent rotavirus vaccine: a systematic review of the experience in industrialized countries. *Hum Vaccin* 2011;**7**:734–48. [SR]

Omenaca F, Sarlangue J, Szenborn L, *et al*. Safety, reactogenicity and immunogenicity of the human rotavirus vaccine in preterm European Infants: a randomized phase IIIb study. *Pediatr Infect Dis J* 2012;**31**:487–93. [RCT]

Steele AD, Madhi SA, Louw CE, *et al*. Safety, Reactogenicity, and immunogenicity of human rotavirus vaccine RIX4414 in human immunodeficiency virus-positive infants in South Africa. *Pediatr Infect Dis J* 2011;**30**:125–30.

Use

A live attenuated rubella virus vaccine was introduced in 1970 to provide active immunity against Rubella in children and in seronegative women of childbearing age. A trivalent measles, mumps and rubella (MMR) vaccine is the product now used in the United Kingdom and many other countries.

Rubella

Rubella (or German measles) is a mild notifiable illness with an incubation period of 14–21 days. Patients are infectious from a week before the rash appears for a period of about 10 days. Symptoms may be minimal, and the rash is often not diagnostic. Diagnosis currently depends on testing paired sera taken 2–3 and 8–9 days after the first appearance of the rash for rubella antibody or a single sample taken 1–6 weeks after the rash first appears tested for the presence of rubella-specific IgM antibody. An alternative is identification of specific IgM in saliva. Natural infection usually causes lasting immunity.

Maternal infection in early pregnancy or just prior to conception can cause serious fetal damage. Infection at 8–10 weeks damages up to 90% of babies. The risk of damage is about 10–20% by 16 week. It is negligible after this. A 750 mg dose of normal immunoglobulin (HNIG) is sometimes given intramuscularly to reduce the chance of clinical infection in pregnant seronegative mothers who do not terminate their pregnancy, but there is no good evidence that it does much good.

Problems associated with congenital infection include cataract, glaucoma, pneumonia, meningoencephalitis, hepatitis, purpuric skin lesions and fetal growth retardation. Cardiac lesions include patent ductus, septal defects and pulmonary artery stenosis. Progressive deafness may develop even in babies who seem normal at birth. Infection in pregnancy is now rare in countries with a policy of universal vaccination in infancy, but such a policy has yet to be instituted in most of Africa, much of Southeast Asia and some parts of Eastern Europe, and it has been estimated that around 100,000 children are probably still born with congenital rubella in the world every year (and even more die of measles).

Product

A vaccine made from an attenuated live virus first came into use in the United Kingdom in 1970. One dose of the vaccine promotes an antibody response in over 95% of recipients, and a second dose has been recommended since 1996. In the United Kingdom, rubella is now only available as part of the MMR vaccine.

The antibody response is well maintained for at least 20 years, and protection against clinical rubella seems to persist even after antibody levels decline. Nevertheless, natural infection does occasionally occur after immunisation (due, presumably, to primary vaccination failure or subsequent loss of immunity), as it can after natural infection, and such infection can cause fetal damage if it occurs in early pregnancy.

Indications in adult life

All women of childbearing age should be made aware of their rubella status and told the outcome of any serological test. Any found to be seronegative during pregnancy should also be offered vaccination with the MMR after delivery and, ideally, before discharge from the maternity unit. It is perfectly acceptable to give a Rubella-containing vaccine and anti-D (Rh$_0$) immunoglobulin at the same time as long as different syringes and different sites are employed. Blood transfusions during delivery blunt the response to vaccination however. In such cases, a test for seroconversion should be undertaken 8 weeks later and revaccination offered if necessary. Short-term contraceptive cover can, if necessary, be offered in the interim using medroxyprogesterone acetate (Depo-Provera®) as long as the mother is counselled appropriately and shown the manufacturer's leaflet first. Give 150 mg in 1 ml once by deep intramuscular (IM) injection.

Vaccination should be avoided in early pregnancy (and patients advised not to become pregnant within a month of vaccination), but there has been no recorded case of fetal damage in the United States, Canada, Costa Rica, Sweden, Germany or the United Kingdom among the significant number of mothers inadvertently immunised with the attenuated virus in early pregnancy. Seronegative male and female health service staff in maternity units should also be vaccinated to prevent their transmitting rubella to pregnant patients. A mild reaction with fever, rash and arthralgia may occur 1–3 weeks after vaccination.

Continued on p. 462

Indications in childhood

All children should be offered one dose of the MMR vaccine when 12 months old unless there is a specific contraindication (see overleaf) and a second dose as part of the preschool programme. Children not immunised at this time should be immunised before they start school (or nursery school) and again 3 months later. Measles, mumps and rubella are all notifiable illnesses. All became very uncommon in the United Kingdom after the MMR vaccine was introduced in 1988, but epidemics of measles and congenital rubella are sure to recur unless the current fall in uptake is soon reversed. Recurring media-fuelled fears that the vaccine could be causing autism or a non-specific colitis still persist even though no study to date has shown any such link.

Interactions

More than one live vaccine can be given at different sites on the same day, but an interval of 3 weeks should be allowed if vaccination is not simultaneous. Do not give within 4 weeks of BCG administration.

Contraindications

Pregnancy, immunodeficiency, immunosuppression, reticuloendothelial malignancy and high-dose corticosteroid treatment (the equivalent of >1 mg/kg of prednisolone a day or 2 mg/kg for >1 week in the last 6 weeks) are generally considered contraindications to vaccination. It should also be avoided in those individuals who have had a confirmed anaphylactic reaction to neomycin or gelatin.

All children with egg allergy should receive the MMR vaccination as a routine procedure in primary care. Anaphylaxis after MMR is extremely rare and is usually due to other components of the vaccine rather than egg antigens. A history of fits is not a contraindication.

Vaccination should be delayed if there is any febrile illness and postponed after immunoglobulin injection (other than Rhesus anti-D) for 3 months.

Administration

Over 95% of patients achieve immunity with a single 0.5 ml deep IM injection of the MMR vaccine with a 25 mm 23 gauge needle, but a two-dose regimen is now generally recommended.

Case notification

All cases of suspected congenital rubella (with or without symptoms) in the United Kingdom should continue to be notified to the National Congenital Rubella Surveillance Programme. This can be done directly (tel: Pat Tookey on 020 7905 2604; e-mail: ptookey@ucl.ac.uk) or via the British Paediatric Surveillance Unit's orange card scheme (tel: 020 7092 6173).

The Immunisation Department of the Health Protection Agency is undertaking surveillance of women given either rubella, human papilloma virus (HPV) or varicella immunisations in pregnancy. For details, see http://www.hpa.org.uk/Topics/InfectiousDiseases/InfectionsAZ/VaccineInPregnancySurveillance/.

Supply

Single-dose vials of the freeze-dried live trivalent (MMR) vaccine are available in the United Kingdom and distributed free. In resource-poor countries, immunisation against measles is the main priority, and this is offered as a monovalent vaccine at 6 and 9 months. Although a simple monovalent rubella vaccine is available in some of these countries, this particular vaccine is no longer obtainable in the United Kingdom. Store vaccines at 2–8 °C and use within an hour of reconstitution with the diluent provided. Do not freeze.

References (See also the relevant Cochrane reviews and UK guidelines **DHUK**)

Anon. Rubella and congenital rubella syndrome control and elimination – global progress, 2012. *Wkly Epidemiol Rec* 2013;**88**:521–7.

Badilla X, Morice A, Avila-Aguero ML, *et al.* Fetal risk associated with rubella vaccination during pregnancy. *Pediatr Infect Dis J* 2007;**26**:830–5.

Best J. Rubella. *Semin Fetal Neonatal Med* 2007;**12**:182–92.

Best JM, O'Shea S, Tipples G, *et al.* Interpretations of rubella serology in pregnancy – pitfalls and problems. *Br Med J* 2002;**325**:147–8.

Bloom S, Rguig A, Berrahp A, *et al.* Congenital rubella syndrome burden in Morocco: a rapid retrospective assessment. *Lancet* 2005;**365**:135–41.

Continued on p. 463

Cooper LZ, Alford CA Jr. Rubella. In: Remington JS, Klein JO, Wilson CB, *et al.*, eds. *Infectious diseases of the fetus and newborn infant.* 6th edn. Philadelphia, PA: WB Saunders, Elsevier, 2006: pp. 893–926.

Mehta NM, Thomas RM. Antenatal screening for rubella – infection or immunity? *Br Med J* 2002;**325**:90–1. (See also pp. 596–7.)

Miller E, Cradock-Watson JE, Pollock TM. Consequences of confirmed maternal rubella at different stages of pregnancy. *Lancet* 1982;**ii**:781–4.

Muscat M, Bang H, Wohlfahrt J, *et al.* Measles in Europe: an epidemiological assessment. *Lancet* 2009;**373**:383–9. (See also pp. 356–8.)

Rolfe A, Sheikh A. Measles, mumps, and rubella vaccination in a child with suspected egg allergy. *Br Med J* 2011;**343**:d4536.

Sheridan E, Aitken C, Jeffries D, *et al.* Congenital rubella syndrome: a risk in immigrant populations. *Lancet* 2002;**359**:674–5. (See also **360**:803–4.)

Tookey P. Pregnancy is contraindication for rubella vaccination still. *Br Med J* 2001;**322**:1489.

Tookey P. Rubella in England, Scotland and Wales. *Euro Surveill* 2004;**9**:21–3.

Tookey PA, Bedford H, Peckham CS. Act now to prevent re-emergence of congenital rubella. *Br Med J* 2013;**347**:f4498.

Tookey PA, Cortina-Borja M, Peckham CS. Rubella susceptibility among pregnant women in North London 1996–1999. *J Publ Health Med* 2002;**24**:211–6.

Vestergaard M, Hviid A, Meldgaard Madsen K, *et al.* MMR vaccination and febrile seizures: evaluation of susceptible subgroups and long-term prognosis. *JAMA* 2004;**292**:351–7.

Use

Salbutamol and terbutaline are β-adrenergic stimulants (β-mimetics) widely used by asthmatics for their bronchodilator activity. Given by intravenous (IV) injection or infusion, they have been used in an attempt to inhibit preterm labour. Use can also temporarily control a sudden rise in plasma potassium by causing influx of potassium into cells.

Pharmacology

Salbutamol is a synthetic sympathomimetic developed in 1967 which, like noradrenaline and isoprenaline (q.v.), has its main effect on bronchial muscle β_2 receptors. High doses can cause tachycardia, tremor and agitation. Headache and nausea have also been reported. Nebulised salbutamol is of short-term benefit in a minority of babies with chronic lung damage, but no trial has shown sustained use to be helpful. Nor is use of much benefit in the majority of 'wheezy' babies in the first year of life. Drug binding to liver and muscle adrenergic receptors stimulates cyclic AMP production causing a rise in intracellular potassium uptake and a fall in plasma potassium.

Use in pregnancy

None of the inhaled steroid or β-adrenergic drugs commonly used to treat asthma during pregnancy or lactation seem to pose a threat to the baby. Under-treatment of maternal asthma is the more common problem. The safety of cromoglycate is less clearly established. β-mimetics can help make external cephalic version easier.

Use in early labour

Atosiban (q.v.), nifedipine (q.v.) and the β-mimetics ritodrine, terbutaline and salbutamol all seem capable of inhibiting uterine contractions (so-called tocolysis) to a comparable degree, but use has not yet been shown to impact on perinatal morbidity or mortality. All can usefully be used to delay delivery long enough to effect antenatal transfer and/or offer antenatal steroids. However, while IV β-mimetic use seems generally safe, there is a risk of pulmonary oedema from IV fluid overload. Use can cause palpitations and an unpleasant tachycardia, particularly in mothers with cardiac disease, hyperthyroidism or diabetes. Mothers with impaired renal function or a multiple pregnancy may also be at increased risk. Atosiban or nifedipine are, for these reasons, generally considered better alternatives. β-mimetics cross the placenta, and while tachycardia is rare, transient neonatal hypoglycaemia and hyperinsulinaemia have been noted.

Neonatal hyperkalaemia

Potassium toxicity (hyperkalaemia) is relatively common in low birthweight babies in the first 3 days of life and seems to correlate with low early post-delivery systemic blood flow. Plasma levels >6.5 mmol/l are quite common. Most babies remain asymptomatic, but cardiac arrhythmia can occur when potassium levels exceed 7.5 mmol/l. Give IV calcium gluconate (q.v.) to stabilise the myocardium, and correct any acidosis with IV sodium bicarbonate (q.v.). An infusion of glucose and insulin (q.v.) will also reduce plasma potassium levels, and the consequential risk of arrhythmia, by encouraging influx into cells, but IV salbutamol offers a simpler and more rapid way of controlling *anuric* hyperkalaemia, *temporarily* lowering the plasma potassium by at least 1 mmol/l. Nebulised salbutamol can be used if the IV drug is unavailable and seems, in older children, to produce a more sustained response. Dialysis, exchange transfusion or polystyrene sulfonate resins (q.v.) are required to remove potassium from the body.

Treatment

Hyperkalaemia: Give an infusion of 4 micrograms/kg IV over 5–10 minutes. Sustained benefit may sometimes require one repeat infusion after a minimum of 2 hours.
Chronic lung disease: A minority of babies show an unequivocal short-term response to nebulised salbutamol. A 1 mg dose is more than enough, but the standard 2.5 mg nebuliser solution can be used once every 6–8 hours, irrespective of age or body weight, because little of the drug enters the bloodstream.

Supply and administration

Salbutamol is available in 5 ml IV ampoules containing 1 mg/ml (costing £2.50 each). To give a 4 micrograms/kg infusion, take 0.2 ml of this product for each kilogram the baby weighs, dilute to 50 ml with 10% glucose saline, and infuse at a rate of 6 ml/hour for just 10 minutes. A less

Continued on p. 465

concentrated solution of glucose or glucose saline can be used if necessary. 2.5 mg (2.5 ml) neb-ules (costing 9p) are available for nebuliser use, and ipratropium (q.v.) can be added to this fluid.

References   (See also the relevant Cochrane reviews, and UK guidelines on tocolytic use **DHUK**)

Barrington KJ, Finer NN. Treatment of bronchopulmonary dysplasia. *Clin Perinatol* 1998;**25**:177–202.

de Heus R, Mol BW, Erwich J-JHM, *et al*. Adverse drug reactions to tocolytic treatment for preterm labour: prospective cohort study. *Br Med J* 2009;**338**:b744 (See also pp. 727–8.)

Helfrich E, de Vries TW, van Roon EN. Salbutamol for hyperkalaemia in children. *Acta Paediatr* 2001;**90**:1213–6.

Impey L, Pandit M. Tocolysis for repeat external cephalic version in breech presentation at term: a ran-domised, double-blind, placebo-controlled trial. *Br J Obstet Gynaecol* 2005;**112**:627–31. [RCT]

Kluckow M, Evans N. Low systemic blood flow and hyperkalemia in preterm infants. *J Pediatr* 2001;**139**:227–32.

Royal College of Obstetricians and Gynaecologists. *Tocolytic drugs for women in preterm labour.* Clinical guide-line. London: RCOG, 2002.

Singh BS, Sadiq HF, Noguchi A, *et al*. Efficacy of albuterol inhalation in treatment of hyperkalaemia in pre-mature neonates. *J Pediatr* 2002;**141**:16–20.

Tata LJ, Lewis SA, McKeever TM, *et al*. Effect of maternal asthma, exacerbations and asthma medication use on congenital malformations in offspring: a UK population-based study. *Thorax* 2008;**63**:981–7. (See also pp. 939–40.)

Use

Sildenafil is used as a pulmonary artery vasodilator in children with primary and post-surgical pulmonary hypertension. It is also being used to treat persistent pulmonary hypertension of the newborn (PPHN) and to wean them from inhaled nitric oxide treatment (q.v.). Efficacy in the preterm baby is not yet established.

Pharmacology

Sildenafil citrate, a type-5 phosphodiesterase (PDE5) inhibitor, was originally developed as a treatment for hypertension and angina, but due to its, then, side effect of inducing penile erection, it first came onto the market in 1998 as a treatment for male erectile dysfunction.

PDE5 is especially highly expressed in the lung, so it is not surprising that sildenafil was soon shown to relax the pulmonary arteries by slowing down the resultant degradation of cyclic guanosine monophosphate in a dose that did not cause troublesome systemic vasodilatation. As a result, the drug was soon put to use in the management of pulmonary hypertension in adults and in the management of post-operative pulmonary hypertension in children with congenital heart disease. The drug is quite rapidly absorbed when given by mouth and then metabolised by cytochrome P450 (CYP3A4 and CYP2C9) to the inactive N-desmethyl metabolite in the liver before excretion in the faeces and, to a lesser extent, in the urine (the terminal half-life in adults being 4 hours). As a result of fairly extension first-pass metabolism, only about half the ingested dose enters the systemic circulation. Intravenous (IV) treatment therefore has twice the potency of oral sildenafil. Drug elimination rises rapidly in the first week of life, and the volume of distribution (V_D 1–4 l/kg) is higher than in adult life, making it important to give an initial loading dose.

In August 2012, the FDA in the United States issued a formal statement limiting its use in childhood (but not adult) pulmonary arterial hypertension after 3-year follow-up data showed dose-dependent increases in mortality. These concerns, shared by regulatory authorities in Europe, related to long-term use of sildenafil argue strongly that further safety and efficacy studies are needed. The manufacturer has yet to endorse use in patients under 1 year of age, and treatment in the neonatal period and in the ex-preterm infant with chronic lung disease is 'off-licence'.

Use in persistent pulmonary hypertension of the newborn (PPHN)

While inhaled nitric oxide (q.v.) is probably the mainstay of treatment of PPHN, this is not always available, especially in resource poor countries, nor is it always effective. Several case reports describe the effectiveness of sildenafil in PPHN and four controlled trials – three versus standard treatment and one versus magnesium sulfate (q.v.) – suggesting that it is beneficial, at least compared to standard treatment or magnesium sulfate. There are, as yet, no randomised trials comparing it against inhaled nitric oxide.

Enteral administration could raise concerns about gastrointestinal absorption, particularly in conditions that may have an element of compromised intestinal perfusion, and hypotension was the most commonly reported adverse effect when the loading dose of sildenafil was given intravenously although giving this over at least 3 hours avoided this in most cases. There is an increasing amount of evidence to suggest that enteral sildenafil may facilitate weaning from inhaled nitric oxide discontinuation in infants after surgery for congenital heart disease or who were critically ill, although the evidence is not robust enough to suggest that it should be used routinely in these situations.

Use in PPHN complicating BPD

Approximately a third of babies with chronic lung disease have coexisting pulmonary hypertension, and a number of case reports suggest that sildenafil may be useful, as monotherapy or in combination with other pulmonary vasoactive drugs such as bosentan (q.v.) in reducing the oxygen that a number of these babies require. Not all babies with chronic lung disease have pulmonary hypertension, and an accurate cardiology assessment is necessary to decide which babies might benefit and then to monitor the progress. There are many unanswered questions regarding use of sildenafil in this situation and until such time that the evidence exists prescribing should be restricted to specialist units and physicians, ideally with experience in dealing with both chronic lung disease and pulmonary hypertension.

Continued on p. 467

Maternal use

Sildenafil use has been reported in a number of pregnancies affected by maternal pulmonary hypertension. It is not known whether sildenafil crosses the placenta. The high molecular weight makes significant transfer unlikely. Rodent studies are reassuring, revealing no evidence of teratogenicity or IUGR despite the use of doses higher than those used clinically.

Obstetric use in pregnancies complicated by placenta dysfunction and growth restriction is now undergoing assessment. Just as with treatment in the neonatal population, the use of sildenafil in the pregnant mother requires careful assessment, and use should probably be restricted to the context of a clinical trial.

Interactions

Sildenafil clearance is reduced with concomitant use of cimetidine, erythromycin, clarithromycin and saquinavir (where there is increased risk of arrhythmias). Dose reductions should be considered when using sildenafil with any of these drugs. Bosentan (a moderate inducer of CYP3A4, CYP2C9 and possibly CYP2C19) reduces plasma concentrations of sildenafil. Both nitrate and alpha-blocking antihypertensives can potentiate the hypotensive effects of sildenafil.

Treatment

Oral treatment: Start by giving 250–500 micrograms/kg once every 6 hours and increase, as required, to no more than 2 mg/kg once every 4 hours. Start with a low dose if there is hepatic or renal impairment. There are a few reports of babies who respond initially and then benefit from sustained oral treatment for some weeks or months.

IV treatment: A loading dose of 400 micrograms/kg infused over 3 hours, followed by a maintenance infusion of 1.6 mg/kg/day, is the dose used in the open-label dose-ranging study of IV treatment.

Supply

While tablets are available on prescription (and were previously crushed and dispersed in water to give a suspension for infant use), an oral suspension that is now available containing 10 mg/ml of sildenafil when reconstituted with water costs £187 (for 112 ml). 20 ml vials of IV preparation containing 800 micrograms/ml of sildenafil cost £45.

References

(See also the relevant Cochrane reviews)

Baquero H, Soliz A, Neira F, *et al*. Oral sildenafil in infants with persistent pulmonary hypertension of the newborn: a pilot randomized blinded study. *Pediatrics* 2006;**117**:1077–83. [RCT] (See also **119**:215–6.)

Barst RJ, Ivy DD, Gaitan G, *et al*. A randomized, double-blind, placebo-controlled, dose-ranging study of oral sildenafil citrate in treatment-naive children with pulmonary arterial hypertension. *Circulation* 2012;**125**:324–34.

Chaudhari M, Vogel M, Wright C, *et al*. Sildenafil in neonatal pulmonary hypertension due to impaired alveolisation and plexiform pulmonary arteriopathy. *Arch Dis Child Fetal Neonatal Ed* 2005;**90**:F527–8.

Croom KF, Curran MP. Sildenafil. A review of its use in pulmonary arterial hypertension. *Drugs* 2008;**68**:383–97. [SR]

Duarte AG, Thomas S, Safdar Z, *et al*. Management of pulmonary arterial hypertension during pregnancy: a retrospective, multicenter experience. *Chest* 2013;**143**:1330–6.

Fernánandez González N, Rodríguez Fernández A, Jerez Rojas J, *et al*. Oral sildenafil: a promising drug for persistent neonatal pulmonary hypertension. [In Spanish] *An Pediatr (Barc)* 2004;**61**:563–8.

George EM, Granger JP. Mechanisms and potential therapies for preeclampsia. *Curr Hypertens Rep* 2011;**13**:269–75.

Herrera TR, Concha GP, Holberto CJ, *et al*. Oral sildenafil as an alternative treatment in the persistent pulmonary hypertension in newborns. *Rev Mex Pediatr* 2006;**73**:107–11. [RCT]

Hon K-IE, Cheung K-I, Siu K-L, *et al*. Oral sildenafil for treatment of severe pulmonary hypertension in an infant. *Biol Neonate* 2005;**88**:109–12.

Juliana AE, Abbad FCB. Severe persistent pulmonary hypertension of the newborn in a setting where limited resources exclude the use of inhaled nitric oxide: successful treatment with sildenafil. *Eur J Pediatr* 2005;**164**:626–9.

Lee JE, Hillier SC, Knoderer CA. Use of sildenafil to facilitate weaning from inhaled nitric oxide in children with pulmonary hypertension following surgery for congenital heart disease. *J Intensive Care Med* 2008;**23**:329–34.

Continued on p. 468

Mukherjee A, Dombi T, Wittke B, *et al*. Population pharmacokinetics of sildenafil in term neonates: evidence of rapid maturation of metabolic clearance in the early neonatal period. *Clin Pharmacol Ther* 2009;**85**:56–63.

Nagdyman N, Fleck T, Bitterling B, *et al*. Influence of intravenous sildenafil on cerebral oxygenation measured by near-infrared spectroscopy in infants after cardiac surgery *Pediatr Res* 2006;**59**:46–25.

Noori S, Friedlich P, Wong P, *et al*. Cardiovascular effects of sildenafil in neonates and infants with congenital diaphragmatic hernia and pulmonary hypertension. *Neonatology* 2007;**91**:92–100.

Schulze-Neick I, Hartenstein P, Stiller B, *et al*. Intravenous sildenafil is a potent pulmonary vasodilator in children with congenital heart disease. *Circulation* 2003;**108**(suppl II):II-167–73.

Shekerdemain LS, Ravn HB, Penny DJ. Interaction between inhaled nitric oxide and intravenous sildenafil in a porcine model of meconium aspiration syndrome. *Pediatr Res* 2004;**55**:413–8. (See also pp. 370–1.)

Sher G, Fisch JD. Vaginal sildenafil (Viagra): a preliminary report of a novel method to improve uterine artery blood flow and endometrial development in patients undergoing IVF. *Hum Reprod* 2000;**15**:806–9.

Steinhorn RH, Kinsella JP, Pierce C, *et al*. Intravenous sildenafil in the treatment of neonates with persistent pulmonary hypertension. *J Pediatr* 2009;**155**:841–7.e1.

Stocker C, Penny DJ, Brizard CP, *et al*. Intravenous sildenafil and inhaled nitric oxide: a randomised trial in infants after cardiac surgery. *Intensive Care Med* 2003;**29**:591–611. [RCT]

Uslu S, Kumtepe S, Bulbul A, *et al*. A comparison of magnesium sulphate and sildenafil in the treatment of the newborns with persistent pulmonary hypertension: a randomized controlled trial. *J Trop Pediatr* 2011;**57**:245–50. [RCT]

Vargas-Origel A, Gomez-Rodriguez G, Aldana-Valenzuela C, *et al*. The use of sildenafil in persistent pulmonary hypertension of the newborn. *Am J Perinatol* 2010;**27**:225–30. [RCT]

Villanueva-García D, Mota-Rojas D, Hernández-González R, *et al* A systematic review of experimental and clinical studies of sildenafil for intrauterine growth restriction and pre-term labour. *J Obstet Gynaecol* 2007;**27**:255–9. [SR]

Wardle AJ, Tulloh RM. Paediatric pulmonary hypertension and sildenafil: current practice and controversies. *Arch Dis Child Educ Pract Ed* 2013;**98**:141–7.

Wardle AJ, Wardle R, Luyt K, *et al*. The utility of sildenafil in pulmonary hypertension: a focus on bronchopulmonary dysplasia. *Arch Dis Child* 2013;**98**:613–7.

Use

Skin care practices play an important role in the health of well newborns and hospitalised neonates, yet many of the protocols used or recommendations made in caring for newborn skin are derived as much from tradition and hearsay as from evidence-based decision making. Gentle twice-daily oiling can improve the appearance and the integrity of the skin in babies of 28–32 weeks' gestation and reduce the risk that skin bacteria will cause an invasive septicaemia. Simply wiping with a cloth impregnated with 0.25% chlorhexidine can reduce sepsis and neonatal death in a third-world setting.

Skin cleansing is critically important before any invasive procedure. Clean hands are just as important, and supplementing hand washing with an alcoholic hand rinse greatly reduces the risk of potential pathogens being passed from one patient to another, especially in a hospital setting. Attempts to keep the healing umbilical stump sterile are misplaced, but heavy bacterial colonisation does need to be controlled.

Physiology

Mature skin creates a barrier to minimise fluid and electrolyte losses, protect against infection, prevent absorption of toxic substances and support thermoregulation. Vernix caseosa covers the fetal skin during the last trimester of pregnancy, but it is almost non-existent in preterm infants. While primarily providing a 'waterproof' barrier for the skin while *in utero*, recent studies suggest that it has important hydration, thermoregulation, bacterial protection and wound healing effects. Bacterial colonisation of newborn skin occurs in the first 2–3 days after birth. The baby's first bath should be delayed for several hours after birth and then use only clear water (later bathing should be based on the parents' cultural practices). It used to be normal routine practice in the 1950s to bathe babies in hexachlorophene (a chlorinated biphenol) to prevent serious staphylococcal infections often seen when hospital-born babies were regularly nursed in cots only inches apart. This ritual was discontinued very rapidly once it was found to be causing toxic brain damage!

The skin of the very preterm baby is extremely delicate and very easily damaged. That of a baby born more than about 8 weeks early is not even waterproof and, in a baby born >12 weeks early, a *lot* of water leaks 'insensibly' out of the body in this way in the first few days of life. Increasing the incubator humidity can halve insensible water loss during this time. However, maturation occurs quite rapidly over a period of 10–14 days after birth as long as the skin is protected from damage during that time and as long as the air is only moderately (~50%) humid. As a result, the skin of a 2-week-old baby born at 24 weeks' gestation is much more waterproof than that of a 2-day-old baby of 27 weeks' gestation.

Prevention is the key ingredient of good skin care. Even minor trauma (such as the brisk removal of adhesive tape) can easily strip the skin of all its surface sheet of keratinised cells, leaving the baby with the equivalent of a third-degree 'skin burn'. Infection can also seriously damage the integrity of the preterm baby's skin.

Pharmacology

Skin that is thin enough to let water out is also thin enough to let drugs in, and the widely used skin disinfectant, hexachlorophene, had to be withdrawn in 1972 when its use was found to have caused brain damage. Alcoholic lotions not only penetrate the skin of the preterm baby but also damage the outer layer causing haemorrhagic surface necrosis. The risk is highest when the skin is left lying in liquid alcohol for several minutes. Absorption of iodine, or povidone iodine, can make the preterm baby hypothyroid (as can the intravenous use of X-ray contrast media containing iodine). Aniline dyes can cause methaemoglobinaemia by penetrating the skin even in the full-term baby.

Hydrocortisone, oestrogens, propylene glycol, urea and lindane have all caused toxicity after absorption through the skin, and absorption of the neomycin in Polybactrin® (a triple antibiotic spray) has been incriminated as a possible cause of profound deafness in the very preterm baby. Regular oil massage is common in many cultural groups; trials have shown that the use of a bland product such as olive oil can be beneficial, but some mustard oil products seem toxic.

Chlorhexidine is a cationic biguanide antiseptic used to cleanse skin and wounds and to disinfect working surfaces and instruments. It is sometimes combined with cetrimide (a quaternary ammonium antiseptic). Both can cause skin hypersensitivity. All are rapidly bactericidal and particularly effective against Gram-positive bacteria. Avoid contact with the eyes. Alcohol is a bactericidal antiseptic, but use as a cord dressing merely delays its separation. Povidone iodine (a loose complex of iodine and carrier polymers) also has a slowly lethal effect on bacteria, fungi, viruses and spores.

Continued on p. 470

Routine skin care

The term baby: Gently towel the baby dry after birth to prevent hypothermia, but do no bathe until body temperature has stabilised (12–24 hours after birth). Washing with 0.25% aqueous chlorhexidine markedly reduces infection in a third-world setting, but soap and water suffices in other settings. Most babies only need to be 'topped and tailed' each day after that. A pectin-based barrier limits the skin damage caused by the tapes used to secure oral and nasal tubing.

The preterm baby: A transparent plastic wrap with an overhead heat source will do more than a blanket to prevent the stressful evaporative heat loss that occurs immediately after birth. A waterproof but water vapour permeable, transparent polyurethane dressing or spray (OPSITE® or Tegaderm®) can also provide a useful protective barrier over the skin during the first week of life. It does not reduce water loss. Applying about 4 g/kg of an emollient cream (aqueous cream BP) or a simple oil (such as sunflower seed oil) twice a day can reduce dermatitis and other signs of minor skin trauma and reduce the risk of skin commensals causing an invasive blood-borne infection in babies of 28–32 weeks' gestation, but repeated use in the *very* preterm baby may actually be harmful.

Neonatal management routines

Intravascular access: Cleansing with 0.5% chlorhexidine is better at reducing the risk of catheter-related sepsis in adults than alcohol or povidone iodine (and an aqueous solution is probably as good as an alcoholic one). The latter two products also pose hazards when used on immature skin. Employ two different swabs, applying each for 10 seconds, and then leave the skin to dry for 30 seconds. A surgical 'keyhole' drape and no-touch technique will reduce the risk of re-contamination. A transparent polyurethane dressing can help to secure the line, reduce gross soiling and minimise skin damage while allowing regular site inspection. Concern that moisture build-up under the dressing could cause catheter colonisation by skin bacteria can be further addressed by placing a chlorhexidine-impregnated disc under the dressing.

Intramuscular injections: While it is sensible to make the skin socially clean, the overenthusiastic 'swabaholics' who insist on trying to achieve sterility with spirit or a 'mediswab' are indulging in a pointless ritual. Indeed, where a live vaccine is to be given, it is said that alcohol should *not* be used.

Umbilical care: Where delivery occurs in hospital, a policy of only treating those stumps that look inflamed reduces true sepsis just as effectively as universal prophylaxis – flucloxacillin (q.v.) is the antibiotic most commonly used for overt infection. In the developing world, the situation is very different. Here, some traditional ways of dressing the cord risk causing clostridial infection and lethal neonatal tetanus. In any such setting, it is now known that the routine use of 4% aqueous chlorhexidine to clean the umbilical stump soon after birth, and then daily for the next few days, greatly reduces the incidence of serious peri-umbilical infection and may even reduce neonatal mortality.

Supply

100 g of the emulsifying ointment Epaderm® costs £3, 100 g of zinc and castor oil ointment £1.30, and 100 g of aqueous cream £1. Zinc and castor oil ointment contains arachis (peanut) oil, and while the oil should not contain proteins, it is best avoided where there is a family history of peanut allergy.

1000 ml of chlorhexidine 0.05% solution costs 77p; a stronger 4% chlorhexidine solution (Hibiscrub®) for cleansing of hands costs £4.25.

References

(See also the relevant Cochrane reviews)

Aitken J, Williams FLR. A systematic review of thyroid dysfunction in preterm neonates exposed to topical iodine. *Arch Dis Child Fetal Neonatal Ed* 2014;**99**:F21–8. [SR]

Darmstadt GL, Saha SK, Ahmed AS, *et al.* Effect of skin barrier therapy on neonatal mortality rates in preterm infants in Bangladesh: a randomized, controlled, clinical trial. *Pediatrics* 2008;**121**:522–9. [RCT]

Dollison EJ, Beckstrand J. Adhesive tape vs pectin-based barrier use in preterm infants. *Neonatal Netw* 1995;**14**:35–39. [RCT]

Donahue ML, Phelps DL, Richter SE, *et al.* A semipermeable skin dressing for extremely low birthweight infants. *J Perinatol* 1996;**16**:20–4. [RCT]

Dyer JA. Newborn skin care. *Semin Perinatol* 2013;**37**:3–7.

Continued on p. 471

Edwards WH, Conner JM, Soll RF, for the Vermont Oxford Network Neonatal Skin Care Study Group. The effect of prophylactic ointment therapy on nosocomial sepsis rates and skin integrity in infants with birthweights 501 to 1000 g. *Pediatrics* 2004;**113**:1195–203. [RCT]

Garland JS, Alex CP, Mueller CD, *et al.* A randomized trial comparing povidone-iodine to a chlorhexidine gluconate-impregnated dressing for prevention of central venous catheter infections in neonates. *Pediatrics* 2001;**107**:1431–6. [RCT]

Girou E, Loyeau S, Legrand P, *et al.* Efficacy of handrubbing with alcohol based solution versus standard handwashing with antiseptic soap: randomised clinical trial. *Br Med J* 2002;**325**: 362–5. [RCT]

Kramer A, Rudolph P, Kampf G, *et al.* Limited efficacy of alcohol-based hand gels. *Lancet* 2002;**359**:1489–90. (See also **360**:1509–11.)

Larson EL. APIC guideline for handwashing and hand antisepsis in health care settings. *Am J Infect Control* 1996;**23**:251–69. [SR]

Mullany LC, Darmstadt GL, Khantry SK, *et al.* Topical applications of chlorhexidine to the umbilical stump for prevention of omphalitis and neonatal mortality in southern Nepal: a community-based, cluster-randomised trial. *Lancet* 2006;**367**:910–8. [RCT]

Mullany LC, Darmstadt GL, Tielsch JM. Safety and impact of chlorhexidine antisepsis interventions for improving neonatal health in developing countries. *Pediatr Infect Dis J* 2006;**25**:665–75. [SR] (See also pp. 676–9.)

O'Grady NP, Alexander M, Dellinger EP, *et al.* Guidelines for the prevention of intravascular catheter-related infections. *Pediatrics* 2002;**110**:e51. [SR]

Pessoa-Silva CL, Hugonnet S, Pfister R, *et al.* Reductions of health care-associated infection risk in neonates by successful hand hygiene promotion. *Pediatrics* 2007;**120**:e382–90. [RCT]

Polin RA, Denson S, Brady MT, and the Committee on Fetus and Newborn and Committee on Infectious Diseases. Clinical Report: Strategies for prevention of health care–associated infections in the NICU. *Pediatrics* 2012;**129**:e1085–93.

Rutter N. Percutaneous drug absorption in the newborn: hazards and uses. *Clin Perinatol* 1987;**14**:911–30.

Smederley P, Lim A, Boyages SC, *et al.* Topical iodine-containing antiseptics and neonatal hypothyroidism in very-low-birthweight infants. *Lancet* 1989;**ii**:661–4.

Timsit J-F, Schwebel C, Bouadma L, *et al.* Chlorhexidine-impregnated sponges and less frequent dressing changes for prevention of catheter-related infections in critically ill adults. *JAMA* 2009;**301**:1231–41. [RCT] (See also pp. 1285–7.)

Use

Sodium benzoate and sodium phenylbutyrate are used to control the hyperammonaemia seen in children with urea cycle defects. A plasma ammonia level above 200 µmol/l needs urgent referral and investigation.

Pharmacology

Sodium benzoate is excreted in the urine as hippurate after conjugation with glycine. As each glycine molecule contains a nitrogen atom, one mole of nitrogen is cleared for each mole of benzoate given, if there is complete conjugation. Phenylbutyrate is oxidised to phenylacetate and also excreted after conjugation with glutamine. Phenylacetate is the intravenous (IV) product normally used in North America. Since phenylacetylglutamine contains two nitrogen atoms, two moles of nitrogen are cleared, if there is complete conjugation, for each mole of phenylbutyrate given. All three drugs can lower plasma ammonia levels in patients with urea cycle disorders. Sodium phenylbutyrate is more effective than sodium benzoate but less palatable.

Hyperammonaemia

Plasma ammonia should be measured in any patient with unexplained encephalopathy (vomiting, irritability or drowsiness), particularly in term neonates who deteriorate after an initial period of good health. Inform the laboratory in advance and send the specimen urgently on ice. Ammonia levels above 200 µmol/l suggest an inborn error of metabolism, but a repeat sample should be sent to check that the result is not an artefact. Severe hyperammonaemia (>500 µmol/l) causes serious neurological damage, and urea cycle defects presenting in the neonatal period have a poor prognosis. Circulating ammonia levels should be lowered as quickly as possible, if treatment is considered appropriate, using haemodialysis (peritoneal dialysis is too slow), and sodium benzoate and sodium phenylbutyrate should also be given while organising dialysis. The main use of these drugs is, however, in the long-term management of urea cycle disorders, including patients with milder defects presenting after the neonatal period. The drugs need to be combined with a low protein diet and other treatment, such as arginine (q.v.) or citrulline (q.v.), appropriate to each disorder.

Specialist advice

Specialist advice on a range of inborn errors of metabolism is available from the British Inherited Metabolic Disease Group (BIMDG), and detailed guidance on the management of hyperammonaemia is available on this Group's website (www.bimdg.org.uk). Click on the red box to access a range of emergency protocols.

Note: Treatment with either of drugs should only be initiated after consultation with a specialist metabolic diseases centre. Long-term treatment should be supervised by a consultant with expertise in metabolic diseases.

Treatment

Acute hyperammonaemia: Begin by giving an IV loading dose of 250 mg/kg of each drug, given over 90 minutes, followed by a continuing maintenance infusion of each drug at 20 mg/kg/hour. Co-infusion is safe. Note that an overdose can cause metabolic acidosis and a potentially fatal encephalopathy. There is a theoretical risk that benzoate could displace bilirubin from albumin, so consider treating any severe jaundice.

Long-term management: Sodium benzoate is given at 50–150 mg/kg three to four times daily, with food, adjusted according to response (maintenance is typically 250 mg/kg/day). Sodium phenylbutyrate is given at doses of 75–150 mg/kg three to four times daily, with food. It is, however, possible to achieve very adequate control in some patients using sodium benzoate without phenylbutyrate. The nausea and vomiting caused by the unpleasant taste of the raw products can be minimised by the use of a savoury or fruit-flavoured solution.

Continued on p. 473

Sodium overload

Note that 500 mg of sodium benzoate contains 3.5 mmol of sodium and 500 mg of sodium phenylbutyrate contains 2.7 mmol of sodium, and take care to avoid sodium overload.

Monitoring

Drug dosages and diet should be adjusted to keep the plasma ammonia concentration <60 μmol/l and the plasma glutamine level <800 μmol/l while maintaining a normal essential amino acid profile.

Supply

Sodium benzoate is available for 'named' patients as a 100 mg/ml sugar-free blackcurrant-flavoured oral liquid from Special Products Ltd. (100 ml costs £5). 500 mg tablets are also available. 10 ml (200 mg/ml) ampoules for IV use cost £4.10; dilute the contents with 40 ml of 5 or 10% glucose to obtain a solution containing 50 mg/ml, and give as a continuous infusion. Sodium phenylbutyrate is available from Swedish Orphan Biovitrum; 100 g of the EU licensed granules (Ammonaps®) cost £325. It is also available for 'named patients' as a 250 mg/ml strawberry-flavoured liquid from Special Products Ltd. (100 ml costs £50). Reconstitute the powder with 80 ml of purified water and use within 28 days. 10 ml (200 mg/ml) ampoules for IV use cost £7; dilute the contents with 40 ml of 5 or 10% glucose to obtain a 50 mg/ml solution, and give this as a continuous infusion. It can be put in the same syringe as sodium benzoate. Ammonul® is a commercially available aqueous solution of sodium phenylacetate and sodium benzoate widely used in North America. 50 ml vials requiring further dilution with 10% dextrose contain 100 mg/ml of sodium phenylacetate and 100 mg/ml of sodium benzoate.

References

Das AM, Illsinger S, Hartmann H, *et al.* Prenatal benzoate treatment in urea cycle defects. *Arch Dis Child Fetal Neonatal Ed* 2009;**94**:F216–7.

Enns GM, Berry SA, Berry GT, *et al.* Survival after treatment with phenylacetate and benzoate for urea-cycle disorders. *N Engl J Med* 2007;**356**:2282–92. (See also pp. 2321–2.)

Wijburg FA, Nassogne M-C. Disorders of the urea cycle and related enzymes. In: Saudubray J-M, van den Berghe G, Walter JH, eds. *Inborn metabolic diseases. Diagnosis and treatment*, 5th edn. Berlin: Springer-Verlag, 2012: pp. 297–310.

Use

Sodium bicarbonate can be used to correct severe metabolic acidosis. Significant respiratory acidosis is more appropriately managed by providing adequate respiratory support.

Pharmacology

Sodium bicarbonate is one of the most important natural buffers of the hydrogen ion (acid) content of the blood, and the body responds to a build-up of metabolic acids by increasing the amount of buffering bicarbonate. The process is controlled by the kidney and is very slow to respond. The neonatal kidney also has a limited ability to excrete acid. Infusing small doses of sodium bicarbonate is a way of maintaining the acid–base balance of the blood by speeding these processes up.

There is much controversy about the role of sodium bicarbonate therapy in neonatal medicine. It was used very liberally for a number of years but is now used less extensively with the recognition that its use can cause sudden osmolar shifts that could be damaging to the brain. Excessive use can also cause hypernatraemia. There is also some largely anecdotal evidence to suggest that it can cause intra-ventricular haemorrhage especially in the preterm baby if administered rapidly. The drug still has a role, however, because there is no doubt that serious acidosis (pH < 7.2) compromises cardiac output and surfactant production as well as causing gastrointestinal ileus. Trometamol, more widely known as 'THAM' (q.v.), is an alternative where there is CO_2 retention or a risk of hypernatraemia.

Use during resuscitation

Although present UK guidelines for resuscitation at birth still include the use of intravenous (IV) sodium bicarbonate, recent updated guidelines from some other countries do not even mention its use in the delivery room. The priority in newborn resuscitation is to ensure adequate ventilation and chest compressions; addressing these aspects effectively means that <0.3% of all term newborn babies will need drugs. Both alkalosis and hyperosmolarity after the use of bicarbonate in cardiopulmonary resuscitation have been associated with increased mortality. There is, perhaps, some justification for use in prolonged resuscitation or in the presence of hyperkalaemia but *only* after the restoration of adequate ventilation and circulation. Most term babies recover unaided from any episode of severe intrapartum asphyxia within 4 hours, and giving bicarbonate does not seem to speed this recovery or have any benefit on the immediate outcome.

Treatment

Newborn Resuscitation: In a prolonged resuscitation, after ventilation and chest compressions have been adequately addressed, and drugs are needed, sodium bicarbonate may be given intravenously (preferably via an umbilical venous catheter) at a dose of 1–2 mmol/kg. 8.4% sodium bicarbonate is usually diluted on a 1:1 basis with 10% dextrose or 0.9% saline.

Correcting acidosis: Give 0.5 mmol/kg IV for each unit (mmol) by which it is hoped to reduce the measured blood–gas base deficit. Do not inject this at a rate of faster than 0.5 mmol/kg/minute or allow it to mix with any other IV drug. Partial correction is normally quite adequate.

Exchange transfusion: The pH of a unit of whole blood or plasma-reduced red cells is around 7.0; however, this does not contribute significantly to acidosis in the infant. Routine 'correction' of pH to physiological levels, which was previously a common practice, by the addition of buffer solutions is not indicated. However, if the donor blood is difficult to obtain and is >7 days old, it may be worth checking the blood pH, and if it is <7.0, then consider correction (as mentioned earlier).

Symptomatic hyperkalaemia: Maintain mild alkalosis by giving 1 mmol/kg of IV sodium bicarbonate.

Late metabolic acidosis: Preterm babies sometimes develop a late metabolic acidosis because the kidney has only a limited ability to excrete acid, and this can inhibit weight gain. Give 1–2 mmol/kg of sodium bicarbonate with feeds once a day for 7 days to any baby with a urinary pH that is consistently <5.4.

Tissue extravasation

Tissue extravasation due to IV administration can be managed with hyaluronidase (q.v.). The use of a dilute preparation reduces the risk of serious tissue damage.

Continued on p. 475

Supply

Stock 10 ml ampoules of 8.4% sodium bicarbonate contain 1 mmol of sodium and 1 mmol of bicarbonate per ml (cost £11). Some units stock ampoules containing 4.2% sodium bicarbonate (costing £11 each). Except for the resuscitation scenario, when 8.4% is best diluted on a 1:1 basis, prior dilution is not necessary as long as any infusion is given slowly (as indicated earlier). Sachets of powder for oral use that can be used for 24 hours after reconstitution (with instructions on their use) are available on request.

References

(See also the relevant Cochrane reviews)

Ascher JL, Poland RL. Sodium bicarbonate: basically useless therapy. *Pediatrics* 2008;**122**:831–5.

Berg CS, Barnette AR, Myers BS, *et al*. Sodium bicarbonate administration and outcome in preterm infants. *J Pediatr* 2010;**157**:684–7.

British Committee for Standards in Haematology. Transfusion guidelines for neonates and older children. *Br J Haematol* 2004;**124**:433–53.

Deshpande SA, Ward Platt MP. Association between blood lactate and acid-base status and mortality in ventilated babies. *Arch Dis Child Fetal Neonatal Ed* 1997;**76**:F15–20.

Kalhoff H, Diekmann L, Stick GJ, *et al*. Alkali therapy versus sodium chloride supplement in low birth weight infants with incipient late metabolic acidosis. *Acta Paediatr* 1997;**86**:96–101. [RCT]

Lokesh L, Kumar P, Murki S, *et al*. A randomized controlled trial of sodium bicarbonate in neonatal resuscitation – effect on immediate outcome. *Resuscitation* 2004;**60**:219–23. [RCT]

Shah PS, Raju NV, Beyene J, *et al*. Recovery of metabolic acidosis in term infants with postasphyxial hypoxic-ischaemic encephalopathy. *Acta Paediatr* 2003;**92**:941–7.

Wyckoff MH, Perlman J. Use of high-dose epinephrine and sodium bicarbonate during neonatal resuscitation: is there proven benefit? *Clin Perinatol* 2006;**33**:141–51.

Use

Sodium is an essential nutrient, and to balance renal loss, many orally fed preterm babies benefit from supplements for the first few weeks. Isotonic (0.9%) sodium chloride is often used to correct hypovolaemia, but compound sodium lactate (Hartmann's) solution is a better option because it does not cause hyperchloraemic acidosis.

Pathophysiology

The kidney of the term newborn infant rapidly develops an ability to conserve salt, and the fractional excretion of sodium falls tenfold in the first few days of life. The preterm infant, however, has a high persisting obligatory salt loss. As a result, most healthy infants of <34 weeks' gestation need at least 3 mmol/kg/day, while many babies of <30 weeks' gestation benefit from getting 6 mmol/kg/day during the first 2 weeks of life. This is greater than the sodium intake provided by any of the standard preterm milk formulae (q.v.). Losses may be even higher after renal tubular damage due to severe hypoxia or hypotension.

While *hypo*natraemia is often caused by excessive renal sodium loss, it can also be dilutional, and limitation of water intake is then appropriate. However, if the serum sodium is <120 mmol/l, water deprivation alone is unlikely to correct the hyponatraemia, and supplementation to increase the serum sodium to above 120 mmol/l may be necessary. Calculation assumes that sodium is distributed through almost all the extracellular space (i.e. through 60% of the body in the very preterm baby and 40% of the term baby). Regular weighing and calculation of fractional sodium excretion (as outlined in the introductory section on renal failure) will help to define the disordered electrolyte and fluid balance.

*Hyper*natraemia is also a risk however because the neonatal kidney's ability to excrete excess sodium is also limited and its maximum ability uncertain. While the apathy and hypotonia caused by serious hyponatraemia (<120 mmol/l) may on occasion render a small baby ventilator dependent, the permanent brain damage caused by severe hypernatraemia (>160 mmol/) is a disaster of an entirely different magnitude. Such hypernatraemia *must* be corrected slowly, by dialysis if necessary.

0.9% saline contains 0.15 mmol of sodium (9 mg of sodium chloride) per ml. Use during the reconstitution or infusion of a drug, to maintain line patency or to 'flush' a drug through, can potentially deliver quite a lot of sodium; a baby receiving an infusion of 1 ml/hour of 0.9% sodium chloride will receive 3.6 mmol of sodium a day. Aim for a serum sodium of 130–145 mmol/l.

Terminology

The term 'normal saline' was previously used to mean 0.9% saline; such terms are best avoided.

Management

Intravenous (IV) intake: A daily IV intake of 150–200 ml/kg of 0.18% sodium chloride provides between 4.5 and 6 mmol of sodium per kg per day (a safe basic minimum intake for the very preterm baby without being a dangerously high intake for the full-term baby). Babies of ≤30 weeks' gestation, especially if they 'fluid restricted' them in the first few days, may require further oral or IV sodium, particularly if renal function is compromised. It is better not to start supplementation, if the baby requires ventilation, until the physiological adjustment of extracellular fluid volume (and weight loss) that normally occurs in the first few days of life has occurred. Giving large bolus volumes during neonatal resuscitation to correct perceived hypovolaemia serves little purpose and may not be risk-free.

Oral intake: Preterm milk formulas (q.v.) contain enough sodium for most babies of >30 weeks' gestation. Babies more immature than this seem to need a further 2 mmol of sodium once a day by mouth for each 100 ml of milk they are given for at least the first couple of weeks of life to optimise both their early growth and their later motor and neuropsychological development. Those fed breast milk should receive a supplement of 3–4 mmol per 100 ml of milk. While such dietary supplements do not need a medical prescription, it is wise to record the existence of any such supplement in the drug prescription chart.

Nebulised use: Hypertonic (3%) saline (4 ml every 2–4 hours) may speed recovery in babies with bronchiolitis, and a solution twice as strong may help to sustained the health of the lung in infants with cystic fibrosis.

Continued on p. 477

Supply

The 2 ml ampoules of 0.9% sodium chloride frequently used to flush IV lines cost 20p each. A 1 mmol/ml oral solution can be provided on request. A range of ampoules and packs are available also containing glucose (q.v.), as are 500 ml packs of 0.9% sodium chloride and of Hartmann's solution (which also contains 0.25% sodium lactate).

Reference

(See also the relevant Cochrane reviews)

Al-Dahhan J, Jannoun L, Haycock GB. Effect of sodium salt supplementation of newborn premature infants on neurodevelopmental outcome at 10–13 years of age. *Arch Dis Child Fetal Neonatal Ed* 2002;**86**:F120–3.

Elkins MR, Robinson M, Rose BR, *et al.* National Hypertonic Saline in Cystic Fibrosis (NHSCF) Study Group. A controlled trial of long-term inhaled hypertonic saline in patients with cystic fibrosis. *N Engl J Med* 2006;**354**:229–40.

Ewer AK, Tyler W, Francis A, *et al.* Excessive volume expansion and neonatal death in preterm infants born at 27–28 weeks gestation. *Paediatr Perinatal Epidemiol* 2003;**17**:180–6.

Kuzik BA, Al Qadhi SA, Kent S, *et al.* Nebulized hypertonic saline in the treatment of viral bronchiolitis in infants. *J Pediatr* 2007;**151**:266–70. [RCT] (See also pp. 235–7.)

Mandelberg A, Amirav I. Hypertonic saline or high volume normal saline for viral bronchiolitis: mechanisms and rationale. *Pediatr Pulmonol* 2010;**45**:36–40.

Nagakumar P, Doull I. Current therapy for bronchiolitis. *Arch Dis Child* 2012;**97**:827–30.

Use

Sodium fusidate is an anti-staphylococcal antibiotic primarily of value in the treatment of penicillin-resistant osteomyelitis. Only limited information is available on its use in the neonatal period.

Pharmacology

Sodium fusidate is a bacteriostatic narrow-spectrum anti-staphylococcal antibiotic first isolated in 1960. Most staphylococci are sensitive, including methicillin-resistant and coagulase-negative strains. It also has activity against *Neisseria* and *Clostridium* species.

Concurrent treatment with a second anti-staphylococcal antibiotic (such as flucloxacillin or vancomycin) is advisable, especially if treatment is prolonged, despite a few reports of antagonism *in vitro*. Monotherapy with fusidate alone carries a serious risk of drug resistance developing. Treatment with two antibiotics is generally considered particularly important when treating methicillin-resistant staphylococci. The frequent use of topical Fucidin® in the management of skin conditions may be one factor behind the recent rise in the proportion of all *Staphylococcus aureus* isolates that are resistant to this antibiotic in the United Kingdom.

Sodium fusidate is relatively well absorbed from the gastrointestinal tract and widely distributed in most body tissues, but it does not penetrate CSF well. Some crosses the placenta and appears in breast milk, but there is no evidence of teratogenicity, and there is no evidence to suggest that breastfeeding is contraindicated. Caution is advised, however, in any baby with jaundice, because the drug is highly bound to plasma proteins, and there may be competitive binding with bilirubin.

Reported toxic effects included skin rashes and jaundice (which can be reversed by stopping treatment). The half-life in adults is 10–15 hours; that in neonates is less certain. The drug is largely excreted in the bile. Very little is excreted by the kidney. Intravenous treatment, now discontinued, cause vasospasm or thrombophlebitis unless the drug is given slowly after suitable dilution into a large vein. Rapid infusion also caused a high concentration of sodium fusidate to develop locally causing red cell haemolysis and jaundice.

Bacterial conjunctivitis responds as rapidly to fusidic acid eye drops as it does to chloramphenicol eye drops, and such treatment has the advantage of only requiring administration twice a day, but such a product is not generally available outside Europe.

Treatment

Oral administration: Sodium fusidate is not available in liquid formulation, instead use the slightly less well absorbed fusidic acid in babies and children who cannot swallow tablets. Give 15 mg/kg of fusidic acid once every 8 hours.

Long-term administration: High blood levels are often encountered when adult patients are given a standard dose (1.5 g a day) for >4–5 days: in the absence of any reliable pharmacokinetic information, it may be advisable to monitor liver function to watch for any rapid rise in liver enzyme levels and/or to reduce the dose used in the neonatal period if treatment is continued for >5 days.

Supply and administration

Intravenous sodium fusidate is no longer available after the pharmaceutical company decided to discontinue the formulation. A sugar-free oral suspension containing 50 mg/ml of fusidic acid (equivalent to 35 mg/ml of sodium fusidate) is available which should not be diluted prior to administration (50 ml bottles cost £6.70).

Two topical preparations (Fucidin®) are available in 15 g quantities: a 2% fusidic acid cream (cost £1.90) and a 2% sodium fusidate ointment (cost £2.20). Both contain cetyl alcohol. An ophthalmic preparation (Fucithalmic®) of 1% fusidic acid in a gel that liquefies on contact with eye is available in 5 g tubes costing £2.70. This contains benzalkonium chloride (see the web commentary for 'eye drops' in relation to this). Sodium fusidate (sodium fucidate = USAN) is not currently available in North America.

References

Bergdahl S, Elinder G, Eriksson M. Treatment of neonatal osteomyelitis with cloxacillin in combination with fusidic acid. *Scand J Infect Dis* 1981;**13**:281–2.
Dobie D, Gray J. Fusidic acid resistance in *Staphylococcus aureus*. *Arch Dis Child* 2004;**89**:74–7.

Continued on p. 479

Grayson A, Wylie K. Towards evidence-based emergency medicine: best BETs from the Manchester Royal Infirmary. BET 3: fucidic acid or chloramphenicol for neonates with sticky eyes. *Emerg Med J* 2011;**28**:634.

Normann EK, Bakken O, Peltola J, *et al*. Treatment of acute neonatal bacterial conjunctivitis: a comparison of fucidic acid and chloramphenicol eye drops. *Acta Ophthalmol Scand* 2002;**80**:183–7. [RCT]

Reeves DS. The pharmacokinetics of fusidic acid. *J Antimicrob Chemother* 1987;**20**:467–76.

Turnidge J, Collignon P. Resistance to fusidic acid. *Int J Antimicrob Agents* 1999;**12**:S35–44.

Use

Sodium valproate has been widely used in the treatment of several epilepsies since 1974, but the risk of liver toxicity due to an unrecognised metabolic disorder has limited its use in early infancy.

Pharmacology

Sodium valproate has a unique chemical structure, and its mode of action is not fully understood although it may involve the modification of gamma-aminobutyric acid behaviour in the brain. It is slowly but completely absorbed by mouth although peak levels are not reached for 3–8 hours in the newborn. It is highly protein bound and undergoes hepatic metabolism. Sodium valproate has a long half-life (10–67 hours) at birth which falls to 7–13 hours by 2 months. It is of particular value in the management of generalised seizures, and the intravenous (IV) preparation is sometimes used to control status epilepticus in older children and adults. Pancreatitis and severe liver toxicity have been reported in infants and young children, and valproate should only be used with great caution in children <2 years old. Nausea, vomiting, lethargy and coma can occur, as can reversible neutropenia and thrombocytopenia. Such problems usually develop soon after treatment is started, but sometimes develop after 3–6 months. Hyperglycinaemia may occur and has been reported in an infant whose mother was treated during pregnancy. Treatment with 100 mg/kg a day of L-carnitine IV improves survival. Respiratory support may be needed in severe cases.

Sodium valproate is a known human teratogen increasing the risk four-fold. Sodium valproate rapidly crosses the placenta (F/M ratio >2). Pregnancy databases suggest sodium valproate is significantly more teratogenic than carbamazepine, and sodium valproate–lamotrigine combinations are particularly teratogenic. The likelihood of the offspring being affected is dose dependent.

A constellation of dysmorphic features (the 'fetal valproate syndrome') has been described consisting of a distinct facial appearance, a cluster of minor and major anomalies and CNS dysfunction. Of affected infants, 10% die in infancy and 25% of survivors are neurologically impaired. Increased nuchal thickening may indicate an affected fetus during first trimester screening and a fetal medicine specialist should evaluate women taking valproate during pregnancy. It is also important to undertake serum α-fetoprotein screening for spina bifida and also to arrange for expert ultrasound screening of the fetal spine at 18-weeks' gestation. Sodium valproate should only be used during pregnancy if the benefit justifies the potential perinatal risk. If it cannot be avoided (especially in the first trimester), monotherapy using the lowest effective dose should be prescribed in divided doses to minimise the peaks. Folate supplementation is essential; the risks of teratogenicity, especially neural tube defects, are otherwise even higher. Sodium valproate enters breast milk, but because the baby will only receive 5% of the weight-adjusted maternal dose, breastfeeding is not associated with the same concerns that are seen with pregnancy use.

Drug interactions

Treatment with valproate substantially increases the half-life of lamotrigine and phenobarbital.

Treatment

Experience with use in the neonatal period remains *extremely* limited. A 20 mg/kg loading dose (given either by mouth or IV) followed by 10 mg/kg every 12 hours has been suggested. Watch for hyperammonaemia during the first week of administration and suspend treatment if the serum ammonia level exceeds 350 μmol/l. Use blood levels to guide dosage because clearance changes over time.

Blood levels

The immediate pre-dose serum concentration will usually be between 40 and 100 mg/l (1 mg/l = 6.93 μmol/l). However, while monitoring may help to identify non-compliance, it seldom helps to optimise treatment.

Supply

Sodium valproate is available as a sugar-free liquid (£3.10 for 100 ml) containing 40 mg/ml. Pharmacies can provide a more dilute syrup, but the shelf life is only 2 weeks. An IV preparation (100 mg/ml) is available in 3 ml vials (£7) and 4 ml vials (cost £11.60). The solution is compatible with IV glucose and glucose saline, but it should not be mixed with any other drug.

Continued on p. 481

References

(See also the relevant Cochrane reviews)

Adab N, Kini U, Vinten J, *et al.* The longer term outcome of children born to mothers with epilepsy. *J Neurol Neurosurg Psychiatry* 2004;**75**:1575–83.

Artama M, Auvinen A, Raudaskoski T, *et al.* Antiepileptic drug use of women with epilepsy and congenital malformations in offspring. *Neurology* 2005;**64**:1874–8. (See also pp. 938–9.)

Bohan TP, Helton E, König S, *et al.* Effect of L-carnitine treatment for valproate-induced hepatotoxicity, *Neurology* 2001;**56**:1405–9.

Jentink J, Loane MA, Dolk H, *et al.* Valproic acid monotherapy in pregnancy and major congenital malformations. *N Engl J Med* 2010;**362**:2185–93.

Meador KJ, Baker GA, Browning N, *et al.* Cognitive function at 3 years of age after fetal exposure to antiepileptic drugs. *N Engl J Med* 2009;**360**:1597–605. (See also pp. 1667–9.)

Thomas SV, Ajakumar B, Sindu K, *et al.* Motor and mental development of infants exposed to antiepileptic drugs in utero. *Epilepsy Behav* 2008;**13**:229–36.

Williams G, King J, Cunningham M, *et al.* Fetal valproate syndrome and autism: additional evidence of as association. *Dev Med Child Neurol* 2001;**43**:202–6. (See also p. 847.)

Use

Sotalol is a non-selective β-adrenoreceptor blocker that also exhibits classes II and III antiar-rhythmic properties by inhibiting potassium channels. Because of this dual action, it prolongs both the PR and the QT intervals and is used to control atrial flutter. It is also being used, under expert supervision, instead of amiodarone (q.v.) or with flecainide (q.v.) in the control of ventricular and supraventricular arrhythmia.

Pharmacology

Many β-adrenoreceptor blocking drugs now exist. Such drugs have been widely used to control hypertension, manage angina and treat myocardial infarction, arrhythmia, heart failure and thyrotoxicosis, and it is now clear that some are better at some things than others. Some, like propranolol (q.v.), the first beta-blocker to be developed, are essentially non-selective and act indiscriminately on receptors in the heart, peripheral blood vessels, liver, pancreas and bronchi. Others, like labetalol (q.v.), are more selective and are used to control hypertension because of their effect on arteriolar tone.

Non-cardioselective β-blockers like sotalol, which are water rather than lipid soluble, are less likely to enter the brain and disturb sleep and are excreted largely unchanged in the urine. All β-blockers slow the heart and can depress the myocardium. Sotalol, in particular, can prolong the QT interval and cause a life-threatening ventricular arrhythmia, especially if there is hypokalaemia. Because of this, it is now *only* used to manage pre-existing arrhythmia. In this, sotalol functions both as a class II antiarrhythmic to decrease heart rate and AV nodal conduction as a result of non-selective β-blockade and as a class III antiarrhythmic by prolonging the atrial and the ventricular action potential and the heart muscle's subsequent refractory period.

Sotalol, which was first synthesised in 1964, is rapidly absorbed when given orally (absorption is good although food, including milk, can decrease this). The terminal half-life (7–9 hours) remains much the same throughout childhood but is seriously prolonged in renal failure. The manufacturers have not done the studies needed to be able to recommend use in children. Furthermore, because the drug can provoke as well as control cardiac arrhythmia, patients should be subject to continuous ECG monitoring when treatment is started, and treatment only initiated by a paediatric cardiologist well versed in the management of cardiac rhythm disorders. Sotalol may be the drug of choice for fetal atrial flutter, but lack of controlled trial evidence makes it impossible to say what drug regimen is best for other fetal arrhythmias.

There is no evidence that β-blockers are teratogenic, but they can cause intermittent mild fetal bradycardia (90–110 bpm). Sustained high-dose use in the second and third trimesters can also be associated with reduced fetal growth. Use in pregnancy can also cause transient bradycardia and hypoglycaemia in the baby at delivery. Sotalol appears in breast milk in high concentrations (milk/plasma ratio 2.8–5.5). Babies so fed have, to date, been asymptomatic, but it has been shown that they are ingesting 20–40% of the weight-adjusted maternal dose. Propranolol is the β-blocker associated with lowest drug exposure during lactation.

Treatment

Mothers: The dose given when trying to control a fetal arrhythmia has usually been between 60 and 160 mg by mouth twice or three times a day. Watch the mother's ECG carefully for QT changes.

Children: Start cautiously with 1 mg/kg by mouth once every 12 hours and increase the dose as necessary once every 3–4 days to no more than 4 mg/kg. Withdraw treatment gradually.

Toxicity

Absorption is reduced in milk-fed children and diarrhoea may cause sudden withdrawal. Extend the dosage interval if renal function is poor, and stop treatment if the QT_c interval exceeds 550 ms. Overdose of *any* β-blocker can cause bradycardia and/or hypotension. Give 40 micrograms/kg of intravenous (IV) atropine, and treat unresponsive cardiogenic shock with IV glucagon (q.v.) and glucose. Monitor the blood glucose level and control ventilation. Isoprenaline (see web archive) may help. Cardiac pacing is occasionally needed.

Supply

40 g and 80 mg tablets of sotalol cost 4p and 5p each, respectively. No oral suspension is available commercially, but tablets may be crushed and dispersed in water.

Continued on p. 483

References

Beaufort-Krol GC, Bink-Boelkens MT. Effectiveness of sotalol for atrial flutter in children after surgery for congenital heart disease. *Am J Cardiol* 1997;**79**:92–4.

Knudson JD, Cannon BC, Kim JJ, *et al.* High-dose sotalol is safe and effective in neonates and infants with refractory supraventricular tachyarrhythmias. *Pediatr Cardiol* 2011;**32**:896–903.

Läer S, Elshoff JP, Meibohm B, *et al.* Development of a safe and effective pediatric dosing regimen for sotalol based on population pharmacokinetics and pharmacodynamics in children with supraventricular tachycardia. *J Am Coll Cardiol* 2005;**46**:1322–30.

Lisowski LA, Verheijen PM, Benatar AA, *et al.* Atrial flutter in the perinatal age group: diagnosis, management and outcome. *J Am Coll Cardiol* 2002;**35**:771–7.

Price JF, Kertesz NJ, Snyder CS, *et al.* Flecainide and sotalol: a new combination therapy for refractory supraventricular tachycardia in children <1 year of age. *J Am Coll Cardiol* 2002;**39**:717–20.

Russell GA, Martin AP. Flecainide toxicity. *Arch Dis Child* 1989;**64**:860–2.

Shah A, Moon-Grady A, Bhogal N, *et al.* Effectiveness of sotalol as first-line therapy for fetal supraventricular tachyarrhythmias. *Am J Cardiol* 2012;**109**:1614–8.

Wagner X, Jouglard J, Moulin M, *et al.* Coadministration of flecainide acetate and sotalol during pregnancy: lack of teratogenic effects, passage across the placenta, and excretion in human breast milk. *Am Heart J* 1990;**119**:700–2.

Use

Spiramycin is used to protect the fetus from infection when a woman develops toxoplasmosis during pregnancy. Infection of the fetus occurs during periods of parasitaemia in the mother. Such parasitaemia occurs before the appearance of any maternal antibodies and before the mother develops any symptoms (if she ever does). Thus infection of the fetus probably occurs before diagnosis is possible in most cases.

Pharmacology

Spiramycin is a macrolide antibiotic, first isolated in 1954, that is related to erythromycin. It is well absorbed when taken by mouth and mostly metabolised in the liver, although biliary excretion is also high. The serum half-life in adults is about 8 hours. Spiramycin crosses the placenta, where it is also concentrated, and there is a belief that early treatment can prevent the transplacental passage of the *Toxoplasma* parasite. Treatment with pyrimethamine (q.v.) and sulfadiazine (q.v.) may be a more effective way of limiting damage once fetal infection has occurred, but termination is often offered if there is ultrasound evidence of cerebral damage even though many children with antenatally detected cerebral calcification or ventriculomegaly seem to develop normally. Spiramycin appears in therapeutic quantities in breast milk, but it is not the treatment of choice after delivery. It can prolong the QT interval and has occasionally caused a dangerous neonatal arrhythmia. CSF penetration is poor.

Toxoplasmosis

Toxoplasma gondii is a common worldwide protozoan parasite that infects many warm-blooded animals. Cats are the main host, replication occurring in the small intestine, but sheep, pigs and cattle become infected if they ingest faecally contaminated material, and infected cysts within the muscles and brain then remain viable almost indefinitely. Humans usually only become infected by ingesting cysts from contaminated soil or by eating undercooked or poorly cured meat (although transplant recipients are at risk of cross infection). Infection normally goes unrecognised, but fever, muscle pain, sore throat and a lymphadenopathy may manifest themselves after 4–21 days. Hepatosplenomegaly and a maculopapular rash are sometimes seen. Although the illness is usually benign and self-limiting, chronically infected immunodeficient patients can (like the fetus) experience reactivated central nervous system disease. Screening cannot be advocated until the benefit of treatment becomes less uncertain.

The risk of a susceptible woman becoming infected during pregnancy is quite low (~0.5%), and congenital infection is uncommon (1:1,000 to 1:10,000 births). The fetus is more likely to become infected if the mother is infected early in pregnancy but more likely to show *signs* of that infection within 3 years of birth if infected early. Overt signs of infection develop in <5% of babies born to mothers infected in the first 16 weeks of pregnancy. Reliable early recognition requires serial testing of all antibody-negative women, since IgM and IgG tests cannot be used to time infection accurately, and often results in mothers receiving unnecessary antenatal treatment even when the baby is not at risk. Fetal infection can be diagnosed by PCR detection of *T. gondii* DNA in amniotic fluid or by mouse inoculation. Persistence of circulating IgG antibodies for a year confirms that the baby was congenitally infected. Most, but not all, have IgM antibodies at birth. Many show no overt sign of illness at birth, but one in four will develop retinochoroiditis, intracranial calcification and/or ventriculomegaly within 3 years. Only a few (<5%) develop severe neurological impairment, but how many develop minor disability is not known. Half of those with retinal lesions eventually develop some visual loss.

Treatment

Mother: It is common practice to give 1 g of spiramycin prophylactically once every 8 hours as soon as maternal infection is first suspected to minimise the risk of placental transmission. This dose is often continued for the duration of pregnancy. Pyrimethamine and sulfadiazine are often given as well, if there is evidence of fetal infection. No controlled trial evidence exists to support this strategy.
Baby: Use pyrimethamine and sulfadiazine to initiate treatment (as outlined in the pyrimethamine monograph). Some clinicians alternate this with 3–4 week courses of spiramycin (50 mg/kg twice a day).

Supply

Spiramycin has a licence for use in Europe (where it has been used for nearly 20 years), but has not yet been licensed for general use in America or the United Kingdom. It can, however, be obtained by the pharmacy from Sanofi-Aventis for use on a 'named-patient' basis on request when needed to treat perinatal toxoplasmosis.

Continued on p. 485

References

(See also the relevant Cochrane reviews)

Gras L, Wallon M, Pollak A, *et al.* Association between prenatal treatment and clinical manifestations of congenital toxoplasmosis in infancy: a cohort study in 13 European centres. *Acta Paediatr* 2005;**94**:1721–31.

Hotop A, Hlobil H, Gross U. Efficacy of rapid treatment initiation following primary *Toxoplasma gondii* infection during pregnancy. *Clin Infect Dis* 2012;**54**:1545–52.

McLoyd R, Boyer K, Karrison T, *et al.* Outcome of treatment for congenital toxoplasmosis. 1981–2004: the National Collaborative Chicago-based Congenital Toxoplasmosis Study. *Clin Infect Dis* 2006;**42**:1383–94.

Montoya JG, Remington JS. Management of *Toxoplasma gondii* infection during pregnancy. *Clin Infect Dis* 2008;**47**:554–66.

Olariu TR, Remington JS, McLeod R, *et al.* Severe congenital toxoplasmosis in the United States: clinical and serologic findings in untreated infants. *Pediatr Infect Dis J* 2011;**30**:1056–61.

Petersen E. Toxoplasmosis. *Semin Fetal Neonatal Med* 2007;**12**:214–23.

Remington JS, McLeod R, Wilson CB, *et al.* Toxoplasmosis. In: Remington JS, Klein JO, Wilson CB, *et al.*, eds. *Infectious diseases of the fetus and newborn infant*, 7th edn. Philadelphia, PA: WB Saunders, Elsevier, 2011: pp. 918–1041.

SYROCOT (Systematic Review on Congenital Toxoplasmosis) study group. Effectiveness of prenatal treatment for congenital toxoplasmosis: a meta-analysis of individual patients' data. *Lancet* 2007;**369**:115–22. [SR]

Use

Spironolactone is used to treat congestive heart failure, primary hyperaldosteronism and ascites due to liver disease. Whether the use of spironolactone, and a thiazide diuretic such as chlorothiazide (q.v.), is of value in babies with bronchopulmonary dysplasia is much less clearly established; however, such use is fairly widespread.

Pharmacology

Spironolactone is a potassium-sparing diuretic developed in 1959 which acts by competitively inhibiting the action of aldosterone (a natural adrenocortical hormone) on the distal part of the renal tubule. It is well absorbed by mouth and mainly excreted (partly metabolised) in the urine. The half-life in adults is 1–2 hours, but several of the metabolic products (including canrenone) that also have diuretic properties have a 12–24 hour half-life. It is not known whether metabolism and excretion differ in early infancy. Benefits may not become apparent for up to 48 hours after treatment is started and may continue for a similar period after the treatment has stopped. Use declined after sustained high-dose use was shown to cause tumours in rats.

A loop diuretic such as furosemide (q.v.) can improve pulmonary compliance in babies with ventilator-induced chronic lung disease. A thiazide, such as chlorothiazide (q.v.), is better for long-term treatment, and it is common practice to give both a thiazide and spironolactone, although the value of this practise has, as yet, only been assessed in one small trial (which found no evidence of benefit). Spironolactone can be of use in the long-term management of Bartter's syndrome, while high-dose treatment can also help to control ascites in babies with chronic neonatal hepatitis. Treatment should always be stopped if there is renal failure because of the risk of hyperkalaemia.

Spironolactone crosses the placenta. Its antiandrogenic properties have been shown to feminise male rats, but no such effects have been reported in humans even when high-dose treatment is used for maternal Bartter's syndrome. Only very small amounts of spironolactone and its major active metabolite (canrenone) enter breast milk, and the amounts received by the breast-fed infant (<0.5% of the maternal dose) are clinically insignificant.

Potassium canrenoate is an aldosterone antagonist with similar indications to spironolactone, but with the advantage that it can be given parenterally as well as orally. Its primary metabolite is, like spironolactone, canrenone. There is suggestion that it also shares the genotoxic and potentially carcinogenic effects seen with high-dose spironolactone. Intravenous (IV) potassium canrenoate (at a dose of 1–2 mg/kg given by slow IV injection or by infusion) is sometimes used when oral spironolactone cannot be given; however, it is not licensed in the United Kingdom. Such use should be short-term only, and to convert to the equivalent oral spironolactone dose, multiply the potassium canrenoate dose by 0.7 to get the dose of spironolactone to be used.

Treatment

Use as a diuretic: Give 1 mg/kg of spironolactone together with 10 mg/kg of chlorothiazide twice a day by mouth in the management of chronic congestive cardiac failure. Congestive failure that fails to respond to this standard dose may sometimes respond if the dose of both drugs is doubled.

Use in hepatic ascites: A dose of up to 3.5 mg/kg by mouth twice a day is sometimes used in ascites secondary to liver disease, although patients need monitoring for possible hyperkalaemia.

Supply

Spironolactone is available as a 2 mg/ml sugar-free oral suspension (costing £10 per 100 ml) although this is a special formulation for which no formal product licence currently exists. Other strength suspensions also exist. It is also widely available in tablet form from a number of pharmaceutical companies.

Potassium canrenoate is available in 10 ml ampoules containing 200 mg through specialist import companies. It can be given undiluted over 2–3 minutes or diluted by taking 1 ml (20 mg) original solution and further diluting to 20 ml with 0.9% sodium chloride or 5% dextrose to give a 1 mg/ml solution.

References

Groves TD, Corenblum B. Spironolactone therapy during human pregnancy. *Am J Obstet Gynecol* 1995;**172**:1655–6.

Continued on p. 487

Hobbins SM, Fower RC, Row RD, *et al.* Spironolactone therapy in infants with congestive heart failure secondary to congenital heart disease. *Arch Dis Child* 1981;**56**:934–8. [RCT]

Hoffman DJ, Gerdes JS, Abbasi S. Pulmonary function and electrolyte balance following spironolactone treatment in preterm infants with chronic lung disease: a double-blind, placebo-controlled, randomized trial. *J Perinatol* 2000;**1**:41–5. [RCT]

Kao LC, Durand DJ, Philliops BL, *et al.* Randomized trial of long-term diuretic therapy for infants with oxygen dependent bronchopulmonary dysplasia. *J Pediatr* 1994;**124**:772–81. [RCT]

Pérez-Ayuso RM, Arroyo V, Planas R, *et al.* Randomized comparative study of efficacy of furosemide versus spironolactone in nonazotemic cirrhosis with ascites. *Gastroenterology* 1983;**84**:961–8. [RCT]

Phelps DL, Karim A. Spironolactone: relationship between concentrations of dethioacetylated metabolite in human serum and milk. *J Pharm Sci* 1977;**66**:1203.

Pitt B, Zannad F, Remme WJ, *et al.* The effect of spironolactone on morbidity and mortality in patients with severe heart failure. *N Engl J Med* 1999;**341**:709–17. (See also pp. 753–5.) [RCT]

Shah PS. Current perspectives on the prevention and management of chronic lung disease in preterm babies. *Pediatr Drugs* 2003;**5**:463–80. [SR]

Suyagh M, Hawwa AF, Collier PS, *et al.* Population pharmacokinetic model of canrenone after intravenous administration of potassium canrenoate to paediatric patients. *Br J Clin Pharmacol* 2012;**74**:864–72.

Use

Streptokinase can be used to lyse arterial thrombi when there is symptomatic vascular occlusion. Take the advice of a vascular surgeon where this is available. See the website commentary for a more detailed discussion of the available options.

Pharmacology

Streptokinase is a protein obtained from certain strains of *Streptococcus equisimilis* (Lancefield Group C). It was first purified in 1962, and its amino acid sequence established in 1982. The half-life on infusion is about 25 minutes. It activates human plasminogen to form plasmin, a proteolytic enzyme with fibrinolytic effects used to dissolve intravascular blood clots. The plasminogen activator alteplase (q.v.) is a more expensive alternative. Start treatment as soon as there is evidence of an obstructive intravascular thrombus and seek confirmation either by ultrasound or, preferably, by angiography. The relative merits of embolectomy, anticoagulation with heparin and treatment with streptokinase remain undetermined, but embolectomy is often impracticable, and treatment with heparin (q.v.) is of more use as a prophylactic measure than as a therapeutic strategy. Documentary evidence of the value of lytic therapy does not exist, and treatment is not risk-free, but treatment is probably merited for arterial lesions that look set to cause tissue necrosis (gangrene). There is no good evidence that thrombosed renal veins benefit from active treatment and even less information on the wisdom of treating other venous thrombi. Streptokinase antibodies develop and persist for 6–12 months after treatment making repeat treatment less effective and adverse reactions more likely. Instillation into the pleural cavity has sometimes been used to speed recovery where there is a particularly severe thoracic empyema in older children, but urokinase (q.v.) has been the lytic agent more widely used in published studies of this condition in children.

Streptokinase does not appear to pose a major risk to the fetus except during the intrapartum period when maternal haemorrhage is greatest. Fetal haemorrhage has not been reported as placental transfer is minimal. One potential implication of maternal therapy is that the fetus will acquire antistreptokinase antibodies as a result of transplacental passage; however, this would *only* pose a clinical risk in the unlikely event that the neonate required therapy. There are no reports of streptokinase use during lactation. The short half-life and indications for use are such that the breastfed infant will receive very little through breast milk.

Treatment

Arterial thrombi: Give a loading dose of 3000 units/kg of streptokinase slowly intravenously as soon as the diagnosis is made, followed by a continuous infusion of 1000 units/kg/hour (1 ml/hour of a solution made up as described under 'Supply and administration'). Higher doses have been used, but there is no evidence, as yet, that they are more effective. Treatment should continue until vascular flow returns, which may only take 4 hours but may be delayed 24–36 hours. Avoid intramuscular injections during treatment and treat any bleeding from puncture sites with local pressure. **Blocked shunts and catheters:** Dilute 10,000 units with enough 0.9% sodium chloride to fill the catheter dead space. Instil and leave for 1 hour before aspirating. Flush with heparinised saline.

Dose monitoring

Monitor the fibrinogen level if treatment is necessary for >6 hours, aiming for a serum fibrinogen level of 1–1.4 g/l. Slow or stop the infusion temporarily if the level falls below 1 g/l.

Antidote

Tranexamic acid can control bleeding by inhibiting the activation of plasminogen to plasmin. Try an intravenous (IV) infusion of 10 mg/kg over 10 minutes and repeat if necessary after 8–12 hours.

Supply and administration

Vials of streptokinase as a powder for reconstitution in 5 ml of 0.9% sodium chloride are available (250,000 unit vials cost £16). Take care to prevent the production of foam. Vials kept at 4°C can be used for 12 hours after reconstitution. For IV use, take 0.4 ml of reconstituted solution for each kilogram the baby weighs, dilute to 20 ml with 10% glucose or glucose saline, and infuse at a rate of 1 ml/hour. This provides 1000 units/kg of streptokinase per hour. (A less concentrated solution of glucose or glucose saline can be used if necessary.) Prepare a fresh solution every 12 hours.

5 ml (100 mg/ml) ampoules of tranexamic acid cost £1.60.

Continued on p. 489

References

(See also the relevant Cochrane reviews)

Cheah F-C, Boo N-Y, Rohana J, *et al.* Successful clot lysis using low dose of streptokinase in 22 neonates with aortic thromboses. *J Paediatr Child Health* 2001;**37**:479–82.

Monagle P, Michelson AD, Bovill E, *et al.* Antithrombotic therapy in children. *Chest* 2001;**119**:344S–70S. [SR]

Nowak-Göttl U, von Kries R, Göbel U. Neonatal symptomatic thromboembolism in Germany: two year survey. *Arch Dis Child Fetal Neonatal Ed* 1997;**76**:F163–7.

Schmidt B, Andrew M. Neonatal thrombosis: report of a prospective Canadian and international registry. *Pediatrics* 1995;**96**:939–43.

Singh M, Mathew JL, Chandra S, *et al.* Randomized controlled trial of intrapleural streptokinase in empyema thoracis in children. *Acta Paediatr* 2004;**93**:1443–5. [RCT]

te Raa GD, Ribbert LS, Snijder RJ, *et al.* Treatment options in massive pulmonary embolism during pregnancy; a case-report and review of literature. *Thromb Res* 2009;**124**:1–5.

Turrentine MA, Braems G, Ramirez MM. Use of thrombolytics for the treatment of thromboembolic disease during pregnancy. *Obstet Gynecol Surv* 1995;**50**:534–41.

Use

Oral sucrose is the most extensively studied reduction strategy for procedure-related pain in neonatal care. Nevertheless, while sweet taste-induced analgesia significantly reduces the physical response to pain, the mechanism by which it works is still not precisely understood.

Pharmacology

Although the use of oral sucrose has been the most extensively studied pain intervention in newborn care to date, the precise mechanism by which it produces its effects have been poorly studied. There has been some suggestion that a concentrated sugar solution may affect the endogenous opioid system in young rats if given shortly before pain is inflicted. However, babies pre-exposed to the opioid antagonist naloxone (q.v.) actually cried for a shorter, rather than a longer, time in one nurse-initiated trial.

Managing brief pain

Some 57 studies included in the Cochrane review provide unequivocal evidence that babies cry less when given sucrose to suck two minutes before being subjected to a painful procedure; however, it has no effect on the rise in heart rate or in oxygen consumption. Bloodletting was the cause of pain investigated in all these studies. A wide range of doses have been used (0.01–1 g), and higher doses do seem to produce a greater effect. Rather fewer studies have yet looked at the efficacy of this strategy in babies more than a month old. Three recent studies suggest that breastfeeding on its own can be just as effective. Efficacy is also enhanced if the baby is also held close (cuddled) throughout the procedure or more impersonally, given a dummy or pacifier to suck. The artificial sweetener aspartame seems as effective as sucrose. So is glucose and breast milk, but formula milk is not. Sucrose only works when given orally – it is ineffective when given direct into the stomach. Preterm babies show less of a reduction in their 'pain score' than term babies.

Sucrose seems as effective in babies as lidocaine–prilocaine (EMLA) cream. However, other studies have shown that while the latter significantly reduces the pain associated with vene-puncture in older children, it has relatively little impact on the way babies respond to this procedure (as discussed in the monograph on lidocaine). No comparison with tetracaine (q.v.) has yet been published.

Sweets possess a 'magical' ability to keep a child of *any* age quiet, but this does not mean that other strategies do not need to be pursued in parallel (see web commentary). The best way to avoid both heel prick pain and iatrogenic anaemia is, of course, not to take the sample at all. When sampling is necessary, much can be done to ensure that all necessary specimens are collected at one and the same time.

Dose

The evidence behind any given dose is limited. Give 0.5–1 ml depending on the size of the baby. The effective range is reported to be as low as 0.05–0.5 ml. Try smaller doses first; more can always be given during or after the procedure. Many units do not give sucrose to infants with a post-menstrual age <30–32 weeks. Infants who are nil by mouth may be given small (0.2–0.5 ml) volumes of sucrose.

Care strategy

The optimum approach is to drop the required 90 amount of a 24% solution of sucrose onto the swaddled baby's tongue two minutes before starting to take blood and then give the baby a pacifier to suck.

Supply

Maternal breast milk should be considered a better alternative if this is available. While most pharmacies can make up a safe stable 25% solution of sucrose at negligible cost (dissolve 25 g of sucrose in water and make up to 100 ml), most units tend to use proprietary solutions. A variety of different proprietary preparations of 24% sucrose are available; TootSweet® is available in vials containing 0.5, 1 or 2 ml (vials also contain methylparaben and potassium sorbate as preserva-tives). Algopedol® is a 24% (preservative-free) sucrose solution available in single use graduated 2 ml vials. Sweet-Ease® is a 24% sucrose solution available in natural (i.e. preservative-free) and preserved formulations. The latter is only available in North America. Sweet-Ease Natural

Continued on p. 491

contains purified water and sugar (24%) only; Sweet-Ease Preserved contains, in addition, potassium sorbate (preservative) and citric acid (buffer). It is available in single use graduated 2 ml vials and a 15 ml cup for dipping the baby's pacifier in (one dip gives a dose of 0.2 ml).

References (See also the Cochrane reviews of pain relief)

Anand KJS and the International Evidence-Based Group for Neonatal Pain. Consensus statement for the prevention and management of pain in the newborn. *Arch Pediatr Adolesc Med* 2001;**155**:173–80.

Bauer K, Ketteler J, Hellwig M, *et al.* Oral glucose before venepuncture relieves neonates of pain, but stress is still evidenced by increase in oxygen consumption, energy expenditure, and heart rate. *Pediatr Res* 2004;**55**:695–700.

Boyle EM, Freer Y, Khan-Orakzai Z, *et al.* Sucrose and non-nutritive sucking for the relief of pain in screening for retinopathy of prematurity: a randomised controlled trial. *Arch Dis Child Fetal Neonatal Ed* 2006;**91**:F166–8. [RCT]

Chermont AG, Falcão LFM, de Souza Silva EH, *et al.* Skin-to-skin contact and/or25% dextrose for procedural pain relief for term newborn infants. *Pediatrics* 2009;**124**:e1101–7. [RCT]

Codipietro L, Ceccarellu M, Ponzone A. Breast feeding or oral sucrose solution in term neonates receiving heel lance: a randomized controlled trial. *Pediatrics* 2008;**122**:e71621. [RCT]

Gradin M, Schollin J. The role of endogenous opioids in mediating pain reduction by orally administered glucose among newborns. *Pediatrcs* 2005;**115**:1004–7. [RCT]

Ismail AQ, Gandhi A. Non-pharmacological analgesia: effective but underused. *Arch Dis Child* 2011;**96**:784–5.

Simonse E, Mulder PG, van Beek RH. Analgesic effect of breast milk versus sucrose for analgesia during heel lance in late preterm infants. *Pediatrics* 2012;**129**:657–63.

Slater R, Cornelissen L, Fabrizi L, *et al.* Oral sucrose as an analgesic drug for procedural pain in newborn infants: a randomised controlled trial. *Lancet* 2010;**376**:1225–32.

Use

Sulfadiazine is used with pyrimethamine (q.v.) and folinic acid in the treatment of toxoplasmosis.

Pharmacology

Sulfadiazine is a sulphonamide antibiotic which inhibits multiplication of bacteria by acting as a competitive inhibitor of the bacterial enzyme dihydropteroate synthetase. This enzyme is needed for the proper processing of para-aminobenzoic acid (PABA) which is essential for bacterial folic acid synthesis.

Bacterial sensitivity is the same for the various sulphonamides, and resistance to one sulphonamide indicates resistance to all. Most sulphonamides are readily absorbed orally. However, parenteral administration is difficult, since the soluble sulphonamide salts are highly alkaline and irritating to the tissues. The sulphonamides are widely distributed throughout all tissues. High levels are achieved in pleural, peritoneal, synovial and ocular fluids. Although these drugs are no longer used to treat meningitis, CSF levels are high in meningeal infections. Their antibacterial action is inhibited by pus.

Most sulphonamides are well absorbed when given by mouth, widely distributed in the body and excreted after partial conjugation by a combination of renal filtration and tubular secretion. Hypersensitivity reactions usually first present with a rash and a fever after about 9 days; treatment should be stopped before more serious symptoms develop. Blood dyscrasias have been reported. Exfoliative dermatitis, epidermal necrolysis (Lyell's syndrome) and a severe, potentially lethal, form of erythema multiforme (Stevens–Johnson syndrome) have occurred in children and adults. Haemolysis is a hazard in patients with G6PD deficiency. The adult half-life of sulfadiazine is 10 hours but double this in the first week of life. Sulfadiazine is not very soluble in urine, so damaging crystal formation in the renal tract (with haematuria) is possible if fluid intake is low. Manufacturers remain reluctant to endorse the use of *any* sulphonamide in a child <6–8 weeks old because of the risk of kernicteric brain damage, but such a generalisation shows disproportionate caution because sulphadiazine does not displace bilirubin from albumin nearly as much as sulphafurazole and there is no published experience to suggest any increase in the risk of kernicterus.

Sulfadiazine crosses the placenta and is used as a treatment for fetal toxoplasmosis in combination with pyrimethamine. Controversy continues as to how effective it is in preventing disease transmission. Since it is effective in the rhesus monkey model, diagnosis and treatment delay may explain the controversy. Transmission occurs before the mother mounts an antibody response or develops symptoms in almost all cases. There is no evidence that any sulphonamide is teratogenic, but maternal use is probably best avoided in the period immediately before delivery. Only small quantities appear in breast milk, so breastfeeding only needs to be avoided in babies who are jaundiced or both premature and ill.

Toxoplasmosis

See the monograph on spiramycin (q.v.) for information on perinatal infection with *Toxoplasma gondii*.

Treatment

Maternal disease: Give 1 g of sulfadiazine every 8 hours by mouth together with 50 mg of pyrimethamine once a day if toxoplasma infection seems to have spread to the fetus. Spiramycin (q.v.) is probably a more appropriate alternative if transplacental spread is not thought to have occurred.

Neonatal disease: Treatment of toxoplasmal infection with pyrimethamine should be augmented by giving 50 mg/kg of sulfadiazine by mouth once every 12 hours. Treatment is continued for 12 months.

Supply

500 mg tablets of sulfadiazine cost £1 each. A sugar-free suspension can be prepared from these with a 1-week shelf life stored at 4°C.

References

(See also the Cochrane reviews of treatment of toxoplasmosis in pregnancy) ◑

Montoya JG, Remington JS. Management of *Toxoplasma gondii* infection during pregnancy. *Clin Infect Dis* 2008;**47**:554–66.

Petersen E. Toxoplasmosis. *Semin Fetal Neonat Med* 2007;**12**:214–23.

Continued on p. 493

Rajapakse S, Chrishan Shivanthan M, *et al.* Antibiotics for human toxoplasmosis: a systematic review of randomized trials. *Pathog Glob Health* 2013;**107**:162–9. [SR]

Remington JS, McLeod R, Wilson CB, *et al.* Toxoplasmosis. In: Remington JS, Klein JO, Wilson CB, Nizet V, Maldonado YA. eds. *Infectious diseases of the fetus and newborn infant*, 7th edn. Philadelphia, PA: WB Saunders, Elsevier 2011: pp. 918–1041.

Schmidt DR, Hogh B, Andersen O, *et al.* Treatment of infants with congenital toxoplasmosis: tolerability and plasma concentrations of sulfadiazine and pyrimethamine. *Eur J Pediatr* 2006;**165**:19–25.

SYROCOT (Systematic Review on Congenital Toxoplasmosis) study group. Effectiveness of prenatal treatment for congenital toxoplasmosis: a meta-analysis of individual patients' data. *Lancet* 2007;**369**:115–22. [SR]

Wallon M, Liou C, Garner P, *et al.* Congenital toxoplasmosis: systematic review of evidence of efficacy of treatment in pregnancy. *Br Med J* 1999;**318**:1511–4. [SR]

Use

Suxamethonium has long been used to provide short-term muscle paralysis (e.g. in endotracheal intubation).

Pharmacology

Suxamethonium was first developed in 1906 but only came into clinical use in 1951. It acts by mimicking acetylcholine, the chemical that normally transmits all nerve impulses to voluntary muscle. However, because suxamethonium is more slowly hydrolysed by plasma and liver cholinesterases (the adult half-life being 2–3 minutes), the nerve terminal becomes blocked for a time to all further stimuli. As a result, suxamethonium produces rapid and complete muscle paralysis. An effect (phase I block) is seen within 30 seconds after intravenous (IV) injection but usually only lasts 3–6 minutes. Recovery is spontaneous but somewhat delayed in patients taking magnesium sulfate. Unlike the *non*-depolarising muscle relaxants, such as pancuronium and rocuronium (q.v.), the action of suxamethonium cannot be reversed.

Large doses cause excessive quantities of suxamethonium to accumulate at the nerve–muscle junction, producing prolonged, competitive (phase II) block. Suxamethonium causes a 0.5 mmol rise in plasma potassium, making its use unwise in babies with existing hyperkalaemia. It also causes prolonged paralysis in patients who have inherited one of the abnormal genes associated with deficient cholinesterase production (about 0.04% of the population).

Suxamethonium crosses the placenta. Under normal circumstances, very little reaches the fetus due to rapid maternal metabolism; however, partial or complete paralysis has been reported in offspring of women with a family history of atypical cholinesterase. It is not known if suxamethonium enters breast milk. However, considering the indication and dosing, one-off use is unlikely to pose a clinically significant risk to the breastfed infant. Children with a parental history of cholinesterase deficiency should probably have their genetic status determined when they are 6 or more months old because the pseudocholinesterase level and type are easily determined.

Use to facilitate tracheal intubation

Trials have shown that prior paralysis can prevent the rise in intracranial pressure and reduce the fall in arterial pO$_2$ usually seen during neonatal intubation, even though it does not prevent some rise in blood pressure. Paralysis alone does nothing to reduce the pain and distress associated with intubation and suxamethonium, because it mimics acetylcholine, often causing an initial transient period of painful muscle fasciculation. Indeed, the rise in blood pressure rather suggests that the babies in these studies were still under stress.

Anaesthetists nearly always administer nitrous oxide, or give a second drug IV, before inducing neuromuscular blockade, to minimise pain. Midazolam, thiopental, methohexital and propofol (q.v.) have all been used for this purpose, but none of these products abolishes pain as effectively as an opiate. Unfortunately, morphine takes 5–10 minutes to become fully effective even though it produces a detectable effect within one minute. In contrast, remifentanil (q.v.) is effective within 90 seconds, and a 3 micrograms/kg dose usually causes enough muscle relaxation to make formal muscle paralysis unnecessary in children less than a year old.

Premedication

A 15 micrograms/kg dose of atropine (q.v.) is traditionally given prior to suxamethonium administration, to reduce any reactive bradycardia and increased salivation. However, problems are so uncommon with neonatal *single*-dose use that this step can be omitted as long as the drug is readily 'to hand'.

Treatment

A 2 mg/kg dose of suxamethonium IV provides 5–10 minutes of muscle paralysis. A 3 mg/kg IV dose provides maximum neuromuscular blockade. A 4 mg/kg intramuscular dose can be used to provide 10–30 minutes of paralysis after a latent period of 2–3 minutes. Staff should **never** paralyse a baby unless they are confident that they can keep the airway open and ventilate the baby without an endotracheal tube when necessary.

Supply and administration

2 ml ampoules containing 100 mg of suxamethonium chloride cost 58p. Pre-filled 2 ml syringes are also available but cost £8.50. Take 0.2 ml from the ampoule and dilute to 1 ml with 5% glucose or glucose saline in a 1 ml syringe to obtain a preparation containing 10 mg/ml for accurate neonatal administration.

Continued on p. 495

References

Cook DR, Windhard LB, Taylor FH. Pharmacokinetics of succinylcholine in infants, children and adults. *Clin Pharmacol Ther* 1976;**20**:493–8.

Guay J, Grenier Y, Varin F. Clinical pharmacokinetics of neuromuscular relaxants in pregnancy. *Clin Pharmacokinet* 1998;**34**:483.

Lemyre B, Cheng R, Gaboury I. Atropine, fentanyl and succinylcholine for non-urgent intubation in newborns. *Arch Dis Child Fetal Neonatal Ed* 2009;**94**:F439–42.

Meakin G, McKiernan EP, Baker RD. Dose-response curves for suxamethonium in neonates, infants and children. *Br J Anaesth* 1989;**62**:655–8.

Schoeffler P, Viallard JL, Monteillard C, *et al.* Congenital anomaly of serum pseudocholinesterase originating in neonatal respiratory distress. *Ann Fr Anesth Reanim* 1984;**3**:225–7.

Venkatesh V, Ponnusamy V, Anandaraj J, *et al.* Endotracheal intubation in a neonatal population remains associated with a high risk of adverse events. *Eur J Pediatr* 2011;**170**:223–7.

Wyllie JP. Neonatal endotracheal intubation. *Arch Dis Child Educ Pract Ed* 2008;**93**:44–9.

Use

Teicoplanin is a useful antibiotic with a similar spectrum of antimicrobial activity to vancomycin (q.v.) but has some advantages in that it only needs to be given once a day, does not need to be given as slowly as vancomycin and can (when necessary) be given by intramuscular (IM) injection. Vancomycin-resistant organisms are sometimes sensitive to teicoplanin.

Pharmacology

Teicoplanin is a complex of five closely related glycopeptide antibiotics with similar antibacterial properties to vancomycin that were first isolated in 1976. Teicoplanin is active against many Gram-positive anaerobes and is particularly potent against *Clostridium* species. It is also active against most *Listeria*, enterococci and staphylococci (including methicillin-resistant strains). By inhibiting bacterial cell wall synthesis, it may work more as a bacteriostatic drug than as a bactericidal drug. Some coagulase-negative staphylococci are now resistant, requiring treatment with linezolid (q.v.) and rifampicin, and acquired vancomycin cross-resistance is also starting to be reported. Teicoplanin cannot be given by mouth, but can be given intramuscularly (unlike vancomycin), and does not usually need to be infused slowly to avoid thrombophlebitis when given intravenously (as vancomycin does). Very few children seem to develop adverse effects, and no reports of ototoxicity or nephrotoxicity have yet appeared. Watch for possible leukopenia, thrombocytopenia and disturbances of liver function. Teicoplanin has been used prophylactically in vulnerable babies with a long line in place, but this, like the prophylactic use of vancomycin, remains controversial. Teicoplanin has a high volume of distribution (making an initial loading dose advisable) and penetrates most tissue fluids well, but penetration into the CSF is unsatisfactory and often unpredictable. Almost all the drug is excreted unchanged in the urine; the half-life in adults is 3–4 days, and in older children, it is about 2½ days due to a higher clearance. The half-life in neonates appears not to have been subjected to study. Teicoplanin is known to bind strongly to serum albumin, and *in vitro* studies show that protein binding affects its antibacterial activity. Teicoplanin crosses the placenta, and little is yet known about the safety of using teicoplanin during pregnancy. Use during lactation is unlikely to be hazardous as uptake from the intestinal tract is limited.

Treatment

Babies <1 month old: Give a 16 mg/kg loading dose by intravenous (IV) injection followed by 8 mg/kg given by IV or IM injection once every 24 hours. Treat proven septicaemia for at least 7 days. Double the dosage interval in renal failure.

Older infants: Little has been published on optimising treatment in later infancy (see web commentary). Give three 10 mg/kg IV doses 12 hours apart. Then give 10 mg/kg once every 24 hours.

Blood levels

Monitoring is not necessary to avoid toxicity (which is seen only with very high trough levels of >60 mg/l), but may sometimes be appropriate to check that the trough level is at least 10 mg/l (and preferably nearer 20 mg/l) in ill babies with overt, deep-seated infection. The trough level should also be checked where possible after a 3-day treatment in babies in renal failure. Although the pharmacokinetics have been poorly studied in neonates, limited data suggest that even with a loading dose, the regime described under section 'Babies <1 month old' may fail to achieve the required trough level of at least 10 mg/l in about one-third of the cases, particularly after 5–7 days of age. Failure to respond to treatment should prompt measurement of levels (where facilities exist).

Supply

Stock 200 mg vials (costing £3.90) come with an ampoule of sterile water. Reconstitute by adding the whole of the ampoule of water (3.2 ml) slowly to the vial, and roll the vial gently between the hands until all the powder has dissolved without foaming. If foam does develop, let the vial stand for 15 minutes until the foam subsides. Then remove some air and add a further 2 ml of 0.9% sodium chloride. The solution so prepared contains 40 mg/ml of teicoplanin. Administer using a 1 ml syringe. The solution can, if economic pressures so dictate, be kept for up to 24 hours if stored at 4 °C, but it contains no preservative. Slow infusion over 30 minutes has sometimes been recommended, especially if the baby is less than a month old, but is not necessary if the administrative procedures outlined in the introduction to this compendium are followed.

Continued on p. 497

References

Degraeuwe PLJ, Beuman GH, van Tiel FH, *et al.* Use of teicoplanin in preterm neonates with staphylococcal late-onset sepsis. *Biol Neonate* 1998;**73**:287–94.

Fanos V, Kacet N, Mosconi G. A review of teicoplanin in the treatment of serious neonatal infections. *Eur J Pediatr* 1997;**156**:423–7.

Kacet N, Dubos JP, Roussel-Delvallez M, *et al.* Teicoplanin and amikacin in neonates with staphylococcal infection. *Pediatr Infect Dis J* 1993;**12**:S10–3.

Lukas JC, Karikas G, Gazouli M, *et al.* Pharmacokinetics of teicoplanin in an ICU population of children and infants. *Pharm Res* 2004;**21**:2064–71.

Möller JC, Nelskamp I, Jensen R, *et al.* Teicoplanin pharmacology in prophylaxis for coagulase-negative staphylococcal sepsis in very low birthweight infants. *Acta Paediatr* 1996;**85**:638–40.

Neumeister B, Kastner S, Conrad S, *et al.* Characterisation of coagulase-negative *staphylococci* causing nosocomial infections in preterm infants. *Eur J Clin Microb Infect Dis* 1995;**14**:856–63.

Reed MD, Yamashita TS, Myers CM, *et al.* The pharmacokinetics of teicoplanin in infants and children. *J Antimicrob Chemother* 1997;**39**:789–96.

Terragna A, Ferrea G, Loy A, *et al.* Pharmacokinetics in teicoplanin in pediatric patients. *Antimicrob Agents Chemother* 1988;**32**:1223–6.

Tobin CM, Lovering AM, Sweeney E, *et al.* Analyses of teicoplanin concentrations from 1994 to 2006 from a UK assay service. *J Antimicrob Chemother* 2010;**65**:2155–7.

Wilson APR. Clinical pharmacokinetics of teicoplanin. *Clin Pharmacokinet* 2000;**39**:167–83.

Use
Tetracaine is a useful, well-absorbed topical anaesthetic.

Pharmacology
Tetracaine is an ester-type local anaesthetic related to para-aminobenzoic acid that first came into clinical use in 1932. It acts to block nerve conduction by inhibiting nerve depolarisation and is destroyed by hydrolysis once it enters the bloodstream. Some hydrolysis also occurs in the liver. Systemic absorption can lead to myocardial depression complicated by arrhythmia, while restlessness, tremor and convulsions can be followed by drowsiness, respiratory depression and coma. However, absorption is minimal when the product is only applied to unbroken skin as described here. The elimination half-life in adults is about 70 minutes; the neonatal rate of elimination is not known. Methaemoglobinaemia has been reported, but such a problem is much more common with the topical anaesthetic prilocaine. Surface application may cause slight oedema and mild itching, possibly due to local histamine release. Some mild erythema is often seen, enough on occasion to delineate the treated area. The manufacturers have not yet endorsed the use of tetracaine gel in preterm babies, or babies <1 month old. The product is, however, available 'over the counter' without a doctor's prescription. There is no evidence that its use in pregnancy is hazardous.

Strategies for surface anaesthesia
Several local anaesthetics have been utilised to anaesthetise the skin of the newborn baby. Lidocaine (q.v.) and bupivacaine (q.v.) work best if injected into the skin but can also be used to infiltrate deep tissues. Lidocaine is more rapidly effective, but bupivacaine provides more sustained pain relief. Lidocaine is less cardiotoxic than bupivacaine if accidentally injected into a blood vessel. Lidocaine gel can be used to anaesthetise the urethra and has also been used during nasal intubation. A eutectic mixture of 2.5% lidocaine and 2.5% prilocaine (EMLA®) can be used to anaesthetise the skin if applied under an occlusive dressing for at least 1 hour before venepuncture, but tetracaine gel may be rather more effective. Tetracaine certainly works more quickly (producing anaesthesia after 30–45 minutes that lasts 4–6 hours), and this is probably because it is more lipophilic and therefore better at penetrating the stratum corneum of the skin. It causes some mild vasodilatation, whereas lidocaine causes mild blanching and vasoconstriction. Further comparative study may well show topical tetracaine to be the better product to use before neonatal venepuncture or lumbar puncture, although the greater toxicity of systemic tetracaine needs to be noted. Some treatment failures seem to occur whichever product is used. Unfortunately, EMLA cream does not seem to reduce the behavioural response to neonatal heel lancing, and tetracaine gel is of little value either.

Ocular use
Tetracaine hydrochloride available in 0.5 and 1% strengths can provide corneal anaesthesia in half a minute, but the manufacturer has yet to endorse their use in neonates (see the monograph on eye drops for alternatives).

Pain relief
To achieve local anaesthesia, apply the whole of a 1.5 g tube of the 4% gel to the skin and cover with an occlusive dressing such as OPSITE® (or one of a range of other, rather cheaper, products). Remove the dressing after 30 minutes (1 hour at most) and *wipe away all the remaining gel* before attempting venepuncture. Never apply the gel to mucous membranes or to damaged or broken skin. Tetracaine gel cannot be recommended as a way to significantly reduce the pain caused by heel prick blood sampling.

Toxicity
Wipe the cream off promptly if signs of blistering develop. The effects of systemic toxicity are reviewed in the monograph on bupivacaine.

Supply
Tetracaine is available as a 4% (40 mg/g) gel in 1.5 g tubes costing £1.10 each designed to deliver about 1 g of gel when squeezed. Although this is enough to anaesthetise a 5×5 cm area of skin, the gel should never be applied to a larger area of skin than is actually necessary.

Continued on p. 499

References

(See also the relevant Cochrane reviews)

Arrowsmith J, Campbell C. A comparison of local anaesthetics for venepuncture. *Arch Dis Child* 2000;**82**:309–10. [RCT]

Guay J. Methemoglobinemia related to local anesthetics: a summary of 242 episodes. *Anesth Analg* 2009;**108**:837–45.

Jain A, Rutter N. Does topical amethocaine gel reduce the pain of venepuncture in newborn infants? A randomised double blind controlled trial. *Arch Dis Child Fetal Neonatal Ed* 2000;**83**:F207–10. [RCT]

Jain A, Rutter N, Ratnayaka M. Topical amethocaine gel for pain relief of heel prick blood sampling: a randomised double blind controlled trial. *Arch Dis Child Fetal Neonatal Ed* 2001;**84**:F56–9. [RCT]

Lawson RA, Smart NG, Gudgeon AC, *et al.* Evaluation of an amethocaine gel preparation for percutaneous analgesia before venous cannulation in children. *Br J Anaesth* 1995;**75**:282–5.

Long CP, McCafferty DF, Sittlington NM, *et al.* Randomized trial of novel tetracaine patch to provide local anaesthesia in neonates undergoing venepuncture. *Br J Anaesth* 2003;**91**:514–8. [RCT]

Maulidi H, McNair C, Seller N, *et al.* Arrhythmia associated with tetracaine in an extremely low birth weight premature infant. *Pediatrics* 2012;**130**:e1704–7.

O'Brien L, Taddio A, Lyszkiewicz DA, *et al.* A critical review of the topical local anesthetic amethocaine (Ametop™) for pediatric pain. *Pediatr Drugs* 2005;**7**:41–54. [SR]

Taddio A, Lee C, Yip A, *et al.* Intravenous morphine and topical tetracaine for treatment of pain in preterm neonates undergoing central line placement. *JAMA* 2006;**295**:793–800. [RCT]

Use

Tetracosactide (widely known by the proprietary name Synacthen®) is used diagnostically in the evaluation of adrenal cortex hormone deficiency. It is also sometimes used in the treatment of infantile spasms.

Pharmacology

Serum cortisol levels may be low in the newborn, particularly in babies born before term, and show no detectable diurnal variation for 8–12 weeks, but stimulation tests can be used to test the functional integrity of the adrenal gland. Treatment with dexamethasone (q.v.) and other steroid drugs can suppress cortisol secretion, and the normal reactivity of the adrenal gland can remain depressed for several weeks after treatment stops. Preterm babies with a low cortisol level despite stress in the first few days of life who require ventilation seem to be at greater risk of developing chronic lung damage.

Tetracosactide is a polypeptide with properties similar to corticotrophin (or ACTH), the hormone produced by the anterior lobe of the pituitary gland, which stimulates the secretion of several adrenal gland hormones, including cortisol (hydrocortisone) and corticosterone. It was first synthesised in 1961. Corticotrophin secretion is, itself, controlled by corticorelin (CRH) release from the hypothalamus in the brain and influenced by circulating glucocorticoid hormone levels. Stress can stimulate corticotrophin release. Tetracosactide can be used to test the adequacy of the adrenocortical response to stress (colloquially known as a 'Synacthen test' because that is the trade name of the product). A 1 microgram/kg intravenous (IV) test dose of corticorelin provides a better test of pituitary function. Both hormones are rapidly metabolised to a range of inactive oligopeptides within an hour or two of administration. While it is difficult to see how administration could cause any harm, these hormones should only be given to a pregnant or lactating mother for good reason.

Adverse reactions

Anaphylactic and hypersensitivity reactions can occur, so tetracosactide should only be administered under the direct supervision of an experienced hospital specialist. Most severe reactions occur within 30 minutes.

Test procedure

Standard test: It has been traditional to measure the plasma cortisol level immediately before and exactly 30 minutes after giving a 36 micrograms/kg test injection of tetracosactide IV. Some advise the collection of a second specimen 60 minutes after the test injection. Tetracosactide administration normally causes a 70 micrograms/l (200 nmol/l) rise in the plasma cortisol concentration unless there is primary adrenal failure, but equivocal results are sometimes obtained, especially in the first month of life. The help and advice of a paediatric endocrinologist should always be sought before undertaking any such test in the neonatal period.

Low-dose tests: The procedure described for the standard test involves a supramaximal test dose. Very much smaller doses have been used to assess the response of the adrenal gland to a more physiological stimulus (doses as low as 500 nanograms have sometimes been used in adults). What constitutes a 'normal' response to such a low stimulus in the preterm baby is not yet clear. A 1 microgram/kg dose causes a two to three-fold rise in the baseline cortisol level within 60 minutes in most, but not all, healthy babies of <30 weeks' gestation in the second week of life (mean peak value 500–700 nmol/l).

The initial control of 'infantile spasms'

The simplest way to stop infantile spasms is to give 10 mg of prednisolone four times a day for 2 weeks and then tail treatment off over the next 2 weeks. Give 20 mg three times a day if fits have not stopped after a week. A few clinicians still prefer to start treatment using 500 micrograms (40 IU) of the Synacthen Depot® preparation on alternate days for the first 2 weeks, but it is still necessary to wean the child off steroids with oral prednisolone (as aforementioned) after that. Use vigabatrin (q.v.) instead for babies with tuberous sclerosis or Down syndrome.

Supply

1 ml ampoules containing 250 micrograms of tetracosactide (as acetate) for IV or intramuscular (IM) use cost £2.90 each. Note that a 1 mg depot preparation (using a zinc phosphate complex) for IM use is also available in 1 ml ampoules costing £4.20 each. The depot preparation should

Continued on p. 501

not be used when conducting the standard diagnostic test described in the previous text. All ampoules should be protected from light and stored at 4 °C.

References

Bolt RJ, van Weissenbruch MM, Popp-Snijders C, *et al.* Maturity of the adrenal cortex in very preterm infants is related to gestational age. *Pediatr Res* 2002;**52**:405–10.

Go CY, Mackay MT, Weiss SK, *et al.* Evidence-based guideline update: medical treatment of infantile spasms. Report of the Guideline Development Subcommittee of the American Academy of Neurology and the Practice Committee of the Child Neurology Society. *Neurology* 2012;**78**:1974–80.

Hingre RV, Gross SJ, Hingre KS, *et al.* Adrenal steroidogenesis in very low birth weight preterm babies. *J Clin Endocrinol Metab* 1994;**78**:266–70.

Karlsson R, Kalllio J, Irjala K, *et al.* Adrenocorticotropin and corticotropin-releasing hormone tests in preterm infants. *J Clin Endocrinol Metab* 2000;**85**:4592–5.

Lux AL, Edwards SW, Hancock E, *et al.* The United Kingdom Infantile Spasms Study comparing vigabatrin with prednisolone or tetracosactide at 14 days: a multicentre, randomized controlled trial. *Lancet* 2004;**364**:1773–8. [RCT]

Oglivy-Stuart A, Midgley P. *Practical neonatal endocrinology.* Cambridge: Cambridge University Press, 2006.

Stafstrom CE, Arnason BG, Baram TZ, *et al.* Treatment of infantile spasms: emerging insights from clinical and basic science perspectives. *J Child Neurol* 2011;**26**:1411–21.

Use

While there are few reasons for using this antibiotic during childhood, it remains the treatment of choice for brucellosis and for rickettsial infection and the most effective treatment for some uncommon erythromycin-resistant mycoplasma infections. Malaria is sometimes treated with quinine (q.v.) followed by a tetracycline.

Pharmacology

Tetracycline is a naturally occurring antibiotic produced by a *Streptomyces* fungus. It was first isolated in 1952. Tetracycline is bacteriostatic, inhibiting bacterial protein synthesis and cell growth. It is only partially absorbed from the gastrointestinal tract, absorption being further affected by the formation of insoluble complexes in milk. Oral administration can also cause adverse gastro-intestinal symptoms, probably as a result of mucosal irritation. CSF penetration is very poor. Most of the drug is excreted in the urine, but substantial amounts appear in bile and faeces. The half-life (8 hours) does not seem to vary with age. Tetracycline can exacerbate any existing renal impairment, and intravenous (IV) treatment should also be avoided where there is hepatic impairment. Tetracycline was once widely used in the management of many Gram-positive and Gram-negative infections, but the emergence of drug-resistant strains, and the development of alternative agents, has led to a decline in the use of this once popular antibiotic. Doxycycline (a semi-synthetic derivative) is sometimes used along with quinine (q.v.) to treat malaria because of its longer half-life.

Systemic tetracycline should normally be avoided during childhood because sustained use causes an unsightly green discolouration of the permanent teeth. It remains of value, however, in the treatment of malaria and brucellosis and of chlamydial, rickettsial, mycoplasma and protozoal infection, and there are situations where efficacy, availability and low cost still make short-term treatment a logical option. Tetracycline is also active against most spirochetes including *Borrelia*, the cause of Lyme disease. Treatment can occasionally provoke a dangerous rise in CSF pressure (so-called benign intracranial hypertension).

Tetracycline crosses the placenta and may cause a yellow-grey/brown tooth discolouration after fetal or early childhood exposure. Rodent teratogenicity studies are generally reassuring. The related drug, oxytetracycline, is associated with increased risk of neural tube defects, cleft palate and cardiovascular abnormalities. More seriously, use in pregnancy has occasionally been associated with fatal maternal hepatotoxicity. Treatment during lactation probably carries little risk: the amount ingested by the baby in breast milk represents <5% of the usual therapeutic dose, and absorption seems to be limited by chelation to calcium. Tetracycline has been shown to retard bone growth in the preterm baby, probably because of its absorption by the epiphyseal plate.

Treatment

Systemic treatment: Treat malaria and erythromycin-resistant mycoplasma infection with 5 mg/kg IV once every 12 hours (or 7.5 mg/kg by mouth once every 8 hours) for at least 7 days.
Topical treatment: Topical chlortetracycline ointment has been used to prevent, or (with oral erythromycin) to treat, *Chlamydia* conjunctivitis, as discussed in the monograph on eye drops, but is not available in the United Kingdom. The only preparation containing chlortetracycline available in the United Kingdom, and used in treatment of severe inflammatory skin disorders, is Aureocort®, a mix of chlortetracycline hydrochloride 3% with triamcinolone acetonide 0.1%. The latter is an extremely potent topical steroid and best avoided in young children and infants.

Supply and administration

500 mg vials for IV use are only available in the United Kingdom on a 'named-patient' basis. They cost £5. Reconstitute the powder with 25 ml of water for injection to obtain a solution containing 20 mg/ml. Take 2.5 ml of this solution, dilute immediately before use to 10 ml with 10% glucose to give a solution containing 5 mg/ml for accurate administration, and give through an IV line that contains a terminal 0.22 μm filter. The IV preparation can also be given by mouth (a fresh vial should be opened daily). A 25 mg/ml suspension is available in the United States (but not in the United Kingdom). Intramuscular injection is painful, and absorption erratic. 250 mg tablets cost 12p each.

Continued on p. 503

References

Hammerschlag MR. Pneumonia due to *Chlamydia pneumonia* in children: epidemiology, diagnosis and treatment. *Pediatr Pulmonol* 2003;**36**:384–90.

Kong YL, Tey HL. Treatment of acne vulgaris during pregnancy and lactation. *Drugs* 2013;**73**:779–87.

Mylonas I. Antibiotic chemotherapy during pregnancy and lactation period: aspects for consideration. *Arch Gynecol Obstet* 2011;**283**:7–18.

Salsky K, Yahav D, Bishara J, *et al.* Treatment of human brucellosis: systematic review and meta-analysis of randomised controlled trials. *Br Med J* 2008;**336**:701–4. (See also 678–9.) [SR]

Theilen U, Lyon AJ, Fitzgerald T, *et al.* Infection with *Ureaplasma urealyticum*: is there a specific clinical and radiological course in the preterm infant? *Arch Dis Child Fetal Neonatal Ed* 2004;**89**:F163–7.

Waites KB, Schelonka RL, Xiao L, *et al.* Congenital and opportunistic infections: Ureaplasma species and *Mycoplasma hominis. Semin Fetal Neonat Med* 2009;**14**:190–9.

Use

Thiopental sodium is most widely used during induction of anaesthesia, but it can also be used to control seizures that do not respond to other anticonvulsants as long as ventilation is supported artificially.

Pharmacology

First used in 1934, thiopental sodium is a hypnotic and anticonvulsant barbiturate, but it does not relieve pain. Because it causes marked respiratory depression, it should only be used in situations where immediate respiratory support can be provided. Large doses also cause a fall in peripheral vascular resistance and cardiac output. It quickly reaches the central nervous system and is then redistributed away from the brain into body fat stores. Clearance is through oxidation (hepatic cytochrome 2C19) and N-glycosylation. The terminal half-life is variable but about 3–8 hours in adults. The half-life in newborn infants is about double this. It is longer still in preterm infants as the half-life is affected by gestation with a marked increase in clearance around term as the CYP2C19 system matures. Drug accumulation (neonatal V_D ~4 l/kg) after a high-dose or a continuing infusion has been given is known to result in slow, delayed, triexponential elimination by the liver. Thiopental crosses the placenta rapidly, but the effect of a single maternal injection is small because the drug only remains briefly in the bloodstream. A continuous infusion could, however, cause fetal accumulation. Only a trace appears in breast milk after use during routine operative anaesthesia.

Thiopental can be very effective in controlling seizures that prove resistant to more conventional treatment, but because the drug acts as a general anaesthetic, its ability to abolish continuing and potentially damaging cerebral discharges can only be reliably confirmed by monitoring the EEG. A cerebral function monitor (aEEG) will suffice for most purposes, but multi-channel EEG recordings will usually be necessary – particularly for important management decisions. Most babies whose immediate post-delivery seizures are only controlled by thiopental anaesthesia die before being discharged home or become severely disabled in later infancy. However, while thiopental cannot be expected to reverse the cerebral damage already done to a baby with hypoxic–ischaemic encephalopathy, use could well minimise the potential for continuing cortical seizure activity to further compound that damage.

Thiopental can also be used to provide sedation during brief but painful neonatal procedures and has been shown to halve the time it takes to intubate the trachea. The absence of analgesic effect means that other drugs, such as remifentanil (q.v.), will be necessary.

Treatment

To achieve brief anaesthesia: 2–3 mg/kg IV, flushed in with saline, produces sleep after about 45 seconds. Further 1 mg/kg doses may be given to a maximum total dose of 4 mg/kg. Recovery begins 5–10 minutes later.

To stop seizures resistant to phenobarbital: Begin with a dose of 2 mg/kg by intravenous (IV) injection over 15–20 seconds and then up to 8 mg/kg/hour by continuous IV infusion, adjusted according to response.

Tissue extravasation

Extravasation can cause severe tissue necrosis because the undiluted product has a very high pH (11.5). Intra-arterial injection should be avoided for the same reason. A strategy for the immediate management of suspected tissue damage is outlined in the monograph on hyaluronidase (q.v.).

Supply and administration

500 mg vials of thiopental cost £5.75. Reconstitute the vial with 20 ml of preservative-free water for injection to give 25 mg/ml solution. Take 125 mg (5 ml) of this solution and dilute to 50 ml with 0.9% sodium chloride to give a solution containing 2.5 mg/ml for accurate, trouble-free administration.

References

Bhutada A, Sahni R, Rastogi E, *et al*. Randomised controlled trial of thiopental for intubation in neonates. *Arch Dis Child Fetal Neonatal Ed* 2000;**82**:F34–7. [RCT]

Bonati M, Marraro G, Celardo A, *et al*. Thiopental efficacy in phenobarbital-resistant neonatal seizures. *Dev Pharmacol Ther* 1990;**15**:16–20.

Continued on p. 505

Gaspari F, Marraro G, Penna GF, *et al.* Elimination kinetics of thiopentone in mothers and their newborn infants. *Eur J Clin Pharmacol* 1985;**28**:321–5.

Hussain N, Appleton R, Thorburn K. Aetiology, course and outcome of children admitted to paediatric intensive care with convulsive status epilepticus: a retrospective 5-year review. *Seizure* 2007;**16**:305–12.

Larsson P, Anderson BJ, Norman E, *et al.* Thiopentone elimination in newborn infants: exploring Michaelis-Menten kinetics. *Acta Anaesthesiol Scand* 2011;**55**:444–51.

Norman E, Malmqvist U, Westrin P, *et al.* Thiopental pharmacokinetics in newborn infants: a case report of overdose. *Acta Paediatr* 2009;**98**:1680–2.

Norman E, Westrin P, Fellman V. Placental transfer and pharmacokinetics of thiopentone in newborn infants. *Arch Dis Child Fetal Neonatal Ed* 2010;**95**:F277–82.

Norman E, Wikström S, Hellström-Westas L, *et al.* Rapid sequence induction is superior to morphine for intubation of preterm infants: a randomized controlled trial. *J Pediatr* 2011;**159**:893–9.e1. [RCT]

Russo H, Bressolle F. Pharmacodynamics and pharmacokinetics of thiopental. *Clin Pharmacokinet* 1998;**35**:95–134. [SR]

Schrum SF, Hannallah RS, Verghese PM, *et al.* Comparison of propofol and thiopental for rapid anesthesia induction in infants. *Anesth Analg* 1994;**78**:482–5.

Tasker RC, Boyd SG, Harden A, *et al.* EEG monitoring of prolonged thiopentone administration for intractable seizures and status epilepticus in infants and young children. *Neuropediatrics* 1989;**20**:147–53.

Use

Tobramycin is an alternative to gentamicin in the management of Gram-negative bacterial infections.

Pharmacology

Tobramycin is a bactericidal antibiotic, related to kanamycin, which is handled by the body in much the same way as netilmicin (q.v.). It first came into clinical use in 1968. All the aminoglycoside antibiotics have a relatively low therapeutic/toxic ratio; there is little to choose between amikacin (q.v.), gentamicin (q.v.), netilmicin and tobramycin in this regard.

Tobramycin crosses the placenta, and while there are reports of total, permanent, bilateral congenital deafness after use of other aminoglycosides, this has not been reported after tobramycin use. Systemic levels are much lower after nebuliser or ophthalmic administration compared to parenteral routes. Rodent teratogenicity studies are reassuring. Monitoring of maternal serum levels is essential to prevent any potential risk to the fetus. Small amounts of tobramycin pass into breast milk; however, as oral bioavailability is poor, no effects would be expected in the breastfed infant.

Tobramycin has certain theoretical advantages over gentamicin in the management of *Pseudomonas* infection because of greater *in vitro* sensitivity, and aggressive high-dose treatment (10 mg/kg once a day in children over 6 months old) is often used when this pathogen colonises the lung of children with cystic fibrosis. Twice daily inhalation (300 mg in 2–5 ml of 0.9% sodium chloride) for 4 weeks is an alternative strategy that has also been used in this condition eliminating both lung infection and pseudomonas carriage. Repeat this, if necessary, after 4 weeks off treatment. Gentamicin is more normally used when treating an undiagnosed Gram-negative infection, while a combination of gentamicin and ceftazidime (or gentamicin and azlocillin) is often thought to be the optimum treatment for neonatal *Pseudomonas* infection.

Like gentamicin, tobramycin may be given either as an 'extended interval dose regimen' or as a 'multiple daily dose regimen' although very few of the studies of once- versus thrice-daily aminoglycoside treatment in neonates have actually involved the use of tobramycin. Check that blood levels can be measured by the local laboratory before starting treatment if monitoring is considered important.

Interaction with other antibiotics

Aminoglycosides are capable of combining chemically with equimolar amounts of most penicillins. Such inactivation has been well documented *in vitro* and is the basis for the advice that these antibiotics should never be mixed together. Problems with combined use have, however, only been encountered in clinical practice when both drugs are given simultaneously to patients with severe renal failure and sustained high plasma antibiotic levels. Leaving a 2–4 hour gap between aminoglycoside and β-lactam antibiotic administration has been shown to enhance bactericidal potency *in vitro* by an unrelated mechanism, but the clinical relevance of this observation remains far from clear.

Treatment

Extended interval dose regimen
Neonates: Give 5 mg/kg by slow intravenous (IV) injection over 3–5 minutes or by IV infusion. Give a dose once every 36 hours in babies with a post-menstrual age <32-weeks' gestation and a dose once every 24 hours in babies more mature than this.
Older infants: Give 7 mg/kg every 24 hours; then adjust according to serum tobramycin concentration.
Multiple daily dose regimen
Neonates: Give 2 mg/kg IV over 3–5 minutes or by IV infusion every 12 hours during the first week of life. Reduce the dosing interval to 8 hours after that.
Older infants: Give 2–2.5 mg/kg IV over 3–5 minutes or by IV infusion every 8 hours.

Blood levels

The trough level is all that usually needs to be monitored in babies on intermittent high-dose treatment, and even this is probably only necessary as a *routine* in babies in possible renal failure or <10 days old. Aim for a trough level of about 1 mg/l (1 mg/l = 2.14 μmol/l). In the multiple daily dose regimen, the 1 hour ('peak') serum concentration should not exceed 10 mg/l, and pre-dose ('trough') concentration should be <2 mg/l.

Continued on p. 507

Supply and administration

1 and 2 ml vials containing 40 mg/ml cost £3.70. For IV infusion, dilute with 5% glucose or 0.9% sodium chloride and administer over 20–60 minutes. 4 ml (300 mg) nebuliser vials cost £21 each.

References

Barclay ML, Begg EJ, Chambers ST, *et al.* Improved efficacy with nonsimultaneous administration of first doses of gentamicin and ceftazidime in vitro. *Antimicrob Agents Chemother* 1995;**39**:132–6.

Bernard B, Garcia-Cazares SJ, Ballard CA, *et al.* Tobramycin: maternal-fetal pharmacology. *Antimicrob Agents Chemother* 1977;**11**:688–94.

Czeizel AE, Rockenbauer M, Olsen J, *et al.* A teratological study of aminoglycoside antibiotic treatment during pregnancy. *Scand J Infect Dis* 2000;**32**:309–13.

Daly JS, Dodge RA, Glew RH, *et al.* Effect of time and temperature on inactivation of aminoglycosides by ampicillin at neonatal dosages. *J Perinatol* 1997;**17**:42–5.

de Hoog M, Schoemaker RC, Mouton JW, *et al.* Tobramycin population pharmacokinetics in neonates. *Clin Pharmacol Ther* 1997;**62**:392–9.

de Hoog M, van Zanten BA, Hop WC, *et al.* Newborn hearing screening: tobramycin and vancomycin are not risk factors for hearing loss. *J Pediatr* 2003;**142**:41–6.

Massie J, Cranswick N. Pharmacokinetic profile of once daily intravenous tobramycin in children with cystic fibrosis. *J Paediatr Child Health* 2006;**42**:601–5.

Ratjen F, Dring G, Nikolaizik WH. Effect of inhaled tobramycin on early pseudomonas aeruginosa colonisation in patients with cystic fibrosis. *Lancet* 2001;**358**:983–4.

Rosenfeld M, Gibson R, McNamara S, *et al.* Serum and lower respiratory tract drug concentrations after tobramycin inhalation in young children with cystic fibrosis. *J Pediatr* 2001;**139**:572–7.

Skopnick H, Heimann G. Once daily aminoglycoside dosing in full term neonates. *Pediatr Infect Dis J* 1995;**14**:71–2.

Smyth A, Tan K H-V, Mulheran M, *et al.* Once versus three-times daily regimens of tobramycin treatment for pulmonary exacerbations of cystic fibrosis – the TOPIC study: a randomised controlled trial. *Lancet* 2005;**365**:473–8. [RCT]

Use

Topiramate is a structurally novel broad-spectrum anti-epileptic drug that has an established efficacy as monotherapy or adjunctive therapy in the treatment of generalised tonic–clonic seizures, partial seizures with or without secondary generalisation and seizures associated with Lennox–Gastaut syndrome. It is used in adults and children, and an increasing amount of 'off-label' use in difficult-to-treat neonatal seizures has been reported.

Pharmacology

Topiramate is a sulphamate-substituted derivative of the monosaccharide D-fructose. Although its precise mechanism of action is unknown, it is thought to produce its anti-epileptic effects by enhancing GABAergic activity, inhibiting kainite or α-amino-3-hydroxy-5-methylisoxazole-4-propionic acid (AMPA) subtype of glutamate receptor, inhibiting voltage-sensitive sodium and calcium channels and inhibiting carbonic anhydrase. Oral topiramate is rapidly absorbed with a bioavailability of ~80%. Protein binding is minimal and there is a linear relationship between the dose and serum concentration. Approximately 20% of topiramate, when used as a mono-therapy, is metabolised by hydrolysis, hydroxylation and glucuronidation. This proportion increases when enzyme-inducing anti-epileptics (e.g. carbamazepine and phenytoin) are used. Most of the drug is excreted unchanged in the urine. Experience with topiramate in neonates is limited and pharmacokinetic data even more so; topiramate has a half-life of about 24 hours in normothermic newborns born to mothers treated with this drug. The drug's pharmacokinetics are affected by administration of other anticonvulsants and by the use of therapeutic hypothermia.

Topiramate readily crosses the placenta (F/M ratio ~1). Topiramate monotherapy may carry an increased risk of oral clefts and hypospadias, and the risk of birth defects is further increased when topiramate is combined with other anticonvulsants. Small amounts enter breast milk, but no side effects have been reported in breastfed infants.

Animal model data suggest that topiramate is neuroprotective and, unlike phenobarbital and phenytoin, does not exacerbate apoptosis after a severe hypoxic–ischaemic insult. This latter finding has led to the suggestion that it may be synergistic with therapeutic hypothermia. The half-life is extended during therapeutic hypothermia due to effects on absorption and elimination. Although topiramate seems a promising therapy, caution is advised; it can cause metabolic acidosis due to inhibition of carbonic anhydrase in the proximal renal tubule and loss of bicarbonate from the kidney. Treatment is with sodium bicarbonate supplementation. More worrying is that studies have reported a relatively high number of infants displaying cognitive and neuropsychiatric adverse events (predominantly anorexia and somnolence), and there is evidence that topiramate causes language impairment, both in normal volunteers and in patients with epilepsy. Further study, particularly of long-term outcomes, is required before neonatal use of this drug can be recommended.

Treatment

Pharmacokinetic and safety data for long-term use has not been reported in neonatal populations. The doses given below are for short-term use only, in newborn infants after a severe hypoxic–ischaemic insult.

Normothermia: Give 5 mg/kg once every 24 hours. Use of 10 mg/kg has also been reported in one study.

Therapeutic hypothermia: Give 5 mg/kg as a loading dose on day 1 and 3 mg/kg once every 24 hours thereafter during the period of hypothermia.

Topiramate is available only as tablets that can be crushed and suspended in water or as capsules (Topamax® Sprinkle) that release enteric-coated granules (the 15 mg capsules cost 32p each). An extemporaneous preparation of 6 mg/ml topiramate oral suspension may be made by crushing six 100 mg tablets and using one of two different vehicles (a 1:1 mixture of Ora-Sweet® and Ora-Plus® or a mixture of Simple Syrup, NF and methylcellulose 1% with parabens). Liquid formulations of topiramate in various strengths (1, 3 and 5 mg/ml) may be purchased from a number of 'specials' manufacturers. 100 ml costs between £37 and £140 depending on the formulation strength and shelf life.

Continued on p. 509

References

Choi JW, Kim WK. Is topiramate a potential therapeutic agent for cerebral hypoxic/ischemic injury? *Exp Neurol* 2007;**203**:5–7.

Filippi L, la Marca G, Fiorini P, *et al.* Topiramate concentrations in neonates treated with prolonged whole body hypothermia for hypoxic-ischemic encephalopathy. *Epilepsia* 2009;**50**:2355–61.

Filippi L, Poggi C, la Marca G, *et al.* Oral topiramate in neonates with hypoxic ischemic encephalopathy treated with hypothermia: a safety study. *J Pediatr* 2010;**157**:361–6.

Hernández-Díaz S, Smith CR, Shen A, *et al.* North American AED Pregnancy Registry; North American AED Pregnancy Registry. Comparative safety of antiepileptic drugs during pregnancy. *Neurology* 2012;**78**:1692–9.

Kim J, Kondratyev A, Gale K. Antiepileptic drug-induced neuronal cell death in the immature brain: effects of carbamazepine, topiramate, and levetiracetam as monotherapy versus polytherapy. *J Pharmacol Exp Ther* 2007;**323**:165–73.

Liu Y, Barks JD, Xu G, *et al.* Topiramate extends the therapeutic window for hypothermia-mediated neuroprotection after stroke in neonatal rats. *Stroke* 2004;**35**:1460–5.

Margulis AV, Mitchell AA, Gilboa SM, *et al.* National Birth Defects Prevention Study. Use of topiramate in pregnancy and risk of oral clefts. *Am J Obstet Gynecol* 2012;**207**:405.e1–7.

Ohman I, Vitols S, Luef G, *et al.* Topiramate kinetics during delivery, lactation, and in the neonate: preliminary observations. *Epilepsia* 2002;**43**:1157–60.

Philippi H, Boor R, Reitter B. Topiramate and metabolic acidosis in infants and toddlers. *Epilepsia* 2002;**43**:744–7.

Use

Trimethoprim is widely used to limit the risk of urinary infection in babies with ureteric reflux or a structural renal tract abnormality. It is also a useful oral antibiotic in the management of many aerobic Gram-positive and Gram-negative infections.

Pharmacology

While trimethoprim is only licensed for neonatal use *under careful medical supervision*, the drug is now very widely used both to prevent and to treat urinary tract infection (UTI) both in infancy and childhood. There is, however, little controlled trial evidence to support prophylaxis.

Trimethoprim works by inhibiting steps in the synthesis of tetrahydrofolic acid, an essential metabolic cofactor in the synthesis of DNA by bacteria. Adverse effects are rare. Prolonged treatment in adults can rarely cause bone marrow changes, but extensive experience confirms that there is no need to subject young children on sustained low-dose prophylaxis to routine blood testing. A combined preparation with sulfamethoxazole, called co-trimoxazole (q.v.), has occasionally proved of value in the management of pneumonia and meningitis. Both drugs are known to penetrate the lung, kidney and CSF extremely well. There is, however, no evidence that co-trimoxazole is better than trimethoprim in the prevention, or treatment, of renal tract infection, and trimethoprim has been marketed for use on its own since 1979.

Trimethoprim is well absorbed by mouth, is widely distributed ($V_D > 1 l/kg$) and is excreted, largely unmetabolised, in the urine, especially in the neonatal period. Dosage should be halved after 2 days' treatment, therefore, in the presence of severe renal failure. The half-life in the neonate is very variable but averages 18 hours at birth, falling rapidly to only 4 hours within 2 months, before increasing once more to about 11 hours in adults.

Trimethoprim is a folate antagonist and folate supplementation during and after use is therefore essential. Transfer of trimethoprim across the placenta is limited. It is teratogenic in the rat at very high doses, but there is no solid evidence that trimethoprim alone (unlike co-trimoxazole) is a human teratogen. Trimethoprim enters human breast milk; the theoretical infant dose can be calculated at 0.8 mg/kg/day (less than that used for UTI prophylaxis in the infant) and should not pose any clinical risk.

Prophylaxis

Give 2 mg/kg once a day. Evening administration in older children will generate a peak drug level at the time when infrequent nocturnal bladder emptying makes infection more likely.

Treatment

A loading dose of 3 mg/kg, by mouth, followed by 1–2 mg/kg twice a day is widely used to treat urinary infection in the neonatal period. One week's treatment is usually enough. By 4–6 weeks of age, babies require 4 mg/kg twice a day (three times a day for non-renal infection).

Supply

A sugar-free oral preparation containing 10 mg/ml that can be stored at room temperature (5–25 °C) is available costing £2 for 100 ml. It remains stable for a fortnight if further diluted with water or sorbitol. The only commercial intravenous preparation has been withdrawn, but a formulation also containing sulfamethoxazole is still available, as outlined in the monograph on co-trimoxazole.

References

(See also the relevant Cochrane reviews)

Braga LH, Mijovic H, Farrokhyar F, *et al*. Antibiotic prophylaxis for urinary tract infections in antenatal hydronephrosis. *Pediatrics* 2013;**131**:e251–61.

Chin KG, McPherson CE III, Hoffman M, *et al*. Use of anti-infective agents during lactation: part 2– Aminoglycosides, macrolides, quinolones, sulfonamides, trimethoprim, tetracyclines, chloramphenicol, clindamycin, and metronidazole. *J Hum Lact* 2001;**17**:54–65.

Hoppu K. Age differences in trimethoprim pharmacokinetics: need for revised dosing in children? *Clin Pharmacol Ther* 1987;**41**:336–43.

Hoppu K. Changes in trimethoprim pharmacokinetics after the newborn period. *Arch Dis Child* 1989;**64**:343–5.

Kozer E, Rosenbloom E, Goldman D, *et al*. Pain in infants who are younger than 2 months during suprapubic aspiration and transurethral catheterization: a randomized controlled study. *Pediatrics* 2006;**118**:e51–6. [RCT]

Continued on p. 511

Mori R, Lakhanpaul M, Verrier-Jones K. Diagnosis and management of urinary tract infection in children: summary of NICE guidance. *Br Med J* 2007;**335**:395.

National Institute for Health and Clinical Excellence. *Urinary tract infection in children: diagnosis, treatment, and long term management*. Clinical guideline 54. London: NICE, 2007.

Shepard TH, Brent RL, Friedman JM, *et al.* Update on new developments in the study of human teratogens. *Teratology* 2002;**65**:153–61.

Smellie JM, Gruneberg RN, Bantock HM, *et al.* Prophylactic co-trimoxazole and trimethoprim in the management of urinary tract infection in children. *Pediatr Nephrol* 1988; **2**:12–7.

Use

Trometamol is more familiarly known as 'TRIS' after the first four letters of the drug's full chemical name, tris-hydroxymethyl-aminomethane, or by the acronym 'THAM'. It is an organic buffer of occasional value in the management of metabolic acidosis where poor renal function and/or the risk of hypernatraemia makes it unwise to use sodium bicarbonate.

Pharmacology

Trometamol was used widely at one time, and is still of some value, in the management of severe *metabolic* acidosis. The drug has to be given intravenously and is normally fairly rapidly excreted by the kidney; some caution needs to be exercised when the drug is used in a baby with impaired renal function. Infusion has also occasionally been reported to cause apnoea, respiratory depression and hypoglycaemia. Extravasation can cause tissue necrosis after intravenous (IV) infusion (see 'Tissue extravasation' for instructions on how best to deal with this).

Metabolic acidosis nearly always corrects itself quite quickly once tissue oxygenation improves. Respiratory acidosis is usually corrected by initiating more vigorous respiratory support. Attempts to keep pH above 7.2 can, however, traumatise the lung. There are, in addition, situations where using trometamol or sodium bicarbonate (q.v.) to induce an alkalosis can do much to combat persisting pulmonary hypertension. Such strategies were, for many years, probably overused, but they are now probably underused. Trometamol should always be used in preference to sodium bicarbonate in patients where CO_2 retention is a problem. Bicarbonate is largely ineffective in such a 'closed' system because the additional CO_2 produced by bicarbonate administration causes respiratory acidosis if it is not eliminated promptly through the lungs. However, because trometamol is only 80% ionised when pH is in the physiological range, it is not as therapeutically effective as an equivalent molar volume of sodium bicarbonate.

A mixture of trometamol and glucose appeared, in a small number of experiments undertaken nearly 50 years ago, to speed the recovery of an effective cardiac output in animals asphyxiated at birth to the point where they were known to be in terminal apnoea. The strategy has never been subjected to further rigorous study, and the long-term outcome for most of the few babies ill enough to really require this sort of intervention at birth is really quite bleak. There is *no* evidence that either the short- or long-term outcome is improved if the severe acidosis (pH ≤ 6.8) present at birth is corrected (using either trometamol or sodium bicarbonate) *after* the circulation has been restored.

Treatment

Give 0.6 mmol/kg for each unit (mmol/l) by which it is hoped to lower the base deficit, giving the infusion slowly at a rate never exceeding 0.5 mmol/kg/minute. Because of the risk of respiratory depression, the drug is usually only given to babies already receiving respiratory support. Partial correction is usually adequate. It is not usually necessary to give >5 mmol/kg but twice as much as this can be given on demand in a real emergency. Birth-related acidosis in the term baby does not merit any such intervention.

Tissue extravasation

Extravasation following IV infusion can cause tissue necrosis; a strategy for the early management of this complication is described in the monograph on hyaluronidase (q.v.). Accidental intra-arterial injection of trometamol is reported to have produced severe haemorrhagic necrosis in some newborn infants (probably because there was circulatory stasis at the time the drug was injected). Localised liver necrosis has also been reported when trometamol is given blind and undiluted into the umbilical vein, but most published reports relate to the use of concentrated solutions containing >0.6 mmol/ml.

Supply

Sterile 5 and 10 ml ampoules containing 3.6% (0.3M) or 7.2% (0.6M) trometamol are prepared by a number of NHS manufacturing units in the United Kingdom using the Addenbrooke's Hospital formula. The isosmotic 3.6% solution contains 0.3 mmol/ml; the hyperosmolar 7.2% solution contains 0.6 mmol/ml (conversion factor: 1 mmol = 120 mg).

Continued on p. 513

References (See also the relevant Cochrane reviews)

Adamsons K, Behrman R, Dawes GS, *et al.* Resuscitation by positive pressure ventilation and TRIS-hydroxymethyl-aminomethane of rhesus monkeys asphyxiated at birth. *J Pediatr* 1964;**65**:807–18.

Blench HL, Schwartz WB. TRIS buffer (THAM): an appraisal of its physiological effect and clinical usefulness. *N Engl J Med* 1966;**274**:782–6.

Daniel SS, Dawes GS, James LS, *et al.* Analeptics and the resuscitation of asphyxiated monkeys. *Br Med J* 1996;**2**:562–3.

Holmdahl MH, Wiklund L, Wetterberg T, *et al.* The place of THAM in the management of acidemia in clinical practice. *Acta Anaesthesiol Scand* 2000;**44**:524–7.

Hoste EA, Colpaert K, Vanholder RC, *et al.* Sodium bicarbonate versus THAM in ICU patients with mild metabolic acidosis. *J Nephrol* 2005;**18**:303–7.

Nahas GG, Sutin KM, Fermon C, *et al.* Guidelines for the treatment of academia with THAM. *Drugs* 1998;**55**:191–224 and 517.

Wyllie J, Niermeyer S. The role of resuscitation drugs and placental transfusion in the delivery room management of newborn infants. *Semin Fetal Neonatal Med* 2008;**13**:416–23.

Use

Ubidecarenone is the recommended International Nonproprietary Name (rINN) for a vitamin-like substance that is found naturally in most eukaryotic cells. It is also known as ubiquinone or coenzyme Q_{10} (CoQ_{10}) and is used, sometimes in combination with other vitamins and cofactors, to treat a number of inherited mitochondrial respiratory chain disorders.

Biochemistry

CoQ_{10} is a fat-soluble quinone that is part of the mitochondrial respiratory chain and transfers electrons from complexes I and II (and the electron transfer flavoproteins) to complex III, a process that is coupled to adenosine 5′-triphosphate (ATP) synthesis. CoQ_{10} is synthesised by a complex pathway and genetic defects at various steps can cause deficiency. CoQ_{10} deficiencies are clinically heterogeneous – six major phenotypes are recognised: (1) encephalomyopathy characterised by the triad of recurrent myoglobinuria, brain involvement and ragged red fibres; (2) severe infantile multi-systemic disease; (3) cerebellar ataxia; (4) Leigh syndrome; (5) steroid-resistant nephrotic syndrome; and (6) isolated myopathy. Unfortunately, some patients do not respond to treatment.

Ubidecarenone has also been used to treat patients with mitochondrial disorders who do not have a deficiency of CoQ_{10}. It has been suggested that it may act as an antioxidant in these patients. A Cochrane review concluded *that there is currently no clear evidence supporting or refuting the use of* [this or other] *agents in mitochondrial disorders.* Given the rarity of the individual diagnoses, there is, however, enormous difficulty in undertaking adequately powered clinical trials in this group of patients to prove once and for all whether this agent (or any other agent) is effective or not.

High doses of ubidecarenone are used as the molecule is extremely hydrophobic, and only a small fraction of oral ubidecarenone is absorbed. Even less reaches the mitochondrion where it is required. Despite the high doses used, side effects (nausea, diarrhoea, heartburn) are extremely rare; given this, there seems little reason not to treat as there is little evidence of harm and there is precious little else we can do for these patients.

Specialist advice

Specialist advice on a range of inborn errors of metabolism is available from the British Inherited Metabolic Disease Group (BIMDG) via their website (www.bimdg.org.uk).

Treatment

> **Note: Treatment with ubidecarenone should only be initiated after consultation with a specialist metabolic diseases centre.**

Neonate: Begin with 5–15 mg/kg/day in three to four divided doses with food. The dose should be adjusted according to response (up to 200 mg daily may be required).
Infant >28 days: Begin with 5–15 mg/kg/day in three to four divided doses with food. The dose should be adjusted according to response (up to 300 mg daily may be required).

Supply and administration

500 ml of an oral solution containing 50 mg of ubidecarenone in 5 ml is available from IDIS, Weybridge, Surrey (cost £144).

References (See also the relevant Cochrane reviews)

Kanabus M, Heales SJ, Rahman S. Development of pharmacological strategies for mitochondrial disorders. *Br J Pharmacol* 2014;**171**:1798–817.
Marriage B, Clandinin MT, Glerum DM. Nutritional cofactor treatment in mitochondrial disorders. *J Am Diet Assoc* 2003;**103**:1029–38.
Quinzii CM, DiMauro S, Hirano M. Human coenzyme Q10 deficiency. *Neurochem Res* 2007;**32**:723–7.

Continued on p. 515

Rahman S, Clarke CF, Hirano H. 176th ENMC international workshop: diagnosis and treatment of coenzyme Q10 deficiency. *Neuromuscul Disord* 2012;**22**:76–86.

Rahman S, Hargreaves I, Clayton P, *et al.* Neonatal presentation of coenzyme Q10 deficiency. *J Pediatr* 2001;**139**:456–8.

Rötig A, Appelkvist E-L, Geromel V, *et al.* Quinone-responsive multiple respiratory-chain dysfunction due to widespread coenzyme Q10 deficiency. *Lancet* 2000;**356**:391–5.

Salviati L, Sacconi S, Murer L, *et al.* Infantile encephalomyopathy and nephropathy with CoQ10 deficiency: a CoQ10-responsive condition. *Neurology* 2005;**65**:606–8.

Suomalainen A. Therapy for mitochondrial disorders: little proof, high research activity, some promise. *Semin Fetal Neonatal Medicine* 2011;**16**:236–40.

Use

Urokinase can clear catheters and shunts that have become blocked by clots and speed the drainage of a pleural empyema. Streptokinase or alteplase (q.v.) is more frequently used to lyse intravascular thrombi.

Pharmacology

Urokinase is an enzyme derived from human neonatal kidney cell cultures that directly converts plasminogen to the proteolytic enzyme plasmin. This then, in turn, converts the fibrin within any clot of blood or plasma into a range of soluble breakdown products. It was first isolated in 1947 and crystallised in 1965. Urokinase is rapidly metabolised by the liver (the circulating half-life is about 15 minutes).

It is often used to clear occluded intravascular catheters and to lyse intraocular thrombi. Streptokinase has been more commonly used to treat intravascular thrombi, even though there is some suggestion that the risk of a hypersensitivity reaction may be higher. Continuous urokinase infusions are relatively expensive, and because plasminogen levels are relatively low in the neonatal period, high-dose treatment may be necessary. A fresh frozen plasma (q.v.) infusion may help by providing additional plasminogen.

The manufacturers do not recommend the use of urokinase during pregnancy or the puerperium because of the possible risk of haemorrhage. It is not known whether urokinase crosses the placenta; however, proteinase inhibitors are found in placental tissue and these likely inactivate urokinase. Rodent teratogenicity studies are reassuring. There are few reports of use during human pregnancy, but placental separation is a recognised complication. Use during breastfeeding has not been reported, but with the short half-life, it is unlikely that urokinase poses a risk to the breastfed infant.

Other strategies for blocked catheters

Instilling enough sterile 0.1 M hydrochloric acid to fill the catheter dead space will usually clear any block caused by calcium or phosphate deposition. A similar quantity of 70% ethanol will often clear a block due to lipid. Alteplase can be used to unblock thrombosed central venous catheters.

Treatment

Blocked catheters: 5000 or 10,000 units of urokinase made up in 2 ml of 0.9% sodium chloride can be used to try to unblock a thrombosed intravascular catheter or shunt. The usual procedure is to instil the urokinase solution into the catheter's dead space and leave in the catheter for up to 2 hours. Aspirate the urokinase before then attempting to flush the catheter with heparinised saline with a view to resuming the original infusion.

Vascular thrombi: Try a dose of 5000 units/kg an hour, and consider increasing the dose two- or even four-fold if blood flow does not improve within 8 hours.

Pleural empyema: Inject 10,000 units in 10 ml saline; drain after 4 hours. Repeat twice daily for 3 days. Open or thoracoscopic surgery may be a better option in selected cases where facilities exist.

Antidote

Tranexamic acid can control bleeding by inhibiting the activation of plasminogen to plasmin. Try an intravenous infusion of 10 mg/kg over 10 minutes and repeat if necessary after 8–12 hours.

Supply and administration

Urokinase is available in vials containing 10,000, 50,000, 100,000, 250,000 and 500,000 units (costing between £34 and £370). For neonatal and infant use, the 10,000 unit vials should suffice. Dissolve the powder in 2 ml of water for injection; the reconstituted solution can be further diluted to the volume required with 0.9% sodium chloride or 10% glucose. 100,000 unit vials are also available and are best suited for use in infusions; they should be reconstituted with 2 ml of water for injection. To give 5000 units/kg/hour, place 1 ml of the reconstituted solution from a 100,000 unit vial for each kilogram the baby weighs in a syringe, dilute to 10 ml with 0.9% sodium chloride, and infuse at a rate of 1 ml/hour.

500 mg (5 ml) ampoules of tranexamic acid are available for £1.55.

Continued on p. 517

References

Ambrus CM, Choi TS, Cunnanan E, *et al.* Prevention of hyaline membrane disease with plasminogen. *JAMA* 1977;**237**:1837–41. [RCT]

Avansino GR, Goldman B, Sawin RS, *et al.* Primary operative versus nonoperative therapy for pediatric empyema: a meta-analysis. *Pediatrics* 2005;**115**:1652–9. [SR]

Balfour-Lynn IM, Abrahamson E, Cohen G, *et al.* BTS guidelines for the management of pleural infection in children. *Thorax* 2005;**60**(suppl 1):i1–21.

Rimensberger PC, Humbert JR, Beghetti M. Management of preterm infants with intracardiac thrombi. *Paediatr Drugs* 2001;**3**:883–98.

Shah SS, DiChristina CM, Bell LM, *et al.* Primary early thoracoscopy and reduction in length of hospital stay and additional procedures among children with complicated pneumonia: results of a multicenter retrospective cohort study. *Arch Pediatr Adolesc Med* 2008;**162**:675–81.

Sonnappa S, Cohen G, Owens CM, *et al.* Comparison of urokinase and video-assisted thoracoscopic surgery for treatment of childhood empyema. *Am J Respir Crit Care Med* 2006;**174**:221–7. [RCT]

Walker W, Wheeler R, Legg J. Update on the causes, investigation and management of empyema in childhood. *Arch Dis Child* 2011;**96**:482–8.

Werlin SL, Lausten T, Jessen S *et al.* Treatment of central venous catheter occlusions with ethanol and hydrochloric acid. *J Parenter Enteral Nutr* 1995;**19**:416–8.

Use

Ursodeoxycholic acid is used to improve biliary acid-dependent bile flow in babies with cholestasis due to biliary atresia and cystic fibrosis. It can relieve the severe itching (pruritus) that can occur in obstetric cholestasis although it does not prevent disease progression. It is less effective in dealing with the cholestasis sometimes caused by parenteral nutrition.

Pharmacology

Ursodeoxycholic acid is a naturally occurring bile acid originally described (*ursocholeinsaure*) in bile obtained from polar bears. It was later crystallised from black bear bile in Japan in 1927 by Shoda who renamed it ursodeoxycholic acid. Ursodeoxycholic acid occurs in all members of the *Ursidae* family, and that obtained from bears is still used in traditional Chinese medicine. Small quantities are excreted in human bile and then reabsorbed from the gastrointestinal tract (enterohepatic recirculation). It suppresses the synthesis and secretion of cholesterol by the liver and the intestinal absorption of cholesterol, and a trial in 1980 showed that it could be used to effect the slow dissolution of symptomatic cholesterol-rich gallstones in patients reluctant to undergo surgery or lithotripsy.

Ursodeoxycholic acid has been used in a number of other conditions, although such use is not endorsed by the manufacturers. They do not recommend use during pregnancy, although treatment with 1 g/day is increasingly being used in patients with obstetric cholestasis. Several reports now attest to the drug's ability to reduce the intense itching and to reverse the laboratory signs of liver damage, although control trial evidence that it improves perinatal outcome is still limited. Safe use has also been reported in a patient with primary biliary cirrhosis who took the drug throughout pregnancy. Ursodeoxycholic acid itself does not appear to cross the placenta, but it does appear to have some beneficial effect on the fetus by inducing placental MRP2 expression and reducing bilirubin and bile acid levels in umbilical cord blood. Ursodeoxycholic acid does not enter human breast milk and thus poses no risk to the breastfed infant.

Reports suggest that the drug is of benefit in some babies with cholestasis due to biliary atresia, alpha-1-antitrypsin deficiency, cystic fibrosis and Alagille syndrome, although it is less clear whether it delays the development of cirrhotic liver damage. Although it may sometimes reduce the serum bilirubin in babies developing cholestasis complicating prolonged parenteral nutrition, liver enzyme levels usually remain high. Side effects are uncommon, although intestinal discomfort may occur initially, and diarrhoea has occasionally been reported. A recent historical cohort review of use in neonatal cholestatic disease has suggested that the drug may not only be ineffective but harmful.

Treatment

In pregnancy: 500 mg twice a day has not yet been shown to slow disease progression but may help in itching.
In infancy: Give 5 mg/kg three times a day by mouth. Double this dose has sometimes been given to help with TPN-induced cholestasis.

Supply

Ursodeoxycholic acid is available as a sugar-free suspension containing 50 mg/ml; 100 ml costs £11. 150 mg tablets (costing 22p) and 250 mg capsules (costing 42p) are also available.

References

(See also the relevant Cochrane reviews and UK guideline on cholestasis in pregnancy **DHUK**)

Arslanoglu S, Moro GF, Tauschel HD, *et al.* Ursodeoxycholic acid treatment in preterm infants: a pilot study for the prevention of cholestasis associated with total parenteral nutrition. *J Pediatr Gastroenterol Nutr* 2008;**46**:228–31.

Bacq Y, Sentilhes L, Reyes HB, *et al.* Efficacy of ursodeoxycholic acid in treating intrahepatic cholestasis of pregnancy: a meta-analysis. *Gastroenterology* 2012;**143**:1492–501. [SR]

Carey EJ, White P. Ursodeoxycholic acid for intrahepatic cholestasis of pregnancy: good for the mother, not bad for the baby. *Evid Based Med* 2013;**18**:e55.

Chen C-Y, Tsao P-N, Chen H-L, *et al.* Ursodeoxycholic acid (UDCA) therapy in very-low-birth-weight infants with parenteral nutrition-associated cholestasis. *J Pediatr* 2004;**145**:317–21

Crofts DJ, Michel VJ-M, Rigby AS, *et al.* Assessment of stool colour in community management of prolonged jaundice in infancy. *Acta Paediatr* 1999;**88**:869–74.

Continued on p. 519

De Bruyne R, Van Biervliet S, Vande Velde S, *et al.* Clinical practice: neonatal cholestasis. *Eur J Pediatr* 2011;**170**:279–84.

Hartley JL, Davenport M, Kelly DA. Biliary atresia. *Lancet* 2009;**374**:1704–13.

Jenkins JK, Boothby LA. Treatment of itching associated with intrahepatic cholestasis of pregnancy. *Ann Pharmacother* 2002;**36**:1462–5. [SR].

Kelly DA, Davenport M. Current management of biliary atresia. *Arch Dis Child* 2007;**92**:1132–5.

Kotb MA. Review of historical cohort: ursodeoxycholic acid in extrahepatic biliary atresia. *J Pediatr Surg* 2008;**42**;1321–7.

Kotb MA. Ursodeoxycholic acid in neonatal hepatitis and infantile paucity of intrahepatic bile ducts: review of a historical cohort. *Dig Dis Sci* 2009;**54**:2231–41.

Palma J, Reyes H, Ribalta J, *et al.* Ursodeoxycholic acid in the treatment of cholestasis of pregnancy: a randomised double-blind study controlled with placebo. *J Hepatol* 1997;**27**:1022–8. [RCT]

Powell JE, Keffler S, Kelly DA, *et al.* Population screening for neonatal liver disease: potential for a community-based programme. *J Med Screen* 2003;**10**:112–6.

Saleh MM, Abdo KA. Consensus on the management of obstetric cholestasis: national UK survey. *BJOG* 2007;**114**:99–103.

Scher H, Bishop WP, McCray PB Jr. Ursodeoxycholic acid improves cholestasis in infants with cystic fibrosis. *Ann Pharmacother* 1997;**31**:1003–5.

Tyler W, McKiernan PJ. Prolonged jaundice in the preterm infant – what to do, when and why. *Curr Paediatr* 2006;**16**:43–50.

Willot S, Uhlen S, Michhaud L, *et al.* Effect of ursodeoxycholic acid on liver function in children after successful surgery for biliary atresia. *Pediatrics* 2008;**122**:e1236–41.

Use

Vancomycin is widely used when staphylococcal infection is caused by an organism resistant to flucloxacillin and/or gentamicin. One alternative is teicoplanin (q.v.). Empiric use is common when nosocomial infection is suspected and the organism is not yet known, but flucloxacillin (q.v.) has the bacteriostatic potential needed to keep most 'resistant' coagulase-negative infection in check.

Pharmacology

The glycopeptide antibiotic, vancomycin, first isolated in 1953, is bactericidal to most Gram-positive organisms, but is inactive against Gram-negative organisms. It crosses the placenta and penetrates most body fluids reasonably well, but only enters the CSF to any extent when the meninges are inflamed. It is very poorly absorbed by mouth, and causes pain and tissue necrosis when given intramuscularly. Vancomycin is excreted virtually unchanged by renal glomerular filtration. This not only means that it has to be given with caution in patients with poor renal function, but that there is at least a two- to threefold difference in vancomycin clearance within the neonatal population, reflecting in part maturation and disease-related renal impairment (including that induced by other drugs) in an individual. The serum half-life is 4–10 hours at birth, later falling to 2–4 hours (6–8 hours in adults). Rapid intravenous (IV) infusion causes erythema and intense pruritus due to histamine release (the so called 'red man syndrome'), and may cause a dangerous arrhythmia.

There is no evidence of toxicity in animals, nephrotoxicity has not been seen with the product currently used, and most patients developing ototoxicity were also taking an aminoglycoside or diuretic (suggesting that damage was wrongly attributed, or that combined use increases the risk). Neutropenia is a rare complication of sustained use.

Use during pregnancy or lactation does not seem hazardous to the baby. Although vancomycin enters breast milk, poor oral absorption means it is unlikely the breast fed neonate will receive clinically relevant amounts. Giving both vancomycin and rifampicin minimises the risk of initially sensitive organisms becoming resistant, and is particularly useful in catheter and shunt-related coagulase-negative staphylococcal infection.

Vancomycin is a time-dependent antibiotic, and activity is highly correlated with the duration of bacterial exposure to the antibiotic rather than being concentration dependent. This has led to the proposition that a continuous infusion, rather than intermittent injection, is the best way to keep levels above the minimal inhibitory concentration (MIC). Trough levels <10 mg/l may lead to inadequate treatment. If an infusion is used, it is essential to give a loading dose at the beginning otherwise it would take almost 2 days to reach a steady state concentration.

Prophylaxis

Oral: Giving 15 mg/kg by mouth once every 8 hours for 7 days can reduce the risk of necrotising enterocolitis (as can an oral aminoglycoside), but might encourage the proliferation of multi-resistant bacteria.

IV: Adding 25 micrograms of vancomycin to each ml of TPN makes catheter-related staphylococcal infection less likely, but such use may not be risk free.

Treatment

Intravenous use

Intermittent treatment:

Post-menstrual age (weeks)	Dose (mg/kg)	Dosing interval (hours)
≤29	20	24
30–33	20	18
34–37	20	12
38–44	15	8
Older infants	10	6

Give the required dose (2–4 ml/kg of the dilute solution made up as described below) IV over one hour piggy-backed onto an existing IV infusion of glucose or glucose saline.

Continued on p. 521

Monitoring: Monitor the trough blood levels (after 3–4 doses or sooner if there is renal impairment). A plasma trough level of 10–15 mg/l (1 mg/l = 0.67 µmol/l) usually suffices, but aim for 15–20 mg/l if endocarditis, a CNS, or a methicillin resistant staphylococcal infection is suspected.

Continuous treatment

For babies who are <7 days old.

Post-menstrual age (weeks)	Loading dose (mg/kg)	Maintenance dose	
		Normal renal function* (mg/kg/day)	Impaired renal function* (mg/kg/day)
<27	10	20	15
27 to <30	10	25	20
30 to <32	15	25	20
≥32	15	30	25

Renal impairment suggested by serum creatinine concentration >90 µmol/l.

For babies older than 1 week:

Post-menstrual age (weeks)	Loading dose (mg/kg)	Maintenance dose	
		Normal renal function* (mg/kg/day)	Impaired renal function* (mg/kg/day)
<27	10	25	20
27 to <30	10	30	25
30 to <32	15	30	25
≥32	15	35	30

Renal impairment suggested by serum creatinine concentration >90 µmol/l.

Begin in all cases by giving the loading dose over 1 hour. Monitor the blood level 24 hours after starting the infusion (the timing is not critical and samples could be drawn at the same time as 'routine' bloods). The target concentration is 15–25 mg/l. If the concentration does not fall within the desired therapeutic range, adjust the dose as follows:

$$\text{New adjusted dose} = \frac{\text{Last maintenance dose} \times 20}{\text{Last measured vancomycin concentration}}$$

Intrathecal use: Give 2 mg/kg of the normal IV preparation once a day, or once every other day, into the ventricles if the CSF is not sterile within 48 hours. Two to four doses will usually suffice. Adjust the initial dose as necessary to achieve a trough CSF level of about 20 mg/l. Consider giving rifampicin as well.

Compatibility

Vancomycin may be added (terminally) to TPN with or without lipid, and mixed (terminally) with caffeine, insulin, midazolam, milrinone, morphine, remifentanil or ≤1 unit/ml heparin. Do not mix vancomycin with IV gelatin.

Continued on p. 522

Supply

Stock 500 mg vials cost £6.25 each. Add 9.7 ml of sterile water for injections to the dry powder to get a solution containing 50 mg/ml. Because concentrated solutions cause thrombophlebitis, individual doses for IV or oral use are prepared by drawing 1 ml of this reconstituted (50 mg/ml) solution into a syringe and diluting to 10 ml with 10% glucose or glucose saline to provide a solution containing 5 mg/ml. The fluid has a pH of 2.8–4.5.

References   (See also relevant Cochrane reviews)

Arnell K, Enblad P, Wester T, *et al*. Treatment of cerebrospinal fluid shunt infections in children using systemic and intraventricular antibiotic therapy in combination with externalisation of the ventricular catheter: efficacy in 34 consecutively treated infections. *J Neurosurg* 2007;**107**(suppl3):213–9.

Cole TS, Riordan A. Vancomycin dosing in children: what is the question? *Arch Dis Child* 2013;**98**:994–7.

de Hoog M, van den Anker JN, Mouton JW. Vancomycin: pharmacokinetics and administration regimens in neonates. *Clin Pharmacokinet* 2004;**43**:417–40.

Elyasi S, Khalili H, Dashti-Khavidaki S, *et al*. Vancomycin-induced nephrotoxicity: mechanism, incidence, risk factors and special populations. A literature review. *Eur J Clin Pharmacol* 2012;**68**:1243–55.

Gemmell CG, Edwards DI, Fraise AP, *et al*. Guidelines for the prophylaxis and treatment of methicillin-resistant *Staphylococcus aureus* (MRSA) infections in the UK. *J Antimicrob Chemother* 2006;**57**:589–608. [SR]

Lodha A, Furlan AD, Whyte H, *et al*. Prophylactic antibiotics in the prevention of catheter-associated bloodstream bacterial infection in preterm neonates: a systematic review. *J Perinatol* 2008;**28**:526–33. [SR]

Nanovskaya T, Patrikeeva S, Zhan Y, *et al*. Transplacental transfer of vancomycin and telavancin. *Am J Obstet Gynecol* 2012;**207**:331.e1–6.

Pacifici GM, Allegaert K. Clinical pharmacokinetics of vancomycin in the neonate: a review. *Clinics (Sao Paulo)* 2012;**67**:831–7.

Plan O, Cambonie G, Barbotte E, *et al*. Continuous-infusion vancomycin therapy for preterm neonates with suspected or documented gram-positive infections: a new dosage schedule. *Arch Dis Child Fetal Neonatal Ed* 2008;**93**:F418–21. (See also 2009;**94**:F233–4).

Reyes MP, Ostrea EM Jr, Cabinian AE, *et al*. Vancomycin during pregnancy: does it cause hearing loss or nephrotoxicity in the infant? *Am J Obstet Gynecol* 1989;**161**:977–81.

Zhao W, Lopez E, Biran V, *et al*. Vancomycin continuous infusion in neonates: dosing optimisation and therapeutic drug monitoring. *Arch Dis Child* 2013;**98**:449–53.

Use

Varicella zoster immunoglobulin (VZIG or ZIG) is used to provide passive immunity to chickenpox.

Pharmacology

This product is prepared from the pooled plasma obtained from donors who are free from infection with HIV, hepatitis B and hepatitis C and who have a recent history of chickenpox or shingles. The product has a minimum potency of 100 units of varicella zoster (VZ) antibody per ml. Normal immunoglobulin offers some protection. No comparable product is available for treating herpes simplex virus (HSV) infection.

Chickenpox

Primary infection with the VZ virus (or human herpes virus 3) causes chickenpox, and reactivation of the latent virus causes herpes zoster (shingles). Spread is by droplet or contact causing infection after an incubation period of 10–21 (usually 14–17) days, subjects with chickenpox being infectious for about a week (from 1–2 days before until about 5 days after the rash first appears). Illness in childhood is usually less severe than illness in adults. 95% of women of childbearing age in the United Kingdom have lasting immunity as a result of natural infection during childhood.

Chickenpox during pregnancy can cause severe pulmonary disease (although selective reporting may have led to the magnitude of the risk being exaggerated). Illness late in the first half of pregnancy also exposes the fetus to a 1–2% risk of embryopathy; lesions include cicatricial skin scarring and limb hypoplasia; CNS and eye lesions also occur. No technique has yet been developed for identifying whether the fetus has been affected or not, nor should it be assumed that exposure in the third trimester incurs no risk. Infection shortly before birth certainly exposes the baby to the risk of severe neonatal infection. The babies at greatest risk are those delivered 2–4 days before or after the onset of maternal symptoms; such babies have been exposed to massive viraemia but have not had time to benefit from transplacentally transferred maternal antibody. These babies are at risk of multi-organ involvement and death from necrotising pneumonia. They need *urgent* treatment with VZIG and careful monitoring for the next 2 weeks. Try to delay labour for at least 3 days if the mother develops a typical rash shortly before delivery is due. Shingles during pregnancy presents little hazard to the baby.

Two vaccines containing attenuated Oka strain live varicella (£27–30/vial) are now available in the United Kingdom, and these should be offered to non-immune children (>1 year old) with leukaemia or a transplant because immunosuppressant drug use puts these children at risk of life-threatening infection. Even post-exposure vaccination seems to work if carried out within 2–3 days of exposure. The vaccines (two doses 6–8 weeks apart) are now also being offered to non-immune UK healthcare workers. Non-immune women contemplating pregnancy should also seek protection if there is a risk of exposure during pregnancy. The vaccines are not yet routinely offered to all children, as it is in other countries such as the United States and Australia.

Prophylaxis

Give an immediate dose of VZIG intramuscular (IM) to:
- Women with no serological immunity to chickenpox who are exposed to the virus while pregnant
- All babies born in the 7-day period before or after their mother first develops signs of chickenpox
- Non-immune term babies exposed to anyone with chickenpox or shingles within a week of delivery
- Preterm babies exposed to chickenpox or shingles before reaching a post-menstrual age of 40 weeks when it is not possible to obtain convincing serological evidence of immunity

The neonatal dose of VZIG is 250 mg IM; the maternal dose is 1 g. It is also worth giving intravenous aciclovir (q.v.) to mothers developing chickenpox around the time of birth, as long as treatment is started within a day of the mother becoming symptomatic. Offer the baby early treatment if symptomatic to limit the severity of the infection. Keep the mother and baby isolated but together.

Continued on p. 524

Supply

VZIG is available from Health Protection Agency and NHS laboratories. 250 mg (1.7 ml) ampoules for IM use should be stored at 4 °C but are stable enough to withstand dispatch by post. Ampoules have a nominal shelf life of 3 years; they must not be frozen.

References

(See also the Cochrane reviews and UK guideline on exposure in pregnancy **DHUK**)

American Academy of Pediatrics. Committee on Infectious Diseases. Prevention of varicella: recommendations for use of varicella vaccines in children, including a recommendation for a routine 2-dose varicella schedule. *Pediatrics* 2007;**120**:221–31.

Chaves SS, Gargiullo P, Zhang JX, *et al*. Loss of vaccine-induced immunity to varicella over time. *N Eng J Med* 2007;**356**:1121–9.

Daley AJ, Thorpe S, Garland SM. Varicella and the pregnant woman: prevention and management. *Aust N Z J Obstet Gynaecol* 2008;**48**:26–33.

Farlow A. Childhood immunization for varicella zoster virus. *Br Med J* 2008;**337**:419–20.

Grote V, von Kries R, Stringer W, *et al*. Varicella-related deaths in children and adolescents – Germany 2003–2004. *Acta Paediatr* 2008;**97**:187–92.

Heininger U, Seward JF. Varicella. *Lancet* 2006;**368**:1365–76. [SR]

Lamont RF, Sobel JD, Carrington D, *et al*. Varicella-zoster virus (chickenpox) infection in pregnancy. *BJOG* 2011;**118**:1155–62.

Smith CK, Arvin AM. Varicella in the fetus and newborn. *Semin Fetal Neonatal Med* 2009;**14**:209–17.

Tebruegge M, Pantazidou A, Curtis N. Towards evidence based medicine for paediatricians. How effective is varicella-zoster immunoglobulin (VZIG) in preventing chickenpox in neonates following perinatal exposure? *Arch Dis Child* 2009;**94**:559–61.

Use

Arginine vasopressin (AVP) and its long-acting analogue desmopressin (DDAVP) act to limit water loss in the urine. Artificially high levels of vasopressin given by intravenous (IV) injection cause arteriolar vasoconstriction. Terlipressin (tricyl-lysine vasopressin) is a long-acting vasopressin agonist which has been reported to decrease pulmonary artery pressure in animal models of hypoxic pulmonary constriction and has been used as rescue therapy in infants with refractory PPHN as well as in infants with refractory hypotension.

Pharmacology

Vasopressin and oxytocin (q.v.) are natural hormones produced by the posterior lobe of the pituitary gland. AVP is a nine-peptide molecule, first synthesised in 1958. It has a structure very similar to that of oxytocin and acts to increase the reabsorption of solute-free water from the distal tubules of the kidney. It is also sometimes known as the antidiuretic hormone (ADH). High (supra-physiological) blood levels cause a rise in blood pressure due to arteriolar vasoconstriction – hence the name vasopressin. Evidence is accumulating that in septic or postoperative shock with hypotension and vasodilatation resistant to treatment with catecholamines such as adrenaline (q.v.), natural AVP levels sometimes become depleted. In this situation, even a modest dose of AVP can re-sensitise the vessels to catecholamine, raising blood pressure without threatening tissue perfusion.

DDAVP is a synthetic analogue of AVP with a longer functional half-life, and enhanced diuretic potency, but little vasoconstrictor potency. DDAVP (unlike AVP) is only partially inactivated when given by mouth, making oral treatment possible (although the dose required varies greatly). Treatment is usually only necessary once or twice a day. DDAVP stimulates factor VIII production, and a 0.4 microgram/kg IV dose is enough to produce a fourfold rise in patients with only moderately severe haemophilia (active factor VIII levels of 1–5%) within 30 minutes. Maternal treatment with AVP, which is inactivated by placental vasopressinase and destroyed by trypsin in the gut, is very unlikely to affect the baby, and reports show that DDAVP can also be used during pregnancy and lactation with confidence when clinically indicated.

Treatment

Vasopressin: Treat severe vasodilatory shock (i.e. hypotension resistant to 200 nanograms/kg/minute of adrenaline with adequate vascular filling and peripheral perfusion and a good cardiac output) with 0.02 units/kg/hour of vasopressin (0.2 ml/hour of a solution made up as described under 'Supply and administration'). Increase this, if hypotension persists, by stages, to no more than 0.1 units/kg/hour (1 ml/hour). One-10th of this dose is enough to control the diabetes insipidus sometimes triggered by brain injury.

Desmopressin: The impact of treatment is difficult to predict, and it is very important to give a low dose to start with. Babies with cranial diabetes insipidus should be given 1–4 micrograms orally, 0.1–0.5 microgram into the nose or 0.1 microgram by intramuscular (IM) injection, irrespective of body weight. A second dose should only be given when the impact of the first has been assessed. Monitor fluid balance with great care and adjust the size (and timing) of further doses as necessary. Avoid changing the route of administration unnecessarily. Get expert endocrine advice, especially if there is coexistent hypoadrenalism.

Terlipressin: The optimal dose of terlipressin required in catecholamine-resistant hypotension and PPHN remains to be determined. In instances of hypotension caused by septic shock, boluses of terlipressin between 7 and 20 micrograms/kg have been used. Similar doses have been used in PPHN. A continuous infusion of 5 micrograms/kg/hour is equally effective and can avoid the swings in blood pressure that bolus administration brings.

Supply and administration

Vasopressin: A 1 ml 20 unit (49 micrograms) ampoule of the synthetic vasopressin, argipressin (rINN), for IV use costs £22.50. Store at 4 °C. To give 0.01 units/kg/hour, take 0.1 ml of this fluid for each kilogram the baby weighs, dilute to 20 ml with glucose or glucose saline, and infuse at a rate of 0.1 ml/hour.

Desmopressin: 1 ml (4 micrograms) ampoules of desmopressin for subcutaneous, IM or oral use cost £1.30. Store ampoules at 4 °C. To obtain a 1 microgram/ml solution for more accurate low-dose administration, take the contents of this ampoule and dilute to 4 ml with 0.9% sodium chloride. If this dilute sugar-free solution is given into the nose or mouth (rather than parenteral use), it can be stored for up to a week at 4 °C. 2.5 ml dropper bottles of a 100 micrograms/ml

Continued on p. 526

multi-dose intranasal solution cost £9.70. These can be kept for 2 weeks at room temperature. Do *not* dilute further. 100 micrograms dispersible tablets cost 52p each.

Terlipressin: 1 mg vials of terlipressin acetate for reconstitution with 5 ml of diluent cost £18. To give an infusion of 5 micrograms/kg/hour, take the reconstituted solution and further dilute to 20 ml with 0.9% sodium chloride. Infuse at a rate of 0.1 ml/kg/hour. The manufacturer has yet to endorse use in children.

References

Bidegain M, Greenberg R, Simmons C, *et al*. Vasopressin for refractory hypotension in extremely low birth weight infants. *J Pediatr* 2010;**157**:502–4.

Cheetham TD, Baylis P. Diabetes insipidus in children. Pathophysiology, diagnosis and management. *Pediatr Drugs* 2002;**4**:785–96.

Filippi L, Gozzini E, Daniotti M, *et al*. Rescue treatment with terlipressin in different scenarios of refractory hypotension in newborns and infants. *Pediatr Crit Care Med* 2011;**12**:e237–41.

Filippi L, Poggi C, Serafini L, *et al*. Terlipressin as rescue treatment of refractory shock in a neonate. *Acta Paediatr* 2008;**97**:500–2.

Ikegami H, Funato M, Tamai H, *et al*. Low-dose vasopressin infusion therapy for refractory hypotension in ELBW infants. *Pediatr Int* 2010;**52**:368–73.

Landry DW, Oliver JA. The pathogenesis of vasodilatory shock. *N Engl J Med* 2001;**345**:588–95.

Masutani S, Senzaki H, Ishido H, *et al*. Vasopressin in the treatment of vasodilatory shock in children. *Pediatr Int* 2005;**47**:132–6.

Papoff P, Caresta E, Versacci P, *et al*. The role of terlipressin in the management of severe pulmonary hypertension in congenital diaphragmatic hernia. *Paediatr Anaesth* 2009;**19**:805–6.

Ray JG. DDAVP use during pregnancy: an analysis of its safety for mother and child. *Obstet Gynecol Survey* 1998;**53**:450–5.

Stapleton G, DiGeronimo RJ. Persistent central diabetes insipidus presenting in a very low birth weight infant successfully managed with intranasal dDAVP. *J Perinatol* 2000;**2**:132–34.

Stathopoulos L, Nicaise C, Michel F, *et al*. Terlipressin as rescue therapy for refractory pulmonary hypertension in a neonate with a congenital diaphragmatic hernia. *J Pediatr Surg* 2011;**46**:e19–21.

Vincent JL, Su F. Physiology and pathophysiology of the vasopressinergic system. *Best Pract Res Clin Anaesthesiol* 2008;**22**:243–52.

Use

Vecuronium is an alternative to pancuronium (q.v.) and can be used to provide sustained muscle paralysis. Atracurium (q.v.) and suxamethonium (q.v.) are better alternatives where only short-term paralysis is required and are more suited to use during intubation.

Pharmacology

Vecuronium bromide is a competitive non-depolarising muscle relaxant that came onto the market in 1980, as an alternative to pancuronium. The duration of action is not as long as that provided by a comparable dose of pancuronium. Vecuronium is slightly more expensive but generates less histamine release and produces few or no adverse cardiovascular effects. It is rapidly taken up by the liver and partially metabolised prior to excretion, largely in the bile. Some of the metabolites, such as 3-desacetyl-vecuronium, which retain considerable neuromuscular blocking activity, are mostly excreted in the urine.

The normal plasma elimination half-life in adults is 30–60 minutes but considerably (and sometimes unpredictably) longer than this in infancy, especially when high-dose treatment is used. Renal failure seems to have relatively little clinical effect on the duration of neuromuscular blockade, but 25% of the drug is renally excreted and atracurium may be the best drug to use in a baby with severe renal failure requiring paralysis. Concurrent treatment with an aminoglycoside or magnesium sulfate may extend the duration of neuromuscular blockade. Use of infusions of vecuronium carries a significant risk of drug accumulation and is best avoided. Placental transfer is limited, and doses of up to 100 micrograms/kg given to mothers requiring caesarean delivery seem to have no significant clinical effect on the baby.

Drug	Onset of action	Duration of action after initial dose
Atracurium	2–3 minutes	20–35 minutes
Cisatracurium	1.5–2 minutes	20–35 minutes
Pancuronium	2–3 minutes	60–100 minutes
Rocuronium	1–2 minutes	22–67 minutes (dose dependent)
Suxamethonium	0.5–1 minutes	4–6 minutes
Vecuronium	2.5–3 minutes	20–40 minutes

Therapeutic hypothermia reduces plasma clearance by about 11% for each degree Celsius reduction in core temperature, and as a result, the action of vecuronium is prolonged compared to that seen in normothermia.

Treatment

First dose: 100 micrograms/kg given by intravenous (IV) injection will cause respiratory paralysis.
Further doses: The standard repeat dose is 30–50 micrograms/kg IV every 2–4 hours as necessary, but some larger and older babies seem to require a higher maintenance dose (up to 150 micrograms has been used). Babies who are paralysed should always be sedated as well.
Infusion: Vecuronium may be given as an infusion at a rate of 0.8–1.4 micrograms/kg/minute; however, due to the risks of accumulation, infusions carry a significant risk of prolonged paralysis and muscle weakness long after the drug has been stopped.

Antidote

Most of the effects of vecuronium can be reversed by giving a combination of 10 micrograms/kg of glycopyrronium (or 20 micrograms/kg of atropine) and 50 micrograms/kg of neostigmine.

Supply

Vecuronium comes as a powder in 10 mg vials, with water for reconstitution. Dissolve the powder with 5 ml of sterile water (as supplied) to give a solution containing 2 mg/ml. Vials can, if necessary, be kept for up to 24 hours after reconstitution, but because the vials contain no preservative, any drug not used promptly is best discarded.

Continued on p. 528

For single doses: Further dilute 0.5 ml of this solution with 0.5 ml of 0.9% sodium chloride or 5% dextrose in a 1 ml syringe to obtain a preparation containing 100 micrograms in 0.1 ml for accurate neonatal administration.

For infusion: Take 2.5 ml (5 mg) of the reconstituted solution for each kilogram body weight and dilute to a final volume of 50 ml with glucose 5% or sodium chloride 0.9%. Running this solution at a rate of 0.5 ml/hour provides a dose of 50 micrograms/kg/hour (0.83 microgram/kg/to minute); running the solution at a rate of 0.8 ml/hour provides a dose of 80 micrograms/kg/hour (which approximates the upper dose of 1.33 micrograms/kg/minute).

References

Björklund LJ. Use of sedatives and muscle relaxants in newborn babies receiving mechanical ventilation. *Arch Dis Child* 1993;**69**:544.

Gravlee GP, Ramsey FM, Roy RC, *et al.* Rapid administration of a narcotic and neuromuscular blocker: a haemodynamic comparison of fentanyl, sufentanil, pancuronium and vecuronium. *Anesth Analg* 1988;**67**:39–47.

Martin LD, Bratton SL, O'Rourke P. Clinical uses and controversies of neuromuscular blocking agents in infants and children. *Crit Care Med* 1999;**27**:1358–68.

Meretoja OA, Wirtavouri K, Neuvonen PJ. Age-dependence of the dose-response curve of vecuronium in pediatric patients during balanced anesthesia. *Anesth Analg* 1988;**67**:21–6.

Playfor S. Neuromuscular blocking agents in critically ill children. *Paediat Perinat Drug Ther* 2002;**5**:35–46.

Scheiber G, Ribeiro FC, Marichal A, *et al.* Intubating conditions and onset of action after rocuronium, vecuronium, and atracurium in young children. *Anesth Analg* 1996;**83**:320–4.

Sparr HJ, Beuafort TM, Fuchs-Buder T. Newer neuromuscular blocking agents. How do they compare with established agents? *Drugs* 2001;**61**:919–42.

Caldwell JE, Heier T, Wright PM, *et al.* Temperature-dependent pharmacokinetics and pharmacodynamics of vecuronium. *Anesthesiology* 2000;**92**:84–93.

Withington D, Menard G, Harris J, *et al.* Vecuronium pharmacokinetics and pharmacodynamics during hypothermic cardiopulmonary bypass in infants and children. *Can J Anaesth* 2000;**47**:1188–95.

Use

Vigabatrin has been used to treat focal (partial) seizures since 1989 and infantile spasms since 1994. While sustained use often causes progressive peripheral visual field damage, this should not inhibit short-term use.

Pharmacology

Vigabatrin is an anticonvulsant that is currently only licensed for use as a secondary *additional* drug in the management of seizures resistant to other anti-epileptic drugs. It is certainly of value in the management of partial seizures with, or without, secondary generalisation and in infantile epileptic encephalopathy (Ohtahara syndrome). There does not appear to be any very clear dose–response relationship, and the plasma level seems to bear no relationship to the concentration in the central nervous system (CNS). It is not, therefore, either necessary or helpful to monitor drug levels.

Vigabatrin has also been used on its own in the management of infantile spasms (West's syndrome) and is now accepted as the treatment of choice if a child developing infantile spasms has Down syndrome or is found to have tuberous sclerosis. The first United Kingdom Infantile Spasms Study suggested that most other children show a better short-term response to prednisolone, but assessment a year later was unable to detect any long-term advantage to the adoption of this approach. If prednisolone *is* used, many would start by giving 2 mg/kg by mouth four times a day and some would then increase this, if necessary, to as much as 5 mg/kg four times a day, before then tailing treatment off over the next 3–4 weeks.

Vigabatrin, (*RS*)-4-aminohex-5-enoic acid, has a structure similar to the potent inhibitory neurotransmitter gamma-aminobutyric acid (GABA). It acts as an irreversible inhibitor of GABA transaminase, the enzyme responsible for degrading GABA. It is rapidly absorbed when given by mouth, achieving good bioavailability because of limited first-pass metabolism in the liver. It is excreted, mostly in the urine, with a plasma elimination half-life of 5–10 hours both in infancy and in adult life. Vigabatrin is given as a racemic mixture, but only the S(+) enantiomer is pharmacologically active. The drug penetrates the CNS where levels seem to stabilise after about 2 weeks. Because the drug is neither plasma protein bound nor metabolised by the liver, it does not interact with, or influence, the metabolism of other anticonvulsants.

Adverse effects in infancy (usually drowsiness, irritability and hypo- or hypertonia) are few and usually transient and mild. Sustained use has been shown to cause progressive, concentric, peripheral visual field damage but seldom with use in the first year of life and only after continuous exposure for at least 6 months and more, usually 2 years (the median time of onset being 5 years). It is almost always bilateral. While this can eventually be disabling, central vision is very seldom affected.

Vigabatrin appears to cross the placenta slowly. In rodents, it was associated with oral clefts, growth restriction and skeletal hypoplasia. Visual field defects, reported during adult and paediatric use, do not seem to occur after *in utero* exposure. The effects of vigabatrin in human studies are difficult to separate from those of other anticonvulsants that are frequent co-prescribed. Limited information indicates vigabatrin passes into breast milk in low levels that would not be expected to cause any adverse effects in breastfed infants. Nonetheless, a degree of caution should be exercised as this drug acts by raising levels of inhibitory GABA in the brain.

Treatment

Start by giving 15–20 mg/kg twice a day by mouth, and increase this, if necessary, over 2–3 weeks to the usual maintenance dose of 30–40 mg/kg twice daily. Further increases to no more than 75 mg/kg twice a day are possible. Double the dosage interval if there is renal failure. Stop treatment if meaningful benefit is not seen after 12 weeks. Sustained benefit is most often seen in children with tuberous sclerosis.

Monitoring treatment

Organise baseline age-appropriate visual field testing if benefit seems to make sustained use appropriate, and repeat this after 3, and subsequently every 6, months looking, in particular, for nasal field changes. Carers should be warned to report any new visual symptoms that develop, and those with symptoms should be referred for an urgent ophthalmological opinion. Gradual withdrawal of vigabatrin should be considered.

Continued on p. 530

Supply

Vigabatrin is available as a white sugar-free powder in 500 mg sachets costing 41p each. The powder dissolves immediately in water, juice or milk, giving a colourless and tasteless solution which is stable for at least 24 hours after reconstitution if kept at 4°C. It can be given into the rectum if oral treatment is temporarily not possible. Dissolve the sachet in 20 ml of water to obtain a solution containing 25 mg/ml.

References   (See also the relevant Cochrane reviews) ⊙

Curatolo P, D'Argenzio L, Cerminara C, *et al.* Management of epilepsy in tuberous sclerosis complex. *Expert Rev Neurother* 2008;**8**:457–67.

Desguerre I, Nabbout R, Dulac O. The management of infantile spasms. *Arch Dis Child* 2008;**93**:462–3.

Dunin WD, Kasprzyk OJ, Jurkiewicz E, *et al.* Infantile spasms and cytomegalovirus infection: antiviral and antiepileptic treatment. *Dev Med Child Neurol* 2007;**49**:684–92.

Gaily E, Jonsson H, Lappi M. Visual fields at school-age in children treated with vigabatrin in infancy. *Epilepsia* 2009;**50**:206–16.

Kroll-Seger J, Kaminska A, Moutard ML, *et al.* Severe relapse of epilepsy after vigabatrin withdrawal: for how long should we treat symptomatic infantile spasms. *Epilepsia* 2007;**48**:612–13.

Lux AL, Edwards SW, Hancock E, *et al.* The United Kingdom Infantile Spasms Study (UKISS) comparing hormone treatment with vigabatrin: on developmental and epilepsy outcomes to age 14 months: a multicentre randomised trial. *Lancet Neurol* 2005;**4**:712–17. [RCT]

Parisi P, Bambardieri R, Curatolo P. Current role of vigabatrin in infantile spasms. *Eur J Paediatr Neurol* 2007;**11**:331–6.

Tran A, O'Mahoney T, Rey E, *et al.* Vigabatrin: placental transfer in vivo and excretion into breast milk of the enantiomers. *Br J Clin Pharmacol* 1998;**45**:409–11.

Tulloch JK, Carr RR, Ensom MH. A systematic review of the pharmacokinetics of antiepileptic drugs in neonates with refractory seizures. *J Pediatr Pharmacol Ther* 2012;**17**:31–44. [SR]

Vanhatalo S, Nousiainen I, Eriksson K, *et al.* Visual field constriction in 91 Finnish children treated with vigabatrin. *Epilepsia* 2002;**43**:748–56.

Vauzelle-Kervroëdan FR, Rey E, Pons G, *et al.* Pharmacokinetics of the individual enantiomers of vigabatrin in neonates with uncontrolled seizures. *Br J Clin Pharmacol* 1996;**42**:779–81.

Willmore LJ, Abelson MB, Ben-Menachem E, *et al.* Vigabatrin: 2008 update. *Epilepsia* 2009;**50**:163–73.

Use
Vitamin A deficiency remains common in developing countries where it contributes significantly to mortality and morbidity in both mothers and infants. By contrast, in more affluent countries, vitamin A deficiency is uncommon and almost exclusively confined to older subjects with significant malabsorption. One exception to this is the preterm baby; they are born with low stores and are usually given insufficient amounts to meet their ongoing needs.

Nutritional factors
Vitamin A is the generic name given to a group of fat-soluble compounds including retinol (the alcohol form), retinyl esters, retinaldehyde and retinoid acid. Deficiency, first recognised in 1912, can damage the epithelial cells lining the respiratory tract. It can also affect immunocompetence, reproductive function, growth and vision (vitamin A is responsible for formation of the retina's photosensitive visual pigment).

Green vegetables, carrots, tomatoes, fruit, eggs and dairy produce all provide vitamin A. Deficiency is rare in the United Kingdom, but in developing countries, it is still a common cause of blindness due to xerophthalmia ('dry eye'); it increases the mortality associated with pregnancy and with measles in the first 2 years of life. Weekly supplements reduced maternal mortality in a trial in Nepal and eliminated anaemia in women also taking iron on one trial in Indonesia, but this finding could not be replicated during trials in Malawi. A 50,000 unit dose at birth by mouth seemed to reduce infant mortality in recent trials in Indonesia and south India, but a systematic review of the data from all the trials that have been done to date failed to show that such supplements generally reduce either infant mortality or serious morbidity.

Vitamin A is toxic in excess and also teratogenic, and women planning to become pregnant should avoid an intake in excess of 8000 units/day. Inappropriate and excessive multivitamin supplementation can be unwittingly hazardous, and women are advised not to eat liver during pregnancy because of its high vitamin A content (650 units/g). The anti-acne drugs tretinoin and isotretinoin are also teratogenic when taken by mouth around the time of conception. Topical use may be safe, but many will not wish to take any such risk. Toxicity might also (in theory) develop in a breastfed baby whose mother was taking an excess of any of these retinoids. The dietary antioxidant precursors of vitamin A, including β-carotene, are not teratogenic.

Human breast milk contains 100–250 IU of vitamin A per 100 ml, and the term baby requires no further supplementation whether artificially or breastfed. However, the fetal liver only accumulates vitamin A in the last third of pregnancy, and plasma levels are low in the newborn preterm baby. Low blood concentrations tend to persist throughout the infant's stay in the nursery and into later infancy.

While overt clinical deficiency has not been detected, additional supplementation has been widely recommended for the very preterm baby. Those who are receiving intravenous nutrition often given a 900 IU/kg daily supplement with their Intralipid® (q.v.). However, this amount falls short of the 2000–3000 IU/kg/day that is currently recommended for preterm babies. A plasma retinol concentration of <0.35 mmol/l (10 mg/dl) in a preterm infant almost certainly indicates depletion of hepatic stores. Supplemental intramuscular vitamin A reduces the incidence of chronic lung disease in ELBW babies, and the roles of vitamin A in fetal and postnatal lung maturation are gradually being understood. Vitamin A is also important for retinal development and may have a protective effect against retinopathy of prematurity.

Most orally fed preterm babies are supplemented – often with a multivitamin product (q.v.). There are, however, variations between the two commonly used vitamin preparations in their vitamin A content: Abidec® contains 1330 IU per 0.6 ml dose, whereas Dalivit® contains 5000 IU per 0.6 ml dose. Formula milks for preterm infants (q.v.) also vary in their vitamin A content; Cow & Gate Nutriprem 1® and Aptamil for Preterm® milks contain ~1190 IU per 100 ml, and SMA Gold Prem 1® contains ~610 IU per 100 ml.

Prophylaxis
Prematurity (early prophylaxis): Babies of ≤28-weeks' gestation who are still receiving IV nutrition may derive some benefit from 5000 units (0.1 ml) of vitamin A given by intramuscular injection three times a week until oral supplementation is tolerated.

Prematurity (enterally fed babies): A daily 4000 unit oral supplement normalises blood levels in the very preterm baby, but whether this is of any functional benefit is less clear.

Liver disease: Counteract malabsorption due to prolonged cholestasis by giving 4000 or 5000 units once a day by mouth. Give babies with complete biliary obstruction 50,000 IU once a month IM.

Continued on p. 532

In communities where dietary deficiency is common: The WHO has long recommended that such women should receive a single 200,000 unit dose by mouth shortly after delivery and that their babies should be given a 100,000 unit dose at 9 months and a 200,000 unit dose 3 months later. In communities where severe deficiency is common, babies should be given 50,000 units at birth.

Supply

2 ml ampoules containing 50,000 units of vitamin A palmitate per ml are available from 'special-order' manufacturers or specialist importing companies (1 unit is equivalent to 0.3 micrograms of preformed retinol). Store ampoules at <15 °C, and protect from light. Do not dilute or use if the yellowish opalescent solution shows signs of flocculation.

References   (See also the relevant Cochrane reviews)

Agostoni C, Buonocore G, Carnielli VP, *et al*, on behalf of the ESPGHAN Committee on Nutrition. Enteral nutrient supply for preterm infants: commentary from the European Society of Paediatric Gastroenterology, Hepatology and Nutrition Committee on Nutrition. *J Pediatr Gastroenterol Nutr* 2010;**50**:85–91.

Ambalavanan N, Tyson JE, Kennedy KA, *et al*. Vitamin A supplementation for extremely low birth weight infants: outcome at 18 to 22 months. *Pediatrics* 2005;**115**:e249–54. [RCT]

Azaïs-Braesco V, Pascal G. Vitamin A in pregnancy: requirements and safety limits. *Am J Clin Nutr* 2000;**71**(suppl):1325S–33S.

Benn CS, Diness BR, Roth A, *et al*. Effect of 50 000 IU vitamin A given with BCG vaccine on mortality in infants in Guinea-Bissau: a randomized placebo controlled trial. *Br Med J* 2008;**336**:1416–20. [RCT] (See also pp. 1385–6.)

Gogia S, Sachdev HS. Neonatal vitamin A supplementation for prevention of mortality and morbidity in infancy: systematic review of randomised controlled trials. *Br Med J* 2009;**338**:b919. [SR]

Kaplan HC, Tabangin ME, McClendon D, *et al*. Understanding variation in vitamin A supplementation among NICUs. *Pediatrics* 2010;**126**:e367–73.

Klemm RSW, Labrique AB, Christian P, *et al*. Newborn vitamin A supplementation reduced infant mortality in rural Bangladesh. *Pediatrics* 2008;**122**:e242–50. [RCT] (See also pp. 180–1.)

Mactier H. Vitamin A for preterm infants; where are we now? *Semin Fetal Neonatal Med* 2013;**18**:166–71.

Mactier H, McCulloch DL, Hamilton R, *et al*. Vitamin A supplementation improves retinal function in infants at risk of retinopathy of prematurity. *J Pediatr* 2012;**160**:954–9.e1.

Mactier H, Mokaya MM, Farrell L, *et al*. Vitamin A provision for preterm infants: are we meeting current guidelines? *Arch Dis Child Fetal Neonatal Ed* 2011;**96**:F286–9.

Miller RK, Hendrickx AG, Mills JL, *et al*. Periconceptional vitamin A use: how much is teratogenic? *Reprod Toxicol* 1998;**12**:75–88.

Rothman KJ, Moore LL, Singer MR, *et al*. Teratogenicity of high dose vitamin A intake. *N Engl J Med* 1995;**333**:1369–73.

Shenai JP. Vitamin A supplementation in very low birth weight neonates: rationale and evidence. *Pediatrics* 1999;**104**:1369–74.

Use

Breastfed babies whose mothers have unrecognised pernicious anaemia occasionally become B$_{12}$ deficient, as do a few whose mothers are on a deficient vegetarian diet. Older children occasionally become deficient because of malabsorption. Pharmacological doses are beneficial in several rare (autosomal recessive) disorders of cobalamin (vitamin B$_{12}$) transport and metabolism.

Nutritional factors

Vitamin B$_{12}$ is a water-soluble vitamin that is actively transported across the placenta. Babies have high serum levels and significant liver stores at birth. Meat and milk are the main dietary sources. Toxicity has not been described. Absorption requires binding to intrinsic factor (a protein secreted by the stomach) recognition of the complex by receptors in the terminal ileum and release into the portal circulation bound to transcobalamin II. Ileal absorption can be affected by surgery for necrotising enterocolitis (NEC), while congenital transcobalamin II deficiency can also affect tissue delivery. The first sign of deficiency is neutrophil hypersegmentation. Megaloblastic anaemia develops, and severe deficiency causes neurological damage that can be irreversible. A high folic acid intake can mask the haematological signs of vitamin B$_{12}$ deficiency. Intrinsic factor failure causes pernicious anaemia which Whipple was first able to cure in 1926 with a liver diet. The active ingredient (cyanocobalamin) was finally isolated in 1948, and a bacterial source of production developed the following year.

Pharmacology

Cobalamin is released from transcobalamin II within target cells and converted to adenosylcobalamin or methylcobalamin, cofactors, respectively, for methylmalonyl mutase and methionine synthase. Rare genetic defects can impair cobalamin metabolism at various stages. Patients can present at any age from 2 days to 5 years with symptoms ranging from vomiting and encephalopathy to developmental delay and failure to thrive. Investigations may show a megaloblastic anaemia, methylmalonic aciduria and/or homocystinuria, depending on the precise defect. A trial of vitamin B$_{12}$ should be undertaken in all patients with methylmalonic aciduria, whether or not this is accompanied by homocystinuria. It needs to be conducted when the patient is well and on a constant protein intake. Hydroxocobalamin 1 mg is given daily by intramuscular (IM) injection for five consecutive days and methylmalonate excretion measured before, during and after the intervention.

Patients with isolated homocystinuria and low or normal plasma methionine concentrations are also likely to have a cobalamin defect and should have a similar trial of vitamin B$_{12}$. Patients with these conditions who are acutely unwell should be started on vitamin B$_{12}$ at once and a formal trial deferred till later. Patients who respond should be started on a 1 mg dose daily IM. Treatment should be accompanied by other measures appropriate to the specific defect, such as protein restriction, carnitine and/or betaine under the guidance of a consultant experienced in the management of metabolic disease.

Treatment

Dietary deficiency: Give a single IM injection of between 250 micrograms and 1 mg, and then ensure that the diet remains adequate (1 micrograms/kg a day is sufficient).

Absorptive defects: Malabsorption is treated with 1 mg of hydroxocobalamin IM at monthly intervals, but 1 mg IM three times a week is usually given in transcobalamin II deficiency during the first year of life, later reducing to 1 mg once a week with haematological monitoring.

Metabolic disease: The initial maintenance dose is 1 mg daily IM irrespective of weight, but this can often be reduced later to one to three injections a week, with biochemical monitoring to ensure that there is no deterioration. Oral hydroxocobalamin (1–20 mg/day) is sometimes substituted but is usually less effective because the intestinal tract's absorptive capacity becomes saturated.

Supply

1 ml ampoules containing 1 mg of hydroxocobalamin for IM use cost 69p.

References

Andersson HC, Shapira E. Biochemical and clinical response to hydroxocobalamin versus cyanocobalamin treatment in patients with methylmalonic acidemia and homocystinuria (cblC). *J Pediatr* 1998;**132**:121–4.
Korenke GC, Hunneman DH, Eber S, *et al.* Severe encephalopathy with epilepsy in infant caused by subclinical maternal pernicious anaemia: case report and review of the literature. *Eur J Pediatr* 2004;**163**:196–201.

Continued on p. 534

Kuhne T, Bubl R, Baumgartner R. Maternal vegan diet causing a serious infantile neurological disorder due to vitamin B$_{12}$ deficiency. *Eur J Pediatr* 1991;**150**:205–8.

Marble M, Copeland S, Khanfar N, *et al.* Neonatal vitamin B$_{12}$ deficiency secondary to maternal subclinical pernicious anemia: identification by expanded newborn screening. *J Pediatr* 2008;**152**:731–3.

Monagle PT, Tauro GP. Long term follow up of patients with transcobalamin II deficiency. *Arch Dis Child* 1995;**72**:237–8.

Prasad C, Cairney AE, Rosenblatt DS, *et al.* Transcobalamin (TC) deficiency and newborn screening. *J Inherit Metab Dis* 2012;**35**:727.

Roschitz B, Plaeko B, Huemer M, *et al.* Nutritional infantile vitamin B$_{12}$ deficiency; pathobiological considerations in seven patients. *Arch Dis Child Fetal Neonatal Ed* 2005;**90**:F281–2.

Watkins D, Rosenblatt DS. Inborn errors of cobalamin absorption and metabolism. *Am J Med Genet C Semin Med Genet* 2011;**157C**:33–44.

Watkins D, Rosenblatt DS, Fowler B. Disorders of cobalamin and folate transport and metabolism. In: Saudubray J-M, van den Berghe G, Walter JH, eds. *Inborn metabolic diseases. Diagnosis and treatment,* 5th edn. Berlin: Springer-Verlag, 2012: pp. 385–404.

Use

These formulations should only be used for babies unable to metabolise dietary vitamin D into alfacalcidol or calcitriol because of renal damage (although some babies with congenital hypoparathyroidism also benefit from taking the more potent active substance). Prematurity does not, in itself, make such use appropriate.

Pharmacology

A range of closely related sterol compounds possess vitamin D-like properties, as outlined in the main monograph on vitamin D (q.v.). Most have to be hydroxylated before becoming metabolically active. Toxicity is more likely with vitamin D than with any other vitamin, and it seems particularly common in infancy. It first manifests as hypercalcaemia, with muscle weakness, nausea and vomiting, pain and even cardiac arrhythmia and, if persistent, with generalised vascular calcification and a progressive deterioration in renal function. Because the metabolically active products have a shorter biological half-life, they need to be given daily, but this also means that any toxicity also resolves rather more quickly. Because patients vary quite widely in the amount of calcitriol or alfacalcidol they require, it is important to monitor the total (and, if possible, the ionised) plasma calcium concentration regularly. Such limited information as there is suggests that if use is necessary to keep the mother well during pregnancy, it will keep the fetus well too but high-dose maternal use during lactation should only be attempted if the baby is monitored with some care.

Pathophysiology

Renal disease: Patients with severe renal disease, and on long-term renal dialysis, often become hypocalcaemic. Many develop secondary hyperparathyroidism if the plasma phosphate level remains high, and some develop renal rickets (osteodystrophy). Management is outlined in the website entry for vitamin D, but all such children need to be managed by an experienced paediatric nephrologist. Use just enough alfacalcidol or calcitriol to keep the ionised plasma calcium concentration in the upper half of the normal range (1.18–1.38 mmol/l in late infancy).

Parathyroid disorders: Deficient parathyroid production (as, e.g., in the DiGeorge and CATCH 22 syndromes) causes hypocalcaemia best controlled by giving a metabolically active form of vitamin D. Adjust the dose used to keep the plasma calcium level in the low normal range (2.0–2.25 mmol/l). Patients with receptor insensitivity to parathyroid hormone (pseudohypoparathyroidism) should be managed in the same way.

Pseudovitamin D deficiency rickets: This is a recessively inherited condition in which the kidney's 1α-hydroxylase enzyme system is defective, causing hypocalcaemia, rickets and secondary hyperparathyroidism. All symptoms can be abolished by giving a physiological dose of one of the metabolically active forms of vitamin D.

Treatment

Alfacalcidol (1α-hydroxycholecalciferol): Start babies on 25 nanograms/kg by mouth or intravenous (IV) injection once a day, and optimise the dose as outlined earlier by measuring the plasma calcium level twice a week. Monitoring needs to continue every 2–4 weeks even after treatment seems to have stabilised.

Calcitriol (1,25-dihydroxycholecalciferol): Start babies on 15 nanograms/kg by mouth or IV once a day, and monitor treatment regularly as indicated earlier.

Supply

Alfacalcidol: 1 microgram (0.5 ml) ampoules for IV or intramuscular use cost £2.20. They contain 207 mg of propylene glycol. 10 ml bottles of a sugar-free oral liquid (100 nanograms/drop) cost £21. This liquid cannot be further diluted, so the only way to give a really low dose is to give treatment less than daily.

Calcitriol: 250 nanograms capsules of calcitriol cost 18p each.

References

Caplan RH, Beguin EA. Hypercalcemia in a calcitriol-treated hypoparathyroid woman during lactation. *Obstetr Gynecol* 1990;**76**:485–9.

Chan JCM, McEnery PT, Chinchilli VM, *et al.* A prospective double-blind study of growth failure in children with chronic renal insufficiency and the effectiveness of treatment with calcitriol versus dihydrotachysterol. *J Pediatr* 1994;**124**:520–8. [RCT]

Continued on p. 536

Hochberg Z, Tiosano D, Even L. Calcium therapy for calcitriol-resistant rickets. *J Pediatr* 1992;**121**:803–8.

Hodson EM, Evans RA, Dunstan CR, *et al.* Treatment of childhood osteodystrophy with calcitriol or ergocalciferol. *Clin Nephrol* 1985;**24**:192–200.

Holick MF. Vitamin D deficiency. *N Engl J Med* 2007;**357**:266–81.

Rigden SPA. The treatment of renal osteodystrophy. *Pediatr Nephrol* 1996;**10**:653–5.

Seikaly MG, Browne RH, Baum M. The effect of phosphate supplementation on linear growth in children with X-linked hypophosphatemia. *Pediatrics* 1994;**94**:478–81.

Thomas BR, Bennett JD. Symptomatic hypocalcaemia and hypoparathyroidism in two infants of mothers with hyperparathyroidism and familial benign hypercalcemia. *J Perinatol* 1995;**15**:23–6.

Vanstone MB, Oberfield SE, Shader L, *et al.* Hypercalcemia in children receiving pharmacologic doses of vitamin D. *Pediatrics* 2012;**129**:e1060–3.

Use
Irrespective of weight, babies need 10 micrograms (400 IU) of vitamin D a day for optimal bone growth. While all artificial milks provide this, breast milk will not do this if the mother herself is subclinically deficient. The case for prophylactic supplementation is widely acknowledged and just as widely ignored.

Pharmacology
Vitamin D (calciferol) is the generic term used to describe a range of compounds that control calcium and phosphate absorption from the intestine, their mobilisation from bone and also possibly their retention by the kidneys. Vitamin D_2 (ergocalciferol) and vitamin D_3 (cholecalciferol) are the main dietary sources. Both have to be hydroxylated to 25-hydroxyvitamin D [25(OH)D] by the liver and finally activated by further hydroxylation to 1,25-hydroxy-D by the kidney and placenta. D_3 is more effectively hydroxylated than D_2. Microgram for microgram, D_3 is also more than three times as effective in raising plasma 25(OH)D levels than is D_2. After a single high-dose intramuscular (IM) injection of D_3, levels take 3 months to respond and even longer after IM D_2. Somewhat surprisingly, the response is much faster (days) if either IM preparation is taken orally.

Nutritional factors
Most breakfast cereals and spreading margarines provide dietary vitamin D, as do oily fish. Exposure to ultraviolet summer sunlight is, however, the main reason why most people avoid becoming vitamin D deficient and clothing can block this, as can use of sunblock cream. Maternal deficiency severe enough to cause congenital rickets or craniotabes is rare, but many women have suboptimal levels rendering their children, if breastfed, vulnerable to the hazards of overt rickets. There is also increasing evidence that subclinical deficiency during pregnancy and the first year of life can have a permanently damaging impact on bone growth in later childhood (see web commentary).

The amount of vitamin D required in infancy is influenced by the adequacy of the stores built up during fetal life and by subsequent exposure to sunlight. If neither can be guaranteed, the case for a regular supplement is overwhelming, and there is no reason not to start this at birth. Many weaning foods are fortified, while all formula milks (q.v.) contain at least 10 micrograms/l, but because breast milk usually contains <1 microgram/l even in women with good nutritional reserves, many breastfed babies continue to become covertly deficient if they are not supplemented, especially in winter.

Maternal prophylaxis
The optimum strategy is to get all women to take a 10 micrograms supplement daily throughout pregnancy, and in the United Kingdom, the 'Healthy Start' women's vitamin tablets now make this possible. An alternative strategy, adopted in some parts of Europe, is to give all women suspected of having suboptimal vitamin D stores (including all veiled women) a 2.5 mg IM dose of vitamin D_3 early in the third trimester of pregnancy, though taking the IM preparation by mouth is much more effective at raising 25(OH)D levels.

Prophylaxis after birth
Breastfed babies: Give 7.5 micrograms once a day until mixed feeding is established.
Preterm babies: Give all preterm babies 7.5 micrograms once a day until they weigh at least 3 kg (or longer if breast fed).
Malabsorption: Give babies with complete biliary obstruction 750 micrograms IM once a month.

Supply
Prophylaxis during pregnancy: 'Healthy Start' women's vitamin tablets containing 10 micrograms of D_3, 70 mg of vitamin C and 400 micrograms of folic acid (but no vitamin A) became available in the United Kingdom to all women who are pregnant or breastfeeding in March 2007.
Prophylaxis during the first year of life: See the multivitamin monograph for various alternatives.
Treatment of established vitamin deficiency: 1 ml (7.5 mg or 300,000 unit) ampoules of D_2 for IM use cost £8.50. 10 micrograms (400 unit) tablets, containing 97 mg of calcium, cost 34p each.

Continued on p. 538

References

(See also the relevant Cochrane reviews)

Armas LAG, Hollis BW, Heaney RP. Vitamin D$_2$ is much less effective than Vitamin D$_3$ in humans. *J Clin Endocrinol Metab* 2004;**89**: 5387–91.

Backström MC, Mäki R, Kuusela A-L, *et al.* Randomised controlled trial of vitamin D supplementation on bone density and biochemical indices in preterm infants. *Arch Dis Child Fetal Neonatal Ed* 1999;**80**:F161–6. [RCT]

Dawodu A, Wagner CL. Mother-child vitamin D deficiency: an international perspective. *Arch Dis Child* 2007;**92**:737–40.

Holick MF. Vitamin D deficiency. *N Engl J Med* 2007;**357**:266–81.

Kovacs CS. Maternal vitamin D deficiency: fetal and neonatal implications. *Semin Fetal Neonatal Med* 2013;**18**:129–35

Misra M, Pacaud D, Petryk A, *et al.* Vitamin D deficiency in children and its management: review of current knowledge and recommendations. *Pediatrics* 2008;**122**:398–417.

Onwuneme C, Carroll A, McCarthy R, *et al.* Towards evidence based medicine for paediatricians. Question 2. What is the ideal dose of vitamin D supplementation for term neonates? *Arch Dis Child* 2012;**97**:387–9.

Pearce SH, Cheetham TD. Diagnosis and management of vitamin D deficiency. *Br Med J* 2010;**340**:b5664.

Romagnoli E, Mascia ML, Cipriani C, *et al.* Short and long-term variations in serum calciotropic hormones after a single very large dose of ergocalciferol (D2) or cholecalciferol (D3) in the elderly. *J Clin Endocrinol Metab* 2008;**93**: 3015–20.

Taylor SN, Wagner CL, Hollis BW. Vitamin D supplementation during lactation to support infant and mother. *J Am Coll Nutr* 2008;**27**:690–71.

Use
Deficiency of vitamin E causing haemolytic anaemia can be seen in nutritionally deficient pre-term babies and in babies with malabsorption due to cholestasis. Pharmacological doses are used in abetalipoproteinaemia.

Pharmacology
Vitamin E is the name given to a group of fat-soluble antioxidant tocopherols of which alpha tocopherol shows the greatest activity. The natural vitamin, first isolated in 1936, is concentrated from soybean oil. Excessive intake (100 mg/kg daily) is toxic to the newborn kitten. Plasma levels in excess of 100 mg/l caused hepatomegaly and levels over 180 mg/l were sometimes lethal. The effect of excessive medication in man is unknown. Vitamin deficiency was first identified as causing fetal death and resorption in the laboratory rat. It is now known to cause enhanced platelet aggregation and also thought to cause a haemolytic anaemia, probably as a result of peroxidation of the lipid component of the red cell membrane (a problem that seems to be exacerbated by giving artificial milk containing extra iron).

Various studies in the 1980s looked to see whether early high-dose intravenous (IV) or intra-muscular use reduced the risk of intraventricular haemorrhage, bronchopulmonary dysplasia or retinopathy of prematurity, but the benefits achieved were marginal, and no study ever looked to see how much long-term benefit such treatment delivered. The preparations used in those studies have, in any case, now been withdrawn from general sale because of concern about one of the stabilisation agents used, while high-dose oral administration has been linked to an increased incidence of necrotising enterocolitis that may (or may not) have been related to the product's high osmolarity. Interest in the vitamin's prophylactic use as an antioxidant has now declined, and one recent meta-analysis has suggested that sustained high dose to limit the risk of cardiovascular disease and cancer in older people may actually be harmful. Neither does high-dose supplementation with vitamins C and E in pregnancy seem to reduce the risk of pre-eclampsia as much as early studies had suggested.

High doses of vitamin E can prevent neuromuscular problems in abetalipoproteinaemia, an autosomal recessive disorder associated with fat malabsorption and acanthocytosis. Such babies should also be treated with a low-fat diet and supplements of vitamin A (7 mg) and vitamin K (5–10 mg) once a day by mouth irrespective of weight.

Nutritional factors
Human milk contains an average of 0.35 mg alpha tocopherol per 100 ml (some four times as much as cows' milk), and formula milks between 0.5 and 4.0 mg/100 ml. Babies are relatively deficient in vitamin E at birth, and plasma levels (2.5 mg/l) are less than a quarter those in the mother. Plasma levels rise rapidly after birth in the breastfed term baby but remain low for several weeks in artificially fed preterm babies (especially those weighing <1.5 kg at birth). Significant anaemia does not develop with artificial feeds that provide a daily intake of 2 mg/kg of D-alpha tocopherol (~3 units/kg vitamin E) as long as the ratio of vitamin E to polyunsaturated fat in the diet is well above 0.4 mg/g even if the milk contains supplemental iron. Haemolytic anaemia, when it does occur, usually becomes apparent 4–6 weeks after birth and is usually associated with a reticulocytosis (>8%), an unusually high platelet count and an abnormal peroxide-induced haemolysis test (>30%).

Treatment
Prophylaxis in the preterm baby: Only a minority of units now offer routine oral supplementation. The optimum IV dose for a parenterally fed baby is probably about 2.8 mg/kg/day.
Nutritional deficiency: 10 mg/kg by mouth once a day will quickly correct any nutritional deficiency.
Malabsorption: Babies with cholestasis may benefit from a 17 mg/kg supplement once a day by mouth.
Abetalipoproteinaemia: Give 100 mg/kg by mouth once a day.

Supply
An oral suspension containing 50 mg/ml of alpha tocopherol (as tocofersolan) costs £55 for 20 ml. No licenced parenteral preparation is commercially available either in the United Kingdom or North America.

Continued on p. 540

References

(See also the relevant Cochrane reviews)

Biesalski HK. Vitamin E requirements in parenteral nutrition. *Gastroenterology* 2009;**137**(5 suppl):S92–104.

Brion LP, Bell EF, Raghuveer TS, *et al.* What is the appropriate intravenous dose of vitamin E for very-low-birth-weight infants? *J Perinatol* 2004;**24**:205–7.

Greer FR. Vitamins A, E, and K. In Tsang RC, Uauy R, Koletzko B, *et al.* eds. *Nutrition in the preterm infant. Scientific basis and practical guidelines*, 2nd edn. Cincinnati OH: Digital Educational Publishing, 2005; pp. 141–72.

Kositamongkol S, Suthutvoravut U, Chongviriyaphan N, *et al.* Vitamin A and E status in very low birth weight infants. *J Perinatol* 2011;**31**:471–6.

Low MR, Wijewardene K, Wald NK. Is routine vitamin E administration justified in very-low-birthweight infants? *Dev Med Child Neurol* 1990;**32**:442–50.

Miller ER, Pastor-Barriuso R, Dalal D, *et al.* Meta-analysis: high-dosage vitamin E supplementation may increase all-cause mortality. *Ann Intern Med* 2005;**142**:37–46. [SR] (See also pp. 75–6.)

Raju TNK, Lagenberg P, Bhutani V, *et al.* Vitamin E prophylaxis to reduce retinopathy of prematurity: a reappraisal of published trials. *J Pediatr* 1997;**131**:844–50. [SR]

Westergren T, Kalikstad B. Dosage and formulation issues: oral vitamin E therapy in children. *Eur J Clin Pharmacol* 2010;**66**:109–18.

Use
Vitamin K is required for the hepatic production of coagulation factors II, VII, IX and X.

Nutritional factors
The term vitamin K refers to a variety of fat-soluble 2-methyl-1,4-naphthoquinone derivatives. Vitamin K$_1$ (isolated in 1939) occurs in green plants, while vitamin K$_2$ (menaquinone) is synthesised by microbial flora in the gut. Human milk contains about 1.5 micrograms/l of vitamin K, while cow's milk contains about three times as much as this. Most formula milks contain over 50 micrograms/l. Vitamin K crosses the placenta poorly, and babies are relatively deficient at birth. Any resultant vitamin-responsive bleeding used to be called 'haemorrhagic disease of the newborn' but is now, more informatively, called 'vitamin K deficiency bleeding' (VKDB) because it can occur at any time in the first 3 months of life. Any unexplained bruise or bleed in a young baby calls for *immediate* attention if catastrophic cerebral bleeding is to be avoided.

Pharmacology
Bleeding in the first week of life is usually mild, except in the babies of mothers on some anticonvulsants. Later VKDB can, however, cause potentially lethal intracranial bleeding, and there is a 1:6000 risk of this in the unsupplemented breastfed baby. Malabsorption, usually due to unrecognised liver disease, accounts for most of this increased risk. A single 1 mg intramuscular (IM) dose provides *almost* complete protection, probably by providing a slow-release IM 'depot', but a dose this large causes some liver overload in the very preterm baby. In North America, a single IM dose at birth is the preferred preventive strategy, but in Europe, the breastfed baby is more commonly given at least three 2 mg oral doses at intervals (see web commentary). Britain is somewhere in 'mid-Atlantic', but the UK Government is committed to ensuring that all families are allowed to choose which strategy they would prefer.

Prophylaxis
IM prophylaxis: 1 mg is the dose traditionally given IM to every baby at birth. Intravenous (IV) administration does NOT give the *sustained* protection provided by IM injection. For babies below 2.5 kg, give 0.3 mg/kg to a maximum dose of 1 mg (and then give those later offered breast milk an oral supplement from 4 weeks).
The oral option: Babies born to mothers on carbamazepine, phenobarbital, phenytoin, rifampicin or warfarin and those too ill for early feeding should be offered IM prophylaxis at birth, but all other babies can, with parental consent, be given a 1 or 2 mg dose by mouth instead. In breastfed babies, it is necessary to give further vitamin K; several options are available to allow this (see 'Supply and administration').
Babies with obstructive liver disease: These need a 1 mg protective IM dose once every 2 weeks.

Diagnosis of vitamin K deficiency
Changes in the prothrombin time and international normalised ratio (INR) are poor indicators of vitamin K deficiency. Low vitamin K states lead to production of abnormal prothrombin (PIVKA-II). In vitamin K-replete neonates, PIVKA-II levels are below 0.2 AU/ml. Levels >1 AU/ml indicate subclinical deficiency and >5 AU/ml a clinically relevant deficiency. As PIVKA-II has a half-life of about 60 hours, deficiency can be confirmed by finding high levels even if the test is done a couple of days after vitamin K treatment.

Treatment
Where bleeding may be due to vitamin K deficiency, give 100 micrograms/kg IV (or subcutaneously).

Supply and administration
A concentrated colloidal (mixed micelle) preparation (Konakion MM® Paediatric) designed to make IV use safe, and containing 2 mg in 0.2 ml, has been the only licensed product available in Europe since 2006. Ampoules cost £1 each. This can be given IV, IM or by mouth. If the oral option is taken and the baby is breastfed, two further 2 mg doses are given at 4–7 days and then at 1 month of age.

An oral preparation of K$_1$ (Neokay®) provides an alternative option in Europe. This is classed as a food supplement, rather than a medicinal product requiring a licence. Oral supplementation

Continued on p. 542

must be continued for the first three months of life in exclusively breastfed infants, either with a once *weekly* 1 mg capsule (12 Neokay® 1 mg capsules cost £3.95) or alternatively with a *daily* lower dose using a convenient multi-dose dropper bottle product (Neokay® Drops 200 micrograms/ml). A 0.25 ml daily dose provides 50 micrograms of vitamin K$_1$, and a 25 ml bottle is available without prescription and provides enough for 3 months (cost ~ £3).

References   (See also the relevant Cochrane reviews)

Busfield A, Samuel R, McNinch A, *et al.* Vitamin K deficiency bleeding after NICE guidance and withdrawal of Konakion Neonatal: British Paediatric Surveillance Unit study, 2006–2008. *Arch Dis Child* 2013;**98**:41–7.

Clarke P. Vitamin K prophylaxis for preterm infants. *Early Hum Dev* 2010;**86**(suppl 1);17–20.

Clarke P, Mitchell S, Wynn R, *et al.* Vitamin K prophylaxis for preterm infants: a randomized, controlled trial of three regimens. *Pediatrics* 2006;**118**:e1657–66. [RCT]

Hansen KN, Minousis M, Ebbesen F. Weekly oral vitamin K prophylaxis in Denmark. *Acta Paediatr* 2003;**92**:802–5.

Strehle EM, Howey C, Jones R. Evaluation of the acceptability of a new oral vitamin K prophylaxis for breastfed infants. *Acta Paediatr* 2010;**99**:379–83.

Van Hasselt PM, de Koning TJ, Kvist N, *et al.* Prevention of vitamin K deficiency bleeding in breastfed infants: lessons from the Dutch and Danish biliary atresia registries. *Pediatrics* 2008;**121**:e857–63. (See also pp. 1048–9.)

von Kries R, Hachmeister A, Göbel U. Oral mixed micellar vitamin K for prevention of late vitamin K deficiency bleeding. *Arch Dis Child Fetal Neonatal Ed* 2003;**88**:F109–12. (See also pp. F80–3.)

Use
Children with malabsorption often develop subclinical fat-soluble vitamin deficiency, and babies on sustained intravenous (IV) nutrition are at similar risk. All breastfed babies benefit from being offered additional vitamins D and K.

Nutritional factors
The UK 'Welfare Food' scheme, as originally introduced in 1940, included liquid milk, national dried milk, concentrated orange juice and cod liver oil, and few disputed Winston Churchill's claim that there could be *no finer investment for any country than putting milk into babies*. Mothers also received special supplements. Because the scheme was generally credited with actually improving the health of children during the war years, the relevant regulations were never repealed, although infant vitamin drops (and maternal tablets) replaced cod liver oil and orange juice in 1975, and commercial formula milks replaced National Dried Milk in 1977. Uptake has, however, declined in recent years. By 2000, <5% of babies were getting a vitamin supplement in the first 6 months of life, and only 10% of babies 8–9 months old.

The scheme was eventually revised in 2006, and pregnant women and children under 4 in the United Kingdom in families on income support, income-based jobseeker's allowance or child tax credit and an income of below £16,190 a year are now legally entitled to vouchers that can be obtained from midwives and health visitors and exchanged for fresh fruit, vegetables and milk worth £3.10 a week. Babies under 1 year of age get two vouchers (£6.20) per week (for details, see www.healthystart.nhs.uk). Children 6 months to 4 years old in these families are also entitled to free 'Healthy Start' vitamin A and D drops, while pregnant women are entitled to free vitamin D tablets (as outlined in the vitamin D monograph).

Unfortunately, the programme has not offered clear guidance on the needs of babies <6 months old. While artificially fed babies seldom have problems because all formula milks are fortified, this does not cover the need of preterm babies on a total intake of <500 ml a day. Many breastfed babies across the world also suffer subclinical vitamin D deficiency – in part because their mothers are, themselves, unknowingly deficient – and serious vitamin D deficiency can cause hypocalcaemic seizures, rickets and even, occasionally, death from cardiomyopathy. It is, therefore, best to give all breastfed babies additional vitamin D *from birth*.

Oral vitamins
'Healthy Start' children's vitamin drops: One 5 drop dose each day provides 233 micrograms of vitamin A and 7.5 micrograms of D_3 and 20 mg of vitamin C.
Abidec® drops: The usual dose is 0.3 ml once a day by mouth throughout the first year of life. Very preterm babies and children with cystic fibrosis and other forms of malabsorption are often given 0.6 ml once a day, a dose that provides 400 micrograms (1333 units) of vitamin A, 10 micrograms (400 units) of D_2, 40 mg of C and some B_1, B_2, B_6 and nicotinamide (but not E or K).
Dalivit® drops: This is normally given in the same way, and in the same dose, as Abidec. The vitamin content is almost the same as for Abidec, but a 0.6 ml dose contains more vitamin A (1.5 mg/5000 units).

Intravenous vitamins
Water-soluble vitamins: Amino acid solutions used to provide parenteral nutrition (q.v.) will have usually had all the more important vitamins added (as Solivito N®) prior to issue by the pharmacy.
Fat-soluble vitamins: The manufacturers say that babies weighing under 2.5 kg should have 4 ml/kg of Vitlipid N® *infant* added to their Intralipid® (q.v.) each day so that they get the D_2 and K_1 they need, but this strategy reduces calorie intake (since Vitlipid is formulated in 10% Intralipid) – a quarter of this dose normally suffices. A dose of 10 ml/day is recommended for all children weighing more than 2.5 kg, but such supplements are only important when sustained IV feeding becomes necessary.

Supply
Oral preparations: 10 ml bottles of the UK Government's 'Healthy Start Children's Drops' (which should last 2 months) are available from chemists, maternity and child health clinics. They cost < £2 but are available free to certain families (see preceding text). 25 ml bottles of Abidec and Dalivit are also available without a prescription and cost £4 and £5, respectively. Both products contain sucrose.

Continued on p. 544

543

IV preparations: 10 ml ampoules of Vitlipid N *infant*, designed for adding to Intralipid, contain 690 micrograms (2300 units) of vitamin A, 10 micrograms (400 units) of D_2, 7 mg of E and 200 micrograms of K_1. They cost £2.30. Any amino acid solution designed for IV use will have normally had a vial of Solivito N (containing small amounts of B_1, B_2, B_6, B_{12}, nicotinamide, sodium pantothenate, C and folic acid) added prior to issue. Such vials also cost £2.30 each. Supplements of Solivito N can, alternatively, be added to Intralipid or to a plain infusion of IV glucose.

References

Arundel P, Ahmed SF, Allgrove J, *et al.* British Paediatric and Adolescent Bone Group's position statement on vitamin D deficiency. *Br Med J* 2012;**345**:e8182.

Committee on Medical Aspects of Food and Nutrition Policy Panel on Child and Maternal Nutrition. *Scientific review of the welfare food scheme*. Report on health and social subjects. Department of Health No. 51. London: The Stationery Office, 2002.

Dall'Agnola A, Beghini L. Post-discharge supplementation of vitamins and minerals for preterm neonates. *Early Hum Dev* 2009;**85**(10 suppl):S27–9.

Ferenchak AP, Sontag MK, Wagener JS, *et al.* Prospective long-term study of fat-soluble vitamin status in children with cystic fibrosis identified by newborn screen. *J Pediatr* 1999;**135**:601–10.

Leaf A. Vitamins for babies and young children. *Arch Dis Child* 2007;**92**:160–4.

Valentine CJ, Wagner CL. Nutritional management of the breastfeeding dyad. *Pediatr Clin North Am* 2013;**60**:261–74.

Use

Warfarin is used in the long-term control of thromboembolic disease. Heparin (q.v.) is better for short-term treatment. There is limited experience of its use in the neonatal period.

Pharmacology

Warfarin is an oral coumarin anticoagulant that works, after a latent period of 1–2 days, by depressing the vitamin K-dependent synthesis of a range of plasma coagulation factors, including prothrombin, by the liver. It was developed as a rat poison in 1948 before later coming into clinical use. Because the half-life is about 36 hours, blood levels only stabilise after a week of treatment. Babies need a higher weight-related dose than adults. Those with chronic atrial fibrillation, dilated cardiomyopathy or certain forms of reconstructive heart surgery benefit from prophylactic warfarin, and it has occasionally been used to manage intravascular or intracardiac thrombi. Treatment could initially precipitate purpura fulminans (a form of tissue infarction) in patients with thromboses due to homozygous protein C or S deficiency.

Warfarin crosses the placenta. Exposure between 6 and 10 weeks gestation is associated with an embryopathy, and exposure at a later gestation is associated with a fetopathy simulating chondrodysplasia punctata. The 'fetal warfarin syndrome' includes hypoplasia of nasal bridge, laryngomalacia, pectus carinatum, congenital heart defects, ventriculomegaly, agenesis of the corpus callosum, stippled epiphyses, telebrachydactyly and growth restriction. Use may not be entirely safe even in later pregnancy because of the risk of fetal and neonatal haemorrhage. Warfarin passes into breast milk in only minimal amounts at most and has not produced any reported clinical effects or anticoagulation effects in infants.

Problems are minimised by not letting the dose exceed 5 mg/day. The small risk of congenital optic atrophy, microcephaly and mental retardation (possibly caused by minor recurrent bleeding) may be of more concern than the more common, but less serious, defects associated with exposure in early pregnancy. Unfortunately, while heparin provides reasonable prophylaxis for most women at risk of thromboembolism during pregnancy, it does not provide adequate protection for mothers with pulmonary vascular disease, atrial fibrillation or an artificial heart valve. Here, the balance of risk is such that warfarin should be given until delivery threatens or the pregnancy reaches 37 weeks and then restarted 2 days after delivery. Always cover the intervening period with enoxaparin (q.v.) or heparin. Babies of mothers taking warfarin at the time of delivery need immediate prophylaxis with at least 100 micrograms/kg of intramuscular vitamin K (q.v.).

Drug interactions

Many drugs increase the anticoagulant effect of warfarin including amiodarone, some cephalosporins, cimetidine, erythromycin, fluconazole, glucagon, metronidazole, miconazole, phenytoin, ritonavir and the sulphonamide drugs; L-carnitine, ciprofloxacin and some penicillins can sometimes have a similar effect. So can high-dose paracetamol. Other drugs including barbiturates, carbamazepine, rifampicin, spironolactone and vitamin K decrease warfarin's anticoagulant effect.

Treatment

Initial anticoagulation: Always seek expert advice before starting anticoagulation. Give 200 micrograms/kg by mouth on day one. Give half this dose on the next 3 days (unless the international normalised ratio [INR] is still <1.5).

Maintenance: Laboratory monitoring is essential to determine long-term needs. Most children need 100–300 micrograms/kg once a day, but babies under 1 year old often need 150–400 micrograms/kg/day, especially if bottle fed (possibly because of the high vitamin K intake that this provides).

Dose monitoring

Testing is only needed every few weeks once treatment has stabilised, but because many drugs affect the half-life of warfarin, additional checks are needed each time other treatment is changed. An INR of between 2 and 3 seems to be the best level to aim for in most adults, but slightly higher values have often been recommended for adults after heart valve replacement. The therapeutic INR range in infants and children is extrapolated from adult studies as clinical trials to establish the optimum therapeutic INR range in children have not been performed.

Parents must be told about the need for monitoring, be given an anticoagulant book with a note of all treatment and have the book's importance explained.

Continued on p. 546

Antidote

Stop treatment if the INR exceeds 4.5. Give fresh frozen plasma (q.v.) if the INR exceeds 7. Also give 1 mg of intravenous vitamin K if there is overt bleeding.

Supply

Warfarin can be provided as a 1 mg/ml sugar-free suspension (cost £100 for 150 ml). 500 micrograms (white), 1 mg (brown) and 3 mg (blue) tablets are available costing 3–5p each.

References

Bradbury MJE, Taylor G, Short P, *et al*. A comparison of anticoagulant control in patients on long-term warfarin using home and hospital monitoring of the international normalised ratio. *Arch Dis Child* 2008;**93**:303–6.

Odén A, Fahlén M. Oral anticoagulation and risk of death: a medical record linkage study. *Br Med J* 2002;**325**:1073–5.

Orme ML, Lewis PJ, de Swiet M, *et al*. May mothers given warfarin breast-feed their infants? *Br Med J* 1977;**1**:1564–5.

Payne JH. Aspects of anticoagulation in children. *Br J Haematol* 2010;**150**:259–77.

Robinson MJ, Pash J, Grimwade J, *et al*. Fetal warfarin syndrome. *Med J Aust* 1978;**1**:157.

Streif W, Andrew M, Marzinotto V, *et al*. Analysis of warfarin therapy in pediatric patients: a prospective cohort study of 319 patients. *Blood* 1999;**94**:3007–14.

Vitali N, de Feo M, de Santo LS, *et al*. Dose dependent fetal complications of warfarin in pregnant women with mechanical heart valves. *J Am Coll Cardiol* 1999;**33**:1637–41. (See also pp. 1642–5.)

Use

Whooping cough (or 'pertussis'), due to *Bordetella pertussis*, remains a potentially devastating illness in children 3–6 months old, and because passive maternal immunity is relatively weak, it is very important to start immunisation 2 months after birth. Babies with lung problems are at particular risk. Toxoids, which also provide protection against diphtheria and tetanus, have long been employed in a range of combined vaccines. Diphtheria, tetanus and whooping cough are all notifiable illnesses in the United Kingdom (and in many other countries).

Clinical factors

More than 100,000 cases of whooping cough were notified every year in the United Kingdom prior to the introduction of a vaccine in 1956. Notifications fell 50-fold after that, but severe infection still occurs in young unimmunised children. Death is now rare, but severe non-fatal infection in early infancy is not that uncommon. Indeed, the problem seems to have become more common in the last 10 years (there was one notified case for every 2000 births in one recent US study). Serology and polymerase chain reaction (PCR) tests can often reveal evidence of infection even when direct culture fails.

Vaccines made from a suspension of dead bacteria were the products first produced, but acellular vaccines have since been developed. They were, at one time, of variable potency but are now preferred in Europe and North America because they trigger fewer hypotonic–hyporesponsive episodes and other adverse reactions. However, serious problems are uncommon with any product in babies <6 months old. No vaccine provides complete lasting immunity, and whooping cough is a more common cause of troublesome cough in school-age children than is generally recognised.

Diphtheria was an even more dreaded disease before the introduction of an effective vaccine in 1940. Only 1–2 cases are now recognised each year in the United Kingdom, but there is no doubt that a policy of universal immunisation remains appropriate, as with polio. Tetanus is an even more common and extremely dangerous condition that can strike at any time. Protection requires a personal immunisation programme with boosters (covered, where necessary, by tetanus immunoglobulin) following any injury if there is any risk that the wound has been contaminated with tetanus spores. Tetanus due to poor attention to umbilical cord care still kills 100,000 babies in the world each year. Skilled care, as outlined in the monograph on diazepam, will save a few lives, but the problem could be totally eliminated by ensuring that all pregnant women are fully immunised.

Indications

Immunisation should be started at 8 weeks after delivery when transplacental immunity starts to wane. Give diphtheria, pertussis and tetanus toxoids, and offer simultaneous protection from *Haemophilus influenzae* type b (Hib) and polio using a five-in-one vaccine where this is available (see the monograph on immunisation).

A personal or family history of allergy is not a contraindication to the use of any of these vaccines. Nor is a congenital abnormality (such as Down syndrome or a cardiac abnormality). While immunisation should not be delayed because of prematurity, it is *never* too late to immunise someone who was not immunised at the optimum time. Because efficacy wins over time, it may also be worth offering a booster dose to parents about to go home with a particularly vulnerable baby. Some would also give the influenza vaccine.

Contraindications

Anaphylaxis, stridor, bronchospasm, prolonged unresponsiveness, persistent unconsolable crying lasting ≥3 hours, an otherwise unexplained temperature of ≥40 °C within 48 hours or seizure within 72 hours of immunisation suggest a general reaction. Redness and induration involving much of the thigh or upper limb are evidence of a serious local reaction. Such events are very rare. If a problem of this nature is encountered, it may be better to complete immunisation using a product that does not protect against whooping cough (or use an acellular product if treatment was started using a whole-cell product). A *brief* period of hypotonia or unresponsiveness is not a reason to withhold further treatment.

The one important relative contraindication to immunisation is the existence of an **evolving** cerebral abnormality. Should any such child develop new signs or symptoms shortly after immunisation starts, diagnostic difficulties might occur and the possibility of litigation might arise. In this situation, the perceived risk of immunisation needs to be balanced against the risk

Continued on p. 548

of whooping cough (a very real risk if there are coexisting pulmonary problems), and a decision on timing reached with the parents that allows immunisation to proceed as soon as the child's neurological condition has stabilised.

Immunisation against whooping cough should also be delayed in any child who is acutely unwell, but the specific contraindications associated with the administration of live vaccines (such as the oral rotavirus vaccine) do not apply, and minor infections that are not associated with fever or systemic symptoms are not a reason to delay immunisation even if the child is on an antibiotic or other medicine.

A personal history of seizures (or, more doubtfully, a history of seizures in a brother, sister or parent) was for some years considered a 'relative' contraindication to pertussis immunisation in the United Kingdom (but not in the United States). Such children may be at increased risk of a febrile seizure if immunised when more than 6 months old, but there is no evidence that such an untoward effect carries with it any long-term risk. Primary care and community staff should *not*, therefore, advise against pertussis immunisation without first discussing the issues with a consultant paediatrician familiar with all the issues and circumstances.

Administration

General guidance: Give 0.5 ml deep into the anterolateral thigh muscle using a 25 mm, 23 gauge needle. Stretch the skin taught and insert the needle, up to its hilt, at right angles to the skin surface. Use deep *subcutaneous* injection for children with haemophilia. A combined five-in-one vaccine that also offers protection against diphtheria, Hib, polio and tetanus is the product now used in the United Kingdom. Simultaneous vaccination against type C meningococcal (MenC) infection (q.v.) is normally undertaken at the same time. Babies given BCG do not need to have the timing of these other procedures modified. The normal vaccine schedule is as laid out in the monograph on immunisation, where brief guidance on documentation and on parental consent is also given.

Prematurity: Immunisation should start 8 weeks after birth even in babies not yet discharged home from hospital. Some preterm babies only develop a limited response to the Hib vaccine and probably merit a dose of the monovalent Hib vaccine (q.v.) or another dose of the five-in-one vaccine at a year.

Systemic steroids: While inactivated vaccines (unlike live virus vaccines) are safe when given to patients on high-dose steroid treatment, such exposure can blunt the immune response. Even brief high-dose treatment shortly before, or after, birth can sometimes reduce the response to vaccine administration at 2 months. However, it would seem that this effect is probably only serious enough for a further 1-year booster dose to be merited in those countries where diphtheria remains endemic.

Abnormal reactions: Fever is uncommon when vaccination is undertaken in the first 6 months of life and usually responds to a single 30 mg/kg dose of paracetamol (q.v.). Such reactions are of no lasting consequence, even when associated with a febrile fit, but parents should be told to seek medical advice if fever persists more than 12 hours. Anaphylaxis (which is extremely rare) should be managed as laid out in the monograph on immunisation. Sudden limpness, with pallor and brief loss of consciousness, can occur in young children especially in the hours after they receive their first dose of vaccine. These babies recover without treatment, and such reactions, though alarming, should not result in further doses of the whooping cough vaccine being withheld. Parents can be told that the episode is not unlike a fainting attack, is unlikely to recur and is of no lasting significance.

Supply

A range of vaccines are now in use round the world, and a new five-in-one vaccine (Pediacel®), in 0.5 ml ampoules, containing purified diphtheria, pertussis and tetanus toxoids, Hib polysaccharide and inactivated polio virus (types 1–3), came into use in the United Kingdom in 2004.

A vaccine that only contains diphtheria and tetanus toxoids (but also contains thiomersal) can be used for the rare infant who suffers a severe reaction to the pertussis component of the five-in-one vaccine.

Vaccines must be stored in the dark at 2–8 °C and shaken well before use. Ampoules should be used as soon as possible once they have been opened. Frozen ampoules must be discarded.

Continued on p. 549

References

(See also the relevant Cochrane reviews and UK guidelines **DHUK**)

Cortese MM, Baughman AL, Zhang R, *et al.* Pertussis hospitalizations among infants in the United States, 1993 to 2004. *Pediatrics* 2008;**121**:484–92.

Dylag AM, Shah SI. Administration of tetanus, diphtheria, and acellular pertussis vaccine to parents of high-risk infants in neonatal intensive care unit. *Pediatrics* 2008;**122**:e550–5.

Frampton JE. DTaP(5)-IPV-Hib vaccine (Pediacel®). *Paediatr Drugs* 2011;**13**:401–15.

Grant CC, Roberts M, Scragg R, *et al.* Delayed immunisation and risk of pertussis in infants: unmatched case-control study. *Br Med J* 2003;**326**:852–3. (See also comment on p. 853.)

Harnden A, Grant C, Harrison T, *et al.* Whooping cough in school age children with persistent cough: prospective cohort study in primary care. *Br Med J* 2006;**333**:174–7. (See also pp. 159–60).

Hoppe JE. Neonatal pertussis. *Pediatr Infect Dis J* 2000;**19**:244–9.

Le Saux N, Barrowman NJ, Moore DL, *et al.* Decrease in hospital admissions for febrile seizures and reports of hypotonic-hyporesponsive episodes presenting to hospital emergency departments since switching to acellular pertussis vaccine in Canada: a report from IMPACT. *Pediatrics* 2003;**112**:e348–53.

Lim SS, Stein DB, Charrow A, *et al.* Tracking progress towards universal childhood immunisation and the impact of global initiatives: systematic analysis of three-dose diphtheria, tetanus and pertussis immunization coverage. *Lancet* 2008;**372**:2013–46. [SR]

Omeñaca F, Garcia-Sicilia J, García-Corbeira P, *et al.* Response of preterm newborns to immunization with a hexavalent diphtheria–tetanus–acellular pertussis-hepatitis B–inactivated polio and *Haemophilus influenzae* type B vaccine: first experiences and solutions to a serious and sensitive issue. *Pediatrics* 2005;**116**:1292–8.

Rank C, Quinn HE, McIntyre PB. Pertussis vaccine effectiveness after mass immunization of high school students in Australia. *Pediatr Infect Dis J* 2009 **28**:152–3

Robbins JB, Schneerson R, Trollfors B. Pertussis in developed countries. *Lancet* 2002;**360**:657–8.

Shiball MC, Peters TR, Zhu V, *et al.* Potential impact of acceleration of the pertussis vaccine primary series for infants. *Pediatrics* 2008;**122**:1021–6.

Surridge J, Segedin ER, Grant CC. Pertussis requiring intensive care. *Arch Dis Child* 2007;**92**:970–5.

Theilen U, Johnson ED, Robinson, PA. Rapidly fatal invasive pertussis in young infants – how can we change the outcome *Br Med J* 2008;**337**:a343.

Use
Zidovudine or azidothymidine (AZT) inhibits the replication of the human immunodeficiency virus (HIV), reducing feto-maternal transmission and slowing the progression of the resultant acquired immunodeficiency syndrome (AIDS).

HIV infection
AIDS is a notifiable disease caused by one of two closely related human retroviruses (HIV-1 and HIV-2) that target T helper (CD4) lymphocytes and macrophages, rendering the patient immunodeficient and vulnerable to a range of chronic infectious illnesses that are not normally lethal. Infection is generally by sexual contact or the use of contaminated needles. Babies born to infected mothers have a 20% chance of becoming infected if actions are not taken to prevent vertical transmission.

Pharmacology
Zidovudine is a thymidine analogue that acts intracellularly, after conversion to triphosphate, to halt retrovirus DNA synthesis by competitive inhibition of reverse transcriptase and incorporation into viral DNA. It inhibits the replication of the HIV virus, but does not eradicate it from the body. It is not, therefore, a cure for the resultant AIDS, but it can delay the progression of the disease, and the drug's arrival in 1987 did much to transform the management of this previously untreatable condition. The most common adverse effects are anaemia and leucopenia (which make regular haematological checks essential), but myalgia, malaise, nausea, headache and insomnia have also been reported. Zidovudine is well absorbed by mouth, but first-pass liver uptake reduces bioavailability. The half-life is 1 hour, but this increases to 3 hours in term babies and 6 hours in preterm babies in the first week of life. Concurrent treatment with ganciclovir (q.v.) increases the risk of toxicity, while fluconazole increases the half-life. Tissue levels exceed plasma levels (neonatal $V_D \sim 2 \, l/kg$). Zidovudine crosses the blood–brain barrier.

Zidovudine and its major metabolites rapidly cross the placenta (F:M ratio ~1). Maternal antiretroviral drug therapy during pregnancy and labour followed by neonatal prophylaxis with zidovudine significantly reduces the risk of vertical transmission. Additional antiretroviral drugs may be needed in some high-risk newborns. Mitochondrial disorders are described in children exposed to zidovudine *in utero*, and the incidence of this and the clinical significance are still unknown. Nonetheless, the benefits of treatment outweigh these risks. Zidovudine passes into breast milk and in situations where hygiene and cost combine to make bottle feeding hazardous reduces the risk of the infant becoming infected after birth. Where formula feeding is readily available, breastfeeding is contraindicated.

Overdose in babies may, as in adults, cause a transient metabolic (lactic) acidosis, derangement of liver transaminases and neutropenia.

Prevention of mother–infant transmission
Treatment of the infant with zidovudine **monotherapy** is recommended if maternal viral load is <50 HIV RNA copies/ml at 36 weeks' gestation or thereafter before delivery (or mother delivered by pre-labour caesarean section while on zidovudine monotherapy). Three-drug infant therapy is recommended for all other circumstances.

New information on optimum management becomes available so frequently that communication with a paediatric HIV/infectious diseases specialist is essential. The diagnosis and management must also be discussed with, and supervised by, someone with extensive experience of this condition.

Mothers: Start giving 300 mg twice a day by mouth, as soon after 28 weeks' gestation as possible. Give this dose once every 3 hours as soon as labour starts (or give 2 mg/kg over an hour by intravenous (IV) infusion and a further 1 mg/kg every hour) until delivery is over.
Term babies: Give 4 mg/kg by mouth twice a day for 4 weeks. Start this within 4 hours of birth.
Preterm babies: Give babies of 30–36 weeks' gestation 2 mg/kg twice a day for 2 weeks and then 2 mg/kg three times a day for 2 weeks. Give babies <30 weeks' gestation 2 mg/kg twice a day for 4 weeks. If oral treatment is not possible, give 1.5 mg/kg IV once every 12 hours (or every 6 hours if a term baby).

Continued on p. 551

Sustained prophylaxis when bottle feeding seems inadvisable

In situations where hygiene and cost combine to make bottle feeding hazardous, *exclusive* breast-feeding for 6 months reduces the risk of the baby becoming infected after birth when compared with infants fed with a combination of breast milk and formula or breast milk and solids. Risk can also be reduced by giving the baby nevirapine once a day by mouth until mixed feeding can be established.

Supply

Dilute the content of a 200 mg (20 ml) ampoule (costing £10.50) to 50 ml with 5% glucose to produce an IV solution containing 4 mg/ml, and give any IV dose slowly (over 30 minutes). 100 and 250 mg capsules cost £1.04. A sugar-free oral syrup (10 mg/ml) is also available (a 200 ml pack costs £21).

References

(See the Cochrane review and UK guideline on managing HIV in pregnancy **DHUK**)

Committee on Pediatric AIDS, American Academy of Pediatrics. HIV testing and prophylaxis to prevent mother-to-child transmission in the United States. *Pediatrics* 2008;**122**:1127–34.

Coovadia HM, Rollins NC, Bland RM, *et al.* Mother-to-child transmission of HIV-1 infection during exclusive breastfeeding in the first 6 months of life: an intervention cohort study. *Lancet* 2007;**369**:1107–16. (See also pp. 1065–6 and 2073–5.)

Gray GE, Saloojee H. Breast-feeding, antiretroviral prophylaxis, and HIV. [Editorial] *N Engl J Med* 2008;**359**:189–91.

Livshits Z, Lee S, Hoffman RS, *et al.* Zidovudine (AZT) overdose in a healthy newborn receiving postnatal prophylaxis. *Clin Toxicol (Phila)* 2011;**49**:747–9.

Palombi L, Pirillo MF, Andreotti M, *et al.* Antiretroviral prophylaxis for breastfeeding transmission in Malawi: drug concentrations, virological efficacy and safety. *Antivir Ther* 2012;**17**:1511–19.

Pilwoz EG, Humphrey JH, Tavengwa NV, *et al.* The impact of safer breastfeeding practices on postnatal HIV-1 transmission in Zimbabwe. *Am J Public Health* 2007;**97**:1249–54.

Taylor GP, Anderson J, Clayden P, *et al.* British HIV Association and Children's HIV Association position statement on infant feeding in the UK 2011. *HIV Med* 2011;**12**:389–93.

Taylor GP, Clayden P, Dhar J, *et al.* British HIV Association guidelines for the management of HIV infection in pregnant women 2012. *HIV Med* 2012;**13**(suppl 2):87–157.

Use

Oral zinc sulfate is used, both diagnostically and therapeutically, to supplement the dietary intake of babies with clinical signs of zinc deficiency. Routine supplementation in infancy seems beneficial in some community settings, but trials of *multiple* micronutrient use in pregnancy have not yet delivered consistent outcomes.

Nutritional factors

Zinc is an essential nutrient, being a constituent of many enzymes. It is also a constituent of the DNA and RNA polymerases involved in cell replication and growth. Overt deficiency causes perioral and perianal dermatitis, symmetrical blistering and pustular lesions on the hands and feet, alopecia, irritability, anorexia, diarrhoea and growth failure. The features are the same as for acrodermatitis enteropathica (a rare, and potentially lethal, condition caused by a recessively inherited abnormality of zinc absorption first recognised in 1973). Enterostomy loss and renal loss due to the use of a thiazide diuretic both make zinc deficiency more likely. While the serum zinc level is usually, but not always, below the normal range (7.6–15 µmol/l at 1–3 months), the diagnosis is clinched by the response to a direct trial of supplementation. Debilitating subclinical deficiency is still common in Central and Southern Africa and in Southeast Asia, particularly where soil zinc levels are low and cereal foods account for much of the daily diet.

An intake of at least 700 micrograms/kg of zinc per day may be necessary for healthy growth in some babies during early infancy, but all the artificial formula milks commercially available in the United Kingdom currently provide more than this minimum amount. Human milk initially contains more zinc than cow's milk (0.2 mg/100 ml), and because much of this is present as zinc citrate rather than bound to casein, absorption may be better, but the zinc content of human milk falls 10fold during the first 6 months of lactation. Reserves of zinc accumulate in the skeleton and liver before birth that help to tide the baby over the unexplained period of negative zinc balance normally seen in the first month of life. Nevertheless, a small number of cases of overt zinc deficiency have been seen in exclusively breastfed babies of less than 33 weeks' gestation 2–4 months after birth that responded to zinc supplementation. Deficiency was due to the milk containing little zinc, rather than a defect of absorption or utilisation. Overt symptoms of acrodermatitis take some time to appear.

Subclinical dietary deficiency is less easily recognised, but the consequences can be equally devastating. A small daily supplement (10 mg of elemental zinc a day) reduced the incidence of pneumonia and of malaria by 40% among babies in one at-risk population. Mortality fell 60% among supplemented light for dates children in another trial in India, while immediate supplementation in those developing diarrhoea halved the risk of death for any reason other than trauma in another trial in Bangladesh. Babies with severe pneumonia recovered quicker when given a 20 mg dose once a day from the day of admission. African children with HIV also fare better with supplementation. Recent trials show that maternal supplementation (30 mg daily from 12 to 16 weeks) can increase birthweight and reduce the risk of subsequent illness among children in areas where subclinical deficiency is common.

Treatment

As little as 1 mg/kg of elemental zinc a day will rapidly cure any symptoms due to simple dietary deficiency. A regular daily 5 mg/kg oral supplement may be necessary in babies with acrodermatitis enteropathica.

Supply

125 mg effervescent zinc sulfate monohydrate tablets contain 45 mg (0.7 mmol) of elemental zinc and cost 14p each. One tablet dissolved in 4.5 ml of water gives a 10 mg/ml solution for accurate low-dose administration. Accurate dosing is not important when correcting acute dietary deficiency; here, it suffices to give most babies and toddlers half of a 45 mg tablet once a day for 2 weeks. Orphan Europe markets 25 mg capsules designed for use in Wilson's disease costing 53p each; open and add the contents to water. The use of 1 ml/kg/day of Peditrace® will meet the elemental zinc requirement of most babies on parenteral nutrition. 10 ml vials for intravenous use cost £4.20.

Continued on p. 553

References

(See also the relevant Cochrane reviews)

Obladen M, Loui A, Kampmann E, *et al.* Zinc deficiency in rapidly growing preterm infants. *Acta Paediatr* 1998;**67**:685–91.

Osendarp SJM, van Raaij JMA, Darmstadt GL, *et al.* Zinc supplementation during pregnancy and effects on growth and morbidity in low birthweight infants: a randomised placebo controlled trial. *Lancet* 2001;**357**:1080–5. [RCT]

Santiago F, Matos J, Moreno A, *et al.* Acrodermatitis enteropathica: a novel SLC39A4 gene mutation found in a patient with an early-onset. *Pediatr Dermatol* 2011;**28**:735–6.

Shrimpton R, Gross R, Darnton-Hill I, *et al.* Zinc deficiency: what are the most appropriate interventions? *Br Med J* 2005;**330**:347–9.

Stephens J, Lubitz L. Symptomatic zinc deficiency in breast-fed term and premature infants. *J Paediatr Child Health* 1998;**34**:97–100.

SUMMIT Trial Study Group. Effect of maternal multiple micronutrient supplementation on fetal loss and infant death in Indonesia: a double-blind cluster-randomised trial. *Lancet* 2008;**371**:215–27. [RCT] (See also pp. 450–2 and 492–9.)

Tielsch JM, Khatry SK, Stoltzfus RJ, *et al.* Effect of daily zinc supplementation on child mortality in southern Nepal: a community-based, cluster randomised placebo-controlled trial. *Lancet* 2007;**370**:1230–9. [RCT] (See also pp. 1194–5.)

PART 3

Maternal medication and its effect on the baby

This section of NNF7 provides information on most drugs commonly used during pregnancy and lactation that do *not* have a full monograph to themselves in Part 2 of this book.

Introduction

No attempt has been made to review the extensive literature that now exists on the impact of medication during early pregnancy on the growing fetus. However, a summary of what is known about placental transfer, teratogenicity (the propensity to cause a malformation), fetal toxicity, and use in the lactating mother is included in the section labelled 'Pharmacology' for each drug listed in the main body of this book. Where the text merely says that treatment during lactation is safe, it can be taken that the dose ingested by the baby is almost certain to be less than 10% of that being taken by the mother on a weight-for-weight basis and that no reports have appeared suggesting that the baby could be clinically affected. The purpose of this section is to summarise what is known about the impact on the baby of those drugs that do **not** receive a mention in the main body of this compendium even though they are commonly given to mothers during pregnancy, labour or the puerperium.

Advice to parents has, in the past, often been too authoritarian. While there are a small number of drugs whose use makes breastfeeding extremely unwise, for most drugs, it is more a matter of balancing the advantages and the disadvantages and of being alert to the possibility that the baby might conceivably exhibit a side effect of maternal medication. It is not enough to just say that a particular drug will appear in the mother's milk – that is true of almost every drug ever studied. Mothers will also question why it should be thought unwise to expose their baby to low levels of a drug during lactation when no reservation was voiced over much greater exposure during pregnancy.

Much of the advice offered to UK clinicians in the *British National Formulary* (BNF) and in its paediatric counterpart, the *British National Formulary for Children* (BNFC), simply reflects, of necessity, the advice offered by the manufacturer in the Summary of Product Characteristics. Such statements are always cautious, seldom very informative and often merely designed to meet the minimum requirement laid down by the licensing authority. The same is true of drug use in pregnancy – the arbitrary classification of drugs into one of five 'risk' categories currently used by the Food and Drug Administration (FDA) in America is increasingly seen to be an over-simple approach to a complex issue.

The task of the clinician, in most of these situations, is to provide parents with the information they need to make up their own minds on such issues. To that end, each statement in this section is backed by at least one or two published references. In certain cases, readers may also wish to refer to the more comprehensive overviews provided in the books by Bennett (1996), by Briggs *et al.* (2011), by Schaefer (2007) and by Hale (2012) (see p. 555).

Neonatal Formulary 7: Drug Use in Pregnancy and the First Year of Life, Seventh Edition. Sean B Ainsworth.
© 2015 John Wiley & Sons, Ltd. Published 2015 by John Wiley & Sons, Ltd.
Companion website: www.neonatalformulary.com

The dose the breastfed baby is likely to receive has been calculated, wherever this is possible, as a percentage of the maternal dose (both calculated on a milligram-per-kilogram basis) using the approach first recommended in Bennett's authoritative text. Particular caution should be observed when this fraction exceeds 10% because drug elimination will initially be much slower in the baby than in the mother. The human milk/plasma (M/P) ratio is also given, where known. However, while this shows the extent to which the drug is concentrated in breast milk, it does not, on its own, reveal how much drug the baby will receive, because some drugs achieve a therapeutic effect even when the blood level is very low. Unfortunately, there are still some commonly used drugs for which no reliable information yet exists. Mothers who are breastfeeding and who are already taking one of these drugs are usually more than willing to help with the collection of some steady-state milk and plasma samples if approached, and the analysis of these would soon diminish many of the residual gaps in our knowledge as long as some care is taken to exclude the residual effect of earlier *in utero* exposure.

It is often said that risks can be minimised if the mother takes any necessary medication immediately after completing a breastfeed so that the baby avoids being exposed to peak maternal plasma levels. This is something of a counsel of perfection however for any mother feeding frequently and on demand and the sort of advice usually offered by someone with more theoretical knowledge than practical bedside experience. In many situations,

> 'the question is not whether a medicated mother should be allowed to nurse, but whether a nursing mother needs to be medicated'.

> *(Sumner Yaffe)*

Further reading

Many excellent reviews of the issues that need to be considered when prescribing medication to a mother who is pregnant or breastfeeding have been published in the last 10 years, and these should be turned to for information on drugs not included in this brief, carefully revised, overview. Much high-quality epidemiological work has also been done to define the risks of drug use during pregnancy. A lot of information on use during lactation is, by contrast, still anecdotal. Isolated reports recording apparent complications of use during lactation need to be interpreted with caution (especially where these relate to drugs that have been used by large numbers of other mothers uneventfully). Reports published before 1990, in particular, frequently lacked any documentary evidence that significant quantities of the offending drug were actually present in the baby's blood.

Reference texts on drug use during pregnancy and lactation

American Academy of Pediatrics. Committee on Drugs. The transfer of drugs and other chemicals into human milk. *Pediatrics* 2001;**108**:776–89.

Bennett PM, ed. *Drugs and human lactation*, 2nd edn. Amsterdam: Elsevier, 1996.

Briggs GG, Freeman RK, Yaffe SJ. *Drugs in pregnancy and lactation*, 9th edn. Philadelphia: Lippincott Williams & Wilkins, 2011.

Friedman JM, Polifka JE. *Teratogenic effects of drugs. A resource for clinicians*, 2nd edn. Baltimore: Johns Hopkins University Press, 2000.

Hale TW. *Medications and mother's milk 2012: A manual of lactational pharmacology*, 15th edn. Amarillo: Pharmasoft Publishing, 2012.

Jones W. *Breast feeding and medication*. Abingdon: Routledge, 2013.

Koren G, ed. *Maternal-fetal toxicology. A clinician's guide*, 3rd edn. New York: Marcel Dekker, 2001.

Lee A, Inch S, Finnigan D. *Therapeutics in pregnancy and lactation*. Abingdon: Radcliffe Medical Press, 2000.

Little BB. *Drugs and pregnancy: a handbook*. London: Hodder Education, 2006.

Rubin R, Ramsay M, eds. *Prescribing in pregnancy*, 4th edn. Oxford: Blackwell Publishing, 2008.

Schaefer C, Peters P, Miller RK, eds. *Drugs during pregnancy and lactation. Treatment options and risk assessment*, 2nd edn. Amsterdam: Elsevier, 2007.

Weiner CP, Buhimschi C. *Drugs for pregnant and lactating women*, 2nd edn. Philadelphia: Saunders, Elsevier, 2009.

Yankowitz J, Niebyl JR. *Drug therapy in pregnancy*, 3rd edn. Philadelphia: Lippincott Williams & Wilkins, 2001.

The publishers of the book by Briggs update this with a quarterly bulletin, and the book by Hale is reissued every 1–2 years. Up-to-date information is available from the Organisation of Teratogen Information Specialists (OTIS) in North America (www.mothertobaby.org) and the European Network of Teratology Information Services (ENTIS) in Europe and Latin America (www.entis-org.com). The UK Breastfeeding Network (www.breastfeedingnetwork.org.uk) has a help line that mothers can ring if

Neonatal Formulary 7: Drug Use in Pregnancy and the First Year of Life, Seventh Edition. Sean B Ainsworth.

© 2015 John Wiley & Sons, Ltd. Published 2015 by John Wiley & Sons, Ltd.

Companion website: www.neonatalformulary.com

they have worries on such issues (0300 100 0212). Leave a phone number where you can be contacted in the evening.

Further information

The information given in the BNF and in the version giving advice on drug use in children (BNFC) is generally authoritative, but this is *not* always true of the advice it offers on drug use during pregnancy and lactation. Further useful information on safe drug use in ***pregnancy*** can, however, be obtained in the United Kingdom through local hospital pharmacies, from the Specialist Advisory and Information Service provided by the Northern and Yorkshire Regional Drug & Therapeutics Centre (RDTC) at the Wolfson Unit, 24 Claremont Place, Newcastle upon Tyne, NE2 4HH (0191 213 7855). This unit also maintains the United Kingdom's main teratology database (see www.uktis.org).

Further detailed information on drugs in ***breast milk*** can be obtained, similarly, from the UK Drugs in Lactation Advisory Service (UKDILAS) by contacting the Trent Drug Information Centre, Leicester Royal Infirmary, Leicester LE1 5WW (0116 258 6491), or the West Midlands Drug Information Service, Good Hope General Hospital, Sutton Coldfield, B75 7RR (0121 311 1974).

Maternal medication and the baby

Acarbose

A single report in which six pregnant women were treated with acarbose saw normalisation of glucose levels and uncomplicated pregnancies (although abdominal cramping was a reported side effect). There are no published reports of use during breastfeeding. It is not known whether acarbose enters breast milk.

Zárate *et al.*: *Ginecol Obstet Mex* 2000;**68**:42.

Acebutolol

While there is no evidence of teratogenicity, this drug (and other β-blockers) can cause neonatal bradycardia, mild hypotension and transient hypoglycaemia when prescribed to a mother immediately before delivery. Renal impairment can occur after chronic *in utero* exposure; infants had a significantly smaller early diuresis and impaired sodium and calcium homeostasis. No complications have been reported following use during lactation, but the drug and its metabolite, diacetolol, accumulate in breast milk. Labetalol appears to be a better drug to use during pregnancy and lactation, especially if the dose exceeds 400 mg a day.

Boutroy *et al.*: *Eur J Clin Pharmacol* 1986;**30**:737.
Yassen *et al.*: *Arch Fr Pediatr* 1992;**49**:351.

Acetazolamide

In some rodents, acetazolamide is teratogenic, but there is no evidence that this is so in humans. Reports of use during pregnancy for glaucoma, intracranial hypertension and altitude sickness have not shown any major adverse effects on either the fetus or the infant. Acetazolamide is not concentrated in the milk, and the neonate receives less than 0.5% of the maternal dose; therefore, it is generally considered compatible with breastfeeding.

Falardeau *et al.*: *J Neuro Ophthalmol* 2013;**33**:9.
Luks and Swenson: *Chest* 2008;**133**:744.
Razeghinejad and Nowroozzadeh: *Clin Exp Optom* 2010;**93**:458.
Söderman *et al.*: *Br J Clin Pharmacol* 1984;**17**:599.

Acetylcysteine – See Part 2, p. 57

Aciclovir – See Part 2, pp. 58–59

Acitretin

Acitretin is a metabolite of etretinate which is a potent teratogen in both animals and humans. The effects of the drug persist for some time after treatment, and pregnancy is not advised within 3 years of cessation of treatment. Multiple organ systems are affected, including NTDs, facial and skull abnormalities, limb and digit malformations and skeletal defects. Acitretin passes into breast milk, and although the amounts the nursing infant would receive are small, the toxic effects are such that breastfeeding should be avoided.

Katz *et al.*: *J Am Acad Dermatol* 1999;**41**:S7.
Maradit and Geiger: *Dermatology* 1999;**198**:3.

Adapalene

Adapalene is a topical retinoid used in the treatment of acne, and while systemic absorption across human skin is low, there are no reports of use during pregnancy. Oral retinoids are contraindicated in pregnancy due to their teratogenic effects, and in keeping with this, women of childbearing age using adapalene should be fully informed of the risks and the importance of effective contraception. Avoidance of the topical retinoids is advised during lactation. Systemic exposure and adverse reactions in nursing infants cannot be ruled out. Excretion into breast milk has not been studied.

Akhavan and Bershad: *Am J Clin Dermatol* 2003;**4**:473.
Anonymous: *Prescrire Int* 2005;**14**:100.
Autret *et al.*: *Lancet* 1997;**350**:339.

Adenosine – See Part 2, pp. 60–61

Adrenaline – See Part 2, pp. 62–63

Alendronic acid

Alendronic acid and bisphosphonates are usually used to treat post-menopausal osteoporosis; however, they can be used to treat severe osteoporosis that occurs in younger women secondary to glucocorticoid use. Adult plasma levels are usually below the level of detection. There was no evidence of teratogenicity in two case series. It is not known

Neonatal Formulary 7: Drug Use in Pregnancy and the First Year of Life, Seventh Edition. Sean B Ainsworth.
© 2015 John Wiley & Sons, Ltd. Published 2015 by John Wiley & Sons, Ltd.
Companion website: www.neonatalformulary.com

whether it enters breast milk; however, any risk to the neonate is probably minimal considering the low maternal plasma levels.

Bhalla: *Best Pract Res Clin Rheumatol* 2010;**24**:313.
Djokanovic *et al*.: *J Obstet Gynaecol Can* 2008;**30**:1146.
Ornoy *et al*.: *Reprod Toxicol* 2006;**22**:578.

Alfentanil

Alfentanil crosses the placenta when given intravenously. Neither human embryotoxicity nor teratogenicity is reported, though first trimester data are limited. The drug's lipophilic and hydrophilic characteristics enhance placental transfer. Neonatal depression – reversed by naloxone – is reported when alfentanil is given shortly before delivery. Remifentanil may be a better option. Alfentanil is excreted into human breast milk, and the BNF advises to 'withhold breast-feeding for 24 hours'; this is probably unnecessary as the amount in breast milk is too small to have any significant effect on the infant.

Evron and Ezri: *Curr Opin Anaesthesiol* 2007;**20**:181.
Mattingly *et al*.: *Paediatr Drugs* 2003;**5**:615.

Alimemazine tartrate (trimeprazine, former BAN)

Alimemazine has been widely used during pregnancy for many years without any reports of teratogenicity. Only small amounts are found in breast milk, and use is probably compatible with breastfeeding (although the manufacturer advises to avoid its use). Any exposed infant should be observed for signs of drowsiness.

Nelson and Forfar: *Br Med J* 1971;**1**:523.
O'Brien: *Am J Hosp Pharm* 1974;**31**:844.

Allopurinol

Experience with allopurinol in pregnancy is scarce. It is mainly used to treat hyperuricaemia due to gout or tumour lysis syndrome, both rare during pregnancy. A number of malformations (microphthalmia, cleft lip and palate and microtia) have been reported after first trimester exposure. Small amounts of allopurinol and its metabolite, oxypurinol, are excreted into breast milk, but use is considered compatible with breastfeeding.

Carey *et al*.: *Birth Defects Res A Clin Mol Teratol* 2009;**85**:63.
Hoeltzenbein *et al*.: *PLoS One* 2013;**8**:e66637.
Kamilli and Gresser: *Clin Investig* 1993;**71**:161.

Almotriptan

There is no published experience with almotriptan during pregnancy. It is unknown whether almotriptan crosses the placenta. Rodent teratogenicity studies are reassuring. It is not known whether almotriptan enters breast milk. Sumatriptan is an alternative for which more safety data is available.

Soldin *et al*.: *Ther Drug Monit* 2008;**30**:5.

Alprazolam

Alprazolam is rarely indicated during pregnancy and there are few published reports of its use during pregnancy. There is no evidence that alprazolam is teratogenic. Neonatal withdrawal symptoms are not uncommon with sustained benzodiazepine use in pregnancy. Alprazolam enters breast milk by passive diffusion with the infant receiving approximately 3% of the weight-adjusted maternal dose. Although the risk is likely small, alprazolam is best avoided during lactation.

Gidai *et al*.: *Toxicol Ind Health* 2008;**24**:53.
Oo *et al*.: *Br J Clin Pharmacol* 1995;**40**:231.

Alteplase

Reports of alteplase use during pregnancy to treat PE, MI and peripheral valvular thrombosis do not show any increased risk of haemorrhage, abruption or preterm labour. It is not known whether it crosses the placenta (due to its high molecular weight, it is unlikely to do so). There is no information regarding its use during breastfeeding.

De Keyser *et al*.: *Stroke* 2007;**38**:2612.
Ozkan *et al*.: *Circulation* 2013;**128**:532.

Amantadine

It is not known if amantadine crosses the placenta, but there are concerns with several reports of cardiovascular abnormalities in exposed fetuses. Amantadine passes into breast milk in trace amounts; nonetheless, mothers should probably be advised against breastfeeding.

Greer *et al*.: *Obstet Gynecol* 2010;**115**:711.
Smith and Evatt: *Neurol Clin* 2004;**22**:783.

Amfetamine

'Amfetamines' are compounds which have structural similarity to ephedrine and include amfetamine, dexamfetamine, metamfetamine and multiple amfetamine analogues. Most are schedule 2 drugs and are rarely indicated in reproductive-age women and should be avoided. Dexamfetamine and its prodrug, lisdexamfetamine, are used to treat ADHD in children and adults (although the latter use is off-licence). Maternal amfetamine abuse has not been conclusively identified with increased teratogenicity, although increased risks of preterm delivery, LBW and SGA have been suggested. Neonatal symptoms are usually mild, even with sustained use, when this is the only drug taken. Antenatal amfetamine exposure is associated with aggressive behaviour and delayed development in children. Amfetamines are concentrated in human breast milk and generally considered incompatible with breastfeeding. If recreational use

does occur during lactation, data suggest that breastfeeding should be withheld for 48 hours.
Bartu *et al.*: *Br J Clin Pharmacol* 2009;**67**:455.
Oei *et al.*: *J Perinatol* 2012;**32**:737.
Oei *et al.*: *Arch Dis Child Fetal Neonatal Ed* 2010;**95**:F36.

Amikacin
Amikacin crosses the placenta and, like other aminoglycosides, can cause fetal nephrotoxicity. There is no evidence of teratogenicity. Use during pregnancy should be avoided unless essential (if given, serum concentration monitoring is mandatory). While amikacin passes into breast milk, low concentrations and poor oral absorption suggest little, if any, risk to the neonate.
Pacifici: *Int J Clin Pharmacol Ther* 2006;**44**:57.
Duff: *Obstet Gynecol Clin North Am* 1992;**19**:511.

Amiloride
Published experience of amiloride during pregnancy is limited to the occasional case report (e.g. in Gitelman's, Conn's or Bartter's syndromes). Amiloride crosses the placenta in modest amounts. Rodent teratogenicity studies are reassuring. Amiloride is concentrated in breast milk and should probably be avoided during breastfeeding.
Deruelle *et al.*: *Eur J Obstet Gynecol Reprod Biol* 2004;**115**:106.

Aminophylline
Aminophylline crosses the placenta rapidly (F/M ratio ~1). While there is no substantive evidence of human teratogenicity and embryotoxicity at standard doses, malformations are reported in rats and rabbits at very high doses. Aminophylline is excreted into breast milk and may cause irritability or other signs of toxicity in breastfed neonates. Nonetheless, it is considered compatible with breastfeeding with the infant receiving approximately 5.8% of the weight-adjusted maternal dose.
Schatz: *Drug Saf* 1997;**16**:342.
BTS & SIGN: British Guideline on the Management of Asthma.

Amiodarone – See Part 2, pp. 72–73

Amitriptyline
Depression is common during and after pregnancy, but despite the fact that tricyclic agents are frequently used, there are no well-controlled studies of amitriptyline during pregnancy. Amitriptyline crosses the placenta and there are case reports of CNS and limb abnormalities and developmental delay. Amitriptyline should be used only if the benefit justifies the potential perinatal risk and utilising the lowest possible dose monotherapy.

Giving in divided doses minimises the peaks, which may reduce the risks. Amitriptyline is excreted into breast milk but the neonatal concentrations are extremely low.
Wen and Walker: *J Obstet Gynaecol Can* 2004;**26**:887.
Erickson *et al.*: *Am J Psychiatry* 1979;**136**:1483.
Yonkers *et al.*: *Gen Hosp Psychiatry* 2009;**31**:403.

Amlodipine
It is not known whether amlodipine crosses the placenta. Rodent teratogenicity studies are reassuring. It is not known whether amlodipine passes into breast milk, but breastfeeding appears to be safe. There are, however, alternative medications for which there is more experience during pregnancy and lactation.
Ahn *et al.*: *Hypertens Pregnancy* 2007;**26**:179.

Amoxicillin – See Part 2, pp. 76–77

Amphotericin B – See Part 2, pp. 78–79

Ampicillin – See Part 2, pp. 80–81

Anagrelide
Anagrelide may be used to treat essential thrombocytosis where an increased risk of first trimester loss is not reduced by aspirin. Rodent teratogenicity studies are reassuring. There is no published experience during lactation, and it is not known whether anagrelide enters breast milk.
Petrides: *Semin Thromb Hemost* 2006;**32**:399.
Sobas *et al.*: *Acta Haematol* 2009;**122**:221.

Aqueous iodine solution (potassium iodide)
Aqueous iodine oral solution (and potassium iodide in particular) is an adjunct for women with hyperthyroidism associated with Graves' disease. It is also effective during pregnancy for the treatment of mild–moderate iodine deficiency. It crosses the placenta and, in excess, causes fetal goitre and hypothyroidism. Iodide salts are secreted into breast milk and can also cause hypothyroidism in the breastfed infant. Iodine solution should be used only with extreme caution, if at all, during lactation.
Ayromlooi: *Obstet Gynecol* 1972;**39**:818.
Postellon and Aronow: *JAMA* 1982;**247**:463.

Ascorbic acid – See Part 2, p. 537

Aspirin – See Part 2, pp. 88–89

Atenolol
Atenolol crosses the placenta but there is no substantive evidence of teratogenicity. As a group, β-blockers are associated with IUGR, though controversy continues as to whether

this is drug or disease related. The evidence of this association is strongest for atenolol and may be due to β-blockade, causing a decrease in cardiac output in the mother. For this reason, atenolol is best avoided especially as there are other alternatives with a greater margin of safety. Breastfeeding should also be avoided. Atenolol is concentrated in breast milk and significant bradycardia has been reported in breastfed infants.

Orbach *et al.*: *Am J Obstet Gynecol* 2013;**208**:301.e1.
Schimmel *et al.*: *J Pediatr* 1989;**114**:476.

Atomoxetine

Animal studies have shown adverse fetal effects after high doses of atomoxetine (decreased fetal survival and cardiovascular abnormalities are reported). In adult trials, three pregnancies were documented; no details were published but two pregnancies resulted in healthy newborns and one was lost to follow-up. There is no published data on the effects of atomoxetine during lactation, nor is it known whether it passes into breast milk

Alessi and Spalding: *J Am Acad Child Adolesc Psychiatry* 2003;**42**:883.

Atorvastatin

It is not known whether atorvastatin crosses the placenta. Statins, as a group, appear to be teratogenic with reports of limb deformities and spina bifida. Others suggest the underlying pathologies leading to statin use might also play a role. There is little doubt however that further study is required. There are no adequate reports or well-controlled studies during lactation, and it is unclear whether atorvastatin enters human breast milk. High protein binding and poor oral absorption suggest that a breastfed infant receives negligible amounts. Because cholesterol and products synthesised from cholesterol are important in fetal and infant development, statins are best avoided during pregnancy. Furthermore, the risks of a temporary cessation in statin therapy during pregnancy and lactation appear to be low.

Edison and Muenke: *Am J Med Genet A* 2004;**131**:287.
Lecarpentier *et al.*: *Drugs* 2012;**72**:773.

Atracurium – See Part 2, pp. 92–93

Atropine – See Part 2, pp. 94–95

Azathioprine

Limited human experience of azathioprine use during pregnancy is largely reassuring – most (including transplant patients) have successful outcomes. Use during the third trimester has been linked with marrow suppression in the neonate, but this can be reduced by modifying the maternal dose. Azathioprine is excreted

into breast milk. Levels of 6-mercaptopurine (a metabolite) suggest that the breastfed neonate ingests less than 0.5% of the maternal dose, and there are no well-documented instances of neonatal effect.

Hou: *Adv Ren Replace Ther* 2003;**10**:40.
Temprano *et al.*: *Semin Arthritis Rheum* 2005;**35**:112.

Azithromycin – See Part 2, pp. 96–97

Aztreonam

Aztreonam crosses the placenta reaching therapeutic concentrations. No fetal effects have been reported and rodent teratogenicity studies are reassuring. Aztreonam is present in breast milk at trace levels only.

Clark: *Obstet Gynecol Clin North Am* 1992;**19**:519.
Fleiss *et al.*: Aztreonam in human serum and breast milk. *Br J Clin Pharmacol* 1985;**19**:509.

Baclofen

Published reports of use during pregnancy are limited to case reports of intrathecal use, and plasma concentrations after administration by this route are less than 1% of those after oral administration. Neonatal seizures were noted in one case where the mother was taking 80 mg/kg/day orally (seizures are reported after withdrawal in adults). Only approximately 0.1% of the maternal dose is excreted into breast milk; thus, the nursing infant is unlikely to be affected.

Eriksson and Swahn: *Scand J Clin Lab Invest* 1981;**41**:185.
Moran *et al.*: *Pediatrics* 2004;**114**:e267.
Ratnayaka *et al.*: *Br Med J* 2001;**323**:85.

Balsalazide

Balsalazide is a prodrug of mesalazine (5-aminosalicylic acid [5-ASA]). There are few data for balsalazide use during pregnancy; but there is more experience with mesalazine. It is not known whether balsalazide crosses the placenta; trace amounts of 5-ASA are found in fetal tissues after mesalazine use. Rodent teratogenicity studies are reassuring. In contrast, poorly controlled inflammatory bowel disease is likely to lead to reduced fecundity, prematurity and low birthweight. While it is not known if balsalazide enters breast milk, trace amounts of 5-ASA may be found but are considered compatible with breastfeeding.

Rahimi *et al.*: *Reprod Toxicol* 2008;**25**:271.

Beclometasone – See Part 2, p. 114

Bendroflumethiazide (bendrofluazide, former BAN)

Thiazide diuretics are diabetogenic in some women, and there are several reports of severe electrolyte imbalance in both mothers and newborns (including a case of fetal bradycardia due to hypokalaemia). Congestive cardiac failure is probably the only indication for this drug during pregnancy, and even then, there are alternatives with a better safety profile. Thiazide diuretics are excreted in low concentrations into breast milk but are generally considered safe during breastfeeding. Bendroflumethiazide has been used to suppress lactation.

Healy: *Lancet* 1961;**277**:1353.
Andersen: *Acta Paediatr Scand* 1970;**59**:659.

Bleomycin

It is not known whether bleomycin crosses the placenta. It is teratogenic in rodents, causing skeletal malformations, hydroureter and vascular abnormalities. Isolated clinical reports of bleomycin (usually in combination with other anti-neoplastic drugs) during the second and third trimesters are generally favourable. Neonatal leucopenia has been reported, but long-term follow-up of children exposed *in utero* has not revealed abnormalities. It is not known if bleomycin is present in breast milk. Bleomycin should only be used during pregnancy and lactation if the benefit justifies the potential risk.

Karimi Zarchi *et al.*: *Arch Gynecol Obstet* 2008;**277**:75.
Williams *et al.*: *J Clin Oncol* 1994;**12**:701.

Bretylium

It is not known whether bretylium crosses the placenta. Hypotension is reported in 50% of patients started on bretylium, and there is the potential to cause placental hypoperfusion. The only case reported had a good outcome after treatment of prolonged QT syndrome during pregnancy and breastfeeding. Experience during breastfeeding is lacking and it is not known if bretylium enters breast milk.

Gutgesell *et al.*: *Am J Perinatol* 1990;**7**:144.

Bumetanide

It is unclear whether bumetanide crosses the placenta. No teratogenic effects were seen in rodent studies. It is also not known if bumetanide enters breast milk.

McClain and Dammers: *J Clin Pharmacol* 1981;**21**:543.

Bupivacaine

Bupivacaine is used widely for epidural or spinal anaesthesia during labour. Bupivacaine crosses the placenta in small amounts that increase when fetal acidosis occurs. Bupivacaine and its major metabolite are found in breast milk at clinically irrelevant levels after epidural administration. Its use is unlikely to pose a clinically significant risk to the breastfeeding neonate.

de Barros Duarte *et al.*: *Eur J Clin Pharmacol* 2007;**63**:523.
Ortega *et al.*: *Acta Anaesthesiol Scand* 1999;**43**:394.

Buprenorphine

Buprenorphine has no apparent teratogenic effects. It has been used to treat withdrawal from opioid abuse. Neonatal outcomes have largely been reassuring when use is closely monitored. Most exposed infants show some signs of opioid withdrawal, with signs appearing 12–48 hours after birth, peaking at 72–96 hours and lasting for 120–168 hours after buprenorphine although other factors impact on this. Buprenorphine is excreted into breast milk in low concentrations only, and interruption of breastfeeding does not cause worsening of NAS symptoms.

Ilett *et al.*: *Breast feed Med* 2012;**7**:269.
Jones *et al.*: *Drugs* 2012;**72**:747.

Bupropion

Bupropion has been used as an antidepressant although it is mainly used in smoking cessation. The manufacturer (and the BNF) advises avoiding use during pregnancy and lactation. Animal and human data suggest low teratogenicity although some do report increased cardiovascular abnormalities. This needs to be weighed against the effects of maternal smoking, which incidentally can also increase CVS malformations. Bupropion is excreted into breast milk. In general, no effects have been seen in exposed breastfed infants; however, one case report documents the onset of seizures in a 6-month-old breastfed infant shortly after the start of maternal bupropion treatment (seizures are known to occur in adults taking the drug).

Alwan *et al.*: *Am J Obstet Gynecol* 2010;**203**:52.e1.
Chaudron and Schoenecker: *J Clin Psychiatry* 2004;**65**:881.
Thyagarajan *et al.*: *Pharmacoepidemiol Drug Saf* 2012;**21**:1240.

Buspirone

Experience of this sedative during pregnancy is limited. It is not known whether buspirone crosses the placenta. Rodent teratogenicity studies are reassuring. It is not known whether buspirone enters breast milk; a single report of use (with other medications) during lactation failed to detect any in the breast milk. Buspirone is found in rodent breast milk. The general advice is that buspirone should be avoided during pregnancy and lactation.

Brent and Wisner: *Clin Pediatr (Phila)* 1998;**37**:41.

Busulfan

The manufacturers (and the BNF) advise that busulfan, an alkylating anti-neoplastic agent, should be avoided during pregnancy, especially during the first trimester. They also advise effective contraception during and for 6 months after treatment. There are no data on busulfan during breastfeeding, and it is not known if the drug enters breast milk (although this is likely given that CNS penetration does occur). Given the potential effects on the infant at a crucial stage, use is best avoided during pregnancy and lactation.

Dugdale and Fort: *JAMA* 1967;**199**:131.

Wiebe and Sipila: *Crit Rev Oncol Hematol* 1994;**16**:75.

Calcipotriol

Only small amounts (5–6%) of this topical psoriatic treatment are absorbed systemically. Rodent teratogenicity has not been reported except when administered at levels >7.5 times than would be expected in humans. Although the manufacturer advises avoiding use during pregnancy, two reviews consider it to be safe. Not only are small amounts absorbed systemically, but transfer of vitamin D into milk is also low and calcipotriol levels in breast milk would be expected to be negligible.

Lebwohl: *J Am Acad Dermatol* 2005;**53**(suppl 1):S59.

Tauscher *et al.*: *J Cutan Med Surg* 2002;**6**:561.

Candesartan

Candesartan is an angiotensin II receptor antagonist with many properties similar to the ACE inhibitors. Transfer across the placenta has not been studied. Related drugs in this class cross the placenta and fetal renal effects (anuria and oligohydramnios) have been reported. Angiotensin II receptor antagonists are considered both teratogenic and fetotoxic. They may cause cranial hypoplasia, renal failure (sometimes irreversible), oligohydramnios, anuria, death, prematurity, IUGR and PDA. There are no reports of use during lactation and it is not known if it enters breast milk. Some ACE inhibitors (e.g. captopril and enalapril) are safe during lactation and may offer a suitable alternative.

Oppermann *et al.*: *Br J Clin Pharmacol* 2013;**75**:822.

Schaefer: *Birth Defects Res A Clin Mol Teratol* 2003;**67**:591.

Captopril

Captopril, like ACE inhibitors, is contraindicated throughout pregnancy unless there is no alternative. Risks are greatest during the second and third trimesters through effects on the fetal kidney, causing renal failure and oligohydramnios, but teratogenesis during the first trimester is also reported. Captopril is embryocidal and causes stillbirths in a variety of animals (sheep, rabbits, rats). Captopril is excreted into breast milk at very low concentrations and is compatible with breastfeeding.

Burrows and Burrows: *Aust N Z J Obstet Gynaecol* 1998;**38**:306.

Hanssens *et al.*: *Obstet Gynecol* 1991;**78**:128.

Kirsten *et al.*: *Clin Pharmacokinet* 1998;**35**:9.

Carbamazepine – See Part 2, pp. 126–127

Carbimazole

There is no evidence of teratogenicity, but there is a small risk of neonatal goitre or hypothyroidism especially when a dose in pregnancy exceeds 30 mg/day. Most authorities consider propylthiouracil preferable to carbimazole, especially during lactation, because of the risk of neonatal hypothyroidism.

Cassina *et al.*: *Birth Defects Res A Clin Mol Teratol* 2012;**94**:612.

Karras *et al.*: *Pediatr Endocrinol Rev* 2010;**8**:25.

Carboprost

Carboprost is an analogue of 15-methylprostaglandin PGF2α. It is used for treatment of postpartum haemorrhage secondary to uterine atony after failure to respond to ergometrine and oxytocin. It is unlikely therefore to be used before delivery of the baby. It is not known if carboprost enters breast milk, but it is reassuring that prostaglandins have short half-lives and that even large parenteral doses give very low plasma concentrations.

Bygdeman: *Best Pract Res Clin Obstet Gynaecol* 2003;**17**:707.

Dildy: *Clin Obstet Gynecol* 2002;**45**:330.

Carvedilol

It is not known whether carvedilol crosses the human placenta (it does in rodents where it causes fetotoxicity and IUGR in doses exceeding those likely to be used in humans). As a group, β-blockers are associated with IUGR, though debate continues as to whether this is drug or disease related. Carvedilol is best avoided especially as there are alternatives (e.g. labetalol) with a greater margin of safety. Experience with carvedilol in lactation is limited. It is not known whether carvedilol enters breast milk.

Shannon *et al.*: *J Hum Lact* 2000;**16**:240.

Cefaclor

It is not known whether cefaclor crosses the placenta (most cephalosporins do). Rodent teratogenicity studies are reassuring. Although there is no data for cefaclor, most cephalosporins pass into breast milk, and cefaclor is considered compatible with breastfeeding.

Chin *et al.*: *Curr Med Res Opin* 1981;**7**:168.

Puapermpoonsiri *et al.*: *Antimicrob Agents Chemother* 1997;**41**:2297.

Cefadroxil

There are few data of cefadroxil use during pregnancy and lactation. It is not known whether cefadroxil crosses the placenta. Rodent teratogenicity studies are reassuring. Like most cephalosporins, cefadroxil is compatible with use during pregnancy and lactation.

Shetty *et al.*: *J Hosp Infect* 1999;**41**:229.

Cefalexin

Cefalexin crosses the placenta in a carrier-mediated fashion. As a result, fetal concentrations are greater than the MIC for most sensitive pathogens. There is no evidence of teratogenicity. Only small amounts of cefalexin are excreted into breast milk, and it is generally considered compatible with breastfeeding.

Ilett *et al.*: *Ann Pharmacother* 2006;**40**:986.
Griffith: *Postgrad Med J* 1983;**59** suppl 5:16.

Cefixime

Cefixime can be detected in amniotic fluid after maternal treatment, so it likely crosses the placenta. Rodent teratogenicity studies are reassuring. Most cephalosporins are excreted into breast milk, and cefixime appears to be no exception. Like all cephalosporins, cefixime is generally considered compatible with breastfeeding.

Halperin-Walega *et al.*: *Drug Metab Dispos* 1988;**16**:130.
Ozyüncü *et al.*: *J Obstet Gynaecol Res* 2010;**36**:484.

Cefotaxime – See Part 2, pp. 136–137

Cefpodoxime

It is not known whether cefpodoxime crosses the placenta. Rodent teratogenicity studies are reassuring. Cefpodoxime is reported in the manufacturer's prescribing information to be excreted in breast milk at modest levels. Although not widely used in neonatal units, cefpodoxime may be used in babies as young as 15 days.

Mikamo *et al.*: *Jpn J Antibiot* 1993;**46**:269.

Ceftazidime – See Part 2, pp. 138–139

Ceftriaxone – See Part 2, pp. 140–141

Cefuroxime – See Part 2, pp. 142–143

Celecoxib

Celecoxib is a COX-2 inhibitor used for analgesia in a number of arthritic conditions. It has also been used as a tocolytic in preterm labour. Celecoxib crosses the placenta and can cause ductal closure. Fetal levels are dependent on the maternal concentrations. Celecoxib increases the incidence of VSD and deformities of the bony chest in fetal rabbits. There is also a dose-dependent increase of diaphragmatic hernia in rats. Although NSAIDs were thought to predispose to PPHN, recent studies do not support this. Celecoxib passes into breast milk in subclinical amounts that have not been reported to have any effects in the breastfeeding infant.

Gardiner *et al.*: *Br J Clin Pharmacol* 2006;**61**:101.
Stika *et al.*: *Am J Obstet Gynecol* 2002;**187**:653.
Van Marter *et al.*: *Pediatrics* 2013;**131**:79.

Cefradine (cefradine - former BAN)

Cefradine rapidly crosses the placenta and is found in the amniotic fluid within hours of maternal administration. There is no evidence of teratogenicity in humans or in rodent studies. Cefradine is excreted into breast milk in small amounts that are compatible with breastfeeding.

Lange *et al.*: *Br J Obstet Gynaecol* 1984;**91**:551.
Mischler *et al.*: *J Reprod Med* 1978;**21**:130.
Philipson *et al.*: *Clin Pharmacokinet* 1987;**12**:136.

Cetirizine

It is not known whether cetirizine crosses the placenta. Neither the first-generation (e.g. chlorphenamine) nor the second-generation (e.g. cetirizine) antihistamines have been found to be teratogenic. Cetirizine enters breast milk but has no effects on the breastfed infant. In general, first-generation antihistamines are preferred to newer ones due to the greater wealth of evidence of safety.

Weber-Schoendorfer and Schaefer: *Reprod Toxicol* 2008;**26**:19.
Keleş: *Am J Rhinol* 2004;**18**:23.

Chloral hydrate – See Part 2, pp. 144–145

Chlorambucil

Some reports of chlorambucil use during the first trimester in humans (and rodent teratogenicity studies) suggest that chlorambucil use causes renal tract abnormalities. In general, use should be avoided during the first trimester when risk is greatest. There are no reports of chlorambucil use during lactation; however, because of the potential adverse effects of alkylating agents on the infant, breastfeeding should be avoided.

Kavlock *et al.*: *Toxicology* 1987;**43**:51.
Steege and Caldwell: *South Med J* 1980;**73**:1414.

Chloramphenicol – See Part 2, pp. 146–147

Chlordiazepoxide

Benzodiazepines are rapidly transferred across the placenta. First trimester exposure to some has been linked to an increased risk of anomalies. The experience with chlordiazepoxide has been reassuring with no increase in malformations or adverse effects on neurobehavioural development. Use in the third trimester may cause neonatal hypotonia or marked withdrawal. Symptoms are variable and

include sedation, hypotonia, poor suck, apnoea and cyanosis. These may persist for hours to months after birth. Chlordiazepoxide enters breast milk in low concentrations, and only high maternal doses might be expected to affect the nursing infant.
Iqbal *et al.*: *Psychiatr Serv* 2002;**53**:39.
Gidai *et al.*: *Toxicol Ind Health* 2008;**24**:41.

Chlorhexidine
It is not known whether chlorhexidine crosses the placenta. Exposure during birth is not associated with any known effects in the infant. It is not known whether chlorhexidine enters breast milk; however, given that chlorhexidine is widely used as skin preparation in neonates, the potential for toxicity is low. Use as a disinfectant in traumatised nipples does not seem to cause problems in the infant.
Herd and Feeney: *Practitioner* 1986;**230**:31.
McClure *et al.*: *Int J Gynaecol Obstet* 2007;**97**:89.

Chloroquine – See Part 2, pp. 148–149

Chlorphenamine – See Part 2, pp. 152–153

Chlorpromazine – See Part 2, pp. 154–155

Chlortalidone
Chlortalidone and related thiazide diuretics (e.g. chlorothiazide) may be diabetogenic and are rarely indicated during pregnancy and lactation. Chlortalidone crosses the placenta (F/M ratio ~0.15). Rodent teratogenicity studies are reassuring, but electrolyte imbalances are reported in both mother and newborn. While chlortalidone is excreted into breast milk, it is generally considered compatible with breastfeeding.
Mulley *et al.*: *Eur J Clin Pharmacol* 1978;**13**:129.

Cholestyramine
Cholestyramine has been used for the treatment of cholestasis of pregnancy. In the only randomised trial comparing it to ursodeoxycholic acid, symptom relief for the mother and pregnancy outcomes were worse for the cholestyramine group. Because cholestyramine is not systemically absorbed, it should not directly affect the fetus; however, it could interfere with the uptake of fat-soluble vitamins. It is safe for use in breastfeeding.
Bacq *et al.*: *Gastroenterology* 2012;**143**:1492.
Kondrackiene *et al.*: *Gastroenterology* 2005;**129**:894.

Ciclosporin
Placenta transfer of ciclosporin is reported to be poor. Most infants exposed *in utero* develop and grow normally. Animal teratogenicity studies are reassuring. There is a suggestion of higher risk of stillbirth, preterm delivery and growth restriction in mothers who are treated with ciclosporin used as an immunosuppressant, but it is not clear whether this is related to the maternal disease or the treatment. Ciclosporin passes into breast milk in low amounts; however, the clearance of ciclosporin by the neonate can be quite variable. Some advise against breastfeeding; however, if breastfeeding is continued, the infant should be monitored closely (including serum ciclosporin levels) for signs of toxicity.
Chaparro and Gisbert: *Curr Pharm Biotechnol* 2011;**12**:765.
Ford *et al.*: *Br Med J* 2013;**346**:f432.

Cimetidine
Studies of the use of cimetidine during pregnancy have shown no increased risk of birth defects. Cimetidine is actively transported into breast milk; but the amounts are unlikely to cause problems in the breastfed infant. The interactions of cimetidine with other medications may preclude its use.
Jonker *et al.*: *Nat Med* 2005;**11**:127.
Ruigómez *et al.*: *Am J Epidemiol* 1999;**150**:476.

Ciprofloxacin
Ciprofloxacin crosses the placenta. Short-term treatment appears safe, but the effect of prolonged exposure (e.g. in inflammatory bowel disease) remains unknown. Treatment of fetal mice, dogs and rabbits with other quinolones is associated with an acute arthropathy of the weight-bearing joints. Ciprofloxacin enters breast milk with range levels being reported. *Clostridium difficile* pseudomembranous colitis has been reported in one breastfed infant, and discoloured teeth have been reported in infants treated with ciprofloxacin as neonates. The AAP considers ciprofloxacin safe for breastfeeding women; however, others advise to either avoid or use with caution; in many cases, there will be alternatives for which there is more experience during pregnancy and lactation.
Cassina *et al.*: *Expert Opin Drug Saf* 2009;**8**:695.
Harmon *et al.*: *J Pediatr Surg* 1992;**27**:744.
Lumbiganon *et al.*: *Pediatr Infect Dis J* 1991;**10**:619.

Cisatracurium
Cisatracurium is one of the isomers of atracurium, which has been used during fetal surgery without problems. Although small amounts of atracurium cross the placenta, use during caesarean section is not associated with neonatal sequelae. There are no published reports of use during lactation, and it is not known whether cisatracurium enters breast milk. Considering its use, cisatracurium is unlikely to affect the breastfeeding newborn.

Pan and Moore: *J Clin Anesth* 2001;**13**:112.
Atherton and Hunter: *Clin Pharmacokinet* 1999;**36**:169.

Cisplatin

Although patients should be advised to avoid pregnancy during cisplatin treatment, good outcomes are possible. Cisplatin is considered to be teratogenic and embryotoxic; however, there is increasing evidence for its relative safety during gestation. Cisplatin enters breast milk in variable concentrations. Advice about breastfeeding during treatment is conflicting; while the AAP considers cisplatin compatible with breastfeeding, Hale and a number of other reputable sources advise against breastfeeding during treatment.

Wiebe and Sipila: *Crit Rev Oncol Hematol* 1994;**16**:75.
Lanowska *et al.*: *J Perinat Med* 2011;**39**:279.
Zagouri *et al.*: *Obstet Gynecol* 2013;**121**:337.

Citalopram

Citalopram crosses the placenta (F/M ratio ~0.66). Early studies of paroxetine (but not citalopram) suggested an association with cardiovascular malformations. Overall use during pregnancy does not seem to cause problems other than during the third trimester when neonatal withdrawal syndrome has been reported. Observation for at least 48 hours should identify infants with SSRI-related symptoms needing intervention. There have been two reports of excessive sleepiness in breastfed neonates, but the majority of studies report no effects. It is not known whether exposure through breast milk ameliorates the symptoms of neonatal abstinence.

Gentile: *Drug Saf* 2005;**28**:137.
Sie *et al.*: *Arch Dis Child* Fetal Neonatal Ed 2012;**97**:F472. (Erratum in: *Arch Dis Child* Fetal Neonatal Ed 2013;**98**:F180.)

Clarithromycin – See Part 2, pp. 160–161

Clemastine

It is not known whether clemastine crosses the placenta. It does enter breast milk and can cause drowsiness in the breastfed infant; therefore, caution is advised. There are, however, alternatives for which there is more experience during pregnancy and lactation.

Kok *et al.*: *Lancet* 1982;**1**:914.

Clindamycin – See Part 2, pp. 162–163

Clobazam

Clobazam has been used as an adjunct in epilepsy. It is known to cross the placenta. Use during the third trimester may cause neonatal hypothermia, hypotonia, respiratory depression and withdrawal. Clobazam passes into breast milk in small quantities. Short-term use during breastfeeding is probably safe; long-term treatment is best avoided due to the risks of tolerance in the breastfed infant.

Bar-Oz *et al.*: *Paediatr Drugs* 2000;**2**:113.
Nandakumaran *et al.*: *Dev Pharmacol Ther* 1982;**4** suppl:135.

Clomiphene

A wide range of fetal abnormalities are reported after clomiphene-induced ovulation, but no discernable pattern has emerged. There are no indications for continuing clomiphene during pregnancy or lactation. It can actually suppress lactation.

Canales *et al.*: *Br J Obstet Gynaecol* 1977;**84**:758.
Shoham *et al.*: *Fertil Steril* 1991;**55**:1.

Clomipramine

Clomipramine (and its major metabolite) crosses the placenta (F/M ratio 0.6). There are no reports of fetal abnormalities, and rodent teratogenicity studies are reassuring. Withdrawal symptoms (jitteriness, tremor and seizures) have been reported in exposed neonates. Only small trace amounts of clomipramine are found in breast milk, and these are unlikely to affect the breastfed infant.

Källén: *Expert Opin Drug Saf* 2007;**6**:357.
Schimmell *et al.*: *J Toxicol Clin Toxicol* 1991;**29**:479.

Clonazepam – See Part 2, pp. 164–165

Clonidine

Clonidine is sometimes used to alleviate drug withdrawal in opiate abusers (particularly those who also use cocaine); however, its main use is as an antihypertensive. Clonidine crosses the placenta (F/M ratio 1). Exposed neonates may become hypotensive. Clonidine is concentrated in breast milk (M/P ratio ~2), although neonatal effects are not usually seen. It may, however, reduce prolactin secretion and thus impact on milk production.

Bunjes *et al.*: *Clin Pharm* 1993;**12**:178.
Rothberger *et al.*: *Am J Hypertens* 2010;**23**:1234.

Clotrimazole

It is not known whether clotrimazole crosses the placenta. There is little systemic absorption after dermal application, and only 3–10% is absorbed after vaginal administration. It is unlikely to affect the fetus; rodent teratogenicity studies are reassuring. Levels in breast milk are likely to be low, and any effect on the breastfed neonate is thus minimal.

Czeizel *et al.*: *Epidemiology* 1999;**10**:437.

Clozapine

It is not known whether clozapine crosses the placenta. Rodent teratogenicity studies are reassuring. In two mothers who attempted suicide by ingesting large doses of clozapine, there was one neonatal death; in both cases, maternal toxic effects were seen. Clozapine enters breast milk (M/P ratio 2.8–4.3). Levels seem to diminish as milk matures. There are no reports of effects on the breastfed infant, but they should be monitored for possible adverse effects.

Barnas et al.: Am J Psychiatry 1994;**151**:945.
Kłys et al.: Forensic Sci Int 2007;**171**:e5.
Novikova et al.: Aust N Z J Obstet Gynaecol 2009;**49**:442.

Co-amoxiclav – See Part 2, pp. 166–167

Codeine

Codeine is contained in many tablets and medicines including those available OTC as well as those prescribed. It is metabolised by the liver to morphine, hydrocodone, norcodeine and other metabolites. Morphine readily crosses the placenta; however, reports of use during pregnancy and rodent studies are reassuring, with no evidence of teratogenicity. Neonatal abstinence syndrome is reported after prolonged use. Both codeine and its metabolite morphine are excreted in breast milk. Codeine was originally classified as a low-risk drug when used during breastfeeding; however, a number of reports highlight a particular risk among women with polymorphisms of the cytochrome P450 2D6 (CYP2D6) genes that make them 'ultrarapid metabolisers' of codeine. Breastfed infants of these women (and the women themselves) are then exposed to higher doses of morphine and may exhibit signs of toxicity (drowsiness, constipation and apnoea). The unpredictability of this has led the MHRA to state that codeine should not be used by breastfeeding mothers. If there is no alternative, codeine should be used for short-term therapy only and be discontinued if either the mother or the infant shows symptoms or signs of opioid toxicity. Screening for the CYP2D6 'ultrarapid metaboliser' polymorphisms is not routinely available in the United Kingdom.

Madadi et al.: Can Fam Physician 2009;**55**:1077.
Nezvalová-Henriksen et al.: Eur J Clin Pharmacol 2011;**67**:1253.
Sistonen et al.: Clin Pharmacol Ther 2012;**91**:692.

Colesevelam

Colesevelam is not absorbed; thus, any direct fetal effects are minimal. However, there are concerns that it might interfere with maternal absorption of fat-soluble vitamins (A, D, E and K) in both pregnancy and lactation.

Marquis et al.: Reprod Toxicol 2006;**21**:197.

Colestipol

Less than 0.17% of the colestipol dose is absorbed systemically; thus, it should not directly cause fetal harm at the recommended dosages. Like other drugs in this class, there are concerns that it might interfere with absorption of fat-soluble vitamins (A, D, E and K) in both pregnancy and lactation.

Webster and Bollert: Toxicol Appl Pharmacol 1974;**28**:57.

Co-trimoxazole (trimethoprim–sulfamethoxazole) – See Part 2, pp. 170–171

Cyclophosphamide

Multiple case reports suggest that use can be compatible with a good pregnancy outcome. Cyclophosphamide crosses the placenta, and while there is no convincing evidence of teratogenicity in humans, rodent studies suggest an increase of fetal malformations. Cyclophosphamide enters breast milk in high concentrations and breastfeeding is best avoided. Neonatal marrow suppression has been reported after use in both pregnancy and lactation.

Matalon et al.: Reprod Toxicol 2004;**18**:219.
Temprano et al.: Semin Arthritis Rheum 2005;**35**:112.

Cyproheptadine

It not known whether cyproheptadine crosses the placenta. Rodent studies show no evidence of teratogenicity. It has been shown to alter pancreatic β-cell function in fetal (but not maternal) rats. There are no data on transfer of cyproheptadine into breast milk. Sedation may be a concern and there are alternative antihistamines for which there is more experience during pregnancy and lactation.

Chow and Fischer: Drug Metab Dispos 1987;**15**:740.

Cytarabine

Cytarabine appears to cross the placenta. Normal outcomes have been reported after treatment, but it has been also associated with brachycephaly, facial deformities, cranial synostoses, growth restriction, leucopenia and disturbances of neonatal hepatic transaminases. It is not known if cytarabine passes into breast milk. The BNF (and the manufacturer) advises against breastfeeding; however, Hale suggests that it may be possible to breastfeed some 24–48 hours after treatment on the basis that cytarabine is rapidly metabolised and oral absorption (assuming it passes into breast milk) is poor. Any breastfed infant will require close monitoring for adverse effects.

Wiebe and Sipila: Crit Rev Oncol Hematol 1994;**16**:75.

Dacarbazine

It is not known if dacarbazine crosses the placenta. Teratogenic effects have not been described in human fetuses, and long-term follow-up studies after first trimester exposure are reassuring. Nonetheless, general advice is to avoid use during this period; dacarbazine is teratogenic and embryotoxic in rodents when given in high doses. It is not known whether dacarbazine enters breast milk. Use should be avoided during lactation due to the potential for marrow suppression in the breastfed infant.

Van Calsteren *et al.*: *Acta Obstet Gynecol Scand* 2010;**89**:1338.

Dalteparin

During pregnancy, LMWHs are increasingly used in treating thrombophilias and antiphospholipid syndrome. Dalteparin does not cross the placenta. Only trace amounts, too small to exert any clinically significant effect, enter breast milk. Limited oral bioavailability further reduces the risks in breastfed infants.

Greer: *J Thromb Thrombolysis* 2006;**21**:57.
Richter *et al.*: *Br J Clin Pharmacol* 2001;**52**:708.

Danazol

There are no indications for danazol use during pregnancy. Danazol can cause virilisation of female fetuses, and many would recommend that those so exposed undergo a detailed postnatal ultrasound examination. Rodent studies reveal no evidence of teratogenicity. Danazol is generally considered contraindicated during breastfeeding. It is not known whether danazol passes into breast milk.

Fedele and Berlanda: *Expert Opin Emerg Drugs* 2004;**9**:167.
Moghissi: *Clin Obstet Gynecol* 1999;**42**:620.

Dantrolene

Dantrolene has been used in life-saving treatment of acute malignant hyperthermia and neuroleptic malignant syndrome in pregnant women. It readily crosses the placenta; however, no adverse fetal or neonatal effects are reported. Dantrolene is excreted in breast milk with the infant receiving approximately 7.9% of the maternal dose. A period of 48 hours is recommended between treatment and resumption of breastfeeding.

Fricker *et al.*: *Anesthesiology* 1998;**89**:1023.
Russell *et al.*: *Obstet Gynecol* 2001;**98**:906.

Dapsone

Dapsone is used to treat *Pneumocystis jirovecii* (*Pneumocystis carinii*) pneumonia, leprosy and, in some areas, malaria. Placental transfer probably occurs, as there are reports of neonatal methaemoglobinaemia and haemolysis after maternal dapsone. It does not appear to cause fetal abnormalities. Folic acid 5 mg daily should be given to the mother throughout pregnancy especially if pyrimethamine is also used. Dapsone is excreted in breast milk, and a dose-dependent haemolytic anaemia is the most commonly reported toxic effect (this may occur whether there is G6PD deficiency or not). The amounts the infants receive in breast milk are insufficient for malarial chemoprophylaxis.

Brabin *et al.*: *Drug Saf* 2004;**27**:633.
Sanders *et al.*: *Ann Intern Med* 1982;**96**:465.

Daunorubicin

There are multiple reports of successful outcomes after daunorubicin use during pregnancy. It crosses the placenta (in isolated perfused models, this was <3%). Bone marrow suppression (a common toxic effect in adults) is a reported fetal complication. It is not known if daunorubicin passes into breast milk (the closely related doxorubicin does in negligible amounts); however, because of the potential for toxic effects, breastfeeding is contraindicated.

Kerr: *Pharmacotherapy* 2005;**25**:438.

Demeclocycline

It is not known whether demeclocycline crosses the placenta. However, use during pregnancy is contraindicated because other tetracyclines may cause a permanent (yellow-grey/brown) discolouration of the teeth when given during the second half of pregnancy and are also associated with delayed bone growth. It is likely that demeclocycline enters breast milk (other tetracyclines do so), and for the same reasons as it is contraindicated in pregnancy, it is generally considered incompatible with breastfeeding.

Johnson and Mitchell: *J Dent Res* 1966;**45**:86.

Desferrioxamine mesilate

It is not known if desferrioxamine crosses the placenta, but there are more than 50 published cases of use in transfusion-dependent homozygous β-thalassaemia with no reports of adverse effects in the fetus. Reports of desferrioxamine after acute iron poisoning also suggest good fetal outcomes. No data are available on transfer into breast milk; however, oral bioavailability is virtually non-existent.

Bailey: *Birth Defects Res A Clin Mol Teratol* 2003;**67**:133.
Singer and Vichinsky: *Am J Hematol* 1999;**60**:24.

Desloratadine

Desloratadine is the active metabolite of loratadine. While there were some concerns about increased prevalence of hypospadias after use of desloratadine and loratadine, recent studies refute the association. Desloratadine passes into breast milk, but the breastfeeding neonate receives a dose of less than 1% of the adult dose.

Gilbert *et al.*: *Drug Saf* 2005;**28**:707.

Desmopressin

There is no detectable placental transfer of desmopressin at normal therapeutic concentrations, and no adverse fetal effects have been reported. One study found minimal desmopressin in breast milk after using the nasal spray. It seems unlikely that the breastfed neonate would ingest clinically significant quantities. In any case, desmopressin is destroyed by trypsin in the intestine.

Hime *et al.*: *Obstet Gynecol Surv* 1978;**33**:375.
Trigg *et al.*: *Haemophilia* 2012;**18**:25.

Dexamethasone – See Part 2, pp. 174–176

Dexamfetamine (dexamphetamine)

Dexamfetamine and its prodrug, lisdexamfetamine, are used to treat ADHD in children and adults (although the use in adults is off-licence). See *amfetamine* for effects during pregnancy and lactation.

Diazepam – See Part 2, pp. 179–180

Diazoxide – See Part 2, pp. 181–182

Diclofenac

Diclofenac rapidly crosses the placenta (F/M ratio ~1). Rodent teratogenicity studies are reassuring, but *in utero* closure of the ductus arteriosus is reported in human pregnancies. Studies also show significant associations between diclofenac and both third trimester vaginal bleeding and the development of childhood asthma. Small amounts of diclofenac enter breast milk, but these are probably too low to have any clinical effect.

Auer *et al.*: *Ultrasound Obstet Gynecol* 2004;**23**:513.
Nezvalová-Henriksen *et al.*: *BJOG* 2013;**120**:948.

Dicyclomine

It is not known whether dicyclomine crosses the placenta. It does not appear to increase the risks of fetal malformations, and rodent studies are reassuring. Dicyclomine appears in breast milk. Because of case reports of apnoea and severe respiratory symptoms in neonates (who are very sensitive to anticholinergics), it is generally considered incompatible with breastfeeding.

Friedman *et al.*: *Obstet Gynecol* 1990;**75**:594.
Hall *et al.*: *J Paediatr Child Health* 2012;**48**:128.

Diethylstilbestrol (stilboestrol)

Diethylstilbestrol use during the first trimester is associated with vaginal carcinoma, urogenital abnormalities (hypoplasia of uterus and cervix, T-shaped uterus and bilateral hydrosalpinges) and reduced fertility in exposed female fetuses and increased risk of hypospadias in exposed male fetuses. For these reasons, diethylstilbestrol is contraindicated during pregnancy and breastfeeding. Some suppression of lactation may occur but it should not be used for this purpose.

Newbold: *Toxicol Appl Pharmacol* 2004;**199**:142.

Digoxin – See Part 2, pp. 186–187

Diltiazem

It is not known whether diltiazem crosses the placenta in humans (it does in rabbits). Rodent teratogenicity studies suggest increased incidence of skeletal and aortic arch malformations. Diltiazem enters breast milk, although its use is generally considered safe.

Baroletti *et al.*: *Pharmacotherapy* 2003;**23**:788.
Lubbe: *N Z Med J* 1987;**100**:121.

Dimenhydrinate

This treatment for motion sickness and vertigo should only be used if the benefit justifies the potential perinatal risk. Passage across the placenta has not been studied, and there are no reports of fetal anomalies associated with its use. Small amounts of dimenhydrinate pass into breast milk, but no effects have been reported in the neonate.

Czeizel and Vargha: *Arch Gynecol Obstet* 2005;**271**:113.

Dinoprostone

Dinoprostone is effective when administered by oral, vaginal or intracervical routes for cervical ripening preceding either vaginal delivery or pregnancy termination. It is not known whether dinoprostone crosses the placenta. Rodent studies reveal evidence of embryotoxicity and skeletal anomalies when used during organogenesis. It is not known whether dinoprostone enters breast milk. Given the reasons for its administration, use is unlikely to have a clinically significant effect on the breastfed infant.

Thorburn: *Early Hum Dev* 1992;**29**:63.

Diphenhydramine

Diphenhydramine crosses the placenta. While there is no evidence of fetal harm, the exposed neonate may be slightly depressed if diphenhydramine is administered during labour. It is not known whether diphenhydramine enters breast milk. A non-sedating antihistamine (e.g. cetirizine or loratadine) would be a preferred option if diphenhydramine is being used to treat allergy.

Werler *et al.*: *Am J Obstet Gynecol* 2005;**193**:771.

Dipyridamole

It is not known whether this antiplatelet agent crosses the placenta. Rodent studies are reassuring, and there are no reports of poor outcomes after use in human pregnancies. According to the manufacturer, dipyridamole enters breast milk; however, there is no evidence of neonatal effects that would prohibit breastfeeding.

Kinouchi et al.: J Anesth 2000;**14**:115.

Disodium etidronate

It is not known if etidronate crosses the placenta. Rodent studies are reassuring. A review of 51 cases of in utero exposure to bisphosphonates found no evidence of toxicity. Transient neonatal hypocalcaemia was reported in some cases, but it is not clear whether this was related to the maternal hypercalcaemia or its treatment. It is not known whether etidronate is excreted into breast milk; however, it has poor oral bioavailability, ensuring that the amounts the breastfed infant would receive are small.

Djokanovic et al.: J Obstet Gynaecol Can 2008;**30**:1146.

Disodium pamidronate

It is not known if disodium pamidronate crosses the placenta (low lipid solubility may limit the amount that does). Limited human experience (of all bisphosphonates) is reassuring. Disodium pamidronate appears to pass into breast milk in only small amounts, and coupled with poor oral absorption, this means that the breastfed infant is unlikely to be affected.

Djokanovic et al.: J Obstet Gynaecol Can 2008;**30**:1146.
Siminoski et al.: J Bone Miner Res 2000;**15**:2052.

Disopyramide

Use of disopyramide during pregnancy carries risks of haemorrhage, hypotension, uterine contractions and preterm labour. It crosses the placenta (F/M ratio ~0.26). Rodent teratogenicity studies are reassuring. It also passes into breast milk but the breastfed infant receives, at most, subtherapeutic amounts. While probably safe during lactation, disopyramide should only be used during pregnancy if the benefit justifies the perinatal risks.

Abbi et al.: J Reprod Med 1999;**44**:653.
Hoppu et al.: Br J Clin Pharmacol 1986;**21**:553.

Disulfiram

Use of disulfiram is increasingly more common in women of reproductive age; however, the safety of this drug during pregnancy remains to be established. Disulfiram is embryotoxic in vitro, affecting both DNA synthesis and morphologic development. It is not known whether disulfiram crosses the placenta, but there are case reports of limb abnormalities in fetus of women treated with disulfiram during pregnancy; however, ongoing alcohol ingestion and use of other drugs complicate the picture. It is not known whether disulfiram enters breast milk, but its low molecular weight makes it likely. The risks to the breastfed infant, who will be exposed to alcohol from a number of products, are appreciable, and for this reason, it should not be used during breastfeeding.

Reitnauer et al.: Teratogenicity 1997;**56**:358.
Helmbrecht and Hoskins: Am J Perinatol 1993;**10**:5.

Dithranol

There are no adequate reports or well-controlled studies of this topical psoriatic treatment in pregnant women. Though it is generally considered safe for use during pregnancy, there are no well-controlled studies in human fetuses. Rodent teratogenicity studies have apparently not been conducted. There is no published experience during lactation, and it is not known whether dithranol enters breast milk.

Tauscher et al.: J Cutan Med Surg 2002;**6**:561.

Dobutamine – See Part 2, pp. 188–189

Docetaxel

It is not known if docetaxel crosses the placenta. While there are several case reports of use during pregnancy with reassuring results and no evidence of teratogenicity, rodent studies suggest embryotoxicity during early gestation. There is no data on the transfer of docetaxel into breast milk, and the effects of exposure in the breastfed infant are unknown.

Potluri et al.: Clin Breast Cancer 2006;**7**:167.
Zagouri et al.: Oncology 2012;**83**:234.

Docusate salts (calcium, potassium and sodium)

Salt forms of docusate are considered clinically interchangeable in terms of therapeutic effect. Docusate salts are not absorbed systemically. Chronic high-dose use has been reported to cause hypomagnesaemia in one mother and her newborn, causing jitteriness in the newborn period. Because there is no systemic absorption, it will not enter breast milk.

Schindler: Lancet 1984;**2**:822.
Shafe et al.: Therap Adv Gastroenterol 2011;**4**:343.

Domperidone – See Part 2, pp. 190–191

Dopamine – See Part 2, pp. 192–193

Dosulepin (dothiepin - USAN)

The manufacturers of dosulepin do not advice use during pregnancy. Fetal tachyarrhythmia was reported during dosulepin use which settled after cessation. Dosulepin is excreted in breast milk in small amounts, and no adverse effects have been reported in the nursing infant.

Ilett *et al.*: *Br J Clin Pharmacol* 1992;**33**:635.
Prentice and Brown: *Br Med J* 1989;**298**:190.

Doxazosin
This α1-adrenergic antagonist may be used to treat hypertension; however, there are many alternatives that can be used during both pregnancy and lactation where there is greater experience. It is not known whether doxazosin crosses the placenta in humans (it does so in rats); however, rodent teratogenicity studies are reassuring. It is not known if doxazosin enters breast milk.

Doxepin
While animal teratogenicity and cohort studies of doxepin use during pregnancy are largely reassuring, breastfeeding appears to carry some risks. Although only small amounts of this drug and its active metabolite (*N*-desmethyldoxepin) pass into breast milk, there are two reports of severe hypotonia and drowsiness with, in one case, near-miss respiratory arrest. In the first case, the baby had a blood level of the metabolite that was inexplicably high if the child's only exposure to the drug was from maternal milk. The onset of symptoms also seemed very sudden. In the second, the blood level was much lower, and the drowsiness rather less clearly related to maternal medication. Uncertainties over use during lactation remain worryingly unresolved.

Frey *et al.*: *Ann Pharmacother* 1999;**22**:690.

Doxorubicin
There are several reports of doxorubicin during pregnancy, but it is usually combined with other neoplastic agents, making it difficult to interpret outcomes. There is no conclusive evidence of teratogenicity, and treatment in the second and third trimesters does not seem to be associated with increased complications or adverse neonatal outcomes. Doxorubicin is concentrated in breast milk, and both it and its metabolite may be detectable up to 72 hours after administration.

Egan *et al.*: *Cancer Treat Rep* 1985;69:1387.
Newcomb *et al.*: *JAMA* 1978;**239**:2691.

Doxycycline
Use of tetracyclines during periods of tooth development (i.e. during the third trimester and infancy and in young children) may cause permanent discolouration of the teeth. Doxycycline is therefore contraindicated during pregnancy. It passes into breast milk in small amounts and could theoretically also cause staining of teeth; in practice, this is probably unlikely as it is bound to calcium in milk and infants have 'undetectable' serum levels. While doxycycline is bound to calcium to a lesser degree than the older tetracyclines, this does not seem to cause problems during short-term use (maximum 3–4 weeks). Nonetheless, the BNF advises against use during lactation.

Czeizel and Rockenbauer: *Obstet Gynecol* 1997;**89**:524.

Droperidol
Droperidol crosses the placenta slowly. Rodent teratogenicity studies are reassuring. No adverse fetal outcomes have been reported when it was used for the treatment of hyperemesis gravidarum or to prevent nausea and vomiting during caesarean section. It is not known if droperidol enters breast milk.

Griffiths *et al.*: *Cochrane Database Syst Rev* 2012;**9**:CD007579.
Nageotte *et al.*: *Am J Obstet Gynecol* 1996;**174**:1801.
Zhdanov and Ponomarev: *Anesteziol Reanimatol* 1980;**4**:14.

Econazole
It is not known whether econazole crosses the placenta. It is usually used as a topical treatment for *Tinea* but can be used for vaginal candidiasis (although clotrimazole seems a better option). With either route, it is unlikely that maternal systemic concentrations reach a clinically relevant level. Rodent teratogenicity studies are reassuring. It is not known whether econazole enters breast milk; however, it seems unlikely to pose a clinically significant risk to the breastfeeding infant.

Czeizel *et al.*: *Eur J Obstet Gynecol Reprod Biol* 2003;**111**:135.

Edrophonium
Edrophonium is used in the diagnosis of myasthenia gravis and occasionally for the reversal of non-depolarising neuromuscular blockade. There is little information on use during pregnancy. It is not known whether edrophonium crosses the placenta. Rodent teratogenicity studies have not been performed. There are no reports of use during lactation, and it is not known whether edrophonium enters breast milk (its unique chemical structure suggests it will not). However, considering the indication and rapid dispersion within peripheral tissues, one-time edrophonium use is unlikely to pose a clinically significant risk to the breastfeeding infant especially if a brief waiting period was used.

Drachman: *N Engl J Med* 1978;**298**:186.

Efavirenz

Efavirenz crosses the placenta (F/M ratio ~1). Use has been associated with CNS malformations in monkeys and with NTDs in humans. Advice about efavirenz use during pregnancy is conflicting; in North America, it is advised that efavirenz should be avoided during pregnancy; in contrast, BHIVA guidelines state that emerging prospective data reports no evidence for teratogenicity. BHIVA guidelines suggest that efavirenz should continue to be used if the woman has conceived while using this as part of HAART. Efavirenz enters breast milk. However, in countries where formula feeds are safe and affordable, it is generally recommended that HIV-infected women do not breastfeed.

Giles: *AIDS* 2013;**27**:857.
Taylor *et al.*: *HIV Med* 2012;**13**(suppl 2):87.

Eletriptan

There is no published experience with this 5HT$_1$-receptor agonist during pregnancy. It is not known whether it crosses the placenta. Rodent studies have shown skeletal abnormalities at high doses. The manufacturer states eletriptan is excreted into breast milk in small amounts. It is unlikely that the maternal dose would cause any clinically significant effect in the breastfed infant.

Hutchinson *et al.*: *Headache* 2013;**53**:614.
Soldin *et al.*: *Ther Drug Monit* 2008;**30**:5.

Enalapril

Enalapril should be avoided during pregnancy if possible. It crosses the placenta and exposure is associated with cranial hypoplasia, anuria, reversible or irreversible renal failure, death, oligohydramnios, prematurity and IUGR. Long-term renal disease is reported in survivors. Trace amounts of enalapril are detectable in breast milk, and breastfed infants should be monitored for hypotension.

Laube *et al.*: *Arch Dis Child* Fetal Neonatal Ed 2007;**92**:F402.
Murki *et al.*: *J Matern Fetal Neonatal Med* 2005;**17**:235.
Tabacova: *Crit Rev Toxicol* 2005;**35**:747.

Enoxaparin

Low molecular weight heparins, like enoxaparin, do not cross the placenta and do not pose a direct risk to the fetus. Both epidemiological and rodent studies are reassuring. Enoxaparin is unlikely to enter breast milk due to its size, and even if it did, limited oral bioavailability means that the breastfed infant receives negligible amounts.

Guillonneau *et al.*: *Arch Pediatr* 1996;**3**:513.
Meneveau: *Expert Opin Drug Saf* 2009;**8**:745.

Eplerenone

Eplerenone is an aldosterone antagonist similar to spironolactone but is much more selective for the mineralocorticoid receptor and has less of an antiandrogenic effect. It is not known if eplerenone crosses the placenta. The manufacturer's SPC states that studies in rodents did not reveal any teratogenicity. Use in humans is limited to case reports where it has been used as an alternative to spironolactone. No adverse fetal effects were noted but experience is very limited. It is not known if eplerenone passes into breast milk.

Cabassi *et al.*: *Hypertension* 2012;**59**:e18.
Muldowney *et al.*: *Expert Opin Drug Metab Toxicol* 2009;**5**:425.

Epoietin alfa and related erythropoietins – See Part 2, pp. 207–208

Epoprostenol – See Part 2, pp. 203–204

Ergotamine

Although useful in migraine treatment, ergotamine is contraindicated during pregnancy for a number of reasons. It is a highly active uterine contractile agonist and may lead to abortion. Epidemiological studies show increased prevalence of preterm birth and IUGR. It is not known whether ergotamine crosses the placenta. It is excreted into breast milk. Theoretically, ergotamine might inhibit lactation but this is not seen in practice. Alternatives exist that have a better safety profile.

Bánhidy *et al.*: *Br J Clin Pharmacol* 2007;**64**:510.
Moretti *et al.*: *Can Fam Physician* 2000;**46**:1753.

Erythromycin – See Part 2, pp. 205–206

Escitalopram

It is not known if escitalopram crosses the placenta. Use during pregnancy does not seem to cause problems, but a variety of neonatal withdrawal symptoms have been reported. Escitalopram enters breast milk and infant plasma levels were very low or undetectable. The manufacturer and the BNF state that escitalopram should be avoided during lactation; however, it is probably safe.

Klieger-Grossmann *et al.*: *J Clin Pharmacol* 2012;**52**:766.
Rampono *et al.*: *Br J Clin Pharmacol* 2006;**62**:316.

Esmolol

Esmolol has been used to control high blood pressure in women with pre-eclampsia or phaeochromocytoma before induction of general anaesthesia. It crosses the placenta and may cause a fetal bradycardia that continues for days. Rodent teratogenicity studies are reassuring. It is not known whether it enters breast milk. In any case, the route of administration (intravenous) and indications for this drug limit exposure in lactating mothers.

Fairley and Clarke: *Br J Anaesth* 1995;**75**:801.
Gilson *et al.*: *J Reprod Med* 1992;**37**:277.
Varon and Marik: *Chest* 2000;**118**:214.

Esomeprazole
Esomeprazole is an enantiomer of omeprazole, and most of the data on safety of esomeprazole in pregnancy are derived from studies of omeprazole. It is not known if it crosses the placenta. Teratology studies in rodents are reassuring, and limited human experience does not suggest an increase in fetal abnormalities. It is not known whether it is excreted into breast milk. While both the manufacturer and the BNF recommend avoiding esomeprazole, there is a growing body of work that suggests PPIs are probably safe during pregnancy and lactation. Omeprazole is the PPI with which there is most experience.
Majithia and Johnson: *Drugs* 2012;**72**:171.
Marshall *et al.*: *Can J Gastroenterol* 1998;**12**:225.
Pasternak and Hviid: *N Engl J Med* 2010;**363**:2114.

Estradiol
There are no indications for estradiol during pregnancy. Estradiol has been used to suppress lactation, so in general, combined oral contraceptive pills are not recommended. Both the BNF and the FDA advise avoidance of use until weaning or until 6 months after birth. Some feel this is somewhat conservative and suggest that if milk supplies are established, then oestrogen-containing contraceptives may be used after the first 6 weeks (when the mother's risk from thrombosis is greatest) with little effect on the breastfed infant.
Jackson: *Thromb Res* 2011;**127**(suppl 3):S35.
Queenan: *Clin Obstet Gynecol* 2004;**47**:734.

Ethambutol
Available evidence suggests that all four first-line drugs for the treatment of tuberculosis (isoniazid, rifampin, ethambutol and pyrazinamide) have excellent safety records in pregnancy. Ethambutol crosses the placenta (F/M ratio ~1). There are no reports of adverse fetal effects and rodent studies are reassuring. Ethambutol passes into breast milk in small amounts and is generally considered compatible with breastfeeding.
Bothamley: *Drug Saf* 2001;**24**:553.
Skevaki and Kafetzis: *Paediatr Drugs* 2005;**7**:219.

Ethosuximide
Ethosuximide crosses the placenta (F/M ratio ~1). Associations between ethosuximide and malformations are unclear. Monotherapy with ethosuximide generally seems safe; however, abnormalities increase when it is used with other anticonvulsants. Hyperexcitability has been reported in infants exposed *in utero*.

Ethosuximide freely enters breast milk but does not appear to cause clinically significant effects in the breastfed infant.
Crawford: *Drug Saf* 2009;**32**:293.
Kuhnz *et al.*: *Br J Clin Pharmacol* 1984;**18**:671.

Etodolac
It is not known whether etodolac crosses the placenta; the low molecular weight suggests that this is possible. Rodent studies have shown an increased prevalence of limb abnormalities. It is not known whether etodolac is excreted into breast milk. There are alternatives for which there is more experience during pregnancy and lactation.

Etretinate
Etretinate is a human and rodent teratogen, with the majority of fetuses affected. The effects of the drug persist for some time after treatment, and pregnancy is not advised within 3 years of cessation of treatment. Multiple organ systems are affected, including NTDs, facial and skull abnormalities, limb and digital malformations and skeletal defects. It is not known whether etretinate enters breast milk (its metabolite acitretin does in small amounts); however, the potential for toxic effects is such that breastfeeding should be avoided.
Geiger *et al.*: *Dermatology* 1994;**189**:109.

Famciclovir
Famciclovir is a prodrug of the active penciclovir and is used for treatment of herpes simplex or varicella zoster infections. It is not known whether famciclovir crosses the placenta. Rodent studies are reassuring. There are no studies of use of famciclovir during lactation, and it is not known if it passes into breast milk. The limited data for famciclovir use during pregnancy and lactation mean that aciclovir and valciclovir are better alternatives for which there is more experience.
Pasternak and Hviid: *JAMA* 2010;**304**:859.

Famotidine
Famotidine crosses the placenta (F/M ratio ~0.40). Rodent studies are reassuring. In general, there is no evidence that any histamine H_2 receptor antagonists pose significant risks to the developing embryo or fetus. Famotidine is concentrated in breast milk to a lesser extent than either cimetidine or ranitidine, and because it does not share the same drug interactions as cimetidine, many consider it the preferred choice during breastfeeding even though the manufacturer (and the BNF) advises avoidance of use.
Hagemann: *J Hum Lact* 1998;**14**:259.
Matok *et al.*: *J Clin Pharmacol* 2010;**50**:81.

Felodipine

It is not known if placental transfer of felodipine occurs, but there are effects on the placental blood supply, and rodent studies showed increased prevalence of digital anomalies. Data on use during lactation is lacking. Nifedipine is an alternative for which there is more experience during pregnancy and lactation.

Casele *et al.*: *J Reprod Med* 1997;**42**:378.
Danielsson *et al.*: *Teratology* 1990;**41**:185.

Fenofibrate

Rodent studies of fenofibrate highlights a concern with evidence of IUGR at normal doses and both embryotoxic and teratogenic effects at high doses. It is not known if the drug passes into breast milk; however, the importance of cholesterol in the infant's neurodevelopment means that they should not be exposed. As hyperlipidaemia is not acutely life-threatening, cessation of medication during pregnancy and lactation is suggested.

Sunman *et al.*: *Ann Pharmacother* 2012;**46**:e5.
Whitten *et al.*: *Obstet Gynecol* 2011;**117**:517.

Fentanyl – See Part 2, pp. 211–212

Fexofenadine

Fexofenadine, a metabolite of terfenadine, is a third-generation antihistamine with non-sedating properties. It is not known whether fexofenadine crosses the placenta, but there is no evidence of teratogenicity in rodents. It is not known whether it enters breast milk (terfenadine does in clinically insignificant amounts). Although probably safe during pregnancy and lactation, there are alternative antihistamines with known safety profiles for these periods.

Buccolo and Viera: *J Reprod Med* 2005;**50**:61.
Loebstein *et al.*: *J Allergy Clin Immunol* 1999;**104**:953.

Filgrastim

Filgrastim has been used to treat severe chronic neutropenia and chemotherapy-induced neutropenia during pregnancy without adverse effect. It is not known whether filgrastim crosses the placenta; limited evidence suggests that it does during the second and third trimesters. There are no reports to suggest it is teratogenic in humans. It is not known whether it enters breast milk; as a glycoprotein, it is likely to be digested in the infant's stomach.

Cottle *et al.*: *Semin Hematol* 2002;**39**:134.

Flavoxate

It is not known whether flavoxate crosses the placenta, but rodent teratogenicity studies are reassuring. There is no information on flavoxate during lactation. Flavoxate should only be used during pregnancy and lactation if the benefit justifies the perinatal risk; however, there are few, if any, indications.

Flecainide – See Part 2, pp. 215–216

Flucloxacillin – See Part 2, pp. 217–218

Fluconazole – See Part 2, pp. 219–220

Flucytosine

Flucytosine (5-fluorocytosine) has been used during pregnancy for the treatment of cryptococcal meningitis and pneumonia and candida septicaemia. It is not known if flucytosine crosses the placenta. Rat (but not mice, rabbit or primate) studies have revealed teratogenicity at doses analogous to human doses. In part, the teratogenicity is thought to relate to conversion of flucytosine to 5-fluorouracil (see following text). Limited case reports of use during the second and third trimesters showed no adverse fetal effects. It is not known whether flucytosine enters breast milk. In view of its potential for adverse effects, flucytosine should be avoided during pregnancy and lactation.

Diasio *et al.*: *Antimicrob Agents Chemother* 1978;**14**:903.
Moudgal and Sobel: *Expert Opin Drug Saf* 2003;**2**:475.

Fludrocortisone

Fludrocortisone has been used for the treatment of adrenal insufficiency during pregnancy. Various corticosteroids appear to cause malformations in animal studies, but this association is less clear in humans. The needs of the mother should be balanced against the risk to the fetus. Infants exposed to high doses *in utero* should be carefully observed for signs of hypoadrenalism. It is not known whether fludrocortisone enters breast milk (other corticosteroids are found in low concentrations).

Lekarev and New: *Best Pract Res Clin Endocrinol Metab* 2011;**25**:959.

Fluorouracil

Fluorouracil is embryotoxic and teratogenic in rodents. Reports of fetal immunosuppression suggest that it crosses the placenta. Little is known about the long-term effects of *in utero* exposure to fluorouracil. When it has been used (usually in combination with other antimetabolites) the malformations are highly variable. Use during second and third trimesters is more likely to result in normal outcomes. A recent case report could not detect any in milk from one mother who expressed milk during her treatment. Although this and the reports of good outcomes after second and third trimester use are somewhat reassuring, fluorouracil should be used during pregnancy and lactation only if the benefit justifies the perinatal risk.

Loibl *et al.*: *Lancet Oncol* 2012;**13**:887.
Peccatori *et al.*: *Ann Oncol* 2012;**23**:543.

Fluoxetine

Fluoxetine crosses the placenta (F/M ratio ~0.9). Use during the first trimester does not seem to carry any major risks – studies of SSRIs have shown a minor increase in congenital heart defects (usually septal defects). Maternal doses in the third trimester correlate with umbilical cord concentrations. Neonatal withdrawal is well described. It passes into breast milk and the manufacturer advises avoiding use during lactation. Low maternal doses (20 mg/day) do not seem to cause any problems. Sertraline and escitalopram are safer alternatives during breastfeeding, but if fluoxetine cannot be discontinued, the breastfed infant should be monitored for side effects of colic, excessive fussiness and crying.

Ellfolk and Malm: *Reprod Toxicol* 2010;**30**:249.
Riggin *et al.*: *J Obstet Gynaecol Can* 2013;**35**:362.
Sie *et al.*: *Arch Dis Child Fetal Neonatal Ed* 2012;**97**:F472. (Erratum in: *Arch Dis Child Fetal Neonatal Ed* 2013;**98**:F180.)

Flupentixol (flupenthixol, former BAN)

Flupentixol crosses the placenta and can be found in breast milk. Because of the lack of published experience, other antipsychotics for which there is greater experience may be preferred during both pregnancy and lactation.

Kirk and Jørgensen: *Psychopharmacology (Berl)* 1980;**72**:107.
Matheson and Skjeraasen: *Eur J Clin Pharmacol* 1988;**35**:217.

Fluphenazine decanoate

It is not known if fluphenazine crosses the placenta. Studies in rodents have shown an increase in skeletal and CNS malformations. Use during pregnancy has been reported to cause withdrawal in the neonate. It is not known whether fluphenazine enters breast milk. Because of the lack of published experience, other antipsychotic agents for which there is greater experience may be preferred if breastfeeding is continued.

Einarson and Boskovic: *J Psychiatr Pract* 2009;**15**:183.
Nath *et al.*: *Ann Pharmacother* 1996;**30**:35.

Flurazepam

Flurazepam crosses the placenta. Studies in rats suggest a negative impact on growth;

other benzodiazepines (e.g. diazepam) have also been associated with an increased risk of malformations after first trimester exposure. Neonatal depression has been reported after use during the third trimester. It is not known whether flurazepam passes into breast milk. Because its metabolites have long half-lives, shorter-acting alternatives (e.g. lorazepam) are preferable if a benzodiazepine is necessary during breastfeeding.

Takzare *et al.*: *Toxicol Mech Methods* 2008;**18**:711.

Flurbiprofen

Flurbiprofen crosses the placenta. Although there are no reports of its effects during pregnancy, other NSAIDs cause constriction of the ductus arteriosus and fetal oliguria – similar effects are seen for flurbiprofen in rats. Small and clinically insignificant amounts of flurbiprofen are found in breast milk, and no adverse effects in the nursing infant are reported.

Smith *et al.*: *J Clin Pharmacol* 1989;**29**:174.

Fluticasone

Case series of fluticasone use during pregnancy are reassuring, showing no adverse effects on the fetus. It is not known whether fluticasone enters breast milk, but any if present would be in such small doses as to be clinically insignificant to the nursing infant.

Lim *et al.*: *Ann Pharmacother* 2011;**45**:931.

Fluvastatin

It is not known if fluvastatin crosses the placenta. The manufacturer's data shows that it enters breast milk. The effect on the breastfeeding neonate is unknown. On current evidence, because cholesterol and products synthesised from cholesterol are important in fetal and infant development, statins are best avoided during pregnancy and lactation. Hyperlipidaemia is a chronic illness, and temporarily discontinuing treatment (or indeed any other related drug) is unlikely to compromise care.

Seguin and Samuels: *Obstet Gynecol* 1999;**93**:847.

Fluvoxamine

Fluvoxamine crosses the placenta but there is no evidence of teratogenicity or any other adverse effect in humans after first trimester exposure. Approximately 20–30% of newborns exposed to SSRI antidepressants in the third trimester can show signs of agitation, altered muscle tone and breathing. Small amounts of fluvoxamine are found in breast milk, but levels in the neonates are below the limit of detection. The manufacturer advises avoidance of use during lactation. Sertraline and paroxetine seem to be safer alternatives during lactation, but if the mother is established on fluvoxamine, it may be used with caution.

Gentile: *Arch Women's Ment Health* 2006;**9**:158.

Sie *et al.*: *Arch Dis Child* Fetal Neonatal Ed 2012;**97**:F472. (Erratum in: *Arch Dis Child* Fetal Neonatal Ed 2013;**98**:F180.)

Folinic acid (leucovorin, USAN)

It is not known whether folinic acid crosses the placenta or whether it has the same preventive effects against neural tube defects that folic acid does. Rodent teratogenicity studies have not been conducted, and most case reports of use during pregnancy relate to coadministration with methotrexate to treat ectopic pregnancy. It is not known whether folinic acid enters breast milk. During pregnancy and lactation, the benefits of 'folinic acid rescue' outweigh any risks to the fetus or breastfed infant.

Barnhart *et al.*: *Fertil Steril* 2007;**87**:250.

Fondaparinux sodium

Fondaparinux is sometimes used when the mother cannot tolerate LMWH. While *in vivo* transfer across the placenta is reported to occur, this does not appear to happen *in vitro*, and limited experience has shown no increased incidence of bleeding in the neonate. It is unclear if fondaparinux enters breast milk in humans (it can be found in breast milk from animal studies). Although it has potential for use in DVT prophylaxis during pregnancy, there are alternatives for which there is more experience during pregnancy and lactation.

Dempfle: *N Engl J Med* 2004;**350**:1914.

Knol *et al.*: *J Thromb Haemost* 2010;**8**:1876.

Formoterol fumarate

There is limited reported experience with formoterol during pregnancy, and slightly more experience has been reported with salmeterol; however, inhaled long-acting β2 agonists are regarded as safe during pregnancy and lactation and should be continued.

BTS & SIGN: British Guideline on the Management of Asthma.

Wilton and Shakir: *Drug Saf* 2002;**25**:213.

Fosamprenavir

Fosamprenavir is a prodrug of amprenavir. Teratogenic effects have been reported in rodents, but no such effects are seen in humans. It is unknown whether amprenavir and fosamprenavir are excreted in breast milk. Breastfeeding is contraindicated in HIV-infected nursing women where formula is available to reduce the risk of neonatal transmission.

Bawdon *et al.*: *Infect Dis Obstet Gynecol* 1998;**6**:244.

Cespedes *et al.*: *J Acquir Immune Defic Syndr* 2013;**62**:550.

Martorell *et al.*: *Pediatr Infect Dis J* 2010;**29**:985.

Foscarnet sodium

Foscarnet is used in the treatment of infections due to the herpes family of viruses, including AIDS-related CMV retinitis. There is scant experience of use during pregnancy – two reports (each of a single case) indicate successful pregnancy outcomes. It is not known if foscarnet either crosses the placenta or enters breast milk (it is apparently concentrated in rodent breast milk). Use during pregnancy and lactation is only advised if the benefit justifies the perinatal risk.

Alla *et al.*: *Rev Med Intern* 1999;**20**:514.

Alvarez-McLeod *et al.*: *Clin Infect Dis* 1999;**29**:937.

Fosinopril sodium

Treatment with fosinopril is rarely, if ever, indicated during pregnancy. It is not known if fosinopril crosses the placenta. However, ACE inhibitors are known to adversely affect the fetal kidney and should be considered contraindicated during pregnancy. The manufacturer reports low levels of fosinopril in breast milk. Enalapril and captopril are alternatives for which there is more experience during pregnancy and lactation.

Grove *et al.*: *Toxicol Lett* 1995;**80**:85.

Fosphenytoin sodium

Fosphenytoin is a prodrug of phenytoin and sometimes used in preference during status epilepticus. There are no reports of fosphenytoin use during pregnancy or lactation; however, given its rapid conversion to phenytoin, it is expected that the risks would be similar (see section on **Phenytoin**).

Frovatriptan

The effects of frovatriptan on the fetus have not been studied. Information about its use during lactation is also lacking. Sumatriptan is an alternative for which there is an increasing amount of information – largely reassuring – of use during pregnancy and lactation.

Soldin *et al.*: *Ther Drug Monit* 2008;**30**:5.

Furosemide – See Part 2, pp. 233–234

Gabapentin

Gabapentin crosses the placenta. While there are no reports of human teratogenicity, rodent studies reveal fetotoxicity and increased skeletal abnormalities and hydronephrosis. Gabapentin is excreted into breast milk and is absorbed by the infant. However, serum levels

are fairly low (~12% of maternal levels) and probably unlikely to cause a significant effect.
Fujii *et al.*: *Neurology* 2013;**80**:1565.
Holmes and Hernandez-Diaz: *Birth Defects Res A Clin Mol Teratol* 2012;**94**:599.

Ganciclovir – See Part 2, pp. 235–236

Gemfibrozil

Gemfibrozil crosses the placenta and achieves fetal levels within the therapeutic range for adults. It has been used during pregnancy when hyperlipidaemia causes maternal illnesses (e.g. pancreatitis), but in general, like other lipid-lowering agents, it should be avoided during pregnancy. It is not known whether gemfibrozil enters breast milk. Gemfibrozil should be used only if the benefit justifies the potential risk.
Morse and Whitaker: *J Reprod Med* 2000;**45**:850.
Saadi *et al.*: *Endocr Pract* 1999;**5**:33.
Tsai *et al.*: *BMC Pregnancy Childbirth* 2004;**4**:27.

Gentamicin – See Part 2, pp. 237–238

Glatiramer

There are few data for glatiramer use during pregnancy and lactation. Preliminary evidence suggests that it is not associated with IUGR, congenital anomaly, preterm birth or spontaneous abortion. Rodent teratogenicity studies are reassuring. It is not known if glatiramer enters breast milk, but limited experience of use suggests that it is safe. Moreover, exclusive breastfeeding has been shown to reduce MS relapse rates, so it should be encouraged. Although evidence is beginning to emerge suggesting that it may be used during both pregnancy and lactation, for the time being, the evidence is too limited, and glatiramer should be used only if the benefit justifies the perinatal risk.
Giannini *et al.*: *BMC Neurol* 2012;**12**:124.
Langer-Gould *et al.*: *Arch Neurol* 2009;**66**:958.
Lu *et al.*: *Neurology* 2012;**79**:1130.

Glibenclamide (glyburide, USAN)

Small amounts of glibenclamide cross the placenta. Rodent studies are reassuring. Studies in humans have not showed any increase in malformations. There is an increased risk of transient neonatal hypoglycaemia. One small study (five women) was unable to detect any in breast milk, and there were no effects on the breastfed infant.
Feig *et al.*: *Diabetes Care* 2005;**28**:1851.
Moretti *et al.*: *Ann Pharmacother* 2008;**42**:483.

Glimepiride

It is not known whether glimepiride crosses the placenta (other second-generation sulphonylureas do so only poorly). Neonatal hyperinsulinaemic hypoglycaemia has been reported after *in utero* exposure. Rodent teratology studies are reassuring. It is not known whether glimepiride enters breast milk in humans (it is reported to do so in rodents). Glimepiride should be used during pregnancy and lactation only if the perinatal risk is justified; better studied agents (metformin and glibenclamide) are preferred if an oral hypoglycaemic is necessary.
Balaguer Santamaría *et al.*: *Rev Clin Esp* 2000;**200**:399.

Glipizide

Small amounts (~6% of the maternal dose) of glipizide cross isolated human placenta. No teratogenic effects were found in rodents. In most cases, if glycaemic control is not achieved with diet±metformin, then insulin is used. Minute quantities of glipizide may be found in breast milk. These are not likely to be of clinical significance in the breastfed infant; however, monitoring of the infant for signs of hypoglycaemia is advised.
Elliott *et al.*: *Am J Obstet Gynecol* 1994;**171**:653.
Feig *et al.*: *Diabetes Care* 2005;**28**:1851.

Glucagon – See Part 2, pp. 239–240

Glycerin

Glycerin may be used to treat constipation during pregnancy, and low maternal systemic absorption means that it is unlikely to affect either the fetus or breastfed infant.
Shafe *et al.*: *Therap Adv Gastroenterol* 2011;**4**:343.

Glyceryl trinitrate (nitroglycerin, USAN) – See Part 2, pp. 243–244

Glycopyrrolate (glycopyrronium)

Glycopyrrolate probably crosses the placenta. Small (and clinically insignificant) amounts of glycopyrronium were found in umbilical blood following intramuscular use during caesarean section. Rodent teratogenicity studies are reassuring. It is not known if glycopyrrolate enters breast milk; however, it has poor oral bioavailability, meaning the breastfed infant is unlikely to be affected.
Ali-Melkkilä *et al.*: *Anaesthesia* 1990;**45**:634.

Granisetron

This selective 5HT$_3$ antagonist is used to prevent emesis after caesarean section and during chemotherapy. It is not known if granisetron crosses the placenta. Rodent teratogenicity studies are reassuring. The related drug, ondansetron, does not appear to cause problems in the human fetus. It is not known whether granisetron enters breast milk. Ondansetron is

an alternative which has been studied slightly more during pregnancy and lactation.
Tan *et al.*: *Int J Obstet Anesth* 2010;**19**:56.

Griseofulvin

Imidazole antifungals have now largely replaced griseofulvin in the treatment of fungal skin infections. Griseofulvin is known to be teratogenic and embryotoxic in some animals and has, as a result, been little used during pregnancy. The manufacturers advise avoiding conception for 6 months after receiving treatment because there is evidence of genotoxicity in mice. No information exists on use during lactation.
Czeizel *et al.*: *Acta Obstet Gynecol Scand* 2004;**83**:827.

Haemophilus influenzae type B vaccine – See Part 2, pp. 251–252

Haloperidol

Haloperidol crosses the placenta. While it is teratogenic in some rodents, there is no clear evidence of this in humans. Overdose was reported to cause neuromuscular depression in the fetus long after the mother had recovered (long-term outcome was not reported). Haloperidol enters breast milk in unpredictable fashion but never at levels that are clinically significant in the breastfed infant, and there are no reports of sedation or impaired development.
Einarson and Boskovic: *J Psychiatr Pract* 2009;**15**:183.
Hansen *et al.*: *Obstet Gynecol* 1997;**90**:659.
Klinger *et al.*: *Pediatr Endocrinol Rev* 2013;**10**:308.

Heparin – See Part 2, pp. 253–254

Hepatitis A vaccine

Hepatitis A virus is rarely transmitted to the fetus and is not a known teratogen. The vaccine consists of inactivated virus. The antibodies produced in response to vaccination are known to cross the placenta and may provide enhanced protection during the neonatal period. It is not known whether hepatitis A vaccine enters human breast milk. It is likely that the resulting antibodies do, but it is not known whether they confer any immunity for the breastfed newborn. The vaccine is generally considered compatible with breastfeeding.

Hepatitis B immune globulin – See Part 2, p. 256

Hepatitis B vaccine – See Part 2, pp. 256–257

Hydralazine

Hydralazine readily crosses the placenta; however, the direct effect on the fetus is unclear.

Use during the first trimester does not seem to cause teratogenic effects. In later pregnancy, hydralazine causes a variable effect on placental blood flow, and this is greatly influenced by the occurrence of maternal hypotension. Hydralazine is excreted into breast milk, but the amount ingested by the breastfeeding infant is clinically insignificant.
Liedholm *et al.*: *Eur J Clin Pharmacol* 1982;**21**:417.
Magee *et al.*: *Br Med J* 2003;**327**:955.

Hydrochlorothiazide

Hydrochlorothiazide appears in a number of combination antihypertensives. It crosses the placenta (F/M ratio ~0.5) but does not appear to be teratogenic. It can cause neonatal electrolyte abnormalities, thrombocytopenia and hyperglycaemia when given in the period before delivery. Hydrochlorothiazide enters breast milk but the infant receives a clinically insignificant amount.
Collins *et al.*: *Br Med J* 1985;**290**:17.
Miller *et al.*: *J Pediatr* 1982;**101**:789.

Hydrocortisone – See Part 2, pp. 260–261

Hydromorphone

Hydromorphone crosses the placenta (F/M ratio ~1). Most reports of its use relate to peripartum analgesia, and as with all opiates, there may be respiratory depression of the exposed infant. Hydromorphone passes into breast milk but appears to do so in small amounts that are not clinically significant. The risks of adverse effects are increased with long-term opiate use as accumulation may occur; it is advisable to limit maternal hydromorphone to short-term use and to supplement analgesia with a non-narcotic analgesic if necessary.
Sauberan *et al.*: *Obstet Gynecol* 2011;**117**:611.

Hydroxycarbamide (hydroxyurea, USAN)

It is not known whether hydroxycarbamide crosses the placenta. It is embryotoxic and teratogenic in animal models. In humans, the risk of teratogenicity is somewhat lower (although in many cases it was discontinued early in pregnancy). Hydroxycarbamide passes into breast milk in small amounts. Due to potential toxicity in the infant, breastfeeding should be discontinued (or at least temporarily suspended for 24–48 hours after the dose).
Stevens: *J Biol Regul Homeost Agents* 1999;**13**:172.

Hydroxychloroquine

There is no evidence of teratogenicity in rodents; however, hydroxychloroquine crosses the placenta and is deposited in pigmented fetal tissues. Large clinical series of its use in pregnant women with either malaria or connective tissue disorders are reassuring. Small amounts enter breast milk, but the drug is considered compatible with breastfeeding.

Abarientos et al.: Expert Opin Drug Saf 2011;**10**:705.
Temprano et al.: Semin Arthritis Rheum 2005;**35**:112.

Hydroxyzine

Hydroxyzine crosses the placenta and neonatal blood levels approximate those in the mother. There have been reports of neonatal withdrawal and seizure. Otherwise, there seems to be no major malformations in exposed infants. It is not known whether hydroxyzine enters breast milk. Cetirizine, which is a metabolite of hydroxyzine, enters breast milk but with no reported effects on the breastfed infant.

Einarson et al.: Ann Allergy Asthma Immunol 1997;**78**:183.
Prenner: Am J Dis Child 1977;**131**:529.
Serreau et al.: Reprod Toxicol 2005;**20**:573.

Hyoscine (scopolamine, USAN)

Hyoscine rapidly crosses the placenta and may cause fetal tachycardia and decreased beat-to-beat variability. Rodent teratogenicity studies are reassuring. Toxicity (fever, tachycardia and lethargy) has been described in the exposed infant after parenteral use in the mother. This was not seen with transdermal patches used to prevent nausea and vomiting during caesarean section. No information is available on the use of hyoscine during breastfeeding. Long-term use (as with other anticholinergics) might reduce milk production.

Evens and Leopold: Pediatrics 1980;**66**:329.
Harnett et al.: Anesth Analg 2007;**105**:764.

Ibuprofen – See Part 2, pp. 262–263

Idarubicin

Idarubicin appears to cross the placenta, causing fetal cardiotoxicity (although it is usually used with other drugs that might contribute to the cardiotoxic effect). It is both embryotoxic and teratogenic in rodents. There are no published reports of its use during lactation. It is not known whether idarubicin enters breast milk; however, considering its impact on DNA synthesis, it is best avoided.

Achtari and Hohlfeld: Am J Obstet Gynecol 2000;**183**:511.

Imipenem with cilastatin – See Part 2, pp. 264–265

Imipramine

Imipramine crosses the placenta but is not associated with teratogenicity in either rodents or humans. Neonatal withdrawal symptoms have been reported. Small amounts appear in breast milk, but there is no evidence that it causes problems in the breastfed infant.

Crombie et al.: Br Med J 1972;**1**:745.
Lanza di Scalea and Wisner: Clin Obstet Gynecol 2009;**52**:483.

Imiquimod

Imiquimod is sometimes used for the treatment of anogenital warts. It is not known whether it crosses the placenta. Rodent studies are reassuring, as are limited data from case studies. There are no published reports of use during lactation. Given the limited systemic absorption, the amounts available for transfer to milk should also be low. Nonetheless, due to the lack of safety data for use during pregnancy and lactation, imiquimod is best avoided.

Ciavattini et al.: J Matern Fetal Neonatal Med 2012;**25**:873.

Indapamide

It is not known whether indapamide crosses the placenta. Rodent studies are reassuring; however, other thiazides have neonatal sequelae. There are no published reports of use during lactation, and the manufacturer's SPC states that indapamide passes into breast milk. There are alternatives for which there is more experience during pregnancy and lactation.

Indinavir

Indinavir crosses the placenta although in vivo fetal exposure appears to be minimal. Although most rodent teratogenicity studies are reassuring, indinavir was associated with delayed growth and skeletal and ophthalmic abnormalities in one study. Limited human experience does not suggest a major fetal risk. Indinavir enters breast milk. Nonetheless, breastfeeding is contraindicated where formula milk is available to reduce the risk of neonatal transmission.

Unadkat et al.: Antimicrob Agents Chemother 2007;**51**:783.

Indomethacin – See archived monograph on website

Infliximab

Infliximab is a monoclonal antibody against tumour necrosis factor alpha (TNF-α) used to treat a number of inflammatory diseases. It crosses the placenta and limited case reports are reassuring, suggesting maternal benefit in the absence of any adverse fetal effects. Rodent teratogenicity studies have not been performed. Infliximab crosses into breast milk in very small amounts which should not cause problems in the breastfed neonate.

Fritzsche *et al.*: *J Clin Gastroenterol* 2012;**46**:718.
Gisbert: *Inflamm Bowel Dis* 2010;**16**:881.

Influenza vaccine – See Part 2, pp. 271–272

Insulin – See Part 2, pp. 273–274

Ipratropium bromide – See Part 2, pp. 275–276

Irbesartan

Irbesartan is an angiotensin II receptor antagonist with many properties similar to the ACE inhibitors. It is not known if it crosses the placenta; however, other drugs in this class do, and adverse fetal renal effects (anuria and oligohydramnios) have been reported. Angiotensin II receptor antagonists are considered both teratogenic and fetotoxic. They may cause cranial hypoplasia, renal failure (sometimes irreversible), oligohydramnios, anuria, death, prematurity, IUGR and PDA. There are no reports of use during lactation, and it is not known if it enters breast milk. Some ACE inhibitors can be used during lactation and may offer a suitable alternative.

Schaefer: *Birth Defects Res A Clin Mol Teratol* 2003;**67**:591.
Velázquez-Armenta *et al.*: *Hypertens Pregnancy* 2007;**26**:51.

Irinotecan

Women of childbearing age are advised to use effective contraception during treatment. Rodent studies reveal that irinotecan is embryotoxic and teratogenic. While there are no studies in human lactation, irinotecan is concentrated in rodent breast milk and should probably be considered incompatible with breastfeeding.

Cirillo *et al.*: *Tumori* 2012;**98**:155e.
Taylor *et al.*: *Obstet Gynecol* 2009;**114**:451.

Isocarboxazid

It is not known whether isocarboxazid crosses the placenta (it does in rats). Rodent teratogenicity studies have not been performed; however, other MAOIs have been associated with fetal malformations. Experience with isocarboxazid during lactation is also lacking, and it is not known if it enters breast milk. Use is best avoided during pregnancy and lactation.

Sato *et al.*: *Jpn J Pharmacol* 1972;**22**:629.

Isoniazid – See Part 2, pp. 280–281

Isosorbide mononitrate and dinitrate

The main use of nitrates is in the treatment of coronary heart disease although it has been reported as being used in hypertension in pregnancy. It is not known whether either drug crosses the placenta. Both have been used for cervical ripening prior to induction of labour, and adverse effects were not reported. It is not known whether either drug enters breast milk. Caution should be employed if it is used during breastfeeding.

Haghighi *et al.*: *J Obstet Gynaecol* 2013;**33**:272.
Hatanaka *et al.*: *Clin Exp Obstet Gynecol* 2012;**39**:175.

Isotretinoin

Isotretinoin is contraindicated during pregnancy. It is a known human teratogen causing abnormalities of the skeleton, central nervous system, and cardiovascular and endocrine organs. There is a well-described retinoic embryopathy. It is not known if isotretinoin enters breast milk (other retinoids do); however, the potential for adverse effects is too high to allow treatment during breastfeeding.

Lammer *et al.*: *N Engl J Med* 1985;**313**:837.

Isradipine

Isradipine has been used as a tocolytic and has also been used to treat pre-eclamptic hypertension. It crosses the placenta (F/M ratio ~0.25) but does not seem to impact on fetal haemodynamics. There are no reported adverse effects after *in utero* exposure. It is not known if isradipine enters breast milk (other calcium channel blockers do so only minimally and may be better alternatives).

Fletcher *et al.*: *J Obstet Gynaecol* 1999;**19**:235.

Itraconazole

While evidence from cohort studies shows brief exposure to this antifungal during early pregnancy is compatible with a normal pregnancy outcome, there is evidence of dose-related toxicity and teratogenicity in animals, and other azoles are known to induce malformations in man. Reports of use, whether inadvertent or otherwise, show low risk of major congenital malformations. Itraconazole enters breast milk in small amounts. In newborn animals, it has been shown to cause bony defects, and for this reason, it is best avoided (fluconazole would be a better alternative).

Bar-Oz *et al.*: *Am J Obstet Gynecol* 2000;**183**:617.

Ivermectin – See Part 2, pp. 282–283

Ketoconazole

Ketoconazole is known to be both embryotoxic and teratogenic in rats, causing syndactyly and oligodactyly (as well as maternal toxicity) when used in very high doses. Limb malformations have also been reported in humans. Ketoconazole is known to cause hepatotoxicity when administered orally (and the MHRA has stated that it should no longer be used for the treatment of fungal infection). It may be used topically; other antifungals should be used if systemic administration is required. Apart from its antifungal activity, ketoconazole is also used in Cushing's syndrome to reduce cortisol production, and case reports of use during pregnancy for this indication show no increase in malformations. Ketoconazole passes into breast milk in small amounts (these are probably negligible when ketoconazole is used topically); moreover, absorption (which is best under acidic conditions) may be reduced by the breast milk. Consequently, although the manufacturer advises avoidance of use, Hale, the AAP and others suggest that it is probably safe and compatible with breastfeeding.

Boronat *et al.*: *Gynecol Endocrinol* 2011;**27**:675.
Kazy *et al.*: *Congenit Anom (Kyoto)* 2005;**45**:5.
Loli *et al.*: *J Clin Endocrinol Metab* 1986;**63**:1365.

Ketoprofen
Ketoprofen rapidly crosses the placenta (F/M ratio ~1). Although rodent studies are reassuring, one case report suggests that ketoprofen, like other NSAIDs, causes fetal oliguria and ductal constriction. Acute renal failure has been reported in preterm infants whose mothers received ketoprofen prior to delivery. Ketoprofen passes into breast milk in small amounts that are unlikely to affect the breastfed infant.

Bannwarth *et al.*: *Br J Clin Pharmacol* 1999;**47**:459.
Jacqz-Aigrain *et al.*: *Ther Drug Monit* 2007;**29**:815.

Ketorolac trometamol
Ketorolac crosses the placenta. Most other NSAIDs cause fetal oliguria and ductal constriction, but it is not known if the same is true of ketorolac. Oligohydramnios was not seen in 45 women treated with ketorolac in a trial looking at its use as a tocolytic. Rodent studies are reassuring, revealing no evidence of teratogenicity or IUGR. Small quantities of ketorolac are found in breast milk but are unlikely to cause any problems in the breastfed infant.

Schorr *et al.*: *South Med J* 1998;**91**:1028.
Walker *et al.*: *Eur J Clin Pharmacol* 1988;**34**:509.

Labetalol – See Part 2, pp. 286–287

Lactulose
Lactulose is a frequently used laxative during pregnancy. Poor maternal absorption (~3% of the dose only) means that it is unlikely the maternal systemic concentration will reach a level that will impact on the fetus. Rodent teratogenicity studies are reassuring. It is not known whether lactulose enters breast milk. Again, because of poor maternal absorption, it is unlikely that the breastfed infant would receive a significant amount.

Shafe *et al.*: *Therap Adv Gastroenterol* 2011;**4**:343.

Lamivudine – See Part 2, pp. 288–289

Lamotrigine – See Part 2, pp. 290–291

Lansoprazole
It is not known if lansoprazole crosses the placenta. Although the manufacturer (and the BNF) advises avoiding use during pregnancy, most epidemiological and post-marketing surveillance studies of proton pump inhibitors (lansoprazole is the least well studied) and rodent teratogenicity studies are reassuring. It is not known whether lansoprazole enters breast milk. Omeprazole is a better studied alternative (it enters breast milk in low levels but has a known safety profile).

Broussard and Richter: *Drug Saf* 1998;**19**:325.
Diav-Citrin *et al.*: *Aliment Pharmacol Ther* 2005;**21**:269.

Levetiracetam – See Part 2, pp. 292–293

Levocetirizine
Levocetirizine is the main active compound in cetirizine. Although there are no reports of levocetirizine use during pregnancy, it is expected that there will be similarities with cetirizine. Neither first- nor second-generation antihistamines have been found to be teratogenic. It is not known if levocetirizine enters breast milk (cetirizine is reported to do so). In general, first-generation antihistamines are preferred to newer ones due to the greater experience of use.

Levodopa
Parkinson's disease symptoms often worsen during pregnancy. Levodopa is usually given with an extracerebral dopa-decarboxylase inhibitor (e.g. benserazide or carbidopa) to counter systemic side effects. Levodopa crosses the placenta (F/M ratio ~1). While it appears to concentrate in the fetal brain, most studies reveal no evidence of teratogenicity, and rodent studies are generally reassuring. Levodopa is excreted into breast milk in small amounts that do not seem to cause problems in the breastfed infant. While it suppresses prolactin release, the suckling stimulus seems to override any inhibitory effect in most women.

Hagell *et al.*: *Mov Disord* 1998;**13**:34.
Thulin *et al.*: *Neurology* 1998;**50**:1920.

Levofloxacin
Animal studies of several quinolones show a juvenile arthropathy, and it is this toxicity that has lead to their restricted use during pregnancy. This has not been seen following use of quinolones in human pregnancy. Rodent studies with levofloxacin are reassuring, and less than 4% of levofloxacin crosses an isolated perfused human placenta, suggesting that it might be safer than

other quinolones. Levofloxacin passes into breast milk, but the breastfed infant receives far less than is used to treat children.

Cahill *et al.*: *Pharmacotherapy* 2005;**25**:116.
Lipsky and Baker: *Clin Infect Dis* 1999;**28**:352.

Levomepromazine (methotrimeprazine, USAN)

Levomepromazine is related to chlorpromazine and used as a sedative and analgesic. It has also been used in hyperemesis when other drugs do not work. It is not known whether levomepromazine crosses the placenta, and rodent teratogenicity studies have not been performed. It is not known whether the drug appears in breast milk.

Callaghan and Zelenik: *Am J Obstet Gynecol* 1966;**95**:636.
Heazell *et al.*: *Reprod Toxicol* 2005;**20**:569.

Levothyroxine sodium

Transplacental transfer of thyroxine is low but is sufficient to prevent the fetus without a thyroid gland from showing overt clinical hypothyroidism. In contrast, even subclinical maternal hypothyroidism in early pregnancy may increase the risk of spontaneous abortion and adversely affect neurodevelopment. The aim of treatment is to keep the maternal TSH less than 2.5 mU/l. Small amounts (too low to treat the hypothyroid baby) are found in breast milk.

Mizuta *et al.*: *Pediatr Res* 1983;**17**:468.
Polak: *Horm Res Paediatr* 2011;**76**(suppl 1):97.

Lidocaine (lignocaine, former BAN) – See Part 2, pp. 296–298

Linagliptin

Linagliptin inhibits dipeptidylpeptidase-4 to increase insulin secretion and lower glucagon secretion. It is not known if linagliptin crosses the placenta. Rodent teratogenicity studies have not been reported. No information is available on the use of linagliptin during breastfeeding or whether it passes into breast milk. Linagliptin is best avoided during both pregnancy and lactation until further information is available.

Linezolid – See Part 2, pp. 299–300

Liothyronine sodium

Liothyronine is a synthetic triiodothyronine (T3). Transplacental transfer of endogenous T3 occurs in low, but physiologically relevant, levels. Dose adjustment of thyroid hormones is frequently needed during pregnancy, and even subclinical hypothyroidism is best avoided. Small amounts of liothyronine are detectable in breast milk. These do not cause any reported adverse effects and are insufficient to act as hormone replacement for the breastfed hypothyroid infant.

Khandelwal and Tandon: *Drugs* 2012;**72**:17.
Varma *et al.*: *J Pediatr* 1978;**93**:803.

Lisdexamfetamine

Lisdexamfetamine is a prodrug of dexamfetamine and both are used to treat ADHD in children and adults (although the latter use is off-licence). See section on *amfetamine* for effects during pregnancy and lactation.

Lisinopril

Lisinopril crosses the placenta. While no adverse effects are reported following first trimester use, exposure during the third trimester is reported to cause fetal renal failure (which may be irreversible) and oligohydramnios. Screening for oligohydramnios may detect the affected fetus and allow cessation of lisinopril therapy. Because the drug is renally excreted, the effects may be prolonged and, in some cases, become irreversible. There are no reports of lisinopril use during lactation, nor is it known if lisinopril enters breast milk. Other ACE inhibitors (e.g. captopril and enalapril) are considered compatible with breastfeeding.

Bhatt-Mehta and Deluga: *Pharmacotherapy* 1993;**13**:515.

Loperamide

Use of loperamide during pregnancy does not seem to be associated with an increased risk of major malformations. Rodent teratogenicity studies are also reassuring. Because it is minimally absorbed, only extremely small amounts may be found in breast milk. No adverse effects in exposed infants have been reported.

Einarson *et al.*: *Can J Gastroenterol* 2000;**14**:185.
Nikodem and Hofmeyr: *Eur J Clin Pharmacol* 1992;**42**:695.

Loratadine

It is not known whether loratadine crosses the placenta. One early study observed a prevalence of hypospadias twice that of the general population; however, this has not been confirmed. Rodent teratogenicity studies are reassuring. Loratadine and its active metabolite, descarboethoxyloratadine (desloratadine), pass into breast milk, but the breastfed infant receives a dose of less than 1% of the adult dose on a milligram-per-kilogram basis.

Hilbert *et al.*: *J Clin Pharmacol* 1988;**28**:234.
Schwarz *et al.*: *Drug Saf* 2008;**31**:775.

Lorazepam – See Part 2, pp. 305–306

Macrogols (polyethylene glycol)

The main use of macrogols during pregnancy is in treatment of constipation. They are becoming the most commonly prescribed laxative in pregnant women. It is not known if macrogols cross the placenta, but there is little if any systemic absorption. Use during pregnancy likely represents little risk to the fetus. It is not known if macrogols enter breast milk. With the lack of systemic absorption, they are unlikely to achieve clinically relevant levels in breast milk.

Shafe et al.: Therap Adv Gastroenterol 2011;**4**:343.
Tytgat et al.: Aliment Pharmacol Ther 2003;**18**:291.

Magnesium sulfate – See Part 2, pp. 307–308

Mannitol – See archived monograph on website

Mebendazole – See Part 2, pp. 309–310

Medroxyprogesterone
While as a contraceptive medroxyprogesterone should not be used during pregnancy, inadvertent exposure does occur especially during the first trimester. Implants should be removed if pregnancy is continued. There is some suggestion that in utero exposure of male fetuses may double the risk of hypospadias. Abnormalities beyond the external genitalia are not noted in either humans or rodents. Trace amounts of medroxyprogesterone are found in breast milk. It does not appear to either suppress lactation or affect the nursing infant. Although not specifically used as a galactagogue, depot medroxyprogesterone is reported to have beneficial effects on milk supply in women using the drug for contraception.

Karim et al.: Br Med J 1971;**1**:200.
Yovich et al.: Teratology 1988;**38**:135.

Mefenamic acid
Mefenamic acid crosses the placenta (F/M ratio ~0.32 in the second trimester). As with other NSAIDs, it can cause ductal closure. Rodent teratogenicity studies are reassuring. If mefenamic acid is to be used during the second and third trimesters, the fetus must be monitored for signs of ductal closure. Small amounts of mefenamic acid pass into breast milk and may be absorbed by the nursing infant. Although the manufacturer advises to avoid its use, in general, it is regarded as being compatible with breastfeeding.

Buchanan et al.: Curr Ther Res Clin Exp 1968;**10**:592.
Menahem: Aust N Z J Obstet Gynaecol 1991;**31**:190.

Mefloquine – See Part 2, pp. 311–312

Meloxicam
Meloxicam crosses the placenta and in high doses is associated with cardiac septal defects and embryotoxicity in rodents. As with most NSAIDs, there is the potential for closure of the fetal ductus arteriosus after maternal use. Third trimester use should only be with fetal monitoring. It is not known whether meloxicam passes into breast milk. Because it has a long half-life, other NSAIDs are preferred.

Nielsen et al.: Br Med J 2001;**322**:266.

Meprobamate
Meprobamate crosses the placenta. Several studies suggest an increased prevalence of malformations associated with first trimester use. There was no clear evidence of teratogenicity or fetotoxicity following attempted maternal suicide when very large doses were ingested. As with many drugs during pregnancy, monotherapy and using the lowest effective dose might minimise the risks. Small amounts of meprobamate enter breast milk, but these do not pose a clinically significant risk to the breastfed infant.

Hartz et al.: N Engl J Med 1975;**292**:726.
Timmermann et al.: Toxicol Ind Health 2008;**24**:97.

Mercaptopurine
Mercaptopurine, the active metabolite of azathioprine, is a commonly used anti-neoplastic and immunomodulatory agent that may be required during pregnancy. It probably crosses the placenta and, as a result, can cause severe, but transient, neonatal pancytopenia. The effects of administration during the first trimester are mixed; some cohort studies report a higher incidence of anomalies, while others do not. Many women are exposed to more than one drug as well as to the effects of the underlying disease. Rodent studies show some evidence of teratogenicity with malformations of the jaw, limbs and gut. In general, treatment should not be withheld if medically indicated, and the risk of neonatal marrow suppression can be minimised by reducing the dose near to term. Mercaptopurine and azathioprine pass into breast milk in small amounts, and although marrow suppression may occur in the breastfed neonate, the risk is very low.

Casanova et al.: Am J Gastroenterol 2013;**108**:433.
Nørgård et al.: Am J Gastroenterol 2007;**102**:1406.

Mesalazine (mesalamine, USAN)
Active inflammatory bowel disease can adversely affect pregnancy outcomes – causing spontaneous abortions, stillbirths and growth restriction. Mesalazine (5-ASA) has been used during pregnancy without any reports of fetal or infant adverse effects. Only trace amounts of 5-ASA can be found in the fetus, and rodent teratogenicity studies are reassuring. Use during lactation also seems safe although diarrhoea has been reported in a few babies.

Cassina et al.: Expert Opin Drug Saf 2009;**8**:695.
Silverman et al.: Gut 2005;**54**:170.

Metformin

Using metformin to control blood sugar during pregnancy in women with either type 2 or 'gestational' diabetes seems as effective as insulin and carries fewer adverse side effects in both mother and fetus. First trimester use also seems safe in polycystic ovary syndrome. Use in late pregnancy does not seem to increase the risk of neonatal hypoglycaemia. Small amounts of metformin are excreted into breast milk without any apparent effect on the breastfed infant.

Briggs et al.: Obstet Gynecol 2005;**105**:1437.
Gui et al.: PLoS One 2013;**8**:e64585.
Sun et al.: Arch Gynecol Obstet 2013;**288**:423.

Methadone – See Part 2, pp. 320–321

Methotrexate

Methotrexate has multiple uses in reproductive-age women (including the medical treatment of ectopic pregnancy). It is not known if methotrexate crosses the placenta. Exposure during the first trimester results in an increased risk of malformations or 'methotrexate embryopathy' (consisting of craniofacial abnormalities and limb and digit deformities). This syndrome seems to be associated with exposures 6–8 weeks after conception and with doses ≥10 mg/week. Most children born to mothers on low-dose treatment (<10 mg/week) seem normal at birth. There does not seem to be any association between later pregnancy exposure and fetal abnormalities. Methotrexate passes into breast milk, and most sources consider breastfeeding to be contraindicated during maternal anti-neoplastic therapy. Where the maternal dose is smaller (<65 mg) and administered either weekly or in single doses, the levels are low enough for some authors to suggest that the risks to the infant are low enough to permit breastfeeding. In this case, monitoring of the infant's blood count and differential is advisable.

Hyoun et al.: Birth Defects Res A Clin Mol Teratol 2012;**94**:187.
Johns et al.: Am J Obstet Gynecol 1972;**112**:978.

Methoxypsoralen

It is not known if 8-methoxypsoralen crosses the placenta. Rodent teratogenicity studies have not been performed. Limited preconception and first trimester use was largely associated with normal pregnancy outcomes. Use of 8-methoxypsoralen during breastfeeding does not appear to have been reported. Because of its role as a photosensitiser, it is recommended that if used during breastfeeding, then feeds should be stopped and the milk discarded for at least 24 hours (by which time ~95% of the dose will be excreted in the maternal urine).

Garbis et al.: Arch Dermatol 1995;**131**:492.

Methyldopa

Methyldopa is perhaps the best studied antihypertensive drug during pregnancy. It crosses the placenta and achieves levels in the fetus similar to those in the mother. There are no reported short- or long-term effects on the fetus or the neonate. Rodent teratogenicity studies are also reassuring. Small amounts of methyldopa are excreted into breast milk, but they have not been shown to cause any adverse effects in the breastfed infant.

Beardmore et al.: Hypertens Pregnancy 2002;**21**:85.
Vest and Cho: Cardiol Clin 2012;**30**:407.

Methylphenidate

It is not known whether methylphenidate crosses the placenta. Limited human data do not indicate a significant risk of structural abnormalities, but rodent teratogenicity studies reveal skeletal abnormalities in rabbits treated with high doses and IUGR in lower doses. Also, rodent studies suggest a possible adverse effect on brain development. Methylphenidate enters breast milk; published cases, however, were in infants several months old. While levels of methylphenidate in breast milk were low and no adverse effects were reported, this may not be the case in younger infants. The manufacturers currently advise to avoid use during breastfeeding, but with careful dosing combined with planned timing of feeding, exposure to the infant may be minimised.

Bolea-Alamanac et al.: Br J Clin Pharmacol 2013 Apr 18. doi: 10.1111/bcp.12138. [Epub ahead of print]
Hackett et al.: Ann Pharmacother 2006;**40**:1890.

Methylprednisolone

Methylprednisolone does not cross the placenta and there are no reports of malformations. There are no data on the excretion of methylprednisolone into breast milk. Despite lack of data, methylprednisolone is generally considered safe during pregnancy and lactation for recognised medical indications.

Pacheco et al.: Am J Perinatol 2007;**24**:79.

Metoclopramide – See Part 2, pp. 326–327

Metolazone

It is not known if metolazone crosses the placenta. Rodent teratogenicity studies are reassuring. Metolazone enters breast milk but there are no clinically significant effects on the infant. While metolazone does appear to be safe during pregnancy and lactation, there are few clinical indications for its use, and if these are present, there are other, better studied, alternatives.

Duffy *et al.*: *J Ir Med Assoc* 1972;**65**:615.

Metoprolol

Metoprolol crosses the placenta; however, it does not seem to cause the IUGR seen with some other β-blockers (e.g. atenolol and propranolol). Rodent teratogenicity studies are reassuring but high doses may cause embryotoxicity. Only small quantities of metoprolol are found in breast milk, and the neonatal plasma levels are very low or undetectable. No adverse effects are seen in the breastfed infant.

Benfield *et al.*: *Drugs* 1986;**31**:376.
Shannon *et al.*: *J Hum Lact* 2000;**16**:240.

Metronidazole – See Part 2, pp. 328–329

Miconazole

It is not known whether miconazole crosses the placenta. It is systemically absorbed in very small amounts after vaginal application. Rodent teratogenicity and post-marketing studies are reassuring, revealing no adverse outcomes. It is not known if miconazole enters breast milk. However, considering the dose and route, it is unlikely that the breastfed infant would ingest clinically relevant amounts.

Kjærstad *et al.*: *Eur J Clin Pharmacol* 2010;**66**:1189.
Timonen: *Mycoses* 1992;**35**:317.

Midazolam – See Part 2, pp. 334–335

Mifepristone

Mifepristone is a potent antiprogestogenic steroid used in 'medical' termination of pregnancy. A small proportion of women do not abort after its use, and while many will then choose to have a 'surgical' termination of pregnancy, some may not. They should be warned that mifepristone is teratogenic in rabbits but not rats or monkeys. Limited experience in humans has not shown any increase in malformations. Small amounts of mifepristone are found in breast milk if the drug is used during lactation. Although there are concerns about the potential for hormonal effects in the breastfed infant, these appear not to be borne out.

Bernard *et al.*: *BJOG* 2013;**120**:568.
Sääv *et al.*: *Acta Obstet Gynecol Scand* 2010;**89**:618.

Milrinone – See Part 2, pp. 338–339

Minocycline

It is not known whether minocycline crosses the placenta. Topical use is unlikely to result in significant maternal systemic concentrations; however, other tetracyclines can cross the placenta, and their use is associated with tooth discolouration. It is not known if minocycline enters breast milk. Black discolouration of breast milk is reported (and was postulated to be an iron chelate of minocycline or one of its derivatives).

Basler and Lynch: *Arch Dermatol* 1985;**121**:417.
Hunt *et al.*: *Br J Dermatol* 1996;**134**:943.

Minoxidil

It is not known whether minoxidil crosses the placenta. Caudal regression syndrome was reported when a mother had used minoxidil before and during her pregnancy. In one other case, multiple vascular malformations were seen in a number of organs and the placenta. Hypertrichosis has been reported in fetuses exposed to minoxidil throughout pregnancy (even when the drug was applied topically). Rodent teratogenicity studies are nonetheless reassuring. Minoxidil enters breast milk at concentrations that are too small to produce a clinically relevant effect. Minoxidil should be avoided in pregnancy but could be considered during lactation.

Rojansky *et al.*: *J Reprod Med* 2002;**47**:241.
Smorlesi *et al.*: *Birth Defects Res A Clin Mol Teratol* 2003;**67**:997.

Mirtazapine

It is not known whether mirtazapine crosses the placenta, although with a low molecular weight and long plasma half-life, transfer might be expected. It does not appear to carry any increased risk of malformations when used during the first and second trimesters. There is one case report of neonatal hypothermia through the first 10 days of life that has been attributed to mirtazapine. Mirtazapine enters breast milk but only small amounts are detected in the breastfed infant. Other drugs are available with a better studied safety profile during both pregnancy and lactation.

Kristensen *et al.*: *Br J Clin Pharmacol* 2007;**63**:322.
Sokolover *et al.*: *Can J Clin Pharmacol* 2008;**15**:e188.

Misoprostol – See Part 2, pp. 340–341

Mitomycin

Mitomycin is used to treat a variety of cancers. It is not known if it crosses the placenta in humans. In rodents (where transplacental transfer does occur), it is a potent teratogen causing embryo loss and bony malformations. There is no experience of use during human pregnancy. Use during lactation has not been reported, and it is not known if mitomycin enters breast milk.

Boike *et al.*: *Gynecol Oncol* 1989;**34**:187.

Mitoxantrone

It is not known whether mitoxantrone crosses the placenta. In the single report of use during the first trimester, there was growth restriction. Rodent teratogenicity studies are reassuring, but the doses studied were lower than those used in human clinical practice. Significant amounts of mitoxantrone enter breast milk. It should probably be considered incompatible with breastfeeding pending additional study.

Baumgärtner et al.: Onkologie 2009;**32**:40.
De Santis et al.: Neurotoxicology 2007;**28**:696.

Modafinil

Modafinil is used to treat narcolepsy. Limited animal data suggest moderate risk of skeletal and renal malformations. It is not known whether modafinil crosses the placenta or whether it enters breast milk – the manufacturer reports that it does so in animal studies. At present, modafinil should only be used during pregnancy and lactation if the benefit justifies the largely unquantified risks.

Williams et al.: Obstet Gynecol 2008;**111**:522.

Moexipril

There are no reports of use of this ACE inhibitor during pregnancy, and it is not known if it crosses the placenta. Other ACE inhibitors can cause fetal renal failure and are generally considered contraindicated during pregnancy. It is not known whether moexipril enters breast milk (captopril and enalapril are better studied alternatives).

Chrysant and Chrysant: J Clin Pharmacol 2004;**44**:827.

Mometasone

It is not known if mometasone crosses the placenta. Inhaled steroids are used widely during pregnancy and are not associated with malformations. Although it is not known whether mometasone enters breast milk, considering the dose and route, it is unlikely that breastfed neonates ingest clinically relevant amounts. Like other inhaled or intra-nasal steroids, mometasone is considered compatible with pregnancy and lactation.

BTS & SIGN: British Guideline on the Management of Asthma.
Keleş: Am J Rhinol 2004;**18**:23.

Montelukast

It is not known if montelukast crosses the placenta. It is not associated with any known teratogenic effect in animals. While a number of malformations have been reported in humans, the association with montelukast is unclear. The main consistent finding in outcomes after use during pregnancy appears to be an effect on fetal growth, with more women having smaller babies. This might be a reflection of their asthma severity rather than a direct drug effect. Use during lactation, although not reported in the literature, appears to be safe.

Nelsen et al.: J Allergy Clin Immunol 2012;**129**:251.
Sarkar et al.: Eur J Clin Pharmacol 2009;**65**:1259.

Morphine – See Part 2, pp. 344–345

Moxifloxacin

Moxifloxacin crosses the placenta in small amounts. Animal studies in rodents and dogs report that fetal exposure is associated with an arthropathy of the weight-bearing joints. This has led to the restricted use of quinolones in pregnant women. It is not known if moxifloxacin enters breast milk in humans (it is reported to do so in rodents, sheep and goats). At present, moxifloxacin should only be used during pregnancy and lactation if the benefit justifies the risk; there are better studied alternatives.

Ozyüncü et al.: J Obstet Gynaecol Res 2010;**36**:484.

Nabumetone

It is not known placental transfer of nabumetone occurs. Rodent studies are reassuring. In general though, NSAIDs should be avoided during the third trimester because of the risk of closure of fetal ductus arteriosus. There is a lack of experience during lactation, and it is not known if nabumetone (or its metabolite 6MNA) enters breast milk.

Hedner et al.: Drugs 2004;**64**:2315.

Nadolol

It is not known if nadolol crosses the placenta (similar drugs in this class do). Propranolol and labetalol are better studied β-blockers that can be used during pregnancy. Rodent teratogenicity studies of nadolol are generally reassuring. There is some evidence of growth restriction in animal studies, and reports of cardiorespiratory depression, mild hypoglycaemia and growth retardation in exposed neonates. Nadolol is excreted into breast milk. Although the breastfed infant receives only small amounts, the long half-life makes it less than ideal during lactation.

Devlin et al.: Br J Clin Pharmacol 1981;**12**:393.
Fox et al.: Am J Obstet Gynecol 1985;**152**:1045.

Nalidixic acid

Nalidixic acid crosses the placenta, and rodent and canine teratogenicity studies report an association of older quinolones, like nalidixic acid, with acute arthropathy of weight-bearing joints. This has led to the restricted use of these agents during pregnancy. A recent meta-analysis did not seem to bear out many of the concerns of previous studies. Nalidixic acid is excreted into breast milk, but only minimal amounts are ingested by the breastfed neonate. Haemolytic anaemia was reported in one infant. In general, the newer quinolones are preferred.

Bar-Oz *et al.*: *Eur J Obstet Gynecol Reprod Biol* 2009;**143**:75.

Belton and Jones: *Lancet* 1965;**2**:691.

Naloxone – See Part 2, pp. 347–348

Naltrexone

Naltrexone crosses the placenta. Rodent teratogenicity studies are generally reassuring, and there appears to be no behavioural problems seen with chronic opiate misuse. Although the manufacturer (and the BNF) states that naltrexone use should be avoided during breastfeeding due to toxicity, one exposed breastfed infant had plasma levels of the active metabolite, 6-beta-naltrexol, that were 'only marginally detectable'.

Chan *et al.*: *J Hum Lact* 2004;**20**:322.

Naproxen

Naproxen crosses the placenta (F/M ratio 0.92), and fetal levels are dependent on the maternal levels. Other NSAIDs can cause premature closure of the fetal ductus arteriosus, but this has not been reported after naproxen use. Rodent teratogenicity studies are reassuring, as are cohort studies in humans. Naproxen appears in breast milk in small quantities that are unlikely to cause any clinical effects in the breastfed infant.

Jamali and Stevens: *Drug Intell Clin Pharm* 1983;**17**:910.

Nezvalová-Henriksen *et al.*: *BJOG* 2013;**120**:948.

Talati *et al.*: *Am J Perinatol* 2000;**17**:69.

Naratriptan

It is not known if naratriptan crosses the placenta. Rodent studies reveal embryotoxicity and skeletal abnormalities at doses that are only just higher than those used in clinical practice. While studies in humans have not shown any major abnormalities, the numbers of reported cases are too few to adequately assess fetal risk. It is not known if it enters breast milk. Sumatriptan (which enters breast milk in small amounts) may be a better alternative to use until more information is available.

Cunnington *et al.*: *Headache* 2009;**49**:1414.

Duong *et al.*: *Can Fam Physician* 2010;**56**:537.

Nateglinide

Published reports of use during pregnancy are limited to a single case report where it was used until 24-week gestation (after which, treatment with insulin was initiated). It is not known if nateglinide crosses the placenta. Rodent studies are generally reassuring, although there is an increase in gallbladder agenesis at high doses. There is no published experience of use during breastfeeding. Glibenclamide and metformin are better studied oral hypoglycaemics used during pregnancy and lactation.

Teelucksingh *et al.*: *Reprod Toxicol* 2004;**18**:299.

Nedocromil sodium

It is not known if nedocromil crosses the placenta. Considering the dose and route, it is unlikely that maternal systemic concentration reaches a clinically relevant level. Rodent teratogenicity studies are reassuring. There is also no published experience in nursing women, and it is not known whether nedocromil enters breast milk. The potential for harm in a nursing infant is probably negligible given the dose and route of administration.

BTS & SIGN: British Guideline on the Management of Asthma.

Nelfinavir – See archived monograph on website

Neomycin sulphate

It is not known whether neomycin crosses the placenta (other aminoglycosides do). As a group, aminoglycosides have been associated with irreversible deafness after *in utero* exposure. They should generally be avoided during pregnancy, and if used, therapeutic monitoring should be undertaken. Rodent teratogenicity studies have not been performed. It is not known if neomycin enters breast milk, but oral bioavailability is poor and it is unlikely that the breastfed infant will receive significant amounts.

Czeizel *et al.*: *Scand J Infect Dis* 2000;**32**:309.

Neostigmine – See Part 2, pp. 349–350

Netilmicin – See archived monograph on website

Nevirapine – See Part 2, pp. 351–352

Nicardipine

Nicardipine crosses the placenta (F/M ratio 0.15–0.17). In animal studies, it adversely affected the fetus through its actions on the maternal uterine blood flow. In humans, there does not appear to be a significant teratogenic risk, and in one systematic review, nicardipine was as safe and as effective as labetalol. Nicardipine passes into breast milk in only tiny amounts that are unlikely to cause any problems in the breastfed infant.

Jarreau *et al.*: *Paediatr Perinat Drug Ther* 2000;**4**:28.

Peacock *et al.*: *Am J Emerg Med* 2012;**30**:981.

Nicotine replacement therapy

Smoking during pregnancy is a major risk factor for spontaneous abortion, preterm placental abruption, IUGR, late fetal death, neonatal polycythaemia and SUDI. Cigarette smoke contains thousands of chemicals, many of which are well-documented toxins (e.g. nicotine, carbon monoxide, lead). Nicotine replacement therapy may prevent exposure to some of the other chemicals and is therefore probably preferable to continued smoking; nonetheless, it carries its own risks. Non-pharmacological approaches to smoking cessation are safest for mother and her fetus, and these should be tried before embarking on nicotine replacement therapy. If treatment is necessary, it should be intermittent rather than continuous to reduce fetal exposure. The long-term effects of nicotine replacement therapy are unknown. Nicotine passes into breast milk (whether from smoking or from nicotine replacement therapy). During breastfeeding, patches, offering sustained lower doses, might be preferable to gum which can result in fluctuations in the maternal nicotine levels and thus breast milk.
Bruin *et al.*: *Toxicol Sci* 2010;**116**:364.
Coleman *et al.*: *Addiction* 2011;**106**:52.

Nifedipine – See Part 2, pp. 353–354

Nimodipine

Nimodipine crosses the placenta (F/M ratio ~1). Rodent studies are conflicting due to variations in placental transfer between species, but embryotoxicity, teratogenicity and IUGR are reported. Nimodipine enters breast milk, but the breastfed newborn ingests clinically insignificant amounts. Although appearing to be safe during lactation, there are alternative agents for which there is more experience regarding their use during pregnancy.
Carcas *et al.*: *Ann Pharmacother* 1996;**30**:148.
Belfort *et al.*: *N Engl J Med* 2003;**348**:304.

Nitrofurantoin

It is not known whether nitrofurantoin crosses the placenta. Rodent teratogenicity studies are reassuring, and there is no evidence of teratogenicity in humans. The manufacturer (and the BNF) advises that it should be avoided at term and in neonates due to risks of haemolytic anaemia; the evidence for this is scant and any haemolytic reactions, if they do occur, tend to be mild. Nitrofurantoin is excreted in breast milk in small amounts. Again, neonatal haemolysis (especially among those with G6PD deficiency) is thought to be a risk; however, there are no published reports of this.
Gait: *DICP* 1990;**24**:1210.
Varsano *et al.*: *J Pediatr* 1973;**82**:886.

Nizatidine

Nizatidine can be purchased OTC for the prevention and treatment of heartburn and indigestion in adult; however, the manufacturer (and the BNF) cautions against use in pregnancy. Rodent studies suggest a low teratogenic risk, and no increased malformations or fetal risks have been identified from limited exposure during human pregnancies. Only small amounts of nizatidine pass into breast milk and are unlikely to affect the breastfed infant.
Garbis *et al.*: *Reprod Toxicol* 2005;**19**:453.
Obermeyer *et al.*: *Clin Pharmacol Ther* 1990;**47**:724.

Norethisterone (norethindrone, USAN)

Norethisterone is found in combined oral contraceptive and progestogen-only pills. Masculinisation (mainly clitoral hypertrophy) is reported in between 0.3 and 18% of exposed female fetuses. A detailed fetal anomaly ultrasound scan at 18–20 weeks is recommended after first trimester exposure. Norethisterone is not teratogenic in rodents. It is thought to appear in breast milk in small quantities. Changes in breast milk volumes and composition have been reported. If hormonal contraceptives are necessary during lactation, then the lowest possible dose should be used.
Fraser: *Reprod Fertil Dev* 1991;**3**:245.
Jacobson: *Am J Obstet Gynecol* 1962;**84**:962.

Norfloxacin

It is not known if norfloxacin crosses the placenta, and while limited human experience is reassuring, there is conflicting data from animal studies. Arthropathy is a concern following use of other quinolones. Studies of use in children have not shown this to be a major problem with norfloxacin. It is not known if norfloxacin passes into breast milk (other quinolones may be found in breast milk). With limited data, it is not possible to determine if use during breastfeeding is safe; alternatives (e.g. ciprofloxacin) are available.
Ball *et al.*: *Drug Saf* 1999;**21**:407.
Loebstein *et al.*: *Antimicrob Agents Chemother* 1998;**42**:1336.

Nortriptyline

Nortriptyline crosses the placenta but fetal exposure is probably limited due to its lipophilicity. Two case reports suggested an association between nortriptyline and limb anomalies, but this has not been found elsewhere (and in one case, exposure was after the critical period for limb development). Rodent teratogenicity studies have yielded conflicting results. Case

series of nortriptyline use during pregnancies have not shown any increase in fetal adverse events. Only small amounts pass into breast milk, and many consider it a drug of choice for breastfeeding women with depression.
Sit *et al.*: *J Clin Psychiatry* 2011;**72**:994.
Weissman *et al.*: *Am J Psychiatry* 2004;**161**:1066.

Nystatin – See Part 2, pp. 365–366

Octreotide – See Part 2, pp. 367–368

Ofloxacin

Ofloxacin crosses the placenta, reaching therapeutic levels in the fetal serum and amniotic fluid. Rodent teratogenicity studies are generally reassuring. Arthropathy is occasionally seen in animal studies; however, this has not been seen following use of quinolones during human pregnancy. While the manufacturers advise that ofloxacin and other quinolones should be avoided in pregnancy because of this, the risk is probably not as great as originally thought. Ofloxacin passes into breast milk but is generally regarded as being compatible with breastfeeding.
Giamarellou *et al.*: *Am J Med* 1989;**87**:49S.
Loebstein *et al.*: *Antimicrob Agents Chemother* 1998;**42**:1336.

Olanzapine

Olanzapine crosses the placenta (F/M ratio ~0.7). Rodent teratogenicity studies are reassuring. A post-marketing surveillance report by the manufacturer of safety data has not identified increased adverse events in exposed fetuses. Small amounts of olanzapine pass into breast milk; most breastfed neonates are unaffected but a small proportion may show disturbed sleep patterns, irritability or tremor.
Brunner *et al.*: *BMC Pharmacol Toxicol* 2013;**14**:38.
Gilad *et al.*: *Breast feed Med* 2011;**6**:55.

Olmesartan medoxomil

Olmesartan probably crosses the placenta. Maternal use is associated with fetal renal failure and oligohydramnios. In those rare instances when angiotensin II receptor antagonists are necessary, women should be informed of the potential hazards and serial ultrasound examinations undertaken. There are no reports of use during lactation; in the absence of any information about transfer into milk and potential effects on the breastfed infant, olmesartan is probably best avoided. The ACE inhibitors captopril and enalapril are alternatives that may be used during breastfeeding.
Celentano *et al.*: *Pediatr Nephrol* 2008;**23**:333.
Sinelli *et al.*: *Pediatr Med Chir* 2008;**30**:306.

Olsalazine sodium

Active inflammatory bowel disease can adversely affect pregnancy outcomes. Olsalazine and its metabolites cross the placenta in small amounts. While high doses can cause poor growth, delayed skeletal and organ maturation in rodent studies, studies of use in human pregnancies are reassuring. The active metabolite, mesalazine, is excreted into breast milk. Use during lactation seems safe although diarrhoea has been reported in a few babies.
Miller *et al.*: *J Clin Pharmacol* 1993;**33**:703.
Rahimi *et al.*: *Reprod Toxicol* 2008;**25**:271.

Omeprazole – See Part 2, pp. 369–370

Ondansetron – See Part 2, pp. 371–372

Orlistat

Orlistat prevents absorption of dietary fats. It is not known if it crosses the placenta; however, there is very little maternal systemic absorption, meaning that at most the fetus will be exposed to small amounts. Only one case report has been published; a successful outcome was seen but orlistat and other medications were stopped early in the first trimester. It is not known if orlistat enters breast milk; however, the low maternal systemic levels suggest that the infant will not receive clinically relevant amounts.
Kalyoncu *et al.*: *Saudi Med J* 2005;**26**:497.

Oseltamivir – See Part 2, pp. 375–376

Oxazepam

Oxazepam crosses the placenta (F/M ratio ~0.5). Effects of benzodiazepines on the fetus are often difficult to assess; maternal denial regarding use and concurrent exposure to other drugs and substances are confounding factors. Long-term follow-up studies are for the most part reassuring with no increase in major malformations. Use during the final weeks of pregnancy may result in neonatal withdrawal. Minimal amounts of oxazepam appear in breast milk and are unlikely to have a significant clinical effect on the breastfed infant.
Jørgensen *et al.*: *Acta Obstet Gynecol Scand* 1988;**67**:493.
McElhatton: *Reprod Toxicol* 1994;**8**:461.
Wretlind: *Eur J Clin Pharmacol* 1987;**33**:209.

Oxcarbazepine

Oxcarbazepine is closely related to carbamazepine. It crosses the placenta and shows evidence of embryotoxicity and teratogenicity in a number of species. Human pregnancy data are limited, but the related drug carbamazepine is considered to be a modest teratogen. The risk of any anticonvulsant medication is magnified if it is used with other anticonvulsants. Oxcarbazepine and its active metabolite, 10-hydroxycarbazepine, pass into breast milk in small amounts and have not been shown to accumulate or cause adverse effects in breast-fed infants.

Lutz *et al.*: *J Clin Psychopharmacol* 2007;**27**:730.
Reimers and Brodtkorb: *Expert Rev Neurother* 2012;**12**:707.
Wegner *et al.*: *Epilepsia* 2010;**51**:2500.

Oxybutynin

It is not known whether oxybutynin crosses the placenta. Rodent teratogenicity studies are reassuring. It is not known whether it enters breast milk, but it is absorbed only poorly after oral administration.

Edwards *et al.*: *Toxicology* 1986;**40**:31.

Oxytetracycline

Oxytetracycline rapidly crosses the placenta and blood–brain barrier. Use during the first trimester is linked with the development of NTDs, cleft palate and cardiovascular malformations. Tetracyclines, in general, cause tooth discolouration when given in the second half of pregnancy and during the neonatal period. It is not known whether oxytetracycline enters breast milk; however, due to the same considerations about discoloured teeth, it is best avoided.

Czeizel and Rockenbauer: *Eur J Obstet Gynecol Reprod Biol* 2000;**88**:27.

Paclitaxel

In animal studies, paclitaxel causes embryo-fetal toxicity and teratogenicity. Use (usually in combination with other chemotherapy agents) during human pregnancy has been limited to the second and third trimesters when there does not appear to be an increased risk of adverse events. Paclitaxel passes into breast milk with one report of a relative infant dose of 16.7%, a level above which effects might be seen in the breastfed infant and which would preclude breastfeeding due to the risks. It is not known whether these risks also apply to the albumin-bound paclitaxel due to the even more limited data.

Cardonick *et al.*: *Ann Oncol* 2012;**23**:3016.
Griffin *et al.*: *J Hum Lact* 2012;**28**:457.

Pancreatin – See Part 2, pp. 387–388

Pancuronium – See Part 2, pp. 389–390

Pantoprazole

The manufacturer and the BNF advise that use of pantoprazole during pregnancy should be avoided due to fetotoxicity in animals. Experience in humans, both because treatment was required and through inadvertent exposure, is more reassuring, and the risks to the embryo–fetus appear low. It is not known if pantoprazole crosses the placenta; the similar drug, omeprazole, does. Pantoprazole passes into breast milk in very small amounts, and it is unlikely that a breastfed infant would ingest significant and clinically relevant quantities.

Diav-Citrin *et al.*: *Aliment Pharmacol Ther* 2005;**21**:269.
Plante *et al.*: *J Reprod Med* 2004;**49**:825.

Paracetamol (acetaminophen, USAN) – See Part 2, pp. 391–393

Paroxetine

Paroxetine crosses the placenta (F/M ratio ~0.5). While rodent teratogenicity studies are reassuring, two early large studies suggested a 1.5–2-fold increase in CV malformations after first trimester exposure (predominantly ASDs or VSDs). Neonatal withdrawal symptoms are documented after use later in pregnancy. Paroxetine passes into breast milk in variable amounts, but most studies report minimal or no effect in the breastfed infant. A recent review suggests that paroxetine and sertraline are the SSRIs of choice in nursing mothers.

Sie *et al.*: *Arch Dis Child Fetal Neonatal Ed* 2012;**97**:F472.
(Erratum in: *Arch Dis Child Fetal Neonatal Ed* 2013;**98**:F180.)

Penciclovir

Penciclovir is the active metabolite of famciclovir and is available as topical applications for the treatment of herpes labialis ('cold sores'). It is not known whether it crosses the placenta; however, considering the dose and (topical) route, it is unlikely that the maternal systemic concentrations reach clinically relevant levels. Rodent teratogenicity studies are reassuring. Use during breastfeeding is also unlikely to be a risk to the breastfed infant.

Moomaw *et al.*: *Expert Rev Anti Infect Ther* 2003;**1**:283.

Penicillamine – See archived monograph on website

Penicillins (benzylpenicillin and phenoxymethylpenicillin) – See Part 2, pp. 396–397

Pentamidine isetionate

Pentamidine isetionate is an antiprotozoal drug used for the treatment and prophylaxis of *P. jirovecii* (*P. carinii*) pneumonia which can follow a more aggressive course during pregnancy with higher morbidity and mortality. Evidence (transport across the isolated human placental cotyledon and rodent studies) suggests that it crosses the placenta. Reports of use during pregnancy are largely reassuring. There is no information on use during lactation, but as most patients receiving it are HIV positive, breastfeeding is contraindicated where formula is available to reduce the risk of neonatal transmission.

Connelly and Lourwood: *Pharmacotherapy* 1994;**14**:424.

Pentoxifylline

Pentoxifylline is generally used to lower blood viscosity in peripheral arterial disease. It has also been reported as an adjunct during assisted conception techniques. One pilot study of use during preterm labour suggested improved fetal cerebral blood flow and neonatal outcomes. Other than this, there are few data regarding use during pregnancy. Pentoxifylline passes into breast milk in small amounts, but its effects on the breastfed infant were not reported. A number of studies suggest that pentoxifylline may be beneficial in neonatal sepsis and NEC.

Harris *et al.*: *Paediatr Drugs* 2010;**12**:301.
Lauterbach *et al.*: *Basic Clin Pharmacol Toxicol* 2012;**110**:342.
Witter and Smith: *Am J Obstet Gynecol* 1985;**151**:1094.

Perindopril erbumine

It is not known if perindopril crosses the placenta. Other ACE inhibitors do and, as a group, cause malformations after first trimester use as well as fetal renal failure (which may be irreversible) when used in later pregnancy. It is not known if perindopril enters breast milk, other ACE inhibitors do so in small amounts (captopril and enalapril are better studied alternatives).

Polifka: *Birth Defects Res A Clin Mol Teratol* 2012;**94**:576.

Permethrin

Permethrin is an effective topical treatment for scabies, and less than 2% is systemically absorbed. It is not known if permethrin crosses the placenta; maternal systemic concentrations are unlikely to reach clinically relevant levels. Rodent teratogenicity studies and large case series are reassuring. Permethrin enters breast milk, but the amounts are far less than those that the WHO consider dangerous to the breastfed infant.

Mytton *et al.*: *BJOG* 2007;**114**:582.

Perphenazine

It is not known whether perphenazine crosses the human placenta. Occasional reports have linked phenothiazines to congenital abnormalities, but most published evidences suggest that use during pregnancy is safe. Perphenazine enters breast milk in small amounts that are unlikely to have any adverse effects on the breastfed infant.

Olesen *et al.*: *Am J Psychiatry* 1990;**147**:1378.
Slone *et al.*: *Am J Obstet Gynecol* 1977;**128**:486.

Pethidine (meperidine, USAN)

Pethidine crosses the placenta rapidly; it can be detected in cord blood 2 minutes after maternal IV injection and remains in the infant's body for at least 24–48 hours. Use during labour attracts some criticism; it is only about one-tenth as potent as morphine, and use can lead to poor feto-maternal gas exchange and fetal acidosis. It frequently causes respiratory depression in infants who are born more than 60 minutes after administration (greatest risk is to those born 2–3 hours after administration). Pethidine is excreted into breast milk, and repeated maternal doses adversely affect the newborn due to accumulation and the long (and variable) half-life of 3–60 hours at that age.

Hogg *et al.*: *Br J Anaesth* 1977;**49**:891.
Jones *et al.*: *Cochrane Database Syst Rev* 2012;**3**:CD009234.

Phenelzine

It is not known whether phenelzine crosses the placenta (the low molecular weight suggests that transfer will occur). As with most psychotropic drugs, monotherapy and the smallest effective quantity given in divided doses may reduce risk by minimising the systemic peaks. Rodent teratogenicity studies have not been performed. There are no published studies of use during lactation, and it is not known if phenelzine enters breast milk. Because of the lack of information, other antidepressants are preferred.

Phenobarbital – See Part 2, pp. 400–402

Phenoxybenzamine

Phenoxybenzamine crosses the placenta and is concentrated in the fetus (F/M ratio 3:1). Rodent teratogenicity studies have not been conducted, but case reports of use during pregnancy are largely reassuring. RDS and hypotension were reported in some infants. There is no published experience of use during breastfeeding, and it is not known if it enters breast milk.

Aplin *et al.*: *Anesthesiology* 2004;**100**:1608.
Miller *et al.*: *Obstet Gynecol* 2005;**105**:1185.

Phentermine

Phentermine is a sympathomimetic similar to *amfetamine* approved as an appetite suppressant. It is not known if it crosses the placenta. Rodent teratogenicity studies have not been performed. Inadvertent use may occur during the first trimester, and to date, no significant increase in major malformations has been reported. There are no indications for use of this drug during lactation. It is not known if it passes into breast milk – it has a low molecular weight so it is likely to do so with the potential to cause adverse CNS effects in the breastfed infant.

Jones *et al.*: *Teratology* 2002;**65**:125.

Phentolamine

Phentolamine is a short-acting α-antagonist which has been used in the treatment of phaeochromcytoma during pregnancy. It is not known if it crosses the placenta. Rodent studies are reassuring. There is no published experience during lactation, and it is not known if it enters breast milk.

Burgess: *Obstet Gynecol* 1979;**53**:266.

Phenylephrine

Many OTC preparations contain phenylephrine as their active ingredient. It is not known whether it crosses the placenta. Epidemiological data suggests an association with endocardial cushion defects. It is not known whether phenylephrine enters breast milk, but no adverse effects have ever been reported in breastfed infants.

Yau *et al.*: *Am J Epidemiol* 2013;**178**:198.

Phenytoin – See Part 2, pp. 403–404

Phytomenadione (vitamin K1) – See Part 2, pp. 541–542

Pilocarpine

Although primarily used topically as a miotic for acute glaucoma, pilocarpine may be given orally to treat xerostomia in Sjögren's syndrome or radiotherapy of head/neck cancer. Animal studies have shown some skeletal abnormalities when used in high doses. It is not known if pilocarpine enters breast milk. It is unlikely that the breastfed infant would receive a large dose after topical treatment in the mother, but with it having a low molecular weight, transfer to breast milk is possible after oral use.

Merlob *et al.*: *Eur J Obstet Gynecol Reprod Biol* 1990;**35**:85.

Pimecrolimus

Pimecrolimus and tacrolimus are immuno-modulators used topically in the treatment of atopic dermatitis. It is not known if pimecrolimus crosses the placenta; reported system concentrations after topical use are less than 0.5 ng/ml, and it is unlikely that this poses a problem for the fetus. Rodent teratogenicity studies of topical application and oral administration are reassuring. Pimecrolimus was found to cross the rodent placenta after oral administration. Topical pimecrolimus is unlikely to result in significant amounts in breast milk; however, use on or around the nipple area should be avoided.

El-Batawy *et al.*: *J Dermatol Sci* 2009;**54**:76.
Scott *et al.*: *Clin Pharmacokinet* 2003;**42**:1305.

Pimozide

It is not known whether pimozide crosses the placenta. Rodent teratogenicity studies are reassuring. Limited human data have not suggested any adverse effects associated with use. Pimozide may cause galactorrhoea. It is not known if it enters breast milk, and currently, there are insufficient data to recommend use during lactation.

Bjarnason *et al.*: *J Reprod Med* 2006;**51**:443.
Delitala *et al.*: *Biomedicine* 1977;**27**:190.

Pindolol

Pindolol is sometimes used as second-line treatment for hypertension during pregnancy. It crosses the placenta (F/M ratio 0.4–4.5). Rodent teratogenicity studies are reassuring. Some β-blockers cause *in utero* growth restriction; pindolol, as a non-selective β-blocker with intrinsic sympathomimetic activity, appears to have less of an effect on the fetus. Use during pregnancy requires careful monitoring of fetal growth. Pindolol enters breast milk, and although there is a risk of neonatal β-blockade, the amounts are probably too small to cause this.

Golightly: *Pharmacotherapy* 1982;**2**:134.
Gonçalves *et al.*: *J Chromatogr B Analyst Technol Biomed Life Sci* 2007;**852**:640.

Pioglitazone

It is not known whether pioglitazone crosses the placenta. There is no published human experience during pregnancy other than in women with polycystic ovary syndrome where it may be used to help with infertility. Rodent teratogenicity studies are for the most part reassuring; but there is some evidence of increased losses post-implantation and growth restriction during the latter stages of pregnancy. There are no published reports of use during lactation, and it is not known whether it enters breast milk.

Waugh *et al.*: *Drugs* 2006;**66**:85.

Piperacillin with tazobactam – See Part 2, pp. 407–408

Piperazine

Long clinical experience of piperazine is largely reassuring; one review – citing communication with the manufacturer – reports one case of

cleft lip and palate and anophthalmia after exposure at 14 weeks and one case of abnormality (not otherwise specified) of the right foot after exposure at 6–8 weeks. It is doubtful whether piperazine was responsible – the exposure in the first case was too late to be causal; nonetheless, the manufacturers and the BNF caution against use during the first trimester. The same review reports that piperazine enters breast milk (although the source of the information is not cited), and as a result, the manufacturers advise discarding any breast milk (i.e. 'pump and dump') for the next 8 hours.
Leach: *Arch Dis Child* 1990;**65**:399.

Piroxicam
Due to a number of adverse events, the Committee for Medicinal Products for Human Use recommended restrictions on the use of piroxicam that included initiation by specialist only and that use be limited to symptomatic relief of osteoarthritis, rheumatoid arthritis and ankylosing spondylitis. Piroxicam, like other NSAIDs, crosses the placenta and is associated in case reports with severe fetal oligohydramnios due to fetal renal impairment. Piroxicam passes into breast milk in only small amounts that are compatible with breastfeeding.
Nezvalová-Henriksen *et al.*: *BJOG* 2013;**120**:948.
Ostensen: *Eur J Clin Pharmacol* 1983;**25**:829.

Polystyrene sulfonate resins (calcium polystyrene sulfonate and sodium polystyrene sulfonate) – See Part 2, pp. 419–420

Pramipexole
It is not known if pramipexole crosses the placenta. In rodents, it reduces implantation and is embryotoxic. Limited published human pregnancy experience is reassuring. There is no published experience during breastfeeding, and it is not known if it enters breast milk. It is, however, known to reduce secretion of prolactin and, theoretically, might interfere with milk production.
Dostal *et al.*: *Eur J Neurol* 2013;**20**:1241.
Schilling *et al.*: *Clin Pharmacol Ther* 1992;**51**:541.

Pravastatin sodium
It is not known if pravastatin crosses the placenta (transfer across an isolated perfused human placenta cotyledon is slow), and it is not known whether it enters breast milk. In general, however, statins should be avoided during pregnancy and lactation – congenital anomalies have been reported, and decreased synthesis of cholesterol has a potential to adversely affect fetal development. The risk to

the mother of a temporary cessation in therapy during this period appears to be low.
Zarek *et al.*: *Placenta* 2013;**34**:719.

Prazosin
Prazosin crosses the placenta (F/M ratio 0.2). Rodent teratogenicity studies are reassuring, but there is an unexplained increased perinatal mortality when used in expectant management of pre-eclamptic hypertension. Small quantities of prazosin are found in breast milk; nonetheless, it is considered compatible with breastfeeding.
Hall *et al.*: *BJOG* 2000;**107**:1258.

Prednisolone
The placenta metabolises prednisolone, reducing fetal exposure to approximately 10% of maternal levels. Evidence that corticosteroids are human teratogens is, at best, weak and confined only to cleft lip and palate when used during the first trimester. Prolonged second and third trimester use may cause *in utero* growth restriction. Use prior to delivery may theoretically cause adrenal suppression in the neonate; however, this is rarely clinically significant and resolves spontaneously. Prednisolone passes in small amounts into breast milk. Maternal doses less than 40 mg daily are unlikely to cause systemic effects in the breastfed infant; an infant whose mother is taking higher doses should be monitored for adrenal suppression.
Ost *et al.*: *J Pediatr* 1985;**106**:1008.
Pacheco *et al.*: *Am J Perinatol* 2007;**24**:79.

Prednisone
Prednisone itself is inactive and is rapidly metabolised to the active drug, prednisolone (see section on ***Prednisolone***).

Prilocaine
Prilocaine crosses the placenta. Rodent teratogenicity studies are reassuring. Although largely safe, there are several reports of methaemoglobinaemia in fetuses and infants after use for obstetric procedures. It is not known whether prilocaine enters breast milk. Based on the low excretion of other local anaesthetics into breast milk, a single dose, such as for a dental procedure, is unlikely to adversely affect the breastfed infant.
Poppers and Mastri: *Acta Anaesthesiol Scand Suppl* 1969;**37**:258.

Primaquine
Primaquine is generally not recommended during pregnancy because of the potential to cause haemolytic anaemia especially in the G6PD-deficient fetus. Rodent teratogenicity studies do not appear to have been performed. Primaquine probably crosses the placenta.

There are no reports of haemolysis in the baby of a mother taking primaquine while breastfeeding, but it remains a theoretical risk if the infant's G6PD status is unknown. It is otherwise safe with expected milk levels lower than the 0.3 mg/kg/day dose given to infants.
WHO Malaria Policy Advisory Committee and Secretariat: *Malar J* 2012;**11**:424.

Primidone
Primidone, which is metabolised to phenobarbital and phenylethylmalonamide (PEMA), can be teratogenic in mice, but there are no convincing reports of human teratogenicity. Studies are difficult to interpret because epilepsy itself may increase the risk of malformation and many epileptic patients are on more than one drug. Although now being debated, any risk of neonatal haemorrhage (as for phenobarbital) is easily corrected by giving vitamin K at birth. Primidone and its metabolites are excreted into breast milk. Treatment during lactation has been associated with reports of transient drowsiness.
Harden *et al.*: *Epilepsia* 2009;**50**:1247.

Procainamide
Procainamide crosses the placenta and there are numerous case reports of use to treat fetal tachyarrhythmia. Rodent teratogenicity studies have not been performed, but use during pregnancy has not been associated with any congenital abnormalities of adverse fetal events. Both procainamide and its metabolite, *N*-acetylprocainamide, pass into breast milk. The levels in milk are subtherapeutic.
Trappe: *J Emerg Trauma Shock* 2010;**3**:153.

Procarbazine
It is not known if procarbazine crosses the placenta. It is usually combined with other antineoplastic agents, and there are case reports of fetal malformations after such use during the first trimester. Rodent studies show evidence of a spectrum of malformations including microcephaly and midline clefts. It is also mutagenic and carcinogenic in animals. It is not known if procarbazine enters breast milk. The potential for adverse effects is high, and breastfeeding is considered contraindicated.
Lee and Dixon: *Mutat Res* 1978;**55**:1.

Prochlorperazine
Prochlorperazine readily crosses the placenta, but extensive clinical experience has shown no substantial evidence of teratogenicity. Prochlorperazine enters breast milk. Short-term maternal treatment is likely safe, but high-dose treatment may cause drowsiness in the breastfed infant and caution is advised.

Einarson and Boskovic: *J Psychiatr Pract* 2009;**15**:183.
Moya and Thorndike: *Am J Obstet Gynecol* 1962;**84**:1778.

Procyclidine
There are no published data pertaining to use during pregnancy, and it is not known if procyclidine crosses the placenta. Rodent teratogenicity studies have not been performed. There is also no published experience of use during lactation, and it is also not known if procyclidine enters breast milk.

Progesterone – See Part 2, pp. 427–428

Promethazine hydrochloride
Promethazine has been used to treat nausea and vomiting; however, ondansetron may be an alternative when symptoms are very severe. Promethazine rapidly crosses the placenta. Rodent teratogenicity and epidemiological studies are reassuring. There are no data on transfer of promethazine into breast milk. While other antihistamines have caused drowsiness in the breastfed infant, promethazine has never been reported to cause such a problem.
Tan *et al.*: *Obstet Gynecol* 2010;**115**:975.

Propafenone
Propafenone is used to treat tachyarrhythmias. The drug crosses the placenta. Rodent teratogenesis studies are reassuring although the drug is embryotoxic in higher doses. The few case reports of use during pregnancy were uneventful. Very small amounts of propafenone enter breast milk, and the infant is unlikely to experience any clinically significant effects.
Brunozzi *et al.*: *Br J Clin Pharmacol* 1988;**26**:489.
Libardoni *et al.*: *Br J Clin Pharmacol* 1991;**32**:527.

Propantheline bromide
Data on the safety of this drug during pregnancy and lactation is lacking. It is not known if propantheline crosses the placenta. Rodent teratogenicity studies do not appear to have been performed. There are no published reports of use during lactation, and it is not known if propantheline enters breast milk.

Propofol
Most of the use of propofol during pregnancy occurs during caesarean section. Propofol crosses the placenta (F/M ratios 0.35–1.0). It appears in breast milk in amounts that are negligible compared to the amounts received via the placenta. Propofol was thought to be the cause for green discolouration of breast milk in one woman.
Birkholz *et al.*: *Anesthesiology* 2009;**111**:1168.

Propranolol – See Part 2, pp. 431–432

Propylthiouracil – See Part 2, p. 433

Protamine sulphate
Protamine is used to correct the anticoagulant effect of heparin. There are no published reports of use during pregnancy, and animal teratogenicity studies have not been conducted.

Pseudoephedrine hydrochloride
It is not known if pseudoephedrine crosses the placenta, and there do not appear to be any rodent teratogenicity studies. Limited human data from first trimester use suggest an increased risk of gastroschisis and small bowel atresia. Pseudoephedrine passes into breast milk in small amounts that are unlikely to affect the nursing infant.
Werler: *Birth Defects Res A Clin Mol Teratol* 2006;**76**:445.

Pyrazinamide – See Part 2, pp. 439–440

Pyridostigmine
Pyridostigmine has been used to treat myaesthenia gravis during pregnancy. It would appear to cross the placenta, but rodent teratogenicity studies appear reassuring. Most reports of use in human pregnancy are similarly reassuring, but arthrogryposis multiplex congenita has been reported after use. Pyridostigmine is excreted into breast milk, but no clinical effects have been reported in breastfed infants.
Chieza *et al.*: *Int J Obstet Anesth* 2011;**20**:79.
Hardell *et al.*: *Br J Clin Pharmacol* 1982;**14**:565.

Pyridoxine (vitamin B6) – See Part 2, pp. 441–442

Pyrimethamine – See Part 2, pp. 443–444

Quetiapine
Quetiapine crosses the placenta (F/M ratio ~0.25). Rodent teratogenicity studies are mostly reassuring as is very limited evidence from studies in human pregnancy. In some women, the psychiatric risks of coming off quetiapine might outweigh the fetal risks. Small amounts are excreted into breast milk. No adverse effects were noted in exposed infants.
Klier *et al.*: *J Clin Psychopharmacol* 2007;**27**:720.
Tényi *et al.*: *Am J Psychiatry* 2002;**159**:674.

Quinapril
In general, ACE inhibitors should be avoided during the second and third trimesters because they can cause fetal renal failure. If quinapril is used, the mother should be monitored closely for oligohydramnios; however, this may not appear until after the fetus has irreversible renal injury. Very low levels of quinapril are found in breast milk; they would not be expected to cause any adverse effects in breastfed infants.
Begg *et al.*: *Br J Clin Pharmacol* 2001;**51**:478.
Kieback *et al.*: *Expert Opin Drug Metab Toxicol* 2009;**5**:1337.

Quinine – See Part 2, pp. 445–446

Rabeprazole
There is no published experience with rabeprazole during pregnancy, and it is not known if it crosses the placenta. Rodent teratogenicity studies are reassuring. It is not known whether rabeprazole enters breast milk. Other proton pump inhibitors (e.g. omeprazole) have been used in pregnancy and lactation and are better studied.
Matok *et al.*: *Dig Dis Sci* 2012;**57**:699.

Ramipril
In general, ACE inhibitors are avoided during pregnancy (especially during the second and third trimesters) because of fetal risks. If ramipril is used in pregnancy, the mother should be monitored closely for oligohydramnios; however, this may not appear until after the fetus has irreversible renal injury. It is not known if ramipril appears in breast milk; low levels of other ACE inhibitors may be found in breast milk when they are used and do not cause any adverse effects in breastfed infants.
Kolagasi *et al.*: *Ann Pharmacother* 2009;**43**:147.

Ranitidine – See Part 2, pp. 447–448

Remifentanil – See Part 2, pp. 449–450

Repaglinide
Repaglinide slowly crosses the isolated human placental cotyledon. Rodent teratogenicity studies are reassuring, but data in humans are too limited to allow meaningful analysis of risk. Metformin, glibenclamide and insulin are all better studied alternatives during pregnancy. There is no published experience during breastfeeding, and it is not known if repaglinide enters breast milk.
Tertti *et al.*: *Eur J Pharm Sci* 2011;**44**:181.

Reteplase
It is not known if reteplase crosses the placenta. Rodent teratogenicity studies were reassuring but showed premature separation of the placenta and placental losses. Limited use during human pregnancy is reassuring.

There is no published experience during lactation; the maternal clinical condition, and not use of reteplase, is likely to dictate when breastfeeding resumes.
Wenk *et al.*: *Anaesth Intensive Care* 2011;**39**:671.

Ribavirin – See Part 2, pp. 452–453

Riboflavin (vitamin B2) – See Part 2, pp. 543–544

Rifabutin

Rifabutin is indicated for prophylaxis against *Mycobacterium avium* complex infections in patients with a low CD4 count; it is also licensed for the treatment of non-tuberculous mycobacterial disease and pulmonary TB. It is not known if rifabutin crosses the placenta. Rodent teratogenicity studies are reassuring. It is not known whether rifabutin enters breast milk. Rifabutin has been used to treat a 3-month-old infant.
Giacchino *et al.*: *Pediatr Infect Dis J* 1994;**13**:164.

Rifampicin (rifampin, USAN) – See Part 2, pp. 455–456

Risedronate sodium

There is no published experience with risedronate during pregnancy (etidronate is a slightly better studied alternative). Rodent teratogenicity studies are generally reassuring. However, it is not known whether risedronate crosses the placenta or enters breast milk.
Djokanovic *et al.*: *J Obstet Gynaecol Can* 2008;**30**:1146.

Risperidone

It is not known if risperidone crosses the placenta (it does in rodents). Rodent teratogenicity studies are generally reassuring, as are reports of exposures during human pregnancies. Neonatal tremor, jitteriness, irritability, feeding problems and somnolence, which may represent a withdrawal-emergent syndrome, are reported. Risperidone enters breast milk in amounts that are not expected to cause effects in the breastfed infant.
Aichhorn *et al.*: *J Psychopharmacol* 2005;**19**:211.
Coppola *et al.*: *Drug Saf* 2007;**30**:247.

Rizatriptan

It is not known whether rizatriptan crosses the placenta. Rodent teratogenicity studies are generally reassuring as is limited use (of all triptans) during pregnancy. There are no data on the transfer of rizatriptan to breast milk. Sumatriptan does pass into breast milk and is generally safe. It is suggested that if rizatriptan is used, breastfeeding is best avoided for the next 24 hours (i.e. 'pump and dump').

Fiore *et al.*: *Cephalalgia* 2005;**25**:685.
Nezvalová-Henriksen *et al.*: *Headache* 2010;**50**:563.

Rocuronium – See Part 2, pp. 457–458

Salbutamol (albuterol - USAN) – See Part 2, pp. 464–465

Salmeterol

Systemic levels of salmeterol are low or undetectable after inhalation. It is not known whether it crosses the placenta in humans (there is low transfer in rats). With low systemic levels and (at best) poor placental transport, it is unlikely that the fetus is exposed to a clinically relevant concentration. There are no reports of adverse fetal outcomes associated with use. It is not known whether salmeterol enters breast milk, but the breastfed infant is unlikely to receive clinical significant amounts.
BTS & SIGN: British Guideline on the Management of Asthma.
Mann *et al.*: *J Clin Epidemiol* 1996;**49**:247.

Saquinavir

Saquinavir, like many protease inhibitors, does not cross the placenta in significant amounts. It is, therefore, unlikely to pose a significant risk to the fetus. Rodent teratogenicity studies are reassuring, as are reports of use during human pregnancies. It is not known whether saquinavir enters human breast milk. Breastfeeding is contraindicated in HIV-infected nursing women where formula is available to reduce the risk of neonatal transmission.
Andany and Loutfy: *Drugs* 2013;**73**:229.

Saxagliptin

Saxagliptin inhibits dipeptidylpeptidase-4 to increase insulin secretion and lower glucagon secretion. It is not known if saxagliptin crosses the placenta. Rodent teratogenicity studies are reassuring, but there is no reported experience during human pregnancy. No information is available on the use of saxagliptin during breastfeeding or whether it passes into breast milk. Saxagliptin is best avoided during both pregnancy and lactation until further information is available.
Lam and Saad: *Cardiol Rev* 2010;**18**:213.

Selegiline hydrochloride

It is not known whether selegiline crosses the placenta. Monoamine neurotransmitters are important for the development of the immature brain, and endogenous levels are highly regulated by monoamine oxidase. Potentially, any change in enzyme activity could have a profound effect on brain development. Some recommend discontinuing monoamine oxidase inhibitors even before conception. There are very limited data on use during lactation, and it is not known if selegiline passes into breast milk.

Kupsch and Oertel: *Mov Disord* 1998;**13**:175.
Suzuki *et al*.: *Dev Neurosci* 1978;**1**:172.

Senna

Limited amounts of senna are absorbed from the GI tract. It is not known if it crosses the placenta; however, it is not teratogenic in animals, and no reports of adverse fetal effects have been published. Very small amounts of senna can be found in breast milk; these are too small to produce a clinical effect in the breastfed infant.

Acs *et al*.: *Reprod Toxicol* 2009;**28**:100.
Shafe *et al*.: *Therap Adv Gastroenterol* 2011;**4**:343.

Sertraline

Sertraline crosses the placenta (F/M ratio ~0.30–0.67). There appears to be a significant association with omphalocoele and septal defects. Neonatal abstinence syndrome may occur in up to one-third of exposed neonates which continues for at least a few months. Sertraline is found in breast milk in amounts that are affected by timing and size of the maternal dose. The breastfed infant should be monitored for possible adverse effects; giving the drug in the lowest effective dose and avoiding feeds at times of peak drug levels (7–10 hours after maternal dosing) may minimise exposure.

Gentile: *Drug Saf* 2005;**28**:137.
Müller *et al*.: *Breast feed Med* 2013;**8**:327.
Sie *et al*.: *Arch Dis Child* Fetal Neonatal Ed 2012;**97**:F472. (Erratum in: *Arch Dis Child* Fetal Neonatal Ed 2013;**98**:F180.)

Sildenafil – See Part 2, pp. 466–467

Simethicone

While it is not known if simethicone crosses the placenta, it is unlikely that maternal systemic concentrations reach clinically relevant levels. Rodent teratogenicity studies have not been conducted. There are no reports of use during lactation, and the low maternal levels mean that even if transfer into breast milk did occur, it would be unlikely that the breastfed infant would be adversely affected.

Hodgkinson *et al*.: *Anesthesiology* 1983;**59**:86.

Simvastatin

It is not known if simvastatin crosses the placenta. Post-marketing studies of exposure in early pregnancy are reassuring, as are rodent teratogenicity studies, and inadvertent exposure would not be a medical indication for pregnancy termination. However, because cholesterol and other products of the cholesterol biosynthesis pathway are essential components for fetal development, treatment with simvastatin should be discontinued during pregnancy and lactation (it is not known if simvastatin enters breast milk). Temporarily discontinuing maternal treatment should have little impact on the long-term therapeutic outcome of primary hypercholesterolaemia and will avoid exposing the fetus/infant to drugs at a critical time.

Godfrey *et al*.: *Ann Pharmacother* 2012;**46**:1419.
Pollack *et al*.: *Birth Defects Res A Clin Mol Teratol* 2005;**73**:888.

Sirolimus

It is not known if sirolimus crosses the placenta. There is no evidence of teratogenicity although one *in vitro* study suggested that it may adversely affect the growth of the fetal and infant heart. No clinically significant cardiac effects have been reported in various case reports. It is not known if sirolimus enters breast milk.

Burton *et al*.: *Pediatr Cardiol* 1998;**19**:468.
Chu *et al*.: *Transplant Proc* 2008;**40**:2446.
Guardia *et al*.: *Transplantation* 2006;**81**:636.

Sitagliptin

Sitagliptin inhibits dipeptidylpeptidase-4 to increase insulin secretion and lower glucagon secretion. It is not known if sitagliptin crosses the placenta in humans (it does in rodents). Rodent teratogenicity studies are reassuring, and extremely limited human use has to date generally been reassuring. No information is available on the use of sitagliptin during breastfeeding or whether it passes into breast milk. Sitagliptin is best avoided during both pregnancy and lactation until further information is available.

Choy and Lam: *Cardiol Rev* 2007;**15**:264.

Sodium aurothiomalate

It is not known whether sodium aurothiomalate crosses the placenta. Rodent studies reveal increased risk of embryo- and fetotoxicity, gastroschisis and umbilical hernia. Reducing the dose may be an option in those women who are unable to stop their treatment. Sodium aurothiomalate is excreted into breast milk, but no convincing cases of infant toxicity have been reported. Sodium aurothiomalate should be used during pregnancy and lactation only if the benefit justifies the potential perinatal risk. It may not be necessary to withdraw if well controlled, but alternatives exist for which there is more experience during both pregnancy and lactation.

Almarzouqi *et al*.: *J Rheumatol* 2007;**34**:1827.
Bennett *et al*.: *Br J Clin Pharmacol* 1990;**29**:777.
Ostensen *et al*.: *Eur J Clin Pharmacol* 1986;**31**:251.

Sodium cromoglicate
It is not known whether sodium cromoglicate crosses the placenta. Rodent studies are reassuring with no evidence of teratogenicity. It is not known whether it enters breast milk. Virtually none of the commonly used asthma medications are contraindicated during pregnancy, and given that breastfeeding protects against food allergies, exclusive breastfeeding should be strongly encouraged for as long as possible in such cases.
Hardy-Fairbanks and Baker: *Obstet Gynecol Clin North Am* 2010;**37**:159.

Sodium nitroprusside
It is not known whether sodium nitroprusside crosses the placenta. Rodent teratogenicity studies have not been performed. Fetal cyanide toxicity occurs in sheep after *prolonged* maternal administration. While maternal cyanide toxicity can be reversed by sodium thiosulphate, this does not cross the placenta, allowing treatment of the fetus. Use in humans is limited to case reports of short-term use (e.g. during aneurysm surgery and severe hypertension). There are no reports of use during lactation, the thiocyanate metabolite has a long life, and breastfeeding is best avoided if the mother has received sodium nitroprusside for longer than 24 hours.
Benitz *et al.*: *J Pediatr* 1985;**106**:102.
Willoughby: *Anaesth Intensive Care* 1984;**12**:351.

Sodium valproate – See Part 2, pp. 480–481

Sotalol
Although sotalol reduces blood pressure, reported use during pregnancy is restricted to its role as an antiarrhythmic agent. Sotalol crosses the placenta (F/M ratio ~1), and it has been used to treat fetal tachyarrhythmia with a moderately high response rate (flecainide and digoxin are perhaps more effective). Rodent teratogenicity studies are reassuring. In one case, it was estimated that a breastfed infant received a 20–23% of the weight-adjusted maternal dose; although there were no adverse events in this infant, it is recommended that any baby exposed to maternal sotalol is closely monitored.
Hackett *et al.*: *Br J Clin Pharmacol* 1990;**29**:277.
Jaeggi *et al.*: *Circulation* 2011;**124**:1747.
Shah *et al.*: *Am J Cardiol* 2012;**109**:1614.

Spironolactone – See Part 2, pp. 486–487

Stavudine
Stavudine inhibits viral reverse transcriptase and DNA synthesis. It crosses the placenta and is concentrated in the fetus (F/M ratio 1.32). It reduces implantation rates in rodent studies but shows no major teratogenicity. Use in humans has not shown any increased fetal risk. Stavudine passes into breast milk; however, breastfeeding is contraindicated in HIV-infected nursing women where formula is available to reduce the risk of neonatal transmission. The concentrations in breast milk are too small to be clinically significant.
Fogel *et al.*: *J Acquir Immune Defic Syndr* 2012;**60**:462.
Wade *et al.*: *J Infect Dis* 2004;**190**:2167.

Streptokinase – See Part 2, pp. 488–489

Sucralfate
Sucralfate is only minimally absorbed across the GI tract and thus should pose no risk to the fetus. Rodent teratogenicity studies are reassuring. It is not known whether sucralfate enters breast milk; low maternal levels means that it should pose no risk to the breastfed infant.
Ali and Egan: *Best Pract Res Clin Gastroenterol* 2007;**21**:793.

Sufentanil
Sufentanil crosses the placenta (F/M 1.0). It is used for fetal analgesia during a variety of procedures. Rodent teratogenicity studies are generally reassuring. Considering the indications and dosing, one-off sufentanil use is unlikely to pose a clinically significant risk to the breastfeeding neonate.
Lilker *et al.*: *J Clin Anesth* 2009;**21**:108.

Sulfasalazine
Bacteria in the gut metabolise sulfasalazine to 5-ASA and sulfapyridine. Both sulfasalazine and sulfapyridine cross the placenta (M/F ratio ~1). Large epidemiologic studies identify no evidence of teratogenicity or an increased prevalence of adverse fetal outcomes. Rodent teratogenicity studies are also reassuring. Insignificant amounts of sulfasalazine and 5-ASA are found in breast milk; sulfapyridine levels are 30–60% of those in maternal serum. Few exposed breastfed infants show any adverse effects.
Moffatt and Bernstein: *Best Pract Res Clin Gastroenterol* 2007;**21**:835.
Mottet *et al.*: *Digestion* 2007;**76**:149.

Sulindac
Sulindac crosses the placenta (F/M ratio ~0.4). Like other NSAIDs, sulindac may cause ductal constriction and oligohydramnios. Rodent studies reveal an increased incidence of cleft palate, and there is an increased risk of IUGR and fetal death. No information is available on the use of sulindac during breastfeeding; other agents may be preferred, especially while nursing a newborn or preterm infant.
Lione and Scialli: *Reprod Toxicol* 1995;**9**:7.

Sumatriptan

Only small amounts of sumatriptan cross the placenta, and it should pose only minimal risk to the fetus. Epidemiological studies of use during pregnancy are reassuring, although rodent teratogenicity studies using high doses revealed embryotoxicity and vascular and skeletal abnormalities (these were not seen at levels equivalent to therapeutic doses used in humans). A small amount of sumatriptan enters breast milk, but the quantity ingested by the breastfed infant will be negligible.

Cassina *et al.*: *Expert Opin Drug Saf* 2010;**9**:937.
Wojnar-Horton *et al*. *Br J Clin Pharmacol* 1996;**41**:217.

Suxamethonium chloride (succinylcholine, USAN) – See Part 2, pp. 493–494

Tacrolimus

It is not known whether tacrolimus crosses the placenta. There are insufficient gestational animal studies. Reports of use in humans do not reveal obvious evidence of teratogenicity. Tacrolimus enters breast milk at very low concentrations with the breastfed infant receiving negligible amounts. This and the poor oral bioavailability would mean that the infant should not experience any adverse effects. Monitoring tacrolimus levels in the infant can add a further degree of reassurance.

Armenti *et al.*: *Expert Rev Clin Immunol* 2013;**9**:623.
Bramham *et al.*: *Clin J Am Soc Nephrol* 2013;**8**:563.
Zheng *et al.*: *Ther Drug Monit* 2012;**34**:660.

Tamoxifen

There are a number of concerns with use of tamoxifen during pregnancy. It is not known whether tamoxifen crosses the placenta. Tamoxifen has effects on genital tract development similar to oestrogen, and several reports of use in human pregnancy suggest an association between first trimester use and craniofacial abnormalities. In rodents, tamoxifen inhibits uteroplacental artery dilation, decreases placental and fetal weights and, as a consequence, increases the risk of fetal demise. Tamoxifen is carcinogenic in rodents, and although this has not been demonstrated in humans, no follow-up study of *in utero* exposure has been long enough to totally discount this. Because both tamoxifen and its major metabolite have a long half-life, use in the 8 weeks preceding conception may also expose the embryo. It is not known whether tamoxifen enters breast milk; the potential long-term effects of exposure of the developing ovaries to this anti-oestrogen are unknown. Tamoxifen also suppresses lactation to a degree.

Amant *et al.*: *Lancet* 2012;**379**:570.
Shaaban: *Eur J Obstet Gynecol Reprod Biol* 1975;**4**:167.

Tazarotene

Tazarotene is a third-generation prescription topical retinoid cream or gel. The maternal systemic concentrations are reported to be low (only 2–3% of the topically applied drug), but it is not known if tazarotene crosses the placenta. The manufacturer reports teratogenic and embryotoxic effects after **oral** administration in rodents, and skeletal alterations and decreased pup weight at birth after topical application. Retinoids are known to be teratogenic in humans and are contraindicated in pregnancy. It is not known if tazarotene enters breast milk; in the absence of further information, use during lactation is best avoided.

Duvic: *Cutis* 1998;**61**(suppl):22.

Telmisartan

There are only two published reports of telmisartan use during pregnancy; one attributes severe microcephaly, growth retardation, dysmorphism, developmental delay and polymicrogyria to concurrent use of a statin, and the other reports renal failure in the neonate. The latter is a recurring feature. At least 15 case reports describe oligohydramnios, fetal growth retardation, pulmonary hypoplasia, limb contractures and calvarial hypoplasia after maternal angiotensin II receptor antagonist treatment during the second or third trimester. If telmisartan treatment cannot be stopped, the pregnancy should be monitored closely for oligohydramnios; however, irreversible fetal renal failure may have already occurred before this appears. There is no information on telmisartan during lactation, and it is not known if it passes into breast milk.

Alwan *et al.*: *Birth Defects Res A Clin Mol Teratol* 2005;**73**:123.
Pietrement *et al.*: *J Perinatol* 2003;**23**:254.
Trakadis *et al.*: *Paediatr Child Health* 2009;**14**:450.

Temazepam

Temazepam crosses the placenta (F/M ratio ~0.38 in the second trimester, increasing in later pregnancy). Studies of outcomes during later pregnancy are unavailable. Rodent teratogenicity studies reveal an increased prevalence of skeletal abnormalities and embryo loss. Limited reports of human use have not shown any increased abnormalities. Temazepam passes into breast milk in small amounts. Any infant so exposed should be monitored for lethargy, sedation and weight loss.

Cooper *et al.*: *Reprod Biomed Online* 2001;**2**:165.
Lebedevs *et al.*: *Br J Clin Pharmacol* 1992;**33**:204.

Temozolomide

Experience of temozolomide during pregnancy is limited to a single case report.

Numerous malformations have been reported during rodent teratogenicity studies. It is also carcinogenic in rodents. There is no information about this drug during lactation, and it is not known if it passes into breast milk. The characteristics of the drug make transfer into milk likely, and because of the potential effects on the infant, breastfeeding should be avoided for at least 7 days after treatment.
McGrane et al.: Clin Oncol (R Coll Radiol) 2012;**24**:311.

Tenecteplase
It is not known whether tenecteplase crosses the placenta. Rodent teratogenicity studies are reassuring. Maternal haemorrhage is a major risk; however, tenecteplase should not be withheld because of pregnancy if the maternal condition warrants treatment. There are no published reports of use during lactation, and it is not known if tenecteplase enters breast milk.
Slaoui et al.: Ann Fr Anesth Reanim 2010;**29**:500.

Tenofovir disoproxil
Transfer of tenofovir across the placenta has not been studied in humans (transfer across the primate placenta is known to occur). While breastfeeding is contraindicated in HIV-infected women where formula is available to reduce the risk of neonatal transmission, it may occur in resource-poor countries and in those HIV-negative mothers being treated for hepatitis B. Very small amounts of tenofovir are found in breast milk, and no adverse effects have been seen in exposed infants.
Gouraud et al.: Fundam Clin Pharmacol 2012;**26**(suppl 1):9.
Kinai et al.: AIDS 2012;**26**:2119.
Kuhn and Bulterys: AIDS 2012;**26**:1167.
Pan and Lee: Semin Liver Dis 2013;33(2):138.

Terazosin
It is not known whether terazosin crosses the placenta. Rodent teratogenicity studies are generally reassuring; however, testicular atrophy is seen in some animals. It is not known whether it enters breast milk. Prazosin is an alternative for which there is more experience regarding use during pregnancy and lactation.

Terbinafine
It is not known if terbinafine crosses the placenta. Rodent teratogenicity studies are reassuring. Systemic absorption of topical therapy is minimal. Oral treatment results in small amounts of terbinafine appearing in breast milk; however, the prolonged duration of maternal therapy carries the potential for accumulation and possibly toxicity in the breastfed infant.
Baran et al.: J Dermatol Treat 2008;**19**:168.

Terbutaline
Terbutaline crosses the placenta (F/M ratio 0.11–0.48 after a single IV dose). Rodent teratogenicity studies are reassuring. At one point, there was a suggestion, now disputed, that terbutaline (used parenterally for tocolysis rather than the inhaled use seen in asthma) might increase the risk of autistic spectrum disorders. Terbutaline increases the frequency of fetal breathing, but this does not cause any long-term problems. When inhaled, less than 10% of the drug is systemically absorbed. Terbutaline passes into breast milk but the breastfed infant ingests only small amounts, and no clinical effects have been reported.
Boréus et al.: Br J Clin Pharmacol 1982;**13**:731.
Rodier et al.: Am J Obstet Gynecol 2011;**204**:91.
Witter et al.: Am J Obstet Gynecol 2009;**201**:553.

Tetracycline
Tetracycline crosses the placenta and may cause a yellow-grey/brown tooth discolouration after fetal or early childhood exposure. Rodent teratogenicity studies are generally reassuring. The related drug, oxytetracycline, is associated with increased risk of neural tube defects, cleft palate and cardiovascular abnormalities. Tetracycline enters breast milk. However, due to binding of the drug to calcium in milk, oral absorption by the breastfed infant is minimised. Short-term use is likely to be safe, but long-term therapy (e.g. that for acne) may cause problems.
Kong and Tey: Drugs 2013;**73**:779.
Mylonas: Arch Gynecol Obstet 2011;**283**:7.

Theophylline – See archived monograph on website

Thiopental sodium – See Part 2, pp. 504–505

Tiagabine
It is not known if tiagabine crosses the placenta. It is teratogenic at high doses in rodents, increasing rates of craniofacial, appendicular and visceral defects. The very limited reports of the use of tiagabine during human pregnancy are insufficient to draw any conclusions.
Bar-Oz et al.: Paediatr Drugs 2000;**2**:113.
Leppik et al.: Epilepsy Res 1999;**33**:235.

Ticarcillin sodium with clavulanic acid
Both ticarcillin and clavulanate cross the placenta. Rodent teratogenicity studies are reassuring, as are reports from use in human pregnancy. Both ticarcillin and clavulanate pass into breast milk; there are no reports of any adverse effects in the breastfed infant.

Matsuda: *Biol Res Pregnancy Perinatol* 1984;**5**:57.
Tasker *et al.*: *J Antimicrob Chemother* 1986;**17** suppl C:225.

Timolol

Although timolol may be used to treat hypertension, most reports of use during pregnancy relate to topical treatment of glaucoma. As a group, β-blockers are associated with IUGR when used to treat hypertension during the second and third trimesters, though controversy continues as to whether this is drug or disease related. Timolol crosses the placenta and can cause fetal bradycardia (even when administered as eye drops). Rodent teratogenicity studies are reassuring. Timolol enters breast milk after both oral and topical use. Untoward effects have not been reported in the breastfed infant.
Madadi *et al.*: *J Glaucoma* 2008;**17**:329.
Wagenvoort *et al.*: *Teratology* 1998;**58**:258.

Tinzaparin sodium

Tinzaparin sodium does not cross the placenta. Rodent teratogenicity studies are reassuring, as is an increasing body of information from use during human pregnancy. It is not known whether tinzaparin enters breast milk; however, other low molecular weight heparins (e.g. dalteparin, enoxaparin) are not excreted into breast milk in clinically relevant amounts and may be a suitable alternative until further information is available.
Nelson-Piercy *et al.*: *Eur J Obstet Gynecol Reprod Biol* 2011;**159**:293.

Tioguanine (thioguanine, former BAN)

Small amounts of tioguanine appear to cross the placenta. It is teratogenic in rats at high doses, leading to embryotoxicity, cranial defects, hydrocephalus, skeletal hypoplasia, situs inversus and incomplete limb development. While most of the reported cases of use during human pregnancy end with a normal outcome, few women receive monotherapy, and it is possible that tioguanine is modestly teratogenic in humans. There is no published experience during breastfeeding, and it is not known if tioguanine enters breast milk.
de Boer *et al.*: *Scand J Gastroenterol* 2005;**40**:1374.
Lilleyman *et al.*: *Cancer* 1977;**40**:1300.

Tizanidine

It is not known whether tizanidine crosses the placenta. Rodent teratogenicity studies are predominantly reassuring but did suggest some evidence of prolonged pregnancy and embryotoxicity. There are no published reports of use during human pregnancy or lactation. It is not known if it passes into breast milk.

Tobramycin – See Part 2, pp. 506–507

Tolbutamide

Tolbutamide crosses the placenta and stimulates the secretion of insulin by the fetal pancreas. It can cause a prolonged, severe hypoglycaemia in exposed neonates of between 4 and 10 days duration. If tolbutamide is used during pregnancy, it should be discontinued at least 2 weeks before the EDD. Tolbutamide is teratogenic in rats, causing ocular and bony abnormalities. Only low levels of tolbutamide enter breast milk; nonetheless, it would be prudent to monitor the exposed neonate for hypoglycaemia.
Garcia-Bournissen *et al.*: *Clin Pharmacokinet* 2003;**42**:303.

Topiramate

Topiramate readily crosses the placenta (F/M ratios ~1). Teratogenicity is seen in three animal species. In humans, monotherapy may carry an increased risk of oral clefts and hypospadias. The risks of birth defects are increased combined with other anticonvulsants and are greatest during the first trimester. Small amounts of topiramate enter breast milk, but it has relatively few side effects and none have been reported in breastfed infants.
Hernández-Díaz *et al.*: *Neurology* 2012;**78**:1692.
Margulis *et al.*: *Am J Obstet Gynecol* 2012;**207**:405.e1.

Torsemide

It is not known whether torsemide crosses the placenta. While rodent teratogenicity studies are reassuring, there is no published experience with torsemide during human pregnancy. It is not known whether torsemide enters breast milk. It may potentially adversely affect milk supply due to effects on plasma volume and blood pressure. Furosemide is a better studied alternative during pregnancy and lactation.

Tramadol hydrochloride

Tramadol crosses the placenta (F/M ratio 0.83). Chronic use during pregnancy may lead to physical dependence and neonatal abstinence syndrome in the newborn. Rodent teratogenicity studies are generally reassuring. The excretion of tramadol into milk is low, and no significant effects are seen in the breastfed infant. Short-term maternal use seems compatible with breastfeeding, but long-term use is best avoided as this carries risks particularly in women with polymorphisms of the cytochrome P450 2D6 (CYP2D6) genes that make them 'ultrarapid metabolisers'.
Hartenstein *et al.*: *J Perinat Med* 2010;**38**:695.
Salman *et al.*: *Eur J Clin Pharmacol* 2011;**67**:899.

Trandolapril

There is no published experience with trandolapril during pregnancy. It is not known whether trandolapril crosses the placenta (other drugs of this class do). Adverse fetal effects are reported from drugs that inhibit the renin–angiotensin system with anuria, reversible or irreversible renal failure, oligohydramnios and death. Oligohydramnios may not appear until after the fetus has sustained irreversible injury. Neonates exposed *in utero* should be closely observed for hypotension, oliguria and hyperkalaemia. It is not known whether trandolapril enters breast milk (there is more experience with captopril and enalapril which can be used during breastfeeding).

Tranylcypromine

There is no published experience with tranylcypromine during pregnancy, and use is best reserved for patients who have failed to respond to more commonly used antidepressants. There is also a lack of data on use during breastfeeding, and other antidepressants are preferable.

Trazodone

It is not known if trazodone crosses the placenta (it does cross the rat placenta). Rodent teratogenicity studies reveal increased risk of malformations only with very high doses. Human pregnancy cohort studies are reassuring, with no increase in the prevalence of adverse outcomes. Trazodone enters breast milk in amounts that, when ingested by the neonate, are not clinically relevant.
Einarson *et al.*: *Can J Psychiatry* 2009;**54**:242.
Verbeeck *et al.*: *Br J Clin Pharmacol* 1986;**22**:367.

Tretinoin

Some retinoid agents can be highly toxic to the fetus, and in general, retinoids are contraindicated during pregnancy. Tretinoin crosses the placenta. It is a known teratogen in rodents and primates when given orally. It may be used topically as well as orally. Outcomes after topical use are largely reassuring with no significant increase in the spontaneous abortions or major structural defects. Fewer than 10 neonates have been born to women treated with oral tretinoin during pregnancy (all after the first trimester) for acute promyelocytic leukaemia. All had normal growth without apparent complications. Inadvertent exposure to topical tretinoin during early pregnancy is unlikely to pose a significant risk to the fetus although detailed ultrasound anomaly screening is warranted. Topical tretinoin has not been studied during breastfeeding, and

because it is poorly absorbed after topical application, it is considered a low risk to the nursing infant.
Leachman and Reed: *Dermatol Clin* 2006;**24**:167.
Loureiro *et al.*: *Am J Med Genet A* 2005;**136**:117.

Triamcinolone

It is not known if triamcinolone crosses the placenta. In several rodent models, triamcinolone causes cleft lip and palate. While there is no evidence suggesting that orally or parenterally administered triamcinolone is a human teratogen, avoiding use during the first trimester seems prudent. Continuous use during pregnancy has been associated with *in utero* growth restriction, and there are concerns about the effects of steroids on the developing brain. It is less likely that maternal systemic concentration will reach a clinically relevant level after either topical or inhalational use. There is no information on passage of triamcinolone into breast milk; topical or inhalational use is unlikely to pose a risk to the breastfed infant, but the breastfeeding mother should probably 'pump and dump' for 12 hours after any oral or parenteral dose.
Bekhor *et al.*: *Cleft Palate J* 1978;**15**:220.
Dombrowski *et al.*: *J Matern Fetal Med* 1996;**5**:310.

Triamterene

In addition to its diuretic effect, triamterene is also a folate antagonist, and epidemiological studies suggest such drugs may increase the risk of neural tube defects, cardiovascular malformations, oral clefts and urinary tract abnormalities. Folate supplementation is therefore essential. Triamterene rapidly crosses the placenta (F/M levels ~1). Rodent teratogenicity studies are reassuring. There is no information regarding use of triamterene during lactation, and it is not known if passage into breast milk occurs. Triamterene should be used only if the benefit justifies the potential perinatal risk and there are alternatives for which there is more experience during pregnancy and lactation.
Hernández-Díaz *et al.*: *Am J Epidemiol* 2001;**153**:961.
Hernández-Díaz *et al.*: *N Engl J Med* 2000;**343**:1608.

Trifluoperazine

Trifluoperazine crosses the placenta. Rodent teratogenicity studies are generally reassuring, as are a limited number of case reports of use during human pregnancy. Trifluoperazine was undetectable in breast milk of women who were taking normal therapeutic doses, and no adverse effects have been reported in exposed infants.
Moriarty and Nance: *Can Med Assoc J* 1963;**88**:375.
Yoshida *et al.*: *Psychol Med* 1998;**28**:81.

Trimethoprim – See Part 2, pp. 509–510

Trimipramine

It is not known whether trimipramine crosses the placenta. Rodent teratogenicity studies are generally reassuring. It is not known whether trimipramine enters breast milk. Because of the lack of data on use during breastfeeding, other antidepressants may be preferred.

Wen and Walker: *J Obstet Gynaecol Can* 2004;**26**:887.

Urokinase

It is not known whether urokinase crosses the placenta; however, proteinase inhibitors are found in placental tissue and these probably inactivate it. Rodent teratogenicity studies are reassuring. There are few reports of use during human pregnancy, but placental separation is a recognised complication. Use during breastfeeding has not been reported, but with the short half-life (~20 minutes), it is unlikely that urokinase poses a risk to the breastfed infant.

La Valleur *et al.*: *Postgrad Med* 1996;**99**:269, 272.
Walker *et al.*: *Thromb Haemost* 1983;**49**:21.

Ursodeoxycholic acid (ursodiol, USAN) – See Part 2, pp. 518–519

Valaciclovir (valacyclovir, USAN)

Valaciclovir is an orally administered prodrug of aciclovir and has been used to treat genital herpes, varicella zoster and CMV infection during pregnancy. After oral administration, it is metabolised and enhances aciclovir bioavailability. Valaciclovir crosses the placenta (it is not known if aciclovir does). Maternal treatment leads to therapeutic concentrations in both maternal and fetal compartments. Rodent teratogenicity studies are reassuring, and post-marketing surveys suggest no increased frequency of birth defects. It is not known if valaciclovir enters breast milk, but aciclovir does in small amounts (<5% of the dose used to treat neonates).

Jacquemard *et al.*: *BJOG* 2007;**114**:1113.
Pasternak and Hviid: *JAMA* 2010;**304**:859.
Sauerbrei and Wutzler: *Med Microbiol Immunol* 2007;**196**:89.

Valganciclovir – See Part 2, pp. 235–236

Valproic acid

Valproic acid is used in treatment of mania. The risks to the embryo, fetus and infant are the same as for sodium valproate (see section on **Sodium Valproate – Part 2, pp. 480–481**).

Yonkers *et al.*: *Am J Psychiatry* 2004;**161**:608.

Valsartan

Valsartan is an angiotensin II receptor antagonist. Adverse fetal outcomes are reported for valsartan, suggesting that it crosses the human placenta. Drugs that inhibit the fetal renin–angiotensin system are now recognised to be potentially teratogenic throughout gestation, especially during the second and third trimesters when they can cause fetal hypotension, reversible or irreversible renal failure, anuria and oligohydramnios. If an alternative drug is not available, the woman should be counselled about the risks and monitored closely for oligohydramnios (which may not appear until after the fetus has sustained irreversible renal failure). Neonates exposed *in utero* should be closely observed for hypotension, oliguria and hyperkalaemia. It is not known whether valsartan enters breast milk (alternatives for which there is more experience during breastfeeding are the ACE inhibitors captopril and enalapril).

Alwan *et al.*: *Birth Defects Res A Clin Mol Teratol* 2005;**73**:123.
Berkane *et al.*: *Birth Defects Res A Clin Mol Teratol* 2004;**70**:547.

Vancomycin – See Part 2, pp. 520–521

Vasopressin – See Part 2, pp. 525–526

Vecuronium – See Part 2, pp. 527–528

Venlafaxine

Venlafaxine and its active metabolites cross the placenta. Rodent teratogenicity studies are generally reassuring. Case–control studies suggest that it is not associated with increased fetal malformations; however, a neonatal withdrawal – tremors, jitteriness, irritability, excessive crying, sleep disturbances, tachypnoea and feeding problems – is sometimes seen. Seizures have been reported. This is usually self-limiting. Venlafaxine passes into breast milk, and although it does not appear to ameliorate withdrawal from *in utero* exposure, breastfed infants do not display any additional adverse effects.

Hoppenbrouwers *et al.*: *Br J Clin Pharmacol* 2010;**70**:454.
Sie *et al.*: *Arch Dis Child Fetal Neonatal Ed* 2012;**97**:F472. (Erratum in: *Arch Dis Child Fetal Neonatal Ed* 2013;**98**:F180.)

Verapamil

Verapamil crosses the placenta (F/M ratio 0.7) and has been used with mixed efficacy to treat fetal SVT (flecainide remains the drug of choice). Rodent teratogenicity studies are generally reassuring but growth restriction may occur. Use during human pregnancies has not

shown any increased risk of adverse effects. Verapamil enters breast milk in very small amounts that do not result in measurable levels or clinical effects in the breastfed infant.
Ito *et al.*: *Clin Perinatol* 1994;**21**:543.
Tan and Lie: *Eur Heart J* 2001;**22**:458.

Vigabatrin – See Part 2, pp. 529–530

Vildagliptin
Vildagliptin inhibits dipeptidylpeptidase-4 to increase insulin secretion and lower glucagon secretion. It is not known if vildagliptin crosses the placenta. The manufacturer reports adverse fetal effects in animal studies when high doses (usually causing maternal toxicity) were used. There have been no reports of experience during human pregnancy. No information is available on the use of vildagliptin during breastfeeding or whether it passes into breast milk. Vildagliptin is best avoided during both pregnancy and lactation until further information is available.
He: *Clin Pharmacokinet* 2012;**51**:147.

Vinblastine sulphate
It is not known whether vinblastine crosses the placenta *in vivo*, but *in vitro*, transfer involves P-glycoprotein, whose back transfer of vinblastine may help protect the fetus. Most exposed fetuses do not have any apparent adverse effects, but evaluation in a fetal medicine unit is recommended. There are no data on transfer of vinblastine into breast milk; however, due to the potential for adverse effects, breastfeeding is not advised.
Sagan *et al.*: *J Obstet Gynaecol Res* 2010;**36**:882.
Ushigome *et al.*: *Eur J Pharmacol* 2000;**408**:1.

Vincristine sulphate
It is not known if vincristine crosses the placenta. *In vitro*, transfer involves P-glycoprotein, whose back transfer may help protect the fetus. Vincristine is teratogenic and embryotoxic in rodents. But most exposed human fetuses do not show any adverse effects. Evaluation of fetal well-being in a fetal medicine unit is recommended. It is not known if vincristine passes into breast milk, and most sources consider breastfeeding to be contraindicated during maternal anti-neoplastic drug therapy.
Ushigome *et al.*: *Eur J Pharmacol* 2000;**408**:1.

Vinorelbine
It is not known whether vinorelbine crosses the placenta; *in vitro* studies suggest a role for P-glycoprotein (see section on **Vincristine**). Evaluation of fetal well-being in a fetal medicine unit is recommended. Case reports of use during pregnancy usually note no adverse effects on the fetus or infant attributable to treatment. It is not known whether vinorelbine enters breast milk, and most sources consider breastfeeding to be contraindicated during maternal anti-neoplastic drug therapy.
Jänne *et al.*: *Oncology* 2001;**61**:175.

Vitamin A – See Part 2, pp. 531–532

Voriconazole
Azoles, including voriconazole, are embryotoxic and teratogenic in rodents. In humans, sustained high-dose fluconazole during the first trimester and beyond is associated with major congenital craniofacial, skeletal and cardiac abnormalities. It is not known if voriconazole crosses the placenta, but it seems likely to do so given its low molecular weight. One case report of use during the second and third trimesters was associated with good outcome. There are no reports of use during lactation, and it is not known if transfer to breast milk occurs.
Moudgal and Sobel: *Expert Opin Drug Saf* 2003;**2**:475.
Shoai Tehrani *et al.*: *Antimicrob Agents Chemother* 2013;**57**:1094.

Warfarin – See Part 2, pp. 545–546

Zafirlukast
It is not known if zafirlukast crosses the placenta. Rodent and primate teratogenicity studies are reassuring, and cohort studies suggest that leukotriene receptor antagonists (zafirlukast and montelukast) are not major human teratogens. The manufacturer reports small amounts of zafirlukast pass into breast milk, and the breastfed infant would be expected to show any effects.
Bakhireva *et al.*: *J Allergy Clin Immunol* 2007;**119**:618.

Zanamivir
Zanamivir was used in pregnant women during the pandemic (H1N1) in 2009, and reports of fetal and infant outcomes from that cohort have not shown any increased incidence of malformations or adverse outcomes. It is not known whether zanamivir crosses the placenta; given the route of administration (inhalation) and that only 4–17% is absorbed systemically, it is unlikely that large quantities are available to cross the maternal–fetal interface. Rodent teratogenicity studies are for the most part reassuring. It is not known if zanamivir enters breast milk. Because of the anti-infective benefits of breast milk, continuation of breastfeeding is recommended even if the mother is receiving treatment for novel H1N1 influenza infection.
Saito *et al.*: *Am J Obstet Gynecol* 2013;**209**:130.e1.
Svensson *et al.*: *Pharmacoepidemiol Drug Saf* 2011;**20**:1030.

Zidovudine – See Part 2, pp. 549–550

Zolmitriptan

It is not known if zolmitriptan crosses the placenta. Rodent studies revealed embryotoxicity and skeletal abnormalities at very high doses. There are no human data to suggest teratogenicity for any of the triptans, although there is considerably more experience with sumatriptan during pregnancy. No published experience exists with zolmitriptan during breastfeeding. Again, sumatriptan is an alternative for which more information is available.

Soldin et al.: Ther Drug Monit 2008;**30**:5.

Zolpidem

Zolpidem crosses the placenta. Rodent teratogenicity studies at normal doses are reassuring although neural tube defects occurred at very high doses. One study reports a higher prevalence of low birthweight, prematurity, small for gestational age and caesarean delivery after zolpidem treatment. Small amounts of zolpidem pass into breast milk, and while most breastfed infants are unaffected, they should be observed for drowsiness and poor feeding.

Pons et al.: Eur J Clin Pharmacol 1989;**37**:245.
Sharma et al.: Curr Drug Saf 2011;**6**:128.
Wang et al.: Clin Pharmacol Ther 2010;**88**:369.

Zonisamide

Zonisamide crosses the placenta (F/M ratio 0.92). Limited human experience does not indicate an increased risk of teratogenicity. Animal studies reveal embryotoxicity and increased malformations at the equivalent of human therapeutic doses. Zonisamide readily passes into breast milk with the average breastfed infant receiving a relative dose that is 33% of the maternal dose. Although no adverse effects are reported in breastfed infants, the levels to which they are exposed are high, and adverse effects are reported in older children treated with the drug.

Oles and Bell: Ann Pharmacother 2008;**42**:1139.
Kawada et al.: Brain Dev 2002;**24**:95.

Index
Including synonyms and abbreviations

Note

Drug names beginning with an upper case letter are proprietary (trade) names.

Where several page references are given, the most important entry is printed in **bold**.

The letter **W** after a page number denotes a linked website guideline or commentary.

Page numbers in *italics* refer to figures and tables.

'WEB archive' indicates that a monograph on this drug is available on the book's website, but not in the current print version of the text.

Neonatal Formulary 7: Drug Use in Pregnancy and the First Year of Life, Seventh Edition. Sean B Ainsworth.
© 2015 John Wiley & Sons, Ltd. Published 2015 by John Wiley & Sons, Ltd.
Companion website: www.neonatalformulary.com